www.leedslibraries.nhs.uk

11 016355

KW-221-864

WITHDRAWN

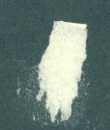

VALENDICK

CLINICAL ENDOCRINE ONCOLOGY

EDITED BY

RICHARD SHEAVES

DPhil MRCP
Division of Medicine
The General Hospital
Jersey

PAUL J. JENKINS

MA BChir MRCP
Department of Endocrinology
St Bartholomew's Hospital
London

JOHN A.H. WASS

MA MD FRCP
Department of Endocrinology
Radcliffe Infirmary
Oxford

FOREWORD BY
MICHAEL O. THORNER

b
Blackwell
Science

© 1997 by
Blackwell Science Ltd
Editorial Offices:
Osney Mead, Oxford OX2 0EL
25 John Street, London WC1N 2BL
23 Ainslie Place, Edinburgh EH3 6AJ
238 Main Street, Cambridge
  Massachusetts 02142, USA
54 University Street, Carlton
  Victoria 3053, Australia

Other Editorial Offices:
Arnette Blackwell SA
  224, Boulevard Saint Germain
  75007 Paris, France

Blackwell Wissenschafts-Verlag GmbH
  Kurfürstendamm 57
  10707 Berlin, Germany

  Zehetnergasse 6
  A-1140 Wien
  Austria

All rights reserved. No part of
this publication may be reproduced,
stored in a retrieval system, or
transmitted, in any form or by any
means, electronic, mechanical,
photocopying, recording or otherwise,
except as permitted by the UK
Copyright, Designs and Patents Act
1988, without the prior permission
of the copyright owner.

First published 1997

Set by Setrite Typesetters, Hong Kong
Printed and bound in Great Britain
at The Bath Press

The Blackwell Science logo is a
trade mark of Blackwell Science Ltd,
registered at the United Kingdom
Trade Marks Registry

DISTRIBUTORS

Marston Book Services Ltd
PO Box 269
Abingdon Oxon OX14 4YN
(*Orders:* Tel: 01235 465500
                 Fax: 01235 465555)
USA
Blackwell Science, Inc.
238 Main Street
Cambridge, MA 02142
(*Orders:* Tel: 800 215-1000
                 617 876-7000
                 Fax: 617 492-5263)
Canada
Copp Clarke Ltd
2775 Matheson Blvd East
Mississauga, Ontario
Canada L4W 4P7
(*Orders:* Tel: 800 263-4374
                 Fax: 905 238-6074)
Australia
Blackwell Science Pty Ltd
54 University Street
Carlton, Victoria 3053
(*Orders:* Tel: 03 9347-0300
                 Fax: 03 9349-3016)

A catalogue record for this title
is available from the British Library

ISBN 0-86542-862-X

Library of Congress
Cataloging-in-Publication Data
Clinical endocrine oncology/edited by Richard Sheaves, Paul J. Jenkins,
   John A.H. Wass; foreword by Michael Thorner.
        p.   cm.
   Includes bibliographical references and index.
   ISBN 0-86542-862-X
   1. Endocrine glands — Tumors. I. Sheaves, Richard.
II. Jenkins, Paul J., MRCP. III. Wass, John A.H.
   [DNLM: 1. Endocrine Gland Neoplasms. 2. Endocrine
Diseases. WK 140 C641 1996]
RC280.E55C567 1997
616.99′24 — dc20
DNLM/DLC
for Library of Congress   96-5659
                                                    CIP

Contents

List of Contributors

A.L. ALBRIGHT MD *Department of Neurological Surgery, University of Pittsburgh School of Medicine, 3705 Fifth Avenue, Pittsburgh, PA 15213-2583, USA*

B. AMBROSI MD *Institute of Endocrine Sciences, University of Milan, Ospedale Maggiore IRCCS, Milan, Italy*

P. ARMSTRONG FRCR *Department of Diagnostic Imaging, St Bartholomew's Hospital, West Smithfield, London EC1A 7BE, UK*

A.B. ATKINSON DSc MD FRCP FRCPEd FRCPGlas FRCPI *Sir George E. Clark Metabolic Unit, Royal Victoria Hospital, Belfast BT12 6BA, UK*

P.H. BAYLIS BSc MD FRCP *Endocrine Unit, Royal Victoria Infirmary, Newcastle upon Tyne NE1 4LP, UK*

G.M. BESSER DSc MD FRCP *Department of Medicine, St Bartholomew's Hospital, West Smithfield, London EC1A 7BE, UK*

R. BICKNELL MA DPhil *ICRF Institute of Molecular Medicine, University of Oxford, John Radcliffe Hospital, Oxford OX3 9DU, UK*

A.E. BISHOP PhD *Department of Histochemistry, Royal Postgraduate Medical School, Du Cane Road, London W12 0NN, UK*

S. BLOOM MA MD DSc FRCP *Division of Endocrinology, Royal Postgraduate Medical School, Hammersmith Hospital, Du Cane Road, London W12 0NN, UK*

J.B. BOMANJI MB BS MSc PhD *Institute of Nuclear Medicine, Middlesex Hospital, Mortimer Street, London W1N 8AA, UK*

P.-M.G. BOULOUX BSc MD FRCP *Department of Endocrinology, Royal Free Hospital Medical School, Rowland Hill Street, London NW3 2PF, UK*

M. BRADA BSc MRCP FRCR *Academic Unit of Radiotherapy and Oncology, Institute of Cancer Research, Royal Marsden Hospital, Downs Road, Sutton, Surrey SM2 5PT, UK*

M. BUCHFELDER MD *Department of Neurosurgery, University of Erlangen-Nürnberg, Schwabachanlage 6 (Kopfklinikum), 91054 Erlangen, Germany*

M. CHARLESWORTH FRCR *Department of Diagnostic Imaging, St Bartholomew's Hospital, West Smithfield, London EC1A 7BE, UK*

M.G. CHEN MD PhD *Division of Radiation Oncology, Mayo Clinic, 200 First Street SW, Rochester, MN 55905, USA*

S.L. CHEW BSc MRCP *Department of Endocrinology, St Bartholomew's Hospital, West Smithfield, London EC1A 7BE, UK*

A.J.L. CLARK BSc FRCP *Department of Endocrinology, St Bartholomew's Hospital, West Smithfield, London EC1A 7BE, UK*

D.S. COOPER MD *Division of Endocrinology, Sinai Hospital of Baltimore, Baltimore, MD 21215, USA*

R.A.F. CRAWFORD FRCS MRCOG *Department of Gynaecology, St Bartholomew's Hospital, West Smithfield, London EC1A 7BE, UK*

H.A. CROCKARD FRCS *Department of Surgical Neurology, National Hospital for Neurology and Neurosurgery, Queen Square, London WC1N 3BG, UK*

J.E. DACIE FRCP FRCR *Department of Diagnostic Radiology, St Bartholomew's Hospital, West Smithfield, London EC1A 7BE, UK*

E. DALY BA *University Department of Public Health and Primary Care, Radcliffe Infirmary, Woodstock Road, Oxford OX2 6HE, UK*

W.H. DAUGHADAY MD *Division of Endocrinology and Metabolism, Department of Medicine, University of California, Irvine, PO Box 157, Balbao Island, CA 92662, USA*

B. DE BERNARDI MD *Department of Paediatric Haematology/Oncology, Giannina Gaslini Children's Hospital, Largo Gerolamo Gaslini 5, 16148 Genova, Italy*

I. DONIACH MD FRCPath FRCP *Department of Histopathology, St Bartholomew's Hospital, West Smithfield, London EC1A 7BE, UK*

F. DUNNE MB BCh MD PhD MRCP *Department of Medicine, University of Birmingham, Queen Elizabeth Hospital, Edgbaston, Birmingham B15 2TH, UK*

C. EDMONDS MD DSc FRCP *Department of Endocrinology, Northwick Park Hospital, Watford Road, Harrow HA1 3UJ, UK*

A.A. EPENETOS PhD FRCP *Department of Clinical Oncology, Royal Postgraduate Medical School, Hammersmith Hospital, Du Cane Road, London W12 0HS, UK*

R. EPSTEIN MD PhD FRACP *CRC Laboratories, Department of Medical Oncology, Charing Cross Hospital, Fulham Palace Road, London W6 8RF, UK*

G. FAGLIA MD *Institute of Endocrine Sciences, University of Milan, Ospedale Maggiore IRCCS, Milan, Italy*

R. FAHLBUSCH MD *Department of Neurosurgery, University of Erlangen-Nürnberg, Schwabachanlage 6 (Kopfklinikum), 91054 Erlangen, Germany*

M. FAKEEH MB BS MRCP(UK) *Department of Endocrinology, Royal Free Hospital Medical School, Rowland Hill Street, London NW3 2PF, UK*

L.A. FITZPATRICK MD *Mayo Clinic, 200 First Street SW, Rochester, MN 55905, USA*

S. FRANKS MD FRCP *Department of Obstetrics and Gynaecology, St Mary's Hospital Medical School, University of London, London W2 1PG, UK*

J. GAWLER MB BS FRCP *Department of Neurology, St Bartholomew's Hospital, West Smithfield, London EC1A 7BE, UK*

S.G. GILBEY MD MRCP *Department of Diabetes and Endocrinology, St James's University Hospital, Leeds LS9 7TF, UK*

N.J.L. GITTOES BSc MB MRCP *Department of Medicine, Queen Elizabeth Hospital, Birmingham B15 2TH, UK*

D.B. GRANT MA MD FRCP DCH *Medical Unit, Division of Clinical Science, Institute of Child Health, Guilford Street, London WC1N 1EH, UK*

A. GROSSMAN BA BSc MD FRCP *Department of Endocrinology, St Bartholomew's Hospital, West Smithfield, London EC1A 7BE, UK*

M. HALL MB BS MRCP *Imperial Cancer Research Fund, 44 Lincoln's Inn Fields, London WC2A 3PX, UK*

D. HAMILTON-FAIRLEY MB BS MRCOG MD *Department of Obstetrics and Gynaecology, St Thomas' Hospital, Lambeth Palace Road, London SE1 7EH, UK*

P.J. HAMLYN BSc MD FRCS FISM *Department of Neurological Surgery, St Bartholomew's Hospital, West Smithfield, London EC1A 7BE, UK*

P. HAMMOND MA MD MRCP *Department of Medicine, St James's University Hospital, Leeds LS9 7TF, UK*

R. HARPER BSc MD MRCP *Sir George E. Clark Metabolic Unit, Royal Victoria Hospital, Belfast BT12 6BA, UK*

K.J. HARRINGTON BSc MRCP FRCR *Department of Clinical Oncology, Royal Postgraduate Medical School, Hammersmith Hospital, Du Cane Road, London W12 0HS, UK*

J.D. HARRIS MSc PhD *Molecular Pathology Laboratory, ICRF Oncology Unit, Royal Postgraduate Medical School, Hammersmith Hospital, Du Cane Road, London W12 0HS, UK*

I.D. HAY MB PhD FRCP *Division of Endocrinology, Mayo Clinic, 200 First Street SW, Rochester, MN 55905, USA*

D.A. HEATH MB ChB FRCP *Department of Medicine, Selly Oak Hospital, University of Birmingham, Raddlebarn Road, Birmingham B29 6JD, UK*

H.J.F. HODGSON DM FRCP *Gastroenterology Unit, Royal Postgraduate Medical School, Hammersmith Hospital, Du Cane Road, London W12 0NN, UK*

J. HONEGGER MD *Department of Neurosurgery, University of Erlangen-Nürnberg, Schwabachanlage 6 (Kopfklinikum), 91054 Erlangen, Germany*

T.J. IVESON MB BS MRCP *Royal Marsden Hospital, Downs Road, Sutton, Surrey SM2 5PT, UK*

J.E. JACKSON MRCP FRCR *Department of Diagnostic Radiology, Royal Postgraduate Medical School, Hammersmith Hospital, Du Cane Road, London W12 0NN, UK*

S. JANMOHAMED BSc MB BS MRCP *Division of Endocrinology, Royal Postgraduate Medical School, Hammersmith Hospital, Du Cane Road, London W12 0NN, UK*

P.J. JENKINS MA BChir MRCP *Department of Endocrinology, St Bartholomew's Hospital, West Smithfield, London EC1A 7BE, UK*

S.W.J. LAMBERTS MD PhD *Department of Medicine, Erasmus University, Dr Molewaterplein 40, 3015 GD Rotterdam, The Netherlands*

E.R. LAWS Jr MD FACS *Department of Neurological Surgery, University of Virginia Health Sciences Center, Box 212, Charlottesville, VA 22908, USA*

N.R. LEMOINE MD PhD MRCPath *Molecular Pathology Laboratory, ICRF Oncology Unit, Royal Postgraduate Medical School, Hammersmith Hospital, Du Cane Road, London W12 0NN, UK*

M.A. LEVINE MD *Division of Endocrinology and Metabolism, The Johns Hopkins University School of Medicine, Baltimore, MD 21205, USA*

A. LEVY PhD MRCP *Department of Medicine, Bristol Royal Infirmary, Bristol BS2 8HW, UK*

J.L. LEWIS Jr MD *Department of Surgery, Memorial Sloan–Kettering Cancer Center, 1275 York Avenue, New York, NY 10021, USA*

D.G. LOWE MD FRCS FRCPath FIBiol *Department of Histopathology, St Bartholomew's Hospital, West Smithfield, London EC1A 7BE, UK*

J. LYNN MS FRCS *Department of Surgery, Royal Postgraduate Medical School, Hammersmith Hospital, Du Cane Road, London W12 0HS, UK*

E.R. MAHER BSc MD FRCP *Division of Medical Genetics, University of Birmingham, Edgbaston, Birmingham B15 2TG, UK*

J.S. MALPAS DPhil FRCP FRCR FFPM *ICRF Department of Medical Oncology, St Bartholomew's Hospital, West Smithfield, London EC1A 7BE, UK*

V. MARKS MA DM FRCP FRCPath *MAE European Institute of Health and Medical Sciences, University of Surrey,*

Guildford GU2 5RF, UK

E.B. MAWER PhD *Department of Medicine, Manchester Royal Infirmary, Oxford Road, Manchester M13 9WL, UK*

V.C. MEDVEI CBE MD FRCP *38 Westmoreland Terrace, London SW1V 3HL, UK*

H. MIKI MD *Mayo Clinic, 200 First Street SW, Rochester, MN 55905, USA*

C. MILANACCIO MD *Department of Paediatric Haematology/Oncology, Giannina Gaslini Children's Hospital, Largo Gerolamo Gaslini 5, 16148 Genova, Italy*

D. MITCHELL MD FRCP *Department of Thoracic Medicine, Royal Brompton National Heart and Lung Hospital, Sydney Street, London SW3 6NP, UK*

M.E. MOLITCH MD *Center for Endocrinology, Metabolism and Molecular Medicine, Northwestern University Medical School, 303 East Chicago Avenue, Chicago, IL 60611, USA*

J. MORRIS BSc MB ChB MD MA *Department of Human Anatomy, South Parks Road, University of Oxford, Oxford OX1 3QX, UK*

I.D. MORRISON MB BS MRCP FRCR *Department of Diagnostic Radiology, St Bartholomew's Hospital, West Smithfield, London EC1A 7BE, UK*

J. NEWELL-PRICE MA MB BChir MRCP *Department of Endocrinology, St Bartholomew's Hospital, West Smithfield, London EC1A 7BE, UK*

A. NICHOLSON MSc MB BS *Department of Epidemiology and Public Health, University College London Medical School, 1–19 Torrington Place, London WC1E 6BT, UK*

F.R.E. NOBELS MD *Department of Endocrinology, Onze Lieve Vrouw Hospital, 164 Moorselbaan, 9300 Aalst, Belgium*

K. ÖBERG MD PhD *Endocrine Oncology Unit, Department of Internal Medicine, University Hospital, S-751 85 Uppsala, Sweden*

M. OCCHI MD *Service of Radiology, Giannina Gaslini Children's Hospital, Largo Gerolamo Gaslini 5, 16148 Genova, Italy*

W.D. ODELL MD PhD *Department of Internal Medicine, University of Utah School of Medicine, 50 North Medical Drive, Salt Lake City, UT 84132, USA*

R.T.D. OLIVER MD FRCP *St Bartholomew's and the Royal London School of Medicine and Dentistry, St Bartholomew's Hospital, West Smithfield, London EC1A 7BE, UK*

D. O'SHEA MB BCh MRCPI *Division of Endocrinology, Royal Postgraduate Medical School, Hammersmith Hospital, Du Cane Road, London W12 0NN, UK*

R.R. PERRY MD *Department of Internal Medicine and Anatomy/Neurobiology, Eastern Virginia Medical School, Norfolk, VA 23510, USA*

D. PETERSON BSc FRCS FRCS(SN) *Department of Surgical Neurology, National Hospital for Neurology and Neurosurgery, Queen Square, London WC1N 3BG, UK*

P.N. PLOWMAN MA MD FRCP FRCR *Department of Radiotherapy, St Bartholomew's Hospital, West Smithfield, London EC1A 7BE, UK*

J.M. POLAK MD DSc FRCPath *Department of Histochemistry, Royal Postgraduate Medical School, Du Cane Road, London W12 0NN, UK*

T.J. POWLES BSc PhD FRCP *Breast Unit, Royal Marsden Hospital, Downs Road, Sutton, Surrey SM2 5PT, UK*

F. RAUE MD *Department of Internal Medicine I, Endocrinology and Metabolism, University of Heidelberg, Bergheimer Straße 58, 69115 Heidelberg, Germany*

N.S. REED FRCP FRCR *Beatson Oncology Centre, Western Infirmary, Dumbarton Road, Glasgow G11 6NT, UK*

R.H. REZNEK FRCP FRCR *Department of Diagnostic Radiology, St Bartholomew's Hospital, West Smithfield, London EC1A 7BE, UK*

V.M. RICCARDI MD MBA *Neurofibromatosis Institute, 5415 Briggs Avenue, La Crescenta, CA 91214, USA*

M.O. SAVAGE MA MD FRCP *Department of Endocrinology, St Bartholomew's Hospital, West Smithfield, London EC1A 7BE, UK*

M.F. SCANLON BSc MD FRCP *Department of Medicine, University of Wales College of Medicine, Heath Park, Cardiff CF4 4XN, UK*

A.B. SCHNEIDER MD PhD *Department of Medicine, Section of Endocrinology and Metabolism, University of Illinois College of Medicine at Chicago, 1819 West Polk Street, Chicago, IL 60612, USA*

W.F. SCHWINDINGER MD PhD *Division of Endocrinology and Metabolism, The John Hopkins University School of Medicine, Baltimore, MD 21205, USA*

D.J. SEBAG-MONTEFIORE MRCP FRCR *Department of Radiotherapy, St Bartholomew's Hospital, West Smithfield, London EC1A 7BE, UK*

M.T. SEYMOUR MA MD MRCP *Department of Medical Oncology, Cookridge Hospital, Leeds LS16 6QB, UK*

S.M. SHALET MD FRCP *Department of Endocrinology, Christie Hospital, Wilmslow Road, Manchester M20 4BX, UK*

R. SHEAVES DPhil MRCP *Division of Medicine, The General Hospital, Jersey JE2 3QS, Channel Islands*

J.H. SHEPHERD FRCS FRCOG *Department of Gynaecology, St Bartholomew's Hospital, West Smithfield, London EC1A 7BE, UK*

S.F. SHEPHERD MRCP FRCR *Academic Unit of Radiotherapy and Oncology, Institute of Cancer Research, Royal Marsden Hospital, Downs Road, Sutton, Surrey SM2 5PT, UK*

M.C. SHEPPARD PhD FRCP *Department of Medicine, Queen Elizabeth Hospital, Birmingham B15 2TH, UK*

M.L. SLEVIN MD FRCP *Department of Medical Oncology, St Bartholomew's Hospital, West Smithfield, London EC1A 7BE, UK*

R.C. SMALLRIDGE MD FACP *Endocrinology Division, Mayo Clinic, Jacksonville, FL 32224, USA*

P.M. STEWART MB ChB MD FRCP *Department of Medicine, University of Birmingham, Queen Elizabeth Hospital, Edgbaston, Birmingham B15 2TH, UK*

M.E. STREET MD *Department of Endocrinology, St Bartholomew's Hospital, West Smithfield, London EC1A 7BE, UK*

S.L. TAYLOR MD PhD *Department of Neurosurgery, Kaiser Hospital, Sacramento, CA 95825, USA*

R.V. THAKKER MD FRCP *MRC Molecular Endocrinology Group, Royal Postgraduate Medical School, Hammersmith Hospital, Du Cane Road, London W12 0NN, UK*

K. THAPAR MD PhD *Division of Neurosurgery, St Michael's Hospital and University of Toronto, Toronto, Ontario M5B 1W8, Canada*

M.O. THORNER MB BS DSc FRCP *Division of Endocrinology and Metabolism, Department of Medicine, University of Virginia Health Sciences Center, Charlottesville, VA 22908, USA*

M.P. VESSEY CBE MD FRS *University Department of Public Health and Primary Care, Radcliffe Infirmary, Woodstock Road, Oxford OX2 6HE, UK*

A.I. VINIK MD MB ChB FCP FACP PhD *Diabetes Institute, Eastern Virginia Medical School, 855 West Brambleton Avenue, Norfolk, VA 23510, USA*

J.A.H. WASS MA MD FRCP *Department of Endocrinology, Radcliffe Infirmary, Woodstock Road, Oxford OX2 6HE, UK*

J. WAXMAN BSc MD FRCP *Department of Clinical Oncology, Royal Postgraduate Medical School, Hammersmith Hospital, Du Cane Road, London W12 0NN, UK*

J. WEBSTER MA MD(Cantab) MRCP(UK) *Department of Medicine, University of Wales College of Medicine, Heath Park, Cardiff CF4 4XN, UK*

D. WILLIAMS MD FRCPath *Department of Histopathology, University of Cambridge, Addenbrooke's Hospital, Cambridge CB2 2QQ, UK*

C.B. WILSON MD *Department of Neurological Surgery, School of Medicine, University of California, San Francisco, CA 94143, USA*

D. WYNFORD-THOMAS MB BCh PhD DSc *CRC Thyroid Tumour Biology Research Group, Department of Pathology, University of Wales College of Medicine, Heath Park, Cardiff CF4 4XN, UK*

Foreword

This text on clinical endocrine oncology is ambitious and is probably the most comprehensive text ever put together on this topic. The editors have divided the work into seven sections: Endocrine Oncology and Therapeutic Options; Thyroid and Parathyroid Tumours; Pituitary and Hypothalamic Lesions; Adrenal and Gonadal Tumours; Neuroendocrine Tumours and their Clinical Syndromes; Medical Syndromes and Endocrine and Neoplasia; and Immunoendocrine-responsive Tumours.

The scope of the book is large and therefore there is little surprise that the book is over 500 pages long. The authors have been carefully selected to provide authoritative and up-to-date reviews in each of the 87 chapters. The book provides not only background information, but also specific and detailed information dealing with basic, clinical, investigative as well as therapeutic information needed for the thorough evaluation of a patient with an endocrine tumour.

The text is well laid out and is liberally illustrated with tables, line drawings and images from radiological and pathological materials.

This book meets a hitherto unmet need for the collection of authoritative information on endocrine oncology, which previously was scattered in textbooks of endocrinology, medicine, oncology, radiology and pathology. It is a pleasure to see this volume come to fruition. This volume will be essential reading and an essential reference source for every endocrine unit. The editors and the publishers are to be commended on undertaking this ambitious project which is certain to be very useful and successful.

Michael O. Thorner
Kenneth R. Crispell Professor of Medicine
Division of Endocrinology and Metabolism
Department of Medicine
University of Virginia Health Sciences Center

Preface

We feel that the management of patients with endocrine tumours provides a basis for studying one of the most fascinating and rewarding patient groups in clinical medicine. Patients are frequently cured, and if not, a large majority are controlled well enough for them to lead near normal lives. Functioning endocrine tumours also result in syndromes with wide ranging symptoms and which conveniently lend themselves to pathophysiological study. However, endocrine tumours are rare in general medical practice and their diagnosis may precipitate a flurry of activity by junior staff towards the medical library while the consultant seeks out an appropriate specialist for expert advice. It would not be unreasonable to assume that such a specialist would already have a significant number of similar patients on a computerized database and would be more than delighted to add to this by taking over the care of an additional case. Specialized units thus create their own melting pot of rare and interesting patients and it is not surprising that the concentrated expertise which grows in these centres become a logical point of patient referral. The planning of this book originated from our work together in such a centre. We have undoubtedly been privileged to participate in the management of a wide range of clinical cases which form the basis of day-to-day clinical and research activities in the Department of Endocrinology at St Bartholomew's Hospital. Our thanks and appreciation are therefore very much due to Professor G. M. Besser who established the department as an international centre of excellence and who continues to attract patients and clinicians alike from all over the world.

A comprehensive plan for the diagnosis and treatment of endocrine tumours requires co-ordination of expertise between clinical specialists and those in laboratory-based disciplines. One of the reasons why a specialist centre may excel in this area is because there is a focus of attention on creating an appropriately high level of radiological and laboratory support. This book has been designed so that contributions from internationally recognized experts in many diverse fields can reflect the multidisciplinary approach to endocrine tumour management.

Our aim in producing this book is to gather together and present a scientifically sound and practical approach to the treatment of endocrine tumours. We have focused considerable effort to ensure adequate representation of the radiology and pathology and where appropriate we have presented a range of illustrations from a wide number of different sources. We hope that we have also been able to integrate a stimulating scientific element to the subject by introducing contributions from experts in other fields including molecular tumour biology. There is no doubt that research in molecular genetics contributes greatly to our understanding of endocrine pathology and doubtless its contribution will grow. We also recognize that the study of endocrine tumour syndromes plays an increasingly important role in enhancing our knowledge of the neoplastic process in general.

We have divided the book into seven sections which is convenient in that each part brings together articles dealing with common endocrine systems and their tumours. It is not our intention, however, that this specialized textbook should solely be a reference manual for endocrinologists. It is inevitable that endocrine tumours present to a wide range of medical specialists and we have invited contributions to reflect this variety. Thus, although patients with pituitary tumours may present to neurologists with headache or to ophthalmologists with visual failure their treatment also notably involves the collaboration of a pituitary neurosurgeon. Investigation of pituitary or hypothalamic lesions occasionally yields unexpected pathologies such as inflammatory or vascular tumours. The initial diagnosis and treatment of the rarer hypothalamic lesions may occur in departments of neurology, neurosurgery or radiotherapy. Our choice of authors from various clinical departments in the pituitary and hypothalmic section represents our view that collaboration across the specialties provides the best possible opportunity for constructive appraisal of the treatment options.

Whereas thyroid disorders are likely to fall into the territory of endocrinologists from the outset, adrenal tumours are often suspected by general physicians, possibly in a hypertension clinic. Similarly, neuro-endocrine tumours although producing syndromes typical for endocrine disorders, may first present with symptoms precipitating referral to a gastroenterologist. Common endocrine problems such as hypercalcaemia may be associated with malignancy in general oncology wards and syndromes of multiple endocrine neoplasia may present to general physicians. The theme of this book therefore is to provide a solid clinical framework for physicians of all specialties to participate in the diagnostic and treatment strategies for endocrine tumour mangement. Although consideration of many of the more common endocrine tumour syndromes are adequately represented in other textbooks we have included and

expanded consideration of the rarer tumours and syndromes. We hope that this more complete guide will offer a source of reference covering most eventual diagnoses in this fascinating area.

Our appreciation is due to our many colleagues for unhesitatingly sharing their own particular expertise in the form of concise articles and clear illustrations. We would particularly like to thank Stuart Taylor, the publisher's project editor, for his invaluable help and expertise. Jane Andrew at Blackwells provided first rate and invaluable support as production editor during the book's gestation as well as one of her own. Excellent secretarial work was provided by Nina MacMillan and Lilian Pallister who we recognize as having surpassed all reasonable expectations by maintaining contact between us and our contributors during our various moves since the start of this project.

Richard Sheaves
Paul Jenkins
John Wass
August 1996

Historical Introduction

V. CORNELIUS MEDVEI

Introduction

Diseases were described long before their causes were understood and therefore before prevention or rational treatment could be contemplated. This is particularly the case in endocrinology [1].

The Egyptians and Babylonians were pioneers of organotherapy and became the teachers of other nations in the Middle East. Homer said of them: '[Egypt] teaming with drugs … the land where each is a physician, skilful beyond all men …' [*The Odyssey*, IV, 230–232]. One of the chapters of the Ebers papyrus deals with anatomy and physiology. The 700-odd prescriptions mentioned appear modern in the sense that they give weights and measures, although not as carefully as those of Hippocrates.

Herodotus' view (in the 5th century BC) of the Egyptians as doctors is interesting: 'Medicine is practised among them on a plan of separation; each physician treats a single disease and not more; thus, the country abounds with physicians, some undertaking to cure the diseases of the eyes, others of the head, others again of the teeth, others of the intestine and some of those which are internal.' They were, obviously, the forerunners of the modern specialists.

Around 400 BC Hippocrates wrote his aphorism number 39 in section V: 'If a woman, who is neither pregnant nor has given birth, produces milk, her menstruation has stopped. …' This was perhaps the first clinical description of prolactinoma.

The gonads

The testes

Historically, the earliest knowledge of glands with endocrine function was of the testes. The results of castration had been known since the dawn of history: castrates and eunuchs were known by the Egyptians and also in the Bible as 'sun castrates'. In the Talmud the same word was used for testis and ovary. When Hippocrates wrote 'On the seed', he knew that mumps could result in sterility.

Aristotle (384–322 BC) thought that the semen was the formative agent or 'soul', the female element being the passive soil to be fertilized. The right testicle produced male offspring, the left female. He too knew of the use of castration in husbandry.

In 1626 Jean Riolan the Younger described the seminiferous tubules. Sixty-two years later de Graaf gave an accurate description of the testicular structure and also ligated the vas deferens. In the late 18th century Lazzaro Spallanzani (1729–99) in Modena, showed in a brilliant filtration experiment in frogs, that spermatozoa are essential for fertilization, the spermatozoon having been discovered in 1677 by van Leeuwenhoek (1632–1723) and Hamen in Delft. Spallanzani also carried out artificial insemination in animals, as did John Hunter in humans.

In 1830, Sir Astley Cooper (1768–1841) of Guy's Hospital in London published his 'Observations on the structure and diseases of the testis', in which he specifically referred to the frequent malignant diseases, which he called 'fungoid'. The cellular origin of the spermatozoon was proved by Rudolph von Koelliker (1817–1905) in 1841 in Germany. About the same time, A.A. Berthold (1803–61) in Goettingen reported in celebrated transplant experiments of a cock's testis that it could prevent atrophy of the comb after castration. In 1850, Franz Leydig (Germany) described the interstitial cells in animal testes. The 'Leydig cells' in humans were described by Koelliker four years later.

Although Charles E. Brown-Sequard (1817–94) in Paris claimed in 1889 the rejuvenating effect of testicular extract on himself, it was not until 1931 that Adolf Butenandt in Germany isolated androsterone in crystalline form, which was synthesized by Leopold Ruzicka in Switzerland three years later. Ernst Laquer's team in Amsterdam isolated testosterone from the testis in 1935. Male infertility due to autoimmunity to sperm was reported by Hendry in London in 1979.

The ovaries

The ovaries have a less intensively explored history, although in ancient Egypt ovariectomy was performed on humans. Aristotle described ovariectomy in sows and camels as a means of increasing growth and strength. Herophilus (4th century BC) called them the 'female testicles'.

In 1561 Fallopio described the tubes, ovaries, corpus luteum, hymen, clitoris and the round ligaments. The term 'corpus luteum' was invented by Malpighi (1628–94) in 1668. The word 'ovarium' was used by Fabricius in 1621, but it was Niels Stensen of Copenhagen who said in 1667 that the female testes of mammals contained eggs and were analogous to the ovaries of oviparous species. William Harvey in 1651 suggested the gradual build up of the embryo from the ovum. Twenty years later, Regnier de Graaf described ovulation and the vesicles now known as the Graafian follicles.

O. Hertwig in Berlin demonstrated the union of sperm and ovum in 1876. The next 50 years saw the isolation of ovarian hormones. Parkes and Bellerby in London extracted oestrin in 1926; a year later, Ernest Laqueur (1880–1947) and his team in Amsterdam discovered a female hormone (menformon) in male urine. Selmar Aschheim and Bernard Zondek (1891–1967) published their pregnancy test produced from female urine in Berlin in 1928. About the same time, George Washington Corner (1889–1981) in the USA described the structure of progesterone. This was followed by Guy Marrian (London, Toronto, Edinburgh) who isolated pregnanediol (1929) and crystalline oestriol a year later. Doisy isolated crystalline oestrone from urine of pregnancy. Adolf Butenandt identified the second ovarian hormone, crystalline progesterone, in 1934. Finally, Sir Edward Dodds (1899–1975) in London and his colleagues produced the first synthetic oestrogen in 1938 (stilboestrol).

In 1773 Percival Pott of St Bartholomew's Hospital in London noted cessation of menstruation and shrinking of the breasts in a young woman of 23 years from whom he had removed herniated ovaries. From this data an American student, John Davidge, concluded in his MD thesis in 1794, that 'menstruation is a peculiar condition of the ovaries'; and this remained the only account of the effect of bilateral oophorectomy on the menses. True, John Hunter in London had reported on the effect on fertility after removing one ovary in a sow in 1786, but it was as late as 1827 that Carl Ernst von Baer (1792–1876) in Koenigsberg discovered the human ovum. In 1896

Joseph Halban and Emil Knauer, both of Vienna and working independently, proved the existence of ovarian hormones by implanting ovarian tissue into spayed rabbits. The zoologist Lataste in Bordeaux observed in 1889 that female laboratory rodents had periods of sexual activity connected with the rhythms of the ovary, and a few years later Marshall and Jolly in the UK noted that ovarian extracts caused oestrus in castrated animals.

Contraception has to be mentioned in this context. In ancient and modern China and in ancient Egypt prolonged lactation by breast feeding was used. Ludwig Haberlandt, physiologist in Innsbruck (Austria), reported in 1921 'On the hormonal (temporary) sterilisation of the female animal'. Independently, he was followed a year later by Otto Fellner of Vienna. Next came Alan Guttmacher of Columbia University in 1961 and, eventually, Gregory Pincus of Worcester, Massachusetts in the USA, 'the father of the Pill', who published in 1965 'The control of fertility', unaware of the works of Haberlandt and Fellner.

Pituitary and hypothalamus

Galen's (129–201 AD) idea (a view still held in 1543 by Vesalius) that the pituitary drains the phlegm from the brain to the nasopharynx was refuted in 1660 by Schneider in Wittenberg. Lieutaud described the pituitary stalk ('tige') in 1742 and in 1859 de Haen (Vienna) mentioned amenorrhoea in connection with a pituitary tumour.

Acromegaly and giants

Giants were repeatedly mentioned in the Old Testament, not only as individuals (Goliath) but also in families and tribes ('Arba was a great man among the Anakim') [*Joshua* XIV, 15]. Interestingly, there were tribes of giants described in Nordic sagas. In many of these individuals there must have been pituitary dysfunction. If there were low gonadotrophin values, the changes of procreation must have diminished, so the occurrence of families and tribes of giants in Nordic and Oriental folklore must have a different explanation to that of growth hormone excess.

Aldred and Sandison studied in detail the monuments of the Pharaoh Akhenaten (approximately 1365 BC) (Fig. 1) and came to the conclusion that Akhenaten had an acromegalic face and eunuchoid obesity, which may have been due to a pituitary adenoma, first with some α cell overactivity, but later leading to hypofunction of the pituitary gland. An alternative but less exciting theory is that his abnormally shaped skull was just a familial trait

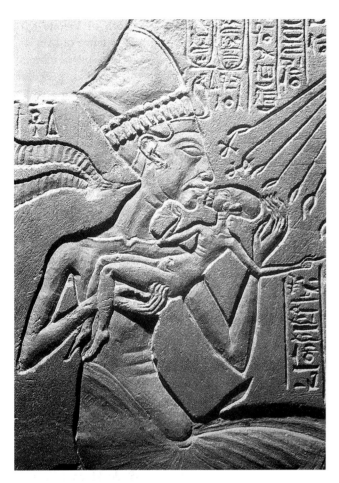

Fig. 1 Pharaoh Akhenaten.

and a marked enlargement of the pituitary gland and of the sella turcica. These important reports appeared before Pierre Marie's (1853–1940) treatise, submitted in September 1885, published in April 1886. Pierre Marie called the disease 'acromegaly'. With his pupil and collaborator, Dr Souza-Leite, Pierre Marie described a great number of other patients, apart from his original two, where the diagnosis was applicable. Pierre Marie did not know the aetiology of his disease. In 1894, Auguso T. Tamburini of Modena (1848–1919) connected acromegaly with hypertrophy and overactivity of the pituitary. In 1900, Carl Benda demonstrated hyperplasia of the eosinophil cells in the anterior lobe of the pituitary in acromegaly.

On the treatment side, Richard Caton and Frank Thomas Paul in Liverpool performed in 1893 a decompression in a married woman of 33 with acromegaly, to relieve cranial pressure, one of the first steps in effective intervention. In 1906, Hermann Schloffer of Innsbruck (1868–1937) first operated successfully on a pituitary tumour by the nasal route, using Oskar Hirsch's (Vienna) endonasal method, which became better known after 1911.

In 1929, Putnam, Benedict and Teel produced experimental acromegaly in dogs by anterior pituitary lobe extract injection. In 1900 and 1901, Joseph Babinski (France), Alfred Froelich (Vienna) and Harvey Cushing (USA) described, independently, dystrophia adiposo-genitalis, Froelich commenting: 'A case of pituitary tumour without acromegaly'.

Prolactinoma

After Hippocrates' first description we jump, as mentioned above, to 1759 to de Haen (Vienna) who mentioned amenorrhoea in connection with a pituitary tumour.

Prolactin itself was not discovered until much later; it was identified only in 1933 by Oscar Riddle (1877–1968). It is interesting that John Hunter (1728–93) discovered that 'pigeon's milk', a substance secreted by the female and the male parent to feed the young pigeon, is so done by the crop, and that Oscar Riddle identified the pituitary-hormone-controlled 'pigeon's milk' as prolactin, which also controls milk secretion in mammals. In 1928, P. Sticker and F. Grueter observed that lactation could be produced in ovariectomized and pseudopregnant rabbits by administration of anterior pituitary extracts (lactogenic hormone). In fact, Walter Lee Gaines (USA) had demonstrated the action of the pituitary in lactation as early as 1915.

Pituitary basophilism (Cushing's disease)

In 1932, Harvey William Cushing (1869–1934) (Fig. 2)

in terms of the skull configuration, which measurements show was similar to that of his relatives.

There were a number of patients who fitted the description of acromegaly prior to its description by Marie: Sancerotte with his description of Sieur Mirbeck in 1772; in 1822, Alibert mentioned 'un géant scrofuleux'; in 1857, Chalk described 'partial dislocation of the lower jaw' from an enlarged tongue. But Johann Jacob Wepfer of Schaffhausen (1620–95) had already recorded in 1681 a pituitary of twice the normal size in a post-mortem examination; also Theophil Bonet (1620–89) referred in his post-mortem material to 'enlargement of the pituitary', as did Raymond Vieussans (1641–1715) in 1705. The Italian Andrea Verga reported in 1864 on a pituitary tumour, which had destroyed the sphenoid and pressed on the optic chiasma. He called the disease 'prosopectasia'. In 1869, Lombroso described 'macrosomia'. In 1877 Brigidi published the autopsy of Ghirlenzoni, an acromegalic actor, including the histology of a pituitary tumour. In 1884, Fritzsche and Klebs (Switzerland) reported on the clinical and post-mortem findings of an alpine cowherd with 'giantism'. Post-mortem examination disclosed a persistent large thymus

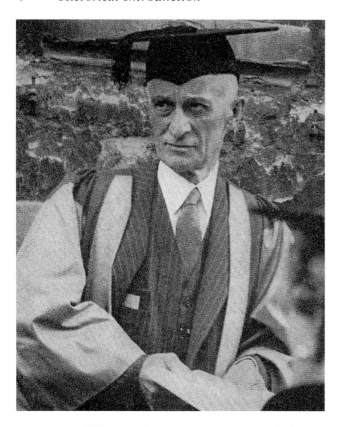

Fig. 2 Harvey William Cushing receiving his degree in Oxford.

described pituitary basophilism [2]. This dated from June 1900, when he gave his celebrated address on 'The hypophysis cerebri: clinical aspects of hyperpituitarism and of hypopituitarism' to the Section of Surgery of the American Medical Association at the 16th Annual Session held at Atlantic City. The first such patient mentioned there was a lady called Minnie of New York, but in 1932, he reported on 12 such patients.

Since then 'Cushing's disease', first so-named by the late P.M.F. Bishop and R.G. Close of Guy's Hospital, London, has been intensively studied and discussed. Cushing had mentioned Minnie briefly in 1912 and thought that her clinical picture resembled that seen in some adrenal tumours.

There is another cause of Cushing's syndrome. Hormones secreted by tissues other than those normally responsible for their synthesis are called 'ectopic', so named by G.W. Liddle (Ann Arbor, Michigan) in the 1960s. The existence of ectopic hormones may be the first indication of the presence of a tumour.

The most important cause may be the ectopic adrenocorticotrophic hormone (ACTH) syndrome. In 1928 W.H. Brown described a patient with Cushing's syndrome and bilateral cortical hyperplasia. Post-mortem examination revealed an oat-cell carcinoma of the bronchus. F.C. Bartter and W.B. Schwarz (USA) described in 1967 bronchial carcinoma, producing excessive vasopressin, causing excretion of hypertonic urine, in spite of hypotonic plasma with expanded extracellular fluid volume and water retention.

The hypothalamus

It gradually emerged that the pituitary gland was a link with the much bigger complex of the hypothalamus, which in itself is part of the brain. In 1742, Joseph Lieutaud (1703–86), professor of anatomy at Aix-en-Provence and Corresponding Fellow of the Royal Society of London, 'stumbled' into the discovery of the pituitary portal system as the hypothalamus–hypophysial connection (in the pituitary stalk). H. von Luschka in Germany described in 1860 the primary capillary loops of the pituitary portal vessels.

In 1913, J. Camus and G. Roussy in France produced experimental diabetes insipidus (DI) in dogs by injury to the hypothalamus. In 1930, G.T. Popa and V. Fielding described the vascular link between the pituitary and the hypothalamic region as a portal circulation.

From 1948–51 G.W. Harris in Oxford published his papers on 'Neural control of the pituitary' and carried out his intensive experimental studies on the hypothalamic control of the pituitary. In the 1950s, 1960s and 1970s came discovery by many researchers, but especially by Harris, Guillemin, Schally and McCann, of the evidence for the presence of the hypothalamic-releasing or -inhibiting factors (hormones).

The pineal

A little-understood gland until recently, the pineal had been mentioned by Ayur-Veda medicine of the Hindus, by Herophilus of Alexandria (about 300 BC) and by Galenos of Pergamon and Rome. It was described by Thomas Wharton (1614–73) of Oxford and Cambridge and St Thomas's Hospital in London in 1659. Rene Descartes in 1661 thought the human body a material machine, controlled by a rational soul, seated in the pineal body. Thomas Willis in Oxford had called it the 'pineal body' (a translation from the Greek for little pine, because of its shape), in his great work *Cerebre Anatome* in 1664.

In 1898, O. Huebner described a 4-year-old boy with precocious sexual and somatic development. He died and at autopsy a teratoma of the pineal was found. By 1907 Otto Marburg in Austria had collected 40 similar cases and called the syndrome 'macrogenitosomia praecox', which he ascribed to hypopinealism. However, removal of the pineal in animals and in man caused no detectable deficiency symptoms.

In 1954, J.I. Kitay and M.D. Altschule published their monumental review: *The Pineal Gland* (Harvard University Press). Their analysis of pineal tumours in the world literature concluded that destructive tumours of the pineal gland are usually associated with advanced sexual development, but tumours of pineal origin (pineocytomas), caused delayed sexual development. In 1958, A.B. Lerner and his group isolated the pineal hormone melatonin, a methoxyderivative of serotonin. They called it melatonin because it is related to melanin and serotonin.

The adrenals

Hydrocortisone

In 1948 Hench and his colleagues discovered the anti-inflammatory effect of cortisone (Kendall's Compound E) and a year later Hench, Kendall and Slocumb described the effects of Compound E and of ACTH on rheumatoid arthritis.

Aldosterone

Between 1953 and 1955 isolation and analysis of the structure of aldosterone was achieved by Simpson and Tait, Wettstein and Neher, Reichstein and van Euw. Aldosterone was finally synthesized by Wettstein and Schmidlin. In 1955, Conn described aldosteronism.

Adrenal medulla

The adrenal medulla, separately from the cortex, was defined by Baron F. Cuvier (1773–1838) in 1805. In 1886, Felix Fraenkel of Freiburg in Breisgau presented the first clinical report of phaeochromocytoma. In 1927 C.H. Mayo first successfully removed a phaeochromocytoma.

The thyroid

The thyroid has an ancient history. In 1600 BC the Chinese used burnt sponge and seaweed for the treatment of goitre. In the 4th century BC the Ayur-Veda (India) discussed goitre. Around 50 BC Caesar spoke of big neck among the Gauls as one of their characteristics.

Caleb Hillier Parry (1755–1822) of Bath (England) gave the first classical description of exophthalmic goitre (Parry's disease), published posthumously in 1825. Two further classic descriptions followed by Robert Innes Graves (1796–1854) of Dublin and by Dr Carl Adolph von Basedow (1799–1854) of Merseburg.

In 1885, Riedel's thyroiditis was described by B.M.K.L. Riedel (1846–1916) originally described by A.A. Bowlby (1855–1929) in London.

In 1907, Charles Mayo first used the term 'hyperthyroidism'.

In 1909 David Marine in New York wrote that iodine is necessary for the function of the thyroid and two years later he proposed treatment of Graves' disease with iodine.

H. Hashimoto (1881–1934) was a surgeon in Japan who from 1908 to 1912 worked in the surgical department of Professor H. Miyake, writing his MD thesis (which he published in Germany) on a hitherto unknown condition 'struma lymphomatosa'. It became known as 'Hashimoto's thyroiditis'.

In 1914, Edward C. Kendall succeeded in isolating thyroxine in crystalline form, but it was another 12 years before Sir Charles Harington in London determined the chemical structure of thyroxine and Harington and Barger actually synthesized it.

The most effective treatment of malignant exophthalmus is orbital decompression, introduced in 1931.

In 1953 Jack Gross and Rosalind Pitt Rivers (London) isolated tri-iodothyronine from the thyroid gland and synthesized it.

In 1956, Roitt and Deborah Doniach demonstrated autoantibodies in Hashimoto's disease.

In 1965 a mass neonatal screening programme was begun for metabolic disorders in Switzerland, which was followed between 1972 and 1978 by screening for congenital hypothyroidism in the USA, Canada, UK and Japan.

The parathyroids

The parathyroids were discovered much later than the thyroid gland. It was when dissecting a rhinoceros at London Zoo in 1852 that Sir Richard Owen noticed these glands in animals. In humans it was the prosector in anatomy in Uppsala (Sweden), Ivar V. Sandstrom (1852–89), who gave an excellent description of them in 1880. He had found them originally in a dog, while still a medical student, and confirmed the gland in a number of other animals and in man. Eugene Gley (1857–1930) in Paris, independently rediscovered the parathyroid glands in 1892, but honestly and generously acknowledged Sandstrom's priority, although it was he who recognized that they are essential for the maintenance of life.

In 1914, Jacob Erdheim in Vienna described compensatory parathyroid hyperplasia in spontaneous rickets in rats (secondary hyperparathyroidism), but it was another nine years before Adolph Hanson in Washington isolated an effective parathyroid extract from cattle.

Two years later, James B. Collip (1892–1965) in Toronto partially purified parathormone and used it successfully in the treatment of tetany. In the same year, the Viennese surgeon Felix Mandl (1892–1957) surgically removed a parathyroid adenoma, curing for the first time hyperparathyroidism (osteitia fibrosa). Between 1934 and 1948 one of Erdheim's American pupils, Fuller Albright (1900–69) at Harvard University described the biochemistry of primary hyperparathyroidism and kidney stones as one of its important features. In 1942 Fuller Albright's group described pseudohypoparathyroidism, in which administration of parathormone does not correct hypocalcaemia. In the 1960s, S.A. Berson and Rosalyn S. Yalow (USA) developed a radioimmunological method for the estimation of parathyroid hormone in serum.

The pancreas

Recent research indicates that the pancreas is not merely an anatomical marriage of endocrine and exocrine tissue. The Egyptian papyrus from *c.* 1550 BC, discovered by Ebers in Thebes, described diabetic polyuria and its treatment. The Ayur-Veda of Susruta mentioned in the 4th century BC sugarcream urine, which attracted rats. Cornelius Celsus described around AD 30 a condition that reminded him of sugar diabetes and Aretaeus of Kappadokia (AD 81–136) offered the first clinical description of the condition, which he called diabetes mellitus (from the Greek 'to pass through'). According to Galen, diabetes was caused by a weakening of the kidneys. In 7th century AD China, Chen Chaun noted sweet urine in diabetes mellitus. Al Razi (Rhazes: AD 860–932) in Baghdad introduced a regimen of treatment for diabetes mellitus. In 1020, Avicenna mentioned the copious amount of urine accompanied by furunculosis and impotence.

Thomas Willis (1621–75) of Oxford and London described the sweet taste of urine in diabetes mellitus. In 1664, Regnier de Graef published some of his experiments on obtaining pancreatic juice similar to salivary gland secretion. *Le Médecin Volant* of Molière tasted the urine for sweetness. Matthew Dobson in Liverpool showed in 1776 that the sweetness of urine was caused by sugar, also present in the blood. Michel Chevreul in Paris showed that the sugar in the urine is glucose. William Prout in England first described diabetic coma. Carl Trommer in Heidelberg published his test for glucose in the urine followed by Christian von Fehling, in 1848. Claude Bernard in Paris discovered in 1849 glycogen in the liver. In 1869, Paul Langerhans in Berlin described the islet cells of the pancreas in his doctoral thesis, but he died in

1888, aged 41, without understanding the function of these cells (beta cells).

In 1874 Adolf Kussmaul in Germany explained that diabetic coma was caused by acetonaemia and described 'Kussmaul's respiration' in acidaemia. In the 1880s Joseph von Mering in Strasbourg produced experimental phloridzin diabetes. He and Oscar Minkowski (1858–1931) removed the pancreas from a dog and created diabetes. Minkowski obtained temporary cure of diabetes in the pancreatectomized dog by subcutaneous reimplantation.

In 1893 Gustave-Edouard Laguesse (1861–1927) suggested that the 'islets of Langerhans' produced a hormone. Nine years later, Sir William Bayliss and Ernest Starling in London discovered secretin. In 1906, Ivar Bang published his method for the estimation of sugar in the blood. In the next year, M.A. Lane in Chicago distinguished between oxyphil and basophil islet cells. In 1909, Jean de Meyer (Brussels) suggested the name 'insuline' for the hormone of the islet cells, but in 1913 J. Homans, one of Cushing's original friends, came to the conclusion that it is the beta cells that produce insulin. In June 1921, Nicolas Constantin Paulesco (1869–1931) of Paris and Bucharest, a pupil of Lancereux reported on his discovery of 'pancreatine', a blood-sugar-lowering extract of the pancreas, discovered by him between 1914 and 1916. He became the 'forgotten man of the discovery of insulin' because in November 1921, Frederick Grant Banting (1891–1941) and J.J.R. Macleod in Toronto reported the discovery of insulin by Banting and Charles Herbert Best (1899–1978).

Clinically, insulin was used for the first time in 1922. It was purified by James Bertrand Collip (1892–1965) of Toronto and crystallized by J.J. Abel in 1926.

In 1927, J. Wilder and his colleagues reported the first case of hyperinsulinism by cancer of the islets of the pancreas. In 1929, Howland, Campbell, Maltby and Robinson could cure hyperinsulinism by surgical removal of an islet cell tumour.

Alloxan hyperglycaemia was described by Jacobs in 1937. In 1942, M.J. Manbon in Montpellier noticed the hypoglycaemic effect of a sulphonamide product; when further investigated, its mode of action was explained by his pupil, Auguste Loubatières. Thus started the use of sulpha drugs for the oral treatment of diabetes. In 1952 Knud Hallas-Moller and J.R. Murlin and his team in Rochester, Minnesota, discovered a hyperglycaemic substance, produced as a second hormone and named it 'glucagon'; its structure was discovered in 1956.

About the same time, Frederic Sanger in Cambridge, England, succeeded in presenting the structure of the bovine insulin molecule. In 1957, S.A. Berson and Rosalyn

Yalow presented their radioimmunological method for the measurement of plasma insulin.

Glucagon was synthesized by E. Wunsch in Munich in the 1960s, after Bromer, Sinn, Staub and Behrens in Indianapolis had synthesized porcine glucagon. Its isolation and crystallization had been achieved by A. Staub and his colleagues by about 1966.

M.H. McGarvan, R.H. Unger and co-workers in the USA first described in 1966 'a glucagon-secreting alpha cell carcinoma of the pancreas'. In 1969 the drug company Boehringer introduced glibenclamide for the oral treatment of diabetes.

In 1978 Deborah Doniach and Gian F. Bottazzo reported on autoimmunity in some cases of diabetes mellitus.

Gut hormones

As already mentioned, Sir William Bayliss and Ernest Starling found in 1902 that crude extract of duodenal mucosa injected into the bloodstream caused pancreatic secretion and they called the agent 'secretin'. However, gastroenterological endocrinology is a fairly recent development. John Sidney Edkins (1863–1940) had first described gastric secretion ('gastrin') in 1906. In 1955, R.M. Zollinger and E.H. Ellison described a syndrome of primary peptic ulceration of the jejunum with islet cell tumours of the pancreas. The isolation of gastrin and definition of its structure was achieved by R. Gregory in 1966; but it was Friedrich Feyrter (1895–1973) in Danzig who described the peripheric (parakrine) endocrine glands of man. He always considered that the cells were 'parakine' in nature, that is to say, acting on their immediate neighbours. In 1969, the APUD concept was introduced by A.G.E. Pearse (*a*mine content, amine *p*recursor, *u*ptake and amine-*d*ecarboxylase content).

In 1959, William Bean summed up our knowledge of the carcinoid syndrome in a postscript to a paper:

This man was addicted to moanin',
Confusion, oedema and groanin',
Intestinal rushes, great tricolored blushes,
And died from too much serotonin.

It was Oberndorfer in 1907 whose first description in the classical publication of carcinoid syndrome was as follows:

1 vasomotor phenomena: flush and telangiectasia;
2 intestinal hyperperistalsis and diarrhoea;

3 right-sided valvular disease with collagen deposits on the endocardium;
4 bronchial constriction.

Since 1975 numerous peptides have been described, located in the islets, the stomach, duodenum, jejunum, ileum and colon. Many of these are now known to be common to the brain and to the gastrointestinal tract.

The kidneys

In 1898 some observations of Robert A. Tigerstedt (1853–1923) of Leipzig and Helsinki suggested that the kidneys formed a pressor agent that entered the circulation by the renal veins. This substance became known as 'renin' and in 1939 it was suggested that it might be secreted by the cells of the juxtaglomerular apparatus and perhaps by other cells of the vascular pole regions of the glomeruli. The discovery of haemopoietin was made by P. Carnot and G. Deflandre of Paris in 1906. The new name 'haemopoietin' was given by the Finnish scientists E. Bondsdorff and E. Jalavista, who felt in 1948 that it was more indicative of its effects on erythroid cells. In 1950, Kurt Reissmann confirmed the existence of an erythropoietic factor.

Conclusion

This historical retrospective is necessarily brief and selective, looking at endocrinology and endocrine oncology over a period of greater than 2000 years. It is impossible to look forward for this length of time, but it is certain that the next 20 years will make great strides forward in our understanding of the development of endocrine tumours, their molecular structure and the mechanisms whereby gene abnormalities affect tumour development, growth and spread and their treatment.

Acknowledgement

I am most grateful to Miss Susanna Johnstone for the great support and help she provided in writing this chapter, which proved invaluable.

References

1. Medvei VC. *The History of Clinical Endocrinology*. Carnforth, UK/ Pearl River, New York: Parthenon Publishing Group, 1993.
2. Medvei VC. The history of Cushing's disease: a controversial tale. *J. Roy. Soc. Med.* 1991;84:363–6.

1

ENDOCRINE ONCOLOGY AND THERAPEUTIC OPTIONS

Structure and Development
of the Endocrine System

JOHN MORRIS

Introduction

Concepts of what comprises the endocrine system are rapidly expanding. Classically thought of as the discrete endocrine glands, the concept has broadened to include the diffuse endocrine systems of the gut, respiratory tract, heart and endothelium. It is now clear that most tissues produce signal molecules that act over longer or shorter distances. To the original concept of an endocrine action via the bloodstream has thus been added paracrine and autocrine modes of action. Indeed, any one hormone may show all three modes of action.

Endocrine cells produce, in addition to their principal hormone, many different compounds in different amounts. Some, such as the neurophysins, are produced as part of the hormone precursor; others, such as the chromogranin group of proteins, are produced rather widely in peptide- and amine-secreting cells; both sorts can serve as useful markers of hormone-producing tumours. Co-secreted molecules, which are not part of the main prohormone, are usually produced in very much smaller (0.1–1.0%) amounts than the main product; the amounts vary physiologically, and their actions are largely autocrine or paracrine. Many molecules produced by endocrine cells are not restricted to one tissue; for example, many 'gut' peptides are also found in the brain. Apparent 'ectopic' production is even more marked in endocrine tumours.

Endocrine tissues are usually divided into those secreting peptide hormones, amines, steroids or iodothyronines. To these can now be added the eicosanoid group (prostaglandins, thromboxanes, leukotrienes, hydroxyeicosatetraenoic acid) and those producing nitric oxide. These compounds are produced by many different cell types and will not be considered further here. It is now clear that most steroid- and amine-secreting endocrine cells also produce peptide/protein products which are secreted. It is also clear that some tissues, especially the brain, can produce and/or modify steroids to new active compounds (neurosteroids).

Our understanding of molecular and developmental endocrinology has mushroomed [1,2]. The genes for most hormones and hormone-producing enzymes have been identified and their chromosomal location determined. Although original concepts of the formation of various glands from ectodermal, endodermal or mesodermal components still largely hold true, we now have a much better understanding of the diverse contributions made by the neural crest, and are beginning to understand the induction processes and molecular switches that lead to the differentiation of endocrine tissues, and thereby determine the tissue-specific production of hormones. Indeed, the concept of dysdifferentiation [3] involving tumour formation by clonal expansion offers perhaps the best explanation of the variety of hormones produced by tumours. Equally, understanding of the receptors and postreceptor mechanisms that lead to hormone release allows insight into how autonomous secretion of hormone can result from defects in these mechanisms.

This basic science, combined with clinical experience of endocrine system dysfunction, now permits a better understanding of the development of endocrine tumours and the products they secrete.

Chemically different hormones: 'regulated' and 'constitutive' release

The chemically different types of hormone necessarily have different cellular mechanisms for their production and release (Fig. 1.1).

The *peptide/protein/glycoprotein* group of hormones are products of genes that usually code for much larger precursors. The mRNAs are translated by ribosomes and simultaneously sequestered in the rough endoplasmic reticulum where the signal sequence is removed, primary glycosylation occurs and disulphide bridges are

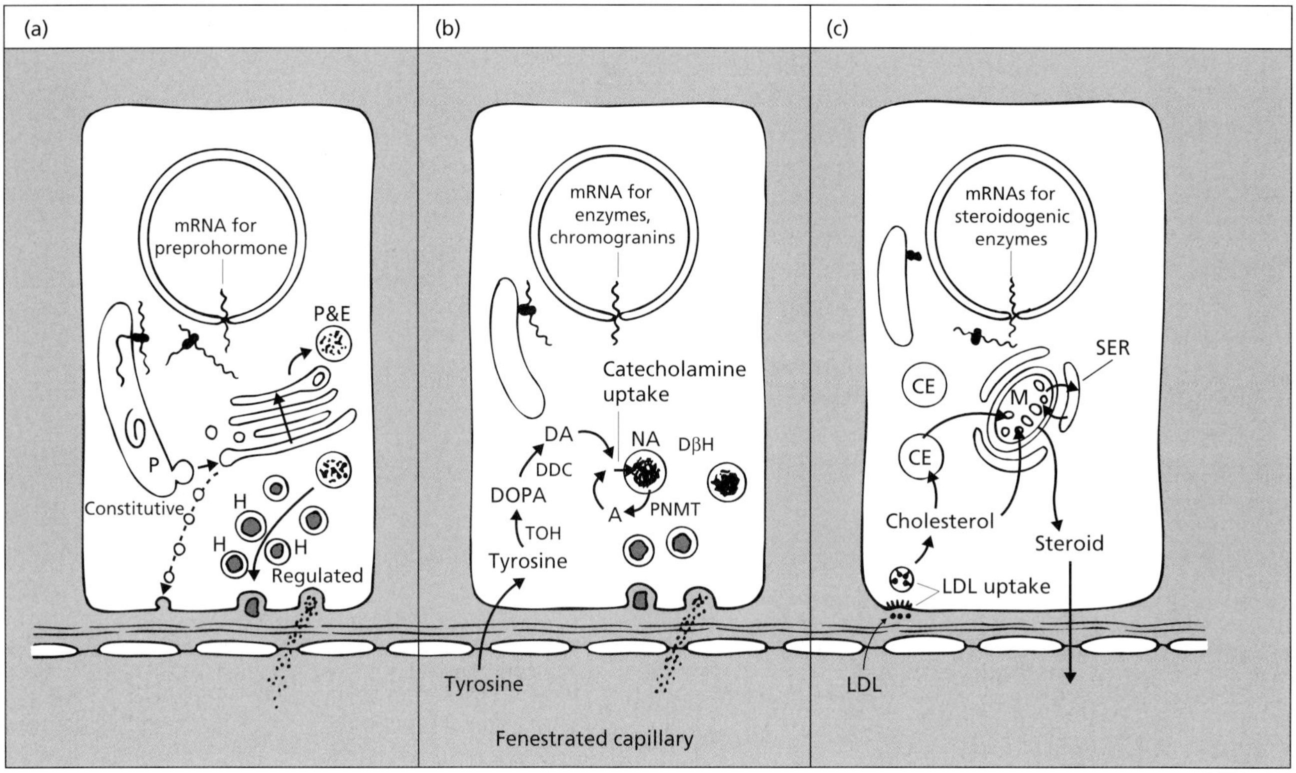

Fig. 1.1 Different cellular mechanisms of hormone secretion.
(a) Production of peptide, protein and glycoprotein hormones (H),
mRNA for the preprohormone and processing enzymes attach first to
free ribosomes, then are translated into the rough endoplasmic
reticulum. The signal is removed to yield the prohormone (P) which
may be core glycosylated; this is passed to the Golgi where the
prohormone is packaged in a concentrated form with processing
enzymes (E), then transported to the plasma membrane or stored
until a secretagogue stimulus is received. Some hormone may be
released by constitutive secretion, especially in tumours. (b) In
catecholamine-secreting cells, granules are produced in the same way,
but the DOPA and dopamine (DA) precursors are produced in the
cytoplasm by the enzymes tyrosine hydroxylase (TOH) and DOPA
decarboxylase (DDC), pumped into the granules where DA is
converted to noradrenaline (NA) by dopamine β-hydroxylase (DβH);
in certain cells the NA which leaks out of the granules is converted
by the enzyme phenylethanolamine *N*-methyl transferase (PNMT) to
adrenaline (A), which is pumped back into the granules, which are
stored prior to release. (c) Steroid-producing cells are characterized
by distinctive mitochondria (M) surrounded by smooth endoplasmic
reticulum (SER). These contain the enzymes which convert
cholesterol derived from low-density lipoprotein (LDL) uptake or
stored cholesterol ester (CE) into steroids which can leave the cell by
diffusion.

formed. The immature products (prohormones) are then translocated to the Golgi apparatus where any terminal glycosylation occurs and proteolytic cleavage of the prohormone commences. The Golgi apparatus packages the prohormones and converts enzymes into vesicles which are then transported to the plasma membrane for release by exocytosis. For the 'regulated' secretory pathway, the prohormones are concentrated within vesicles, and greater or smaller numbers of the dense-cored vesicles are stored in the cytoplasm, awaiting the signal for release (or if not released, for degradation). Other peptide hormones, in particular the growth factors and cytokines, are not concentrated or stored but pass directly in ill-defined vesicles to the plasma membrane via the 'constitutive' pathway for immediate release. In the 'regulated' pathway, the extracellular concentration of the hormone is controlled by signals that stimulate release from the stored

pool of hormone, usually within seconds of the stimulus; at the same time, synthesis is stimulated more slowly to replenish the cytoplasmic stores. By contrast, the extracellular concentration of peptides released by the 'constitutive pathway' is determined by control of their synthesis and usually takes several hours to reach peak levels.

In cells that normally release hormone by the regulated pathway, the number of hormone-containing vesicles that are stored in the cytoplasm varies depending on the demand for the acute release of large amounts of hormone. Thus, for hormones controlling parameters that vary only slowly (e.g. parathyroid hormone (PTH) controlling plasma calcium) the store is small and hormonal vesicles are sparse; by contrast, where the demand can be large (e.g. for insulin) the dense-cored vesicles are plentiful. All endocrine cells have the cellular machinery for both

Table 1.1 Cellular characteristics of hormone-secreting cells

Organ	Principal hormones: cell types	Cellular characteristics	Granules: diameter, form
Hypothalamus Magnocellular	Oxytocin, vasopressin	Large neurones (50 μm), prominent RER, Golgi; beaded axons, Herring bodies in neural lobe	Spherical, 160–200 nm
Parvocellular	CRH (+AVP), TRH, GHRH, GnRH, VIP, somatostatin; dopamine	Small neurones (15 μm), modest RER, Golgi; fine beaded axons to median eminence	Spherical, 100–110 nm
Adenohypophysis	Growth hormone: somatotroph (50%*)	Rounded cells (acidophil), often perivascular; perinuclear RER, Golgi	Profuse, spherical, 350–600 nm
	Prolactin: lactotroph (10–25%; proliferate in pregnancy)	Rounded or irregular (acidophil) cells, modest RER, prominent Golgi. Sparsely and profusely granulated types	Spherical or ovoid; 275–350 nm; 150–700 nm in adenomas
	TSH; thyrotrophin: thyrotroph (< 10%)	Small, irregular (basophilic) cells, sparse, peripheral granules	Small spherical; 100–150 nm
	LH, FSH; gonadotrophins: gonadotroph (10–15%)	Type 1: large oval (basophilic) cells; plentiful RER, Golgi; many large granules Type 2: smaller (basophilic) cells; scant RER, Golgi; fewer, smaller granules	Type 1: mostly 300–400 nm, some smaller Type 2: 200 nm
	ACTH; corticotrophin (with other POMC products): corticotroph (15–20%)	Medium-sized (basophilic) cells; perinuclear bundles of cytokeratin filaments; peripheral granules	Spherical, 250–350 nm
Thyroid	T₄, T₃ (thyroxine, tri-iodothyronine): follicular cells	Cuboidal (normal), columnar (active) or flattened (inactive) cells around follicular lumen containing, respectively, modest, little, or much colloid. Cells have basal RER, supranuclear Golgi, active apical membrane with microvilli, phagocytosis of colloid, fusion with lysosomes	Vesicles of thyroglobulin exocytosed at apical membrane
	Calcitonin: parafollicular 'C' cells (a few also in parathyroids, thymus)	Large, ovoid cells between, or in base of follicular epithelium; rich in mitochondria and secretory granules, which also contain 5-HT	Spherical, 150 nm
Parathyroid	PTH: chief cells	Chief cells, round or polygonal (8–12 μm), glycogen-rich; rather small numbers of peripherally-placed granules. Oxyphil cells (10–18 μm), cytoplasm rich in mitochondria, with scanty glycogen, RER	Chief
Pancreatic islets	Insulin (and IAPP): B or β cells (70%)	Large cells with well developed RER and Golgi; numerous pale (immature) or crystalloid (mature) content	300 nm; dense crystalloid core; or pale core
	Glucagon: A or α cells (20%)	Similar to B cells; more peripherally placed in islet	Spherical, 200 nm granules, eccentric core
	Somatostatin: D or δ cells (5–10%)	Scattered cells, well developed RER, Golgi	350 nm granules; rather pale core

continued over page

Table 1.1 (*Continued*)

Organ	Principal hormones: cell types	Cellular characteristics	Granules: diameter, form
	Pancreatic polypeptide: F or PP cells (1–2%)	Sparse in dorsal pancreas; the predominant cell in ventral pancreas	Spherical, 150–170 nm; dense-cored vesicles with wide halo
	VIP: EC cells	Occasional scattered cells in islets and exocrine tissue	
	Gastrin: G cells	In fetus and in gastrinomas only	Spherical, 250 nm, variable electron-density
Gastro-intestinal tract†	Different peptide or/and amine hormones produced in different parts of the GI tract	Cells stain less than most enterocytes. All contact basal lamina, most ('open') also contact GI tract lumen with receptive microvillous border. Prominent RER and Golgi; granules located basally	
	Gastrin: G cells	Pyriform cells in neck and middle third of pyloric antral glands; 'open'. Also numerous in duodenal crypts, villi and Brunner's glands. Also in fetal pancreas	Spherical, 200–400 nm, variable electron-density
	Secretin: S cells	Scattered in duodenal and jejunal mucosa	Spherical, 200 nm
	Cholecystokinin: I cells	Cells in duodenum and jejunum; also in neurones in distal intestine	Spherical, or slightly irregular, 250 nm
	GIP: K cells	In duodenum and jejunum, a few in ileum	Irregular, 350 nm
	Enteroglucagon, (glicentin): L cells	In ileum and colon	Spherical, 260 nm
	VIP	In neurones in non-epithelial layers of the gastrointestinal and respiratory tract	Dense-cored vesicles in nerves, 150 nm
	Somatostatin: D cells	In stomach and small bowel. Fundic D cells are 'closed', antral are 'open'. Cells often have basal processes which contact other endocrine cells. Also in gut neurones	Spherical, 260–370 nm weakly electron-dense
	Serotonin, substance P, motilin: enterochromaffin cells	EC_1 and EC_2 forms throughout bowel	EC_1: large, very pleomorphic; EC_2: irregular, large
	Histamine, 5-HT: enterochromaffin cells	Widely distributed through bowel. In stomach, the source of histamine	
Adrenal medulla	Adrenaline and noradrenaline (also chromogranins, encephalins)	Large polarized, columnar cells, moderate RER and Golgi. Cholinergic synapses contact apical pole; granules concentrated toward capillary pole. Noradrenaline granules more dense than those containing adrenaline	250–300 nm noradrenaline often ellipsoidal

Table 1.1 (*Continued*)

Organ	Principal hormones: cell types	Cellular characteristics	Granules: diameter, form
Adrenal cortex	Adrenal corticosteroids	Large cells. Characteristic mitochondria with distinctive cristae; abundant SER often encircling mitochondria. 'Lipid' droplets of cholesterol ester more prominent in inactive than active cells	Dense-cored vesicles in some steroid-secreting cells reflect co-secretion of peptides
Zona glomerulosa	Aldosterone	Small polyhedral cells arranged in spherical clusters; dense nuclei, little cytoplasm, few lipid droplets, elongated mitochondria	
Zona fasciculata	Cortisol	Larger polyhedral cells arranged in sheets, two cells thick, between vascular sinusoids; spherical mitochondria with tubular cristae; abundant lipid droplets	
Zona reticularis	Androgens (DHEA)	Rounded cells arranged in a network; abundant SER, lysosomes and pigment granules, possibly indicating senescence	–
Fetal zone	DHEA-sulphate	The major part of the gland in the fetus	
Testis	Androgens (testosterone): Leydig cells	Angular-shaped cells in interstices of seminiferous tubules. Scanty cytoplasm filled with SER, lipid droplets, 20-μm-long crystals of Reinke	–
	Inhibin, steroid interconversion: Sertoli cells	Variable shape and nuclear configuration, long cytoplasmic processes among developing germ cells. Abundant cytoplasmic organelles including RER, SER, but very few secretory vesicles	
Ovary	Androgens (mainly androstenedione): theca interna cells	Vascularized layer of spindle-shaped steroid-secreting cells clustered around the follicle basal lamina	–
	Inhibin, follistatin, steroid conversion to form oestrogen: granulosa cells	Non-vascularized layer within basal lamina of follicle. Regionally variable cells with abundant organelles including RER, SER, but few secretory vesicles	
	Progesterone, oestrogen; relaxin, oxytocin, progesterone-binding protein: corpus luteum	Vascularized steroid-secreting cells produced by luteinization of the follicle Type I: small cells (< 25 μm), irregular nuclei, abundant SER, mitochondria, lipid; no secretory granules Type II: very large (up to 40 μm) polyhedral cells with abundant SER, variously shaped mitochondria, but sparse lipid droplets; extensive RER, Golgi, secretory granules	Type II (large) 250–450 μm

*Proportion of total endocrine cells in the gland.

† Only the major gastrointestinal hormones are listed, in particular those which give rise to tumours. Gastrinomas usually are located in the pancreas.

ACTH, adrenocorticotrophic hormone; AVP, arginine vasopressin; CRH, corticotrophin-releasing hormone; DHEA, dehydroepiandrosterone; EC, enterochromaffin; GHRH, growth-hormone-releasing hormone; GI, gastrointestinal; GnRH, gonadotrophin-releasing hormone; 5-HT, 5-hydroxytryptamine; IAPP, islet-associated polypeptide; POMC, pro-opiomelanocortin; PTH, parathyroid hormone; RER, rough endoplasmic reticulum; SER, smooth endoplasmic reticulum; TRH, thyrotrophin-releasing hormone; TSH, thyroid-stimulating hormone; VIP, vasoactive intestinal polypeptide.

secretory pathways and so it is not surprising that, in some endocrine tumours, a peptide normally released by the regulated pathway can be released constitutively, with virtually no store within the tissue. In tumours that do contain dense-cored vesicles, these may be of a different size to the vesicles that characterize the normal tissue. However, the peptide produced may be abnormal in some way so that, even if it is detected in normal levels by radioimmunoassay of plasma, it may not be bioactive. Finally, tumour cells may have secretory mechanism defects such that hormone can be detected within the cells, but is not released in detectable amounts.

Cells secreting *catecholamine* hormones also contain numerous dense-cored vesicles. However, the synthetic pathway is very different. Tyrosine is converted in the cytoplasm first to dihydroxyphenylalanine (DOPA) and then to dopamine. This amine is then pumped into Golgi-derived vesicles which already contain proteins such as chromogranin, co-packaged peptides such as cortico-trophin-releasing hormone (CRH) and encephalin, the enzyme dopamine β-hydroxylase, together with ATP and calcium accumulated from the cytoplasm. Dopamine is converted to noradrenaline within the vesicles, but the amines leak slowly through the vesicle membrane and, in adrenaline-secreting cells, the noradrenaline is converted to adrenaline by the cytoplasmic enzyme phenylethanolamine *n*-methyl transferase. The amine pump on the vesicles ensures that only 1% of any amine is free within the cytoplasm. Mature amine-containing vesicles are released by exocytosis as in the regulated pathway for peptide hormones.

Cells secreting *steroid* hormones are characterized by mitochondria with tubulo-vesicular cristae, surrounded by large amounts of smooth endoplasmic reticulum. These organelles contain the enzymes of the steroid-synthetic pathways. Cholesterol, derived from low-density lipo-protein (LDL) uptake or from cholesterol esters stored as lipid droplets in the cytoplasm, is transported into the mitochondria where the rate-limiting side-chain cleavage enzyme converts it to pregnenolone. Which other steroids are produced from pregnenolone depends on which other enzymes the cells express. Steroids can diffuse out through the plasma membrane; they are not stored to any extent (though a small amount may be retained in the cell in sulphated form). Some steroid-producing cells also secrete proteins (e.g. some corpus luteum cells secrete both oxytocin and a progesterone-binding protein), which are packed within dense-cored vesicles. Steroids can cross vesicle membranes so that inevitably in protein/steroid-secreting cells some steroid must be associated with hydrophobic regions of the secreted proteins.

Many hormones of all types are secreted in pulses and the amplitude and frequency of these pulses is often critical for the action of the hormone.

The normal histological characteristics of endocrine cells are given in Table 1.1.

Hypothalamus and pituitary gland

The hypothalamus is the forebrain tissue on either side of the lower part of the cerebral third ventricle. Its floor comprises the optic chiasm and tracts, the pituitary stalk, mamillary bodies and posterior perforated substance; anteriorly it is limited by the lamina terminalis and anterior commissure; posteriorly it blends with the midbrain; superiorly it is continuous with the thalamus and epithalamus, and laterally it blends with the zona incerta and internal capsule. Its neuroendocrine neurones are situated in its medial zone (Fig. 1.2): magnocellular neurones secreting vasopressin and oxytocin are mostly in the supraoptic and paraventricular nuclei; parvicellular neurones secreting the releasing factors are more widely distributed but many are located in the paraventricular nucleus (CRH, thyrotrophin-releasing hormone (TRH)), arcuate nucleus (dopamine, growth-hormone-releasing hormone (GHRH)) and adjacent medial basal hypothalamus (gonadotrophin-releasing hormone (GnRH)) and periventricular zone (somatostatin). Central branches of the internal carotid artery enter the ventral surface of the hypothalamus; superior hypophysial branches form the capillary plexus in the neurohaemal contact zone of the median eminence from which the hypophysial portal veins pass down the pituitary stalk to perfuse the anterior pituitary.

The pituitary gland is situated in the pituitary fossa of the sphenoid. Below is the sphenoid air sinus, on either side the internal carotid artery and cavernous sinus, and above the posterior pituitary is continuous with the pituitary stalk of the basal hypothalamus, which, with the pituitary portal vessels, passes down through the dura mater which roofs the pituitary fossa. The pituitary is a composite gland composed of two very different types of endocrine tissue: the individual endocrine cells of the adenohypophysis; and the axonal terminals of magnocellular hypothalamic neurones which (with glial cells) form the neurohypophysis. The posterior pituitary is supplied by inferior hypophysial branches of the internal carotid artery; the anterior by the hypothalamohypophysial portal veins. Both parts drain into the internal jugular venous system.

The hypothalamus is formed from the diencephalic forebrain vesicle (Fig. 1.3). However, the GnRH neurones are now known to originate in the nasal placode and to migrate centrally into the hypothalamus (failure of this

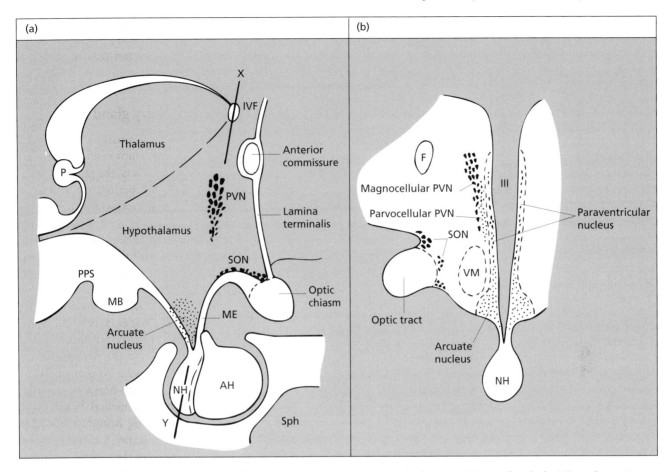

Fig. 1.2 Location of cells producing hypothalamic hormones. (a) midline and (b) near coronal (along line X–Y in (a)) sections through the human diencephalon. PVN, paraventricular nucleus; SON, supraoptic nucleus; AH, adenohypophysis; F, fornix; IVF, interventricular foramen; MB, mamillary body; ME, median eminence (infundibulum); NH, neurohypophysis; P, pineal; PPS, posterior perforated substance; Sph, sphenoid air sinus; III, third ventricle; VM, ventromedial nucleus.

migration is the origin of the hypogonadism of Kallmann's syndrome). The neurohypophysis develops from the neuroectodermal floor of the forebrain vesicle which, at 3.5 weeks' development, lies adjacent to the roof of the ectodermal stomodeum, just anterior to the oropharyngeal membrane. The forebrain induces this ectoderm to form an adenohypophysial (Rathke's) pouch, which then forms a vesicle that separates from the roof of the developing mouth. The anterior wall of the vesicle forms trabeculae of proto-endocrine cells, which interact with surrounding mesoderm to form the pars distalis, an extension of which grows up around the developing neurohypophysial stalk as the pars tuberalis; the posterior wall apposed to the developing neurohypophysis remains small and free of blood vessels to form the pars intermedia; and the original cavity of the vesicle becomes the pituitary cleft. Terminals of the hypothalamic magnocellular neurones grow to contact systemic capillaries in the posterior pituitary part of the neurohypophysis. This is continuous with a similar neurohaemal contact zone in the base of the hypothalamus where parvicellular neurosecretory neurones, which secrete the various releasing factors and thereby control the adenohypophysial cells, end on the portal capillaries that perfuse the adenohypophysis. The anterior pituitary and neurosecretory systems become active around the middle of prenatal life.

The first marker of anterior pituitary differentiation is expression of the α subunit of the glycoprotein hormones, which is expressed in a posterior to anterior gradient in cells making contact with the neuroectoderm. Tissue-specific expression of growth hormone (GH), prolactin (PRL) and thyroid-stimulating hormone (TSH) in definitive anterior pituitary cells and proliferation of these cells is controlled by the POU-domain transcription factor Pit-1; other as yet unknown factors must act to restrict hormone expression to single-cell types [4]. Humans with mutations in the Pit-1 gene have a syndrome of dwarfism, PRL deficiency and congenital hypothyroidism.

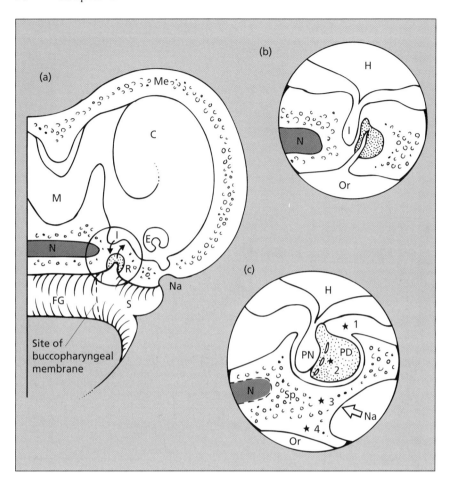

Fig. 1.3 Development of the pituitary gland and sites of associated tumours. Diagrams showing the progressive development of the infundibular process (I) downward from the floor of the forebrain vesicle and of Rathke's pouch (R) upward from the roof of the ectodermal stomodeum (S) to form, respectively, the pars nervosa (PN) and pars distalis (PD) of the pituitary gland. (a) A low power view of early stage; (b, c) area circled in (a) at progressively later stages. Developing structures: C, cerebral cortex; E, eye; F, foregut; H, hypothalamus; M, midbrain; Me, mesenchyme destined to form skull; N, notochord; Na, nasal cavity; Or, oral cavity; Sp, sphenoid bone. Asterisks mark the position of (1) suprasellar; (2) intrasellar; (3) intrasphenoid; and (4) palatal cysts or tumours attributed to Rathke's pouch remnants.

Somatotrophs and prolactotrophs develop from a common stem cell and differentiate to form the two 'acidophil' cell types. It is therefore not surprising that many acidophil tumours produce both GH and PRL. Other pituitary tumours produce TSH, gonadotrophins, pro-opiomelanocortin (POMC) products, or peptides with no apparent endocrine effects. It is possible that a few arise as a result of hyperstimulation from the hypothalamus, but once tumorous, the secretion of hormone is autonomous.

Asymptomatic cystic remnants of Rathke's pouch are found in 13–23% of autopsies, and traces of the oral end of the pouch may be found at the junction of the nasal septum and palate. Tumours (craniopharyngiomas) containing epithelial cells and a brown fluid rich in cholesterol have been thought to derive from such remnants. However, the fact that > 75% occur in a suprasellar position rather than within the sella casts doubt on this origin. Rathke's pouch tumours signal their presence by pressure on the optic chiasm or hypothalamus. The tip of the notochord lies near the developing adenohypophysial pouch; chordomas can therefore occur in the pituitary region.

Because the vasopressin- and oxytocin-secreting cells are non-dividing hypothalamic neurones, neurohypophysial tumours only form from the glial cells (pituicytomas). However, tumours in other sites, particularly the lung, can secrete vasopressin.

Thyroid gland and parafollicular C cells

The thyroid gland is normally situated in the neck and comprises a midline isthmus which lies anterior to the second and third tracheal rings, and two lateral lobes that extend upward over the lower half of the thyroid cartilage laminae. The gland lies deep to the strap muscles of the neck, enclosed in pretracheal fascia which anchors it to the trachea, so that the thyroid moves upwards on swallowing. Its lateral lobes receive the superior thyroid branches of the external carotid artery and inferior thyroid branches from the subclavian artery; a small thyroidea ima artery from the arch of the aorta may pass up to the isthmus. Superior and middle thyroid veins follow, respectively, the superior and inferior thyroid arteries; inferior thyroid veins drain downwards within the pretracheal fascia to the left brachiocephalic vein. Histologically the thyroid is a unique endocrine gland as its epithelial cells form follicles. They secrete a protein (thyroglobulin) into the follicular lumen, where it is complexed with iodine that has been pumped into the cells as iodide. The iodothyronines (principally T_4) are produced by proteolytic (lysosomal) cleavage of endocytosed iodinated colloid. The system contains huge reserves of iodinated colloid and secretion of iodothyronines is slow, starting only about 30 minutes after stimulation by TSH. The T_4 is converted peripherally to the metabolically active T_3, or to inactive rT_3.

The thyroid gland develops at 3–4 weeks from thickened endoderm in the midline of the floor of the pharynx between pharyngeal arches 1 and 2 (Fig. 1.4). Its cells form a bilobed mass connected to the pharynx by a stalk (thyroglossal duct) which, at 6 weeks, migrates caudally through the mesoderm anterior to (sometimes through) the developing hyoid bone, thyrohyoid membrane, thyroid

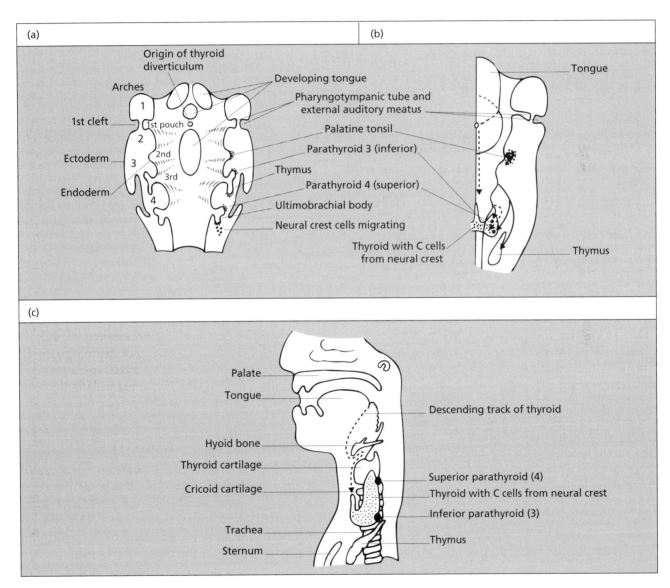

Fig. 1.4 Development of the thyroid, parathyroid and thymus.
(a) Schematic drawing of the floor of the mouth showing the first four branchial arches and corresponding endodermal pouches. Note that the 4th and more caudal pouches open as a single complex.
(b) Right side of the floor of the mouth at a later stage of development. The thymus has migrated caudally carrying parathyroid 3 caudal to parathyroid 4. Neural crest cells have entered the thyroid gland, which has also migrated caudally, where they will produce C cells.
(c) Lateral view to show the course of descent of the thyroid gland. Ectopic thyroid and tumours can appear anywhere along this tract; the thymus and parathyroid 3 are most likely to be ectopic and can be either more cranially or more caudally situated.

and cricoid cartilages to reach its adult position. During development its posterior aspect becomes associated with the parathyroid glands (and sometimes thymic tissue), and parafollicular (C) cells derived from the ultimo-branchial body become incorporated into its substance. In the seventh week the epithelial cells organize themselves into follicles; colloid formation starts 1 week later and iodothyronines are formed.

The gland or its remnants may be found at any position along this route; that is in the tongue (lingual thyroid), as a pyramidal lobe (thyroglossal duct remnant), or it can descend too far to reach the anterior mediastinum. The thyroid may fail to form (congenital cretinism), thyroglossal cysts may form along the duct, and the duct may persist to form a thyroglossal fistula that develops an opening in the midline of the neck. Accessory thyroid tissue may be found elsewhere in the neck, presumably as a result of anomalous attachment to adjacent developing organs, though the possibility that apparently ectopic thyroid tissue is really a secondary deposit of a well differentiated thyroid tumour must always be kept in mind. For unknown reasons, thyroid tissue may rarely also develop in the ovary.

Hyperplasia, and benign or malignant tumours can develop in thyroid tissue at any location. In the neck there is usually plenty of room for enlargement. However, if thyroid tissue behind the hyoid or behind the manubrium expands, it will compress the larynx or trachea. Hyperplastic adenomatoid nodules are organized like normal thyroid follicles. They may secrete autonomously and cause thyrotoxicosis but never become malignant. Their distinction from true adenomas is difficult, as is the distinction between true adenomas (which are of a number of different morphological subtypes) and well-differentiated follicular carcinomas. Invasion of the capsule or blood vessels distinguishes the carcinomas. Follicular and papillary carcinomas obviously originate from malignant change in thyroid epithelial cells and the epithelial markers low molecular weight (cyto) keratin and lactoferrin are usually expressed. The very aggressive, undifferentiated anaplastic thyroid carcinomas probably share the same origin as they may express the same markers and anaplastic areas can be found in otherwise well-differentiated carcinomas; also, about 50% produce iodothyronines and thyroglobulin. The so-called 'small-cell carcinomas' are not of thyroid origin, but probably represent either thyroid lymphomas or occasionally thyroid metastases of small cell lung carcinomas [5,6].

The parafollicular C cells form isolated or small groups of cells associated with the thyroid follicles. They secrete calcitonin. They are derived from neural crest cells, which become incorporated into the ultimobranchial body of the caudal pharyngeal complex (Fig. 1.4) and thus into the thyroid gland in which they disperse, principally in the upper two-thirds of the lateral lobes.

Tumours of parafollicular cells (medullary thyroid carcinoma) can occur sporadically or as part of multiple endocrine neoplasia (MEN)-2a or -2b associated with a mutation in chromosome 10.

Parathyroid glands and thymus

There are usually four parathyroid glands (two superior and two inferior) embedded in the posterior aspect of the lateral lobes of the thyroid gland close to the anastomotic vessel linking the superior and inferior thyroid arteries. Each is a ball of cells: principal cells which secrete parathyroid hormone (PTH) and oxyphil cells of unknown function.

The adult thymus gland comprises two more or less joined lobes of lymphoid tissue in the upper part of the anterior mediastinum, above the pericardium and usually extending into the neck. In addition to its key role in the development and maintenance of cell-mediated immune responses, the thymus also produces a number of associated hormones (e.g. thymosin, thymopoietin). The thymus grows in size until puberty but thereafter atrophies progressively and continuously. This age-associated involution is accelerated by corticosteroids.

The parathyroids develop in the region of the third and fourth pharyngeal pouches (Fig. 1.4). They are usually said to arise from the pouch endoderm but more recently it has been suggested that they arise from the adjacent cleft ectoderm. Parathyroid 3 arises as a cellular mass from the dorsal and the thymus from the ventral part of the third pouch. As the thymus descends into the anterior mediastinum parathyroid 3 is carried partway with it so that it forms the inferior parathyroid gland. As such, it is much more variable in position than parathyroid 4 which becomes the superior parathyroid. The number of parathyroids varies from 2 to 6; they frequently contain cysts. In the DiGeorge syndrome, the thymus and parathyroids are absent, apparently as a result of agenesis of the third and fourth pharyngeal pouches; this results in hypocalcaemia and immunological incompetence. The frequently associated aortic arch and facial defects are probably of neural crest origin (see below).

Tumours of the parathyroids may be restricted to the parathyroids or be associated with tumours of the pancreatic islets and pituitary (MEN-1; autosomal dominant, chromosome 11) or with medullary carcinoma of the thyroid and phaeochromocytoma (MEN-2a; chromosome 10). In MEN-1 two mutations are involved: the first leads to hyperplasia, the second to tumour formation. Of the tumour-prone tissues in MEN-2, the C cells and adrenal medulla derive from the neural crest, whereas the parathyroids are of endodermal origin. However, occipital neural crest cells migrate through the third and fourth arches, and all three tissues express the *ret* (receptor-type tyrosine kinase) proto-oncogene.

Parathyroid hormone-related protein

This molecule, which acts like PTH on the PTH receptor and which causes hypercalcaemia of malignancy, is produced by a wide variety of tumours (particularly lung and breast). It is also secreted constitutively by a similarly wide variety of fetal and adult tissues. Its physiological autocrine and paracrine function in these tissues has yet to be determined. It has been suggested that it helps to activate the placental calcium pump.

Adrenal glands

The adrenal glands are situated on the medial aspect of the upper pole of each kidney. Each comprises a steroid-secreting cortex and a catecholamine-secreting medulla. Each receives a profuse blood supply from the adjacent aorta, phrenic and renal arteries and drains by a large central vein into the inferior vena cava (left) or renal vein (right). Each also receives a profuse innervation largely composed of preganglionic cholinergic sympathetic fibres from the thoracic splanchnic nerves and coeliac plexus; some postganglionic fibres also enter the gland. Many of the preganglionic sympathetic fibres control the secretion of catecholamines from the chromaffin cells of the adrenal medulla, and it is now clear that splanchnic nerve fibres also modulate the secretion from and sensitivity of the adrenal cortex, at least in part by controlling blood flow through the gland. In sympathetic arousal, when most of the splanchnic vascular bed is constricted, blood flow through the adrenals is increased.

The adult adrenal cortex comprises an outer zone (approximately 5%) of balls of cells, the zona glomerulosa; a large mid-zone (approximately 65%) with radially arranged sheets of cells, the zona fasciculata; and an inner network of cells (approximately 30%), the zona reticularis. Cells of the zona glomerulosa express the enzyme 18-hydroxylase and secrete aldosterone; cells of the fasciculata secrete largely cortisol in humans; and cells of the reticularis secrete androgens, principally dehydroepiandrosterone (DHEA). The medulla is composed of the adrenaline- and noradrenaline-secreting chromaffin cells and their associated cholinergic innervation; adrenaline-secreting cells predominate. Chromaffin cells also secrete numerous peptides including met-encephalin, CRH and chromogranins.

The cortex and medulla develop from quite different primordia (Fig. 1.5). The cortical cells develop from the intermediate mesoderm which forms the coelomic epithelium between the mesonephros and the mesogastrium. Cords of endocrine cells form between the developing vascular sinuses. The first cells to develop form the large *fetal zone* of the cortex; this then becomes surrounded by cells that will form the definitive cortex. The fetal cortex cells do not express 3β-hydroxysteroid oxidoreductase and therefore produce largely DHEA. At birth the adrenal glands are relatively very large (about 30% of the size of the kidneys). This is because the fetal zone is very large; the definitive zone and medulla are both small. The fetal cortex decreases in size during the first 2–3 postnatal months due to a non-inflammatory involution process; the definitive cortex increases rapidly at first, then more slowly up to 20 years of age. The chromaffin cells of the medulla are derived from the neural crest and are the equivalent of sympathetic ganglion cells (without neuritic processes). At 5–6 weeks' development, neural crest cells migrate into the developing adrenal cortex and eventually become surrounded by them. The cortical cells probably induce the neural crest cells to form typical chromaffin cells; also, cortisol stimulates expression of the enzyme phenylethanolamine-*N*-methyl transferase (PNMT) which converts noradrenaline to adrenaline. Other neural crest cells migrate anteriorly to form the midline sympathetic ganglion cells and the chromaffin cells of the organ of Zuckerkandl, which is thought to be a major source of catecholamine in the first postnatal year.

Considering the extent to which neural crest cells migrate it is not surprising that ectopic clusters of chromaffin cells can be found outside the adrenal glands along the abdominal aorta and almost anywhere that sympathetic ganglion cells are located. Accessory cortical tissue is also common near the kidneys and along the track of the descending gonads (all of which form from intermediate mesoderm). Abdominal accessory chromaffin and cortical tissue often coexists. Very occasionally suprarenal (cortex and medulla) tissue is found intracranially; the cause is unknown.

Developmental defects in most of the steroid-processing enzymes of the adrenal cortex are known. The most common (an autosomal recessive defect in 21-hydroxylase) leads to the failure of cortisol and aldosterone production; shunting of precursors into androgen production and resultant virilization; the lack of corticosteroid feedback causes increased adrenocorticotrophic hormone (ACTH) secretion and thus congenital adrenal hyperplasia.

Tumours of cortical tissue can secrete aldosterone

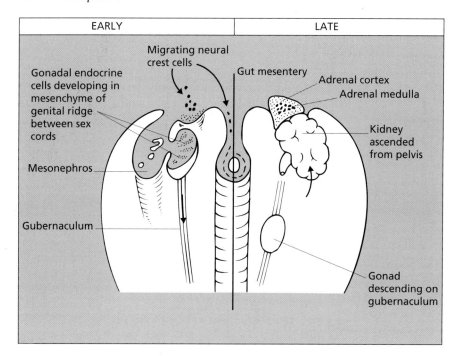

Fig. 1.5 Development of the suprarenals and gonads. Diagrammatic views of early (left) and late (right) stages in the development of the adrenal glands and gonads. Coelomic epithelium between the mesonephros and the gut mesentery develops to form adrenal cortical tissue which comes to surround neural crest cells which have migrated into the region. Other neural crest cells migrate into the gut mesentery where they form sympathetic ganglion cells. Endocrine cells of the gonads develop in the mesenchyme of the genital ridge between the sex cords.

(Conn's syndrome), cortisol (Cushing's syndrome) or sex steroids, and steroid intermediates. Well differentiated tumours usually secrete only one major steroid; carcinomas frequently secrete multiple steroids.

Tumours of adrenal medullary or ectopic chromaffin tissue (phaeochromocytomas) secrete catecholamines (mostly adrenaline) and a wide variety of normally co-secreted (e.g. met-encephalin, ACTH, vasoactive intestinal polypeptide (VIP)), neural crest-associated (e.g. calcitonin, substance P) and unexpected (e.g. gastrin) peptides. The tumours may be isolated, or associated with the MEN-2a (medullary thyroid carcinoma, parathyroid tumours, phaeochromocytomas) or MEN-2b (medullary thyroid carcinoma, phaeochromocytomas, mucosal neuromas) syndromes. Ganglioneuromas (usually well differentiated) and neuroblastomas (malignant) are tumours of neural-crest-derived sympathetic ganglion or more primitive adrenal neuroblast cells; dopamine is the major catecholamine secreted.

Endocrine tissue of the gonads

In the adult male, each testis is an ovoid organ normally located in a pouch of peritoneum within the scrotum. Each consists of a mass of seminiferous tubules comprising the germ cells and the sustentacular (Sertoli) cells connected to the rete testis, epididymis and vas deferens. Between the seminiferous tubules are the interstitial (Leydig) cells, and blood and lymph vessels derived from

the spermatic cord. Leydig cells secrete androgens, particularly testosterone; Sertoli cells secrete inhibin, müllerian-inhibiting factor (MIF), and convert testosterone to both dihydrotestosterone and oestrogen.

The testes develop at about 6 weeks from indifferent gonadal primordia formed when primordial germ cells migrate from the yolk sac wall into the thickened coelomic epithelium on the medial aspect of the intermediate mesoderm (Fig. 1.5). If the DNA-binding protein coded for by the Y-specific gene (*SRY*) for the testis-determining factor is expressed, the epithelium becomes organized around the germ cells to form primary testicular cords which separate from the surface epithelium, the mesodermal cells becoming differentiated to form pre-Sertoli cells. and, later, Leydig cells. Other genes implicated in testis formation include one on the short arm of the X chromosome, the autosomal Wilms' tumour-suppressor gene *WT1*, the gene for the 'orphan receptor' steroidogenic factor 1 (SF-1), and the gene for osteochondrodysplasia. Mesonephric tubules in the hilus of the developing testis form the rete tissue but do not fuse with the developing seminiferous tubules till mid-gestation, and the fusion is not complete until puberty. The Sertoli cells produceMIF, which directs the involution of the paramesonephric ducts in the male and assists in testicular descent; later they also produce inhibin and androgen-converting enzymes. The interstitial (Leydig) cells develop in two waves. The first form at 8 weeks' gestation when testosterone secretion starts and promotes the development of the mesonephric system into the epididymis and vas deferens; later most of these cells degenerate, but a second wave of Leydig cell formation gives rise to the definitive interstitial cells of the adult. Male differentiation of the external genitalia (at 9–11 weeks' gestation) is dependent on 5α-dihydrotestosterone (DHT) production in those tissues. Testicular descent down the gubernaculum on the posterior abdominal wall and into the scrotum is partly the product of differential growth; descent from the pelvic brim and into the scrotum requires androgens and MIF. The current increased incidence of undescended testes is thought to be due to oestrogenic compounds in the environment. The absence of any functional hormonal ligand or receptor will result in defects of the masculinization process.

In the adult, the ovaries are small ovoid organs lying on the posterior aspect of the broad ligament in the recto-uterine pouch, close to the opening of the fallopian tube. The ovarian artery, pampiniform plexus of veins, and some nerves reach the ovary from the pelvic brim in the 'suspensory ligament', and the ovary is attached to the uterotubal junction by the ovarian ligament component of the gubernaculum.

If *SRY* is not present, the coelomic epithelial cells do not separate from the surface as primary sex cords, but differentiate a little later to form pre-granulosa cells which surround the germ cells to form primordial ovarian follicles. Their origin is a little uncertain and they appear to be of two types (which either induce or inhibit the meiosis of the germ cells). The female internal and external genitalia develop independently of any ovarian hormone production, provided MIF and testosterone are not present. Oestrogen secretion starts at about 8 weeks' gestation but in very small amounts and its cellular origin is unclear. At puberty the androgen-producing theca interna cells become apparent around the follicles and the definitive granulosa cells of the follicles produce inhibins, growth factors such as insulin-like growth factor 1 (IGF-1), and aromatase to convert androgens from the theca to oestradiol. After ovulation, cells of both theca and granulosa origin contribute to the formation of the corpus luteum.

In males, tumours can form from both Leydig and Sertoli cells. Leydig cell tumours can produce androgens, oestrogens and progestins; the very rare Sertoli cell tumours usually cause feminization; presumably because of increased aromatase activity. Likewise, in females, tumours can form from granulosa or thecal cells and also from hilus cells; these can produce androgens (especially hilar cell tumours), oestrogens or progestins.

Endocrine tissues of the gut and pancreas

Endocrine cells are found scattered throughout the epithelium of the gut from the stomach to colon, and collected as the islets of Langerhans in the pancreas.

The islets of Langerhans comprise about 2×10^6 roughly spherical balls of endocrine cells surrounded by a capsule of glia-like cells and are distributed widely throughout the pancreas. Those in the body and tail of the pancreas contain 60% Insulin-producing B cells located mainly centrally, 15% glucagon-secreting A cells located peripherally, and 10% somatostatin D cells scattered between. Islets in the uncinate process, which develops from the ventral pancreatic rudiment, also contain pancreatic polypeptide-secreting F cells. Each islet has a rich blood supply which enters it centrally, and a rich innervation from both sympathetic and parasympathetic (vagus) nerves.

The endocrine cells of the gut epithelium are normally found within the crypts. In the body of the stomach enterochromaffin (ECL) cells produce the histamine that controls gastric acid secretion; gastrin(G) cells are located in the gastric pyloric antrum and in the duodenum; secretin (S) cells occur from duodenum to distal ileum; cholecystokinin (I) cells in the duodenum and jejunum; GIP (gastric inhibitory peptide/glucose-dependent insulin-otropic peptide) (K) cells are located in the duodenum and, to a lesser extent the jejunum; enteroglucagon is produced by gastric A cells and colonic L cells and neurotensin is produced by N cells of the distal ileum. Somatostatin (D) cells, motilin cells and VIP (H) cells are distributed throughout the tract. Enterochromaffin cells producing serotonin are also distributed throughout the tract and are the largest single endocrine cell group; they are a heterogeneous group in terms of the peptides (e.g. Substance P, motilin) produced.

It was at one time thought that gut endocrine cells originate from the neural crest, but transplant studies in animal fetuses have now shown the origin to be from endodermal cells of the developing gut. Development of the early pancreatic bud requires expression of the homeobox gene *IPF-1*. Endocrine cells of the islets of Langerhans differentiate early as cells budding off the branching endodermal tubules which will also form the exocrine ducts and acini of the pancreas [7]. It is therefore not surprising that exo-endocrine cells with characteristics of both acinar and endocrine cells can be found. Co-expression of different hormones is also common in early stages. During fetal life activin A- and gastrin-producing cells are prominent in the islets, but these disappear after birth. Abnormal multifocal proliferation of islet cells during development (nesidioblastosis) causes profound uncontrolled hypoglycaemia in infants. The pattern of development of the other gut peptides is beyond the scope of this chapter [8].

Most, if not all these endocrine cells can form tumours. Interestingly, most gastrinomas arise in the pancreas not the stomach. Also, the original discovery of GHRH in a pancreatic tumour emphasizes the apparent ectopic expression that can occur in tumours. Tumours secreting somatostatin, enteroglucagon, and VIP and serotonin all produce characteristic syndromes. Pancreatic endocrine tumours occur in MEN-1; insulinomas produce characteristic hypoglycaemic episodes.

References

1. Baulieu E-E, Kelly PA. *Hormones. From Molecules to Disease.* London: Chapman and Hall, 1990.

2. Greenspan FS, Baxter JD (eds). *Basic and Clinical Endocrinology,* 4th ed. Norwalk: Appleton and Lange, 1994.

3. Baylis SB, Mendelsohn G. Ectopic (inappropriate) hormone production by tumors: Mechanisms involved and the biological and clinical implications. *Endocr. Rev.* 1980;**1**:45–77.

4. Andersen B, Rosenfeld M. Pit-1 determines cell types during development of the anterior pituitary gland. *J. Biol. Chem.* 1994;**269**: 29335–8.

5. Mazzaferri EL. Classification of thyroid tumours. In Mazzaferri EL, Samaan MA (eds). *Endocrine Tumours.* Oxford: Blackwell Science, 1993: 223–7.

6. Mazzaferri EL. Undifferentiated thyroid carcinoma and unusual thyroid malignancies. In Mazzaferri EL, Samaan MA (eds). *Endocrine Tumours.* Oxford: Blackwell Science, 1993: 378–97.

7. Slack JM. Developmental biology of the pancreas. *Development* 1995;**121**:1569–80.

8. Oldham KT, Thompson JC *et al.* In Thompson JC, Greeley GH Jr, Rayford PL, Townsend CM Jr (eds). *Gastrointestinal Endocrinology.* New York: McGraw Hill, 1987:158–77.

2

Epidemiology of Endocrine Tumours

AMANDA NICHOLSON

Introduction

Epidemiology is the quantitative study of distribution, determinants and control of disease in human populations. It seeks to describe the burden of disease; distribution by time, person and place; causes and how it might be prevented. Two measures are commonly used to describe the burden of disease in a population. *Incidence* is the number of new cases occurring in a given population in a given period of time, often described as x cases/100 000 per year. For diseases with a high case fatality rate, mortality may be used as a measure of incidence. *Prevalence* is the number of cases (both old and new) in a given population at a given point in time. Incidence is used most commonly to describe the frequency of neoplasms.

The epidemiology of endocrine tumours is poorly investigated and documented since many of these questions are difficult to answer for some diseases. The problems encountered are threefold. First, for many conditions there is almost certainly a large proportion of undiagnosed disease in the community so that hospital-based studies will only assess the tip of the iceberg. Issues of case definition and completeness of ascertainment arise in nearly all published work and account for large variations in estimates of incidence and prevalence. Second, endocrine disease is rare, necessitating large studies, but investigations are costly, thus precluding true community-based work. Third, since many of these tumours are, fortunately, amenable to treatment, mortality statistics cannot be used as a measure of incidence as they can, for example, for lung cancer so that cancer registries must be used which are not universal and vary in completeness. International comparisons become difficult under these circumstances as apparent differences in incidence may reflect register deficiencies. Data are most reliable for the life-threatening tumours affecting the ovary, testes and thyroid and useful comprehensive review articles are available for each [1–3].

Discussion of other tumours (such as adrenal, parathyroid and of the neuroendocrine system) is severely hampered by the sparse and sometimes poor quality data available.

Scale of the problem

Endocrine tumours are rare. Only ovarian cancer features in estimates of worldwide incidence of 18 major cancers where it is the sixth most frequent cancer in women [4]. Figure 2.1 gives the incidence of some cancers in England and Wales between 1968 and 1985. Some endocrine malignancies show marked geographical variation but even in countries with high incidence, endocrine tumours represent a small fraction of the burden of malignant disease. Cancers of the lung, gastrointestinal tract and breast pose a far greater challenge to health services.

Ovarian cancer

Ovarian cancer is the most common endocrine malignancy. There are three types of ovarian neoplasm: epithelial, germ-cell and sex-cord stromal tumours. The vast majority of malignant tumours are epithelial.

There is a modest degree of geographical variation with a fourfold difference in incidence rates. It is generally more common in developed countries, with incidence rates in northern Europe and north America of between 8 and 12/100 000 per year. Rates are lower in southern Europe. The lowest rates are seen in Japan and the developing world. There is an extremely high incidence in Hawaiian and Pacific Island Polynesians of 26/100 000 per year. When ovarian cancer is considered as a percentage of all incident cancer cases in women, less marked differences are seen, with ovarian cancer contributing 4–6% of all incident cancers in women in most areas. Within countries, ovarian cancer is more common in urban populations and in earlier studies was found to be more common in

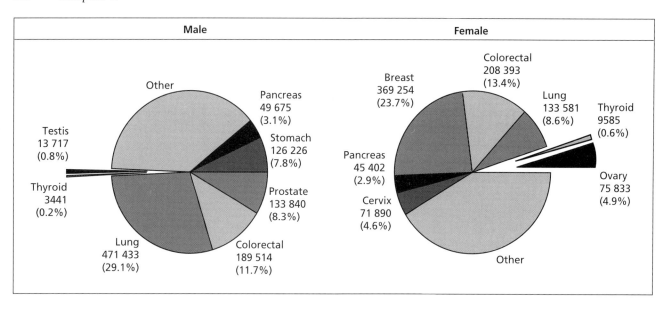

Fig. 2.1 Number of cancer cases in England and Wales, 1968–85 (figures in brackets are percentages of the total number of incident cancers). After [5].

women of higher social status. The incidence rate rises with age to reach a peak at 75 years. Incidence rates appear to be fairly stable in developed countries but are rising in developing countries.

The causes of ovarian cancer remain unclear. Hormonal factors appear to be most important with lifetime number of ovulations related to risk. Nulliparity or low parity increase risk, whereas use of the oral contraceptive pill is protective. Late age at menopause also increases risk. International differences suggest a link with low-fat diet but, other than international correlation studies, there is no epidemiological evidence. Similarly a role for talc or asbestos has not been proven. Social variation appears to be largely explained by differences in hormonal risk factors by social grouping.

Testicular cancer

Testicular cancer is uncommon, with incidence rates of between 3 and 9/100 000 per year in white men and much lower rates in Africans and Asians. Rates are highest in northern Europe, notably in Switzerland and Denmark, with rates of 7/100 000 per year. African Americans have much lower rates than white Americans (1.1 versus 4.1/100 000 per year) and there is no evidence of migration increasing risk, suggesting a genetic component. Indeed white race is one of the strongest risk factors for the disease. There are several different histological groupings of testicular cancer, but epidemiologically the most useful is seminoma and non-seminoma (the majority of which

are germ-cell tumours). Testicular cancer has a distinct pattern with age, with few cases before puberty, followed by a peak for non-seminoma in the late 20s and for seminoma in the 30s. These peaks are followed by a marked fall and then a modest increase after the age of 65. In older men non-germ-cell tumours predominate. This age distribution suggests aetiological factors operating early in life. Testicular cancers have been increasing in white populations and calculations suggest that the rate is doubling every 25 years. Both seminoma and non-seminoma are increasing, although advances in treatment mean that mortality is falling despite this rise.

The major established risk factor is undescended testis. The mechanism is unknown and epidemiological data are lacking but it appears that risk is raised only in the maldescended testis and not in the opposite testis. Previous testicular cancer also raises risk. Based on the descriptive epidemiology, exposures in prenatal life or early postnatal factors have been suggested and are supported by the intriguing finding that men born during the second world war in Denmark have lower risk than those born just before or after [6]. No satisfactory explanation is available for the rise in incidence rates in recent decades. Increased exposure to environmental oestrogens has been proposed but at present there is, as yet, no definite evidence to support this hypothesis [7].

Thyroid cancer

There are four different histological types of thyroid cancer, which have distinct epidemiological features. The vast majority are derived from follicular cells and are differentiated and undifferentiated (anaplastic). The differentiated cancers are subdivided into papillary

(40–70% of reported series) and follicular (10–40% of reported series). The ratio of papillary to follicular carcinoma varies geographically but in Europe papillary carcinomas are most common and show a peak incidence in women in middle age. The incidence of follicular carcinomas rises steadily with age in men and women. Anaplastic carcinomas are less common (approximately 10%) and usually only occur in men and women over 50 years old. Medullary carcinoma derived from the parafollicular cells is rare (less than 5%) and may be sporadic or familial (in approximately 25% of cases) when it is normally associated with multiple endocrine neoplasia type 2 (MEN-2).

Thyroid cancer shows a marked geographical variation (Fig. 2.2) with a tenfold variation in incidence rates. Rates are high in Iceland, Switzerland and the Nordic countries. Exceptionally high rates are seen in Filipino women in Hawaii but incidence is also high in Filipinos in the USA. Mortality patterns are similar to those for incidence.

Thyroid cancer incidence has increased in many countries (mainly those with sophisticated medical services) up until the late 1970s, with some evidence of levelling off since then. The rise seems to be largest in papillary carcinoma in younger women and is not accompanied by rising mortality. One possible explanation is that increased investigation of solitary thyroid nodules is leading to increased diagnosis of occult papillary tumours. By contrast, mortality, largely due to anaplastic tumours, has risen slightly in southern and eastern European countries.

Radiation, perhaps in very low doses, is clearly related to thyroid cancers, particularly papillary. Benign thyroid disease is probably associated with a higher risk of developing a malignancy. Genetic factors are important in the development of medullary cancer, related to MEN-2. Other possible risk factors include high parity and iodine deficiency. The striking geographic differences remain unexplained.

Parathyroid tumours

Issues concerning case ascertainment and the extent of undiagnosed disease are of paramount importance in parathyroid tumours, where the introduction of automated biochemistry has led to a rise in the number of cases of primary hyperparathyroidism (PHP) being treated. Primary hyperparathyroidism is due to an adenoma in 85% of cases and therefore PHP can be used as a marker for

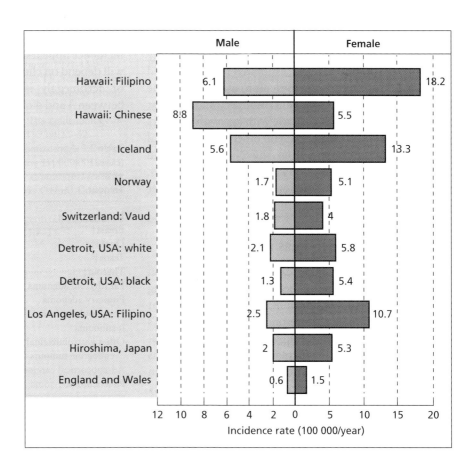

Fig. 2.2 Geographical variation in the incidence of thyroid cancer. After [8], data from *c*. 1980. □, males; ■, females.

Table 3.2 Postulated mechanisms for inherited susceptibility to endocrine tumours

Type of inherited gene defect	Mode of action	Effect	Tumour LOH	Example
Function mutation	Growth stimulation through feedback control	Hyperplasia development of multiple tumours	No	Dyshormonogenesis of thyroid
Oncogene mutation	Direct growth stimulation of cells expressing gene	Hyperplasia development of multiple tumours	No	MEN-2
Tumour-suppressor gene mutation	No action without loss of function of normal gene	Multiple tumours without hyperplasia	Yes	Neurofibromatosis
Oncogene mutation with low level effect?	Direct growth stimulation of cells expressing gene	Hyperplasia development of multiple tumours	Yes	(MEN-1)*

* Gene not yet identified, nature of gene not established, but LOH common in tumours.
LOH, loss of heterozygosity; MEN, multiple endocrine neoplasia.

Tumour-suppressor genes and DNA repair genes are predicted to act in a recessive fashion, that is, the function of both alleles must be abolished to produce a full effect. While this normally requires a mutation in the gene in each allele, it can also be achieved by a dominant-negative effect, in which the product of the mutated gene interferes with the effect of the product of the normal gene. DNA repair genes can have widespread effects, as in the Li Fraumeni syndrome, or can be surprisingly tissue specific as in hereditary non-polyposis colon cancer. Neither repair genes nor genes for invasion or metastasis have yet been shown to be responsible for inducing inherited endocrine tumour syndromes.

Inheritance of a mutated oncogene would be expected to lead to hyperplasia of all those cells where it is normally expressed, with subsequent tumour development at varying times, depending on the chance of acquisition of further mutations, probably in tumour-suppressor genes. Loss of heterozygosity for the appropriate gene locus would not be expected in the tumour if the affected allele was producing a maximal or near maximal effect through the appropriate growth pathway. The paradigm for this is the mutated *ret* oncogene in MEN-2, where hyperplasia of C cells and phaeochromocytes is present from an early age, and tumours develop from the hyperplastic cells at varying intervals. Both thyroid and adrenal medullary tumours are often multiple, and it is probable that mutations giving more potent growth stimulation are associated with a greater degree of hyperplasia, the earlier development of tumours, and more rapidly growing

tumours, than are mutations giving less active growth stimulation. The average age at which tumours develop is related to the nature of the inherited *ret* mutation, but because of the chance element involved in the acquisition of the appropriate further mutations it cannot be predicted with certainty in the individual. Loss of heterozygosity for the centromeric region of chromosome 10, where the *ret* oncogene is located, is not found in the majority of MEN-2 tumours.

Inheritance of a mutated tumour-suppressor gene would not be expected to show any direct effect other than the liability to multiple tumour formation, unless it produced a dominant-negative effect. One of the events needed for tumour development in these patients is therefore somatic mutation leading to loss of function of the normal allele. This second event can be a point mutation, or any mechanism such as deletion or rearrangement affecting the function of the normal gene. Loss of heterozygosity (LOH) for the locus involved is therefore a common feature of tumours in such syndromes, indeed LOH may be the feature providing the evidence for the location of the gene. Hyperplasia of the tissue in which the gene is expressed would not be expected, as the unaffected gene maintains normal function. The classic example of inheritance of a mutated tumour-suppressor gene is inherited retinoblastoma, in which LOH for chromosome 13, the site of the *rb* gene, is common in the tumours that arise. Von Hippel–Lindau syndrome and neurofibromatosis are both examples of inheritance of mutated tumour-suppressor genes; both are associated with a low incidence of endocrine tumours. Given the very low growth rate of endocrine cells in adult life few second mutations would be expected in the absence of hyperplasia; in addition, loss of tumour-suppressor gene function will provide little or no growth advantage in the absence of a stimulus to growth. It is therefore possible that the initial somatic mutation conferring a clonal advantage in an endocrine cell in a patient with an inherited defect in a tumour-suppressor gene would be in an oncogene, and a later step would be loss of heterozygosity. This sequence of events is suggested for neural tumours in neurofibromatosis, as LOH for chromosome 17 appears to be more common in malignant than benign tumours.

Current theories of carcinogenesis are based on the proposal that somatic mutations occur throughout the genome, and a process akin to Darwinian natural selection leads to the propagation of those clones, where the mutation confers a relative growth advantage. If an inherited gene defect is in a tumour-suppressor gene, somatic mutation leading to loss of the function of the normal gene in one cell will allow the resultant clone to continue to divide when other cells have stopped, providing a growth stimulus continues. Under these circumstances, tumour LOH will be frequently observed. If the inherited gene defect is in an oncogene, and provides maximal growth stimulation, there will be no advantage in acquiring a similar defect in the gene on the normal allele, either through point mutation or non-disjunction or some other mechanism; so tumour LOH will not occur or will be infrequent. If the inherited oncogene mutation stimulates the growth of the endocrine cell, but does

not provide maximum stimulation through that growth pathway, then non-disjunction leading to two functional copies of the mutated oncogene will provide a growth advantage, and tumour LOH would be predicted to occur. A syndrome due to such a gene would show mild hyperplasia and multiple tumour formation with LOH. This situation is seen in MEN-1, but the mechanism has not yet been proven.

Classic multiple endocrine tumour syndromes

The classic multiple endocrine syndromes of MEN-1 and MEN-2 were named by Steiner in 1968 [2], the first clear description of MEN-1 having been made by Wermer in 1954, and of MEN-2a and -2b by Williams in 1965 and 1966 [3] respectively. Both MEN-1 and -2 are dominantly inherited and in both the tumours arise against a background of hyperplasia, but the affected endocrines differ, overlapping only in the parathyroids (Table 3.3). MEN-1 involves the pituitary, parathyroids and islets, with less frequently carcinoid tumours of the foregut, and occasionally lipomas and other connective-tissue tumours. The gene, which is present on chromosome 11, has not yet been identified. The type of gene involved is also not clear; a mutated tumour-suppressor gene would not be expected to cause hyperplasia and the possibility that the syndrome results from a mutation in a growth-control gene, which causes more effective growth stimulation when two copies of the mutated gene are present rather than one, is discussed above. An alternative explanation would be one in which there is a tumour-suppressor gene close to the MEN-1 gene, so that the functional effect of

Table 3.3 Classic multiple endocrine tumour syndromes

Type	Tumours	Pathology	Gene/chromosome	LOH in tumour
MEN-1	Pituitary of parathyroid; islets of Langerhans; foregut carcinoids	Hyperplasia and neoplasia of parathyroid and pancreatic islets	Chromosome 11	Common
MEN-2a	Thyroid (C cells); adrenal medulla; parathyroid	Hyperplasia and neoplasia of C cells, phaeochromocytes and less commonly parathyroids	*ret*/chromosome 10	Uncommon
MEN-2b	Thyroid (C cells); adrenal medulla; neuromas	Hyperplasia and neoplasia of C cells and phaeochromocytes. Mucosal neuromas and ganglioneuromatosis of gut	*ret*/chromosome 10	Uncommon

LOH, loss of heterozygosity; MEN, multiple endocrine neoplasia.

the loss of heterozygosity of the MEN-1 gene region relates to the tumour-suppressor gene rather than the oncogene.

MEN-2, like MEN-1, will be discussed more fully in a later chapter; however some points are worth stressing here because of their general importance to inherited endocrine tumour syndromes. The gene responsible for MEN-2a and -2b is the *ret* oncogene, on chromosome 11. *ret* is a gene that regulates growth and development of the enteric neural system, together with the C cells and adrenal medulla. Germline mutations in the transmembrane region of the gene are found in nearly all MEN-2a cases, while germline mutations at position 918 in the tyrosine kinase portion of the gene are found in nearly all MEN-2b cases. The role of *ret* mutation in stimulating C cell growth is also shown by the presence of somatic mutations in many sporadic medullary carcinomas, here the mutation is usually in the 918 position. The relationship between the nature of the mutation and the phenotype of the inherited syndrome is clear for the difference between MEN-2a and MEN-2b, but within MEN-2a there is a relationship between the site of the mutation and the phenotype [4]. The 634 mutation is the most common overall in MEN-2a, but the spectrum of mutations differs in patients with parathyroid disease, and parathyroid involvement does not occur in MEN-2b in association with the 918 mutation. The mechanism of the genotype–phenotype relationship is not clear but there are multiple forms of the *ret* peptide and mutation may influence the ligand–receptor interaction, the post-translational processing, receptor dimerization or the interaction of the receptor and its substrate.

Single endocrine gland syndromes

Families with two or more members with tumours have been described for each major endocrine gland. For the pituitary, parathyroid glands, thyroid C cells, pancreatic islets, adrenal cortex and adrenal medulla care must be taken before accepting such reports as evidence of a distinct syndrome because tumours of each of these glands are found as part of the classical MEN syndrome, or as part of well defined, primarily non-endocrine syndromes. In both groups the chance of developing a tumour depends on the variable penetrance of the gene probably related to the nature of the germline mutation, which, in turn, may influence the chance of the acquisition of the somatic mechanisms needed for tumorigenesis. It is not surprising that some family members may show tumours of only one endocrine gland, or that occasionally it may appear that tumours of one endocrine gland are being inherited, whereas in reality the condition is part of a broader syndrome.

Conditions that do give rise to an inherited susceptibility to endocrine neoplasia restricted to a single endocrine gland (Table 3.4) include two that cause a functional defect in the endocrine gland concerned. These, dyshormonogenesis of the thyroid and adrenal virilism, are

Table 3.4 Single endocrine gland syndromes

Gland	Syndrome	Pathology	Other involvement	Mechanism
Thyroid	Dyshormonogenesis	Hyperplasia and neoplasia of follicular cells	–	Function defect, feedback growth stimulation
	Multiple adenomas	Multiple adenomas without hyperplasia	–	Unknown, possibly tumour-suppressor gene
	Familial papillary carcinomas	Papillary carcinoma, no hyperplasia	–	Unknown
	Familial MTC	Bilateral medullary carcinoma	–	Mutation in *ret* gene (chromosome 10)
Parathyroid	Hereditary hyperparathyroidism/jaw tumours	Multiple adenomas or carcinomas, no hyperplasia	Jaw fibromas	Unknown, gene on chromosome 1
Adrenal	Carcinoma and hemihypertrophy	Carcinomas	Hemihypertrophy	Unknown, possibly related to Beckwith's syndrome
	Adrenal virilism	Adenoma/carcinoma	–	Function defect, feedback growth stimulation

MTC, medullary thyroid carcinoma.

not normally thought of as inherited tumour syndromes because of the clinical importance of the functional effects rather than the tumours. Follicular adenomas are regularly found in dyshormonogenesis, and when carcinoma occurs, it is usually follicular in type. Cortical adenomas and even carcinomas have been described in adrenal virilism, but unlike dyshormonogenesis these are not consistently found. The significance of these two conditions is that they illustrate the role that growth stimulation alone can play in the development of endocrine tumours.

The other thyroid conditions are less well understood; multiple adenomas may occur in a familial setting without dyshormonogenesis and familial papillary carcinomas have been recorded. Some families with medullary thyroid carcinoma (MTC) but without evidence of other tumours show the 634 mutation, which is the commonest in MEN-2a, but over a third of the families show a 618 mutation, which is rare in MEN-2a. The familial MTC-only syndrome may represent a variant of MEN-2a in which the mutation confers a very low liability to tumours of other endocrines.

In the parathyroid gland a liability to hereditary adenomas and carcinomas without other endocrine tumours has been thought to be related to MEN-1 or -2. However there is a clearly distinct syndrome in which the parathyroid tumours do not arise against a background of hyperplasia, show a high chance of progression to carcinoma, and are often linked with the development of jaw tumours [5]. These are not the brown tumours of hyperparathyroidism, but fibromas. The gene for this syndrome has now been mapped to the long arm of chromosome 1 [6].

Adrenal cortical carcinoma in children is occasionally found in association with hemihypertrophy of the body. The cause of the association is not known, but it may be allied to or be a forme fruste of the Beckwith–Wiedemann syndrome.

Non-endocrine syndromes with a minor endocrine component

Three conditions are included here, each is a dominantly inherited well defined syndrome, which is recognized mainly by its effects on non-endocrine tissues (Table 3.5). In each there is an increased liability to endocrine tumours, but these usually affect only a minority of patients with the syndrome. Neurofibromatosis is associated with an increased liability to phaeochromocytomas and a carcinoid tumour of the ampulla of Vater [7]. The carcinoid tumours show morphological differences from the typical carcinoid, and have strong immunocytochemical positivity for somatostatin. The mechanism by which the mutated NF_1 gene in chromosome 17 leads to the development of the tumours is not known; NF_1 is thought to be a tumour-suppressor gene, and heterozygosity for chromosome 17 has been shown to be lost in a minority of neurofibromas. The endocrine tumours have not been linked to a particular mutation of the NF_1 gene, and have not been shown to be particularly frequent within families, although family studies are difficult because of the high proportion of cases of neurofibromatosis that are new mutations. Phaeochromocytoma and duodenal carcinoid have been found in the same patient. While this may in part be due to the fact that laparotomy for one may reveal the other, they are normally such uncommon features of the disease that a co-occurrence suggests that a particular mutation in the NF_1 gene may determine their occurrence.

Von Hippel–Lindau syndrome includes a variety of defects, especially haemangioblastomas in the cerebellum, retinal angiomas and renal cell carcinomas. The endocrine component is composed of phaeochromocytomas and islet cell tumours; the islet cell tumours may be of differing cell types, and somatostatinoma of the ampulla of Vater is not a feature. Islet cell tumours and phaeochromocytoma may occur in the same patient, and islet cell tumours have occurred in more than one family

Table 3.5 Non-endocrine syndromes with minor endocrine involvement

Syndrome	Frequency of endocrine tumours	Type of endocrine tumour	Gene/chromosome
Neurofibromatosis	Rare	Phaeochromocytoma; duodenal carcinoid	NF_1, tumour-suppressor gene, chromosome 17
Von Hippel–Lindau	Rare	Phaeochromocytoma; islet cell tumours	Tumour-suppressor gene; chromosome 3
Familial adenomatous polyposis	Rare	Thyroid carcinoma; colon carcinoid	APC; tumour-suppressor gene; chromosome 5

member [5]. The von Hippel–Lindau gene on chromosome 3 is also thought to be a tumour-suppressor gene.

Familial polyposis is another dominantly inherited autosomal condition and is of course characterized by the development of very large numbers of colonic adenomas in affected individuals. A small proportion of the adenomas progress to carcinomas, but although the progression is infrequent, there are so many adenomas that the majority of patients develop one or more colorectal carcinomas, often at a young age. Some polyposis cases develop a variety of other tumours including desmoid tumours, and a small proportion show thyroid carcinomas. These have generally been described as papillary carcinomas, but a recent review shows that they are of an unusual morphological type, often multiple, and occur in young women. The gene for polyposis, *APC*, is found on chromosome 5; it is thought to be a tumour-suppressor gene, and it is presumed, but not yet demonstrated, that loss of heterozygosity will be present in the thyroid tumours.

Miscellaneous syndromes

The final group of syndromes includes those that do not fall into the other groups (Table 3.6). Many examples of individual endocrine tumours occurring with other syndromes or other tumours have been described; it must be remembered that the coincidental occurrence of two or more tumours in one patient is more likely to be observed with slowly growing tumours than with rapidly fatal tumours, and also that rare combinations are more likely to be reported than a combination of common tumours.

Cowden's syndrome includes goitre with an increased incidence of thyroid carcinoma, and also breast cancer and facial and oral skin tags. The genetic basis is not established.

The Beckwith–Wiedemann syndrome affects children, and has a complex presentation and a complex genetic basis. The main features are macroglossia, nephromegaly and a variety of other observations, including a liability to tumours. The endocrine component is the occurrence of islet cell hyperplasia and of adrenal cortical carcinomas in a minority of cases. The genetic background is complex, involving two genes on chromosome 11, *IGF-2* and *H19*, both of which are regulated by imprinting.

The McCune–Albright syndrome is another syndrome with a complex genetic background. A minority of cases are familial, the majority arise from mutations in a G protein gene, occurring in the early stages of embryonic development, so that mosaicism results. A variety of endocrine glands may show hyperfunction, and nodular adrenal hyperplasia, nodular thyroid hyperplasia and pituitary adenomas have all been described.

Carney's syndrome consists of atrial or other myxomas, spotty pigmentation of the face and legs, with an endocrine component of tumours of the adrenal cortex and Leydig cells. The gene involved is not known.

Conclusion

This brief overview of inherited susceptibility to endocrine tumours has classified the main described syndromes into groups and discussed the mechanisms that are involved in those syndromes with or without hyperplasia. The role of growth in neoplasia of stable cell tissues is stressed; most of the conditions discussed are dominantly inherited, and can be regarded as inheritance of one of the mutations

Table 3.6 Miscellaneous and ill-defined syndromes

Syndrome	Non-endocrine component	Endocrine tumours	Gene/chromosome
Cowden	Breast carcinoma	Thyroid tumours	
Beckwith–Wiedemann	Macroglossia; nephromegaly	Adrenal carcinoma; islet hyperplasia	*IGF-2* and *H19*; chromosome 11, imprinting
McCune–Albright	Polyostotic fibrous dysplasia	Adrenal and thyroid nodules; pituitary adenoma (rare)	GSα (mosaicism)
Carney	Atrial and other myxomas, spotty pigmentation	Adrenal nodules; Leydig cell tumours	

that can form part of the sequence of somatic mutations that lead to neoplasia in the tissue concerned. Fewer somatic mutations are therefore needed than in individuals without the inherited defect, so that tumours tend to be multiple and to occur at an earlier age in inherited tumour syndromes. A genetic component should be considered in any patient with multiple endocrine tumours, or any patient in whom an endocrine tumour is found at a particularly early age.

There are doubtless more syndromes with an inherited susceptibility to endocrine neoplasia awaiting discovery. Genes that confer only a low level risk of developing a tumour of one or more endocrines are difficult to identify without large family studies, as many gene carriers will never develop the tumour. The chance of identifying such families will be increased if exposure to mutagenesis is widespread, such as has happened after Chernobyl. Under these circumstances the general incidence of tumours can be expected to rise, but there may be a particular increase in families with an inherited susceptibility.

Recognition of the syndromes that confer an inherited susceptibility to endocrine tumour is important for several reasons. It benefits patient care by allowing earlier diagnosis of other lesions in the patient concerned, and by allowing screening and earlier diagnosis of family members. A good example of these benefits is with MEN-2; the recognition that medullary carcinoma and phaeochromocytoma were inherited led to investigation of patients with medullary carcinoma for the presence of phaeochromocytoma pre-operatively, reducing the chances of operative mortality and of subsequent complications relating to phaeochromocytoma. It also led to the introduction of family screening, with diagnosis and treatment of medullary carcinoma before metastasis had occurred. Delineation of a syndrome allows identification of the gene responsible, and study of its expression and its effects. These add to our understanding of the normal mechanisms that control growth and function in the involved tissues, and provide information that will aid the development of new therapies in the future.

References

1. Wynford-Thomas D, Stringer BMJ, Williams ED. Dissociation of growth and function in the rat thyroid during prolonged goitrogen admin-istration. *Acta Endocrinol.* 1982;**101**:210–16.
2. Steiner AL, Goodman AD, Powers SR. Study of a kindred with phaeochromocytomas, medullary thyroid carcinoma, hyperparathyroidism and Cushings disease, multiple endocrine neoplasia type II. *Medicine (Baltimore)* 1968;**47**:371–409.
3. Williams ED. Medullary carcinoma of the thyroid. *J. Clin. Pathol.* 1967; **20**(Suppl.): 395–8.
4. Mulligan LM, Marsh DJ, Robinson BG *et al.* Genotype–phenotype correlation in multiple endocrine neoplasia type 2. *J. Int. Med.* 1995; **238**:343–6.
5. Dinnen JS, Greenwood RH, Jones JH, Walker DA, Williams ED. Parathyroid carcinoma in familial hyperparathyroidism. *J. Clin. Pathol.* 1977; **20**: 722–4.
6. Szabo J, Heath B, Hill VM *et al.* Hereditary hyperparathyroidism–jaw tumour syndrome; the endocrine tumour gene HRPT2 maps to chromosome 1q21–q31. *J. Hum. Genet.* 1995;**56**:944–50.
7. Griffiths DFR, Williams GT, Williams ED. Duodenal carcinoid tumours, phaeochromocytoma and neurofibromatosis; islet cell tumours, phaeochromocytoma and the von Hippel–Lindau complex; two distinct neuroendocrine syndromes. *Q. J. Med.* 1987;**245**:769–82.

4

Hormones, Growth Factors and Tumour Growth

RICHARD EPSTEIN

Introduction

Most common human tumours — lung, breast, gastro-intestinal and genitourinary — are carcinomas. Experimental analysis of these epithelial tumours remains hampered by technical problems relating to stromal cell admixture, difficulty disaggregating tissue specimens, and interpretational limitations of adapting primary epithelial cell cultures to long-term growth *in vitro*. Such problems are directly related to the 'tight junction' morphology of epithelial tissue, which reflects epithelial cell dependence on intercellular contact for maintaining intimate chemical communication networks. These networks transmit signals via low (often picomolar) tissue concentrations of signalling molecules termed polypeptide growth factors.

Growth factors have no intrinsic biological activity. Rather, they act as binding molecules (ligands) which trigger a conformational change in large transmembrane *receptor* molecules that transduce intracellular signals using a variety of catalytic mechanisms. Polypeptide growth factors activate two main receptor subclasses, the receptor tyrosine kinases and the cytokine (haematopoietin) receptors; the latter receptors activate cytosolic (non-receptor) tyrosine kinases. Peptide hormones, in contrast, usually activate transmembrane molecules termed G-protein-coupled receptors which interact with cyclic AMP-dependent signalling pathways. Most of these signalling pathways culminate in a substrate phosphorylation cascade coupled to mobilization of intracellular calcium stores, with the latter leading to activation of calcium-dependent cytosolic enzymes. Indeed, transmembrane calcium influx may closely mimic the effects of growth factors [1], raising the possibility that extracellular calcium may have been the first 'growth factor' prior to evolution of multisubunit receptors.

Growth factors overlap with hormones in several important functional respects. Some, such as insulin, share both classifications, being secreted in an 'endocrine' fashion on the one hand while activating a receptor tyrosine kinase on the other. Others such as insulin-like growth factor-1 (IGF-1) may circulate in the peripheral blood bound to carrier proteins, reminiscent of steroid/sterol hormones. Still others may interact with hormones either upstream or downstream, the best example again being IGF-1 which mediates growth hormone action. Like all peptides, those growth factors when used therapeutically (for example, insulin, erythropoietin and granulocyte colony-stimulating factor), must be administered parenterally to avoid gastrointestinal proteolysis. Selective enhancement of tumour cell growth using appropriate mitogens has yielded major improvements in cytotoxic cell kill *in vitro* [2], though routine therapeutic application of this approach has not yet been validated by clinical trials.

So-called growth factors do not always stimulate growth, and are therefore more accurately termed peptide signalling molecules. Epidermal growth factor (EGF), for example, is associated with many physiological functions unassociated with mitogenesis. Some of these functions, such as regulation of gastric acid secretion [3] are difficult to reconcile with a strictly mitogenic mechanism of action. Conversely, the way in which EGF stimulates growth remains unclear: EGF-induced mitogenesis is tightly linked to cell migration in some experimental systems, consistent with a primary effect of the signal on pericellular proteolysis [4]. This raises the possibility that EGF and other growth factors may contribute directly to tumour invasion independently of proliferative effects. Another signalling peptide, platelet-derived growth factor (PDGF), stimulates growth in susceptible target cells while also promoting chemotaxis, cell adhesion, collagenase synthesis and lysosomal granule release. In addition, PDGF morphologically transforms normal fibroblasts *in vitro* (the criteria for which are summarized in Table 4.1), while the viral oncogene v-*sis* acts by encoding an isoform of PDGF. Yet another multifunctional growth

38

Table 4.1 Criteria for cell transformation

1 Reduction in *serum-/growth factor-dependence* of cell growth compared to normal cells *in vitro*
2 Loss of *density-dependent inhibition* of cell growth *in vitro* (monolayer cells continue to proliferate postconfluence)
3 Confluent monolayers form *foci* of aggregated proliferating cells
4 Cells acquire *anchorage-independent growth* (monolayer cells begin to grow in suspension)
5 Cells undergo *immortalization* (cells fail to senesce after finite number of divisions)
6 Cells form *tumours* when injected into nude (athymic) mice

factor family, the fibroblast growth factors (FGFs), are not only fibroblast mitogens but also potent stimuli of endothelial cell proliferation and, hence, neovascularization. The role played by 'growth factors' in determining the neoplastic phenotype thus appears far more interesting than simple stimulation of tumour cell DNA synthesis.

Clonal escape and cancer growth

The term 'tumour marker' is usually reserved for secreted molecules, which are assayed in peripheral blood as an index of host tumour burden. Measuring such peptides can be clinically useful in either diagnosis or follow-up of cancer patients (see Chapter 60); for example, non-seminomatous germ-cell tumours often secrete the 'oncofetal antigen' α-fetoprotein (α-FP) and/or the peptide hormone β-human chorionic gonadotrophin (β-hCG). The half-lives of these molecules (5 days and 30 hours, respectively) are routinely used to predict the curativity of surgical resection or systemic therapy by analysing the marker's rate of decay [5]. Ectopic tumour synthesis of such molecules may be either phenotypically silent (as with α-FP) or symptomatic, as occasionally seen with high levels of β-hCG inducing gynaecomastia.

Why should cancer cell clones expressing such tumour markers survive better than clinically inapparent marker-negative clones? What growth advantage could there be for tumour cells that produce clonal proteins such as CALLA (common ALL antigen, or CD10), a cell-surface neutral endopeptidase that represses cytokine activation during B-cell differentiation? Why do neuroblastomas express neuropeptide Y, an embryogenic peptide implicated in adrenal medullary development? And why do many epithelial tumours express carcinoembryonic antigen (CEA), a cell-surface glycoprotein? The answers to most of these questions are unknown. Instructively, CEA has been shown to be an *intercellular adhesion molecule* which mediates homotypic tumour cell aggregation within heterogeneous cell populations [6], a function which could

well be critical for modulating tumour invasion. For the majority of tumour markers, however, mechanisms for mediation of a neoplastic growth advantage remain undefined.

This uncertainty holds true even for those tumours overexpressing hormones, growth factors, or their receptors. For example, overexpression of oestrogen receptors in many human breast tumours was traditionally regarded as a marker of residual differentiation [7]. This viewpoint was modified when it was found that human oestrogen receptors are encoded by a gene homologous to the v-*erb*A oncogene [8], a steroid receptor superfamily member. The observation that oestrogen receptors and EGF receptors are reciprocally expressed in human breast tumours [9] raises the possibility of two distinct molecular pathways of tumorigenesis. Intriguingly, recent work has suggested that oestrogen receptors play a tumour-suppressive role in some experimental systems [10].

Human tumours consist of heterogeneous subclones which lack negative-feedback growth controls, and one popular model of tumour growth suggests that clinically apparent tumour deposits represent only the clonal outgrowth of a mitogenically dominant tumour cell subpopulation. Such heterogeneity poses a daunting obstacle to therapeutic responsiveness, since: (i) few if any molecular targets distinguish tumours from normal tissues; and (ii) treatment rapidly selects for the survival of resistant tumour subclones. While the search for a 'magic bullet' targeting a tumour-specific antigen is compromised by the likelihood of progressive genetic instability, a further problem may relate to the presence of functionally distinct tumour cell subpopulations defined by growth state rather than by antigenic or mutational subtypes. Hence, slow-growing human neoplasms may exhibit *de novo* drug resistance, which reflects G_o tumour cell subpopulations with ample time for repairing DNA damage prior to reaching critical cell-cycle 'decision points' [11]. Increasing knowledge of tumour cell growth-regulatory molecules may provide viable strategies for recruiting such resistant cancer cell subsets into the cycle, thus improving the therapeutic ratio of cytotoxic drug treatment [12].

Autocrine and paracrine growth

Transformed cells generally require less *in vitro* supplementation with *exogenous* growth factors than do normal cells. This phenomenon can sometimes be explained by *endogenous* growth factor overproduction by transformed cells expressing homologous growth factor receptors. Such autocrine growth stimulation can be illustrated experimentally: transfection of non-tumorigenic EGF-receptor-bearing cells with the gene encoding EGF, for example, can induce both the transformed phenotype *in vitro* and tumorigenicity *in vivo* [13]. More dramatically, creation of transgenic mice overexpressing the EGF-homologous ligand transforming growth factor-α (TGF-α) results in hyperplasia, metaplasia and neoplasia of the breast, pancreas and liver [14], although the pathogenetic implications of these findings for sporadic human disease remain unclear.

Tumours that overexpress growth factors can be plausibly assumed to do so for one of two reasons: either because they express their own receptors for the ligand (*autocrine* growth; see Table 4.2); or because they cause surrounding cells to provide tumour cells with an indirect *paracrine* growth advantage. The latter possibility is consistent with the finding that tumour cells may secrete fibroblast/monocyte chemoattractants [15]. *In vitro sis*-mediated cell transformation occurs due to autocrine stimulation [16]; an analogous *in vivo* mechanism may contribute to the pathogenesis of human cerebral glioblastomas, sarcomas and other mesenchymal tumours. Similarly, human breast cancer cell lines often secrete PDGF without expressing PDGF receptors [17], raising the possibility that breast cancers acquire a growth advantage from PDGF-stimulated fibroblasts that could conceivably release tumour cell mitogens (e.g. IGF-1) in response.

Does constitutive growth factor production occur in real life? In *sis*-transformed cells, PDGF-β receptors are profoundly down-regulated at the cell surface; receptor activation in this context may occur intracellularly [18]. Physiological adaptations such as receptor down-regulation do not always occur in the setting of constitutive expression in tumour cells, however; defective down-regulation of EGF receptors with mutant extracellular domains, for example, may be associated with ligand-dependent transformation [19]. Hence,

autocrine growth may result from abnormal feedback regulation of receptor activity as well as from primary mutations of ligand production and receptor activity.

Cells may be transformed either by inappropriate exposure to an activating ligand or by inappropriate expression of cell-surface receptors. Since growth factor secretion *in vivo* may occur in a paracrine fashion, there is no theoretical requirement for an abnormal cell clone to complete the autocrine loop by synthesizing its own growth factor. Consider, for example, the transforming viruses. A receptor for macrophage colony-stimulating factor (M-CSF) is encoded by the v-*fms* oncogene, and this receptor differs from the wild-type c-*fms*-encoded receptor mainly in the structure of its cytoplasmic domain which lacks a negative regulatory region. Although both receptors bind M-CSF, the tyrosine kinase moiety of the v-*fms* variant remains constitutively activated even in the absence of ligand; for this reason v-*fms*-containing retroviruses will efficiently transform normal cells, while high-level expression of transfected wild-type c-*fms* will not [20]. Similarly, the v-*erb*B oncogene of the avian erythroblastosis virus (AEV) induces polycythaemia in chickens by encoding an EGF receptor which is truncated in its *extracellular* domain and which is also constitutively activated. An additional deletion of the tyrosine autophosphorylation site within the cytoplasmic domain causes the v-*erb*B oncogene to induce *sarcomas* as well as erythroblastosis, while 'cooperation' with the v-*erb*A oncogene yields more aggressive leukaemias.

Cell-surface receptors encoded by v-*kit* are likewise characterized by a truncated extracellular domain and constitutive activation. The transforming ability of viruses like AEV implies that an altered growth factor receptor can mimic and override the effect of its normal ligand. Human cancers are not known to be induced by these oncogene-encoding transforming viruses, but aberrant expression of cell-surface growth factor receptors is commonly found. EGF receptor overexpression occurs in human squamous cell carcinomas of the upper digestive tract, renal cell carcinoma, glial tumours and breast cancer. Such malignancies often co-express the homologous activating ligand TGF-α (but not EGF). Amplification of the encoding gene occurs commonly in brain tumours [21]; as many as 30% of human gliomas have multiple copies of this gene detected by Southern blotting, as do a smaller proportion of primary squamous cell tumours. Breast tumours, in contrast, seldom exhibit amplification of this gene despite frequent overexpression at the protein level.

Approximately 20–30% of primary human breast cancers exhibit amplification of the closely related c-*erb*B-2 (*neu*, HER2) gene with associated overexpression at the

Table 4.2 Human cancers in which autocrine mitogens are implicated

Small-cell lung cancer:
  bombesin

Gliomas:
  PDGF
  TGF-α

Sarcomas:
  PDGF

Breast cancer:
  IGF-1
  TGF-α

IGF, insulin-like growth factor; PDGF, platelet-derived growth factor; TGF, transforming growth factor.

cell surface [22]. The latter gene is also commonly amplified in ovarian cancer and gastric cancer. It is currently not understood why *erb*B-2 overexpression occurs frequently in adenocarcinomas, while the structurally related EGF receptor is preferentially expressed in gliomas and squamous cell cancers. Experimentally mimicking such gene amplification by transfecting and overexpressing wild-type *neu* receptor induces transformation *in vitro*, although less efficiently than when the constitutively activated transmembrane mutant is used. EGF receptor, in contrast, will usually only transform cultured cells in the presence of activating ligand. Overexpression of either EGF receptor or c-*erb*B-2 is a predictor of poor prognosis in human breast cancer, while coexpression of both receptors is even more ominous. Although the transforming activity of *erb*B-2 suggests that this receptor plays a role in the malignant phenotype, overexpression occurs more commonly in the context of *in situ* disease than in invasive breast cancer [23]. Similarly, c-*erb*B-2 is overexpressed in preneoplastic colonic polyps relative to established carcinomas [24]. These anomalies raise the possibility that growth factor receptor dysregulation may be an early event in the natural history of human malignancies.

It is important to appreciate that the 'autocrine hypothesis' remains just that — a hypothesis. As neat as the theory may seem, the evidence that autocrine growth plays a key role in either the genesis or phenotype of human malignant disease remains conjectural. But is there any other way that growth factors could affect human tumour behaviour?

Inhibitory growth factors

The best characterized inhibitory growth factors are those belonging to the TGF-β superfamily. A bifunctional growth regulator, TGF-β exerts an antiproliferative effect on epithelial cells and on some human carcinoma cell lines; for example, MCF-7 (Michigan Cancer Foundation breast isolate number) breast cancer cells have been reported by one group to secrete this growth factor following treatment with the anti-oestrogen tamoxifen [25]. TGF-β also brings about a potent immunosuppressant effect by inhibiting cytokine-induced lymphocyte activation and proliferation. Fibroblasts, on the other hand, see TGF-β as a mitogen and chemotactic stimulus; in addition, these cells respond by reducing protease secretion and increasing extracellular matrix formation.

Epithelial cell transformation has been associated with loss of TGF-β-inducible growth inhibition, both with and without receptor loss. Since the biological activity of the secreted (latent) ligand is regulated at the level of postsecretory activation [26], normal transcriptional and translational activity remains compatible with decreased autocrine growth inhibition by this regulatory peptide. Some tumours express TGF-β: indeed, the development of tumours in Rous sarcoma virus-infected chickens appears critically dependent on TGF-β release [26]. In carcinoma cells that produce the activated form of the ligand, stimulation of stromal cell growth may confer a paracrine growth advantage such as that discussed previously for PDGF and FGF.

Activation of the c-*erb*B-2 receptor tyrosine kinase has more recently been associated with cell growth arrest [27]. Several groups have reported *in vitro* differentiation of human tumour cells in response to treatment with c-*erb*B-3/4 ligands or heregulins, which have also been termed *neu* differentiation factors (NDF) [28]. Other groups have reported mitogenic activity of this ligand, however, and it currently seems likely that receptor heterodimerization will emerge as a key regulatory variable determining the response to this 'growth factor' family.

The *interferons* (IFNs) comprise another family of growth inhibitors. IFN-α, for example, has proven an effective therapeutic agent in hairy cell leukaemia, and has been credited with anecdotal success in other malignancies. Unlike conventional cancer chemotherapeutic agents, interferons appear to exert their maximal antiproliferative effect on non-dividing (G_o) cells rather than on dividing cells, perhaps involving an inverse relationship between cell proliferation and expression of the interferon-inducible enzyme 2′,5′ oligoadenylate synthetase.

Ectopic peptide hormone production

Tumour-induced symptoms may occur in the absence of direct spread. Remote non-metastatic manifestations of human tumours are clinically known as *paraneoplastic syndromes* (see also Chapter 76), most of which result from the inappropriate secretion of a peptide hormone. Such ectopic hormone production is surprisingly common: as many as 60–70% of small-cell lung cancers (SCLC) have been found to synthesize and secrete any one of adrenocorticotrophic hormone (ACTH), neurophysin, calcitonin and neurone-specific enolase, while peptides less commonly produced include β-hCG, antidiuretic hormone (ADH, vasopressin) and parathyroid hormone-related peptide (PTHrP; see below). The multiplicity of these peptides reflects the clonal origin of small-cell lung tumours from a pulmonary neuroendocrine cell lineage. Many ectopic peptides (e.g. calcitonin, neurophysin and neurone-specific enolase) have not been associated with recognizable clinical syndromes.

Peptides secreted by tumours are not necessarily

identical to 'wild-type' peptides. Indeed, many tumours synthesize either biologically inactive subunits of the mature peptide or high-molecular-weight precursor molecules of variable potency. An example of the latter is big ACTH (pro-opiomelanocortin), a pro-hormone commonly secreted by SCLC and occasionally responsible for ectopic Cushing's syndrome. In addition to the usual signal peptides, proteolytic sequences and regulatory domains, big ACTH comprises γ-MSH (melanocyte-stimulating hormone), 'classic' ACTH (which contains within it both α-MSH and corticotrophin-like intermediate peptide, CLIP), β-lipotrophin (which contains within it both γ-lipotrophin and β-MSH), met-encephalin and β-endorphin. Hence the active fragments of this molecule may induce hyperadrenalism, hyperpigmentation and, at least theoretically, opiate-like activity.

Clinical and molecular overlap between paraneoplastic syndromes is extensive. Ectopic ACTH syndrome can be mimicked by ectopic corticotrophin-releasing factor (CRF) synthesis, for example, while the hyponatraemia of inappropriate ADH secretion may be mimicked by tumour-induced stimulation of atrial natriuretic peptide (ANP) production. Similarly, the non-specific hyper-metabolic state often seen in cancer patients may, rarely, be induced by secondary thyrotoxicosis in patients with trophoblastic tumours and high levels of β-hCG, since this hormone may share agonist activity with the structurally related thyroid-stimulating hormone (TSH) (thyrotrophin) glycoprotein hormone. Even rarer is the secretion of thyroid hormone itself by ovarian teratomas. Insulinoma-like hypoglycaemia is seen most frequently with large abdominal mesenchymal tumours (especially mesotheliomas), which secrete IGF-1 and/or IGF-2 [29]. More common, however, are paraneoplastic syndromes which have not yet been associated with a secreted peptide: limbic encephalitis (Ophelia syndrome), dermatomyositis, acanthosis nigricans and finger clubbing are just a few that remain in this category despite some interesting leads.

Paraneoplastic hypercalcaemia, seen especially with squamous cell carcinomas (lung, oesophagus, head and neck) and adult T-cell leukaemia/lymphoma, has been linked to ectopic production of PTHrP, although prostaglandins (PGE_1, PGE_2), 1,25-dihydroxyvitamin D and osteoclast-activating factor (OAF, lymphotoxin) have occasionally been implicated. Wild-type parathyroid hormone (PTH) exhibits homology in only 13 of 141 amino acids near the N-terminal of PTHrP [30], but the organizational pattern of the encoding genes is virtually identical [31], and PTHrP appears to interact with normal PTH receptors [32]. The two hormones are encoded on the short arms of chromosomes 11 and 12 amidst a cluster of mutually related genes [33], suggesting that these chromosomal fragments arose from an ancient DNA duplication event. Although expressed and regulated in several non-parathyroid tissues, including pancreas, lactating breast and uterus, the physiological function(s) of PTHrP remains unknown.

Growth factors, tumour progression and metastasis

Metastasis is the terminal determinant of clinical cancer. Observations in both experimental animals and human patients suggest that *in vivo* induction of malignancy is a 'multi-hit' process in which endogenous mitogens play a promotional role throughout tumour progression [34], and some of the stages involved in this multi-step process have been phenomenologically characterized. First, a growing tumour needs to increase its blood supply (angiogenesis). Peptides implicated in angiogenesis include both acidic and basic FGF; acidic FGF binds to collagen I (a component of interstitial stroma) and collagen IV (a basement membrane constituent), suggesting that direct interactions with extracellular matrix mediate FGF-induced new vessel formation. Tumours also need to invade peri-tumoural stroma, to extravasate into the bloodstream and/or lymphatics, to adhere to metastatic target organs, and to proliferate within such target organs. With respect to the latter, soluble growth factors have been implicated in the organ-specificity of bone marrow [35] and peritoneal [36] metastases, while membrane-bound factors have been linked to liver-specific spread in experimental models [37].

Little is known concerning the exact steps involved in systemic dissemination of tumour cells. Tumour cell motility factors (such as the so-called autocrine motility factor (AMF) [38], and the c-*met* ligand, variously called scatter factor or hepatocyte growth factor) are secreted by certain tumour cells, raising the possibility that such ligands could contribute directly to cancer dissemination. Moreover, just as tumour cells produce chemotactic factors for stromal tissues, so may fibroblasts secrete 'migration stimulating factors' for human tumour cells *in vivo*. Similarly, co-cultivation studies have revealed that EGF stimulates human glioma cell migration and invasiveness [39] in addition to its recognized mitogenic effect, while FGF-dependent interaction of human melanoma cells with laminin may be prevented by a putative inhibitor of growth factor-receptor binding, suramin [40], which has recently entered clinical trials as a biological response modifier. Stromal cell-surface proteins implicated in paracrine tumour growth may therefore come to provide novel molecular targets for anticancer therapy [41].

The preceding summary inevitably omits many fascinating areas of research, but the inescapable conclusion is that abnormalities of growth factors and their receptors play a key role in governing neoplastic cell growth control.

References

1. Epstein RJ, Druker BJ, Jones SD *et al*. Extracellular calcium mimics the effects of platelet-derived growth factor. *Cell Growth Differ.* 1992;3:157–64.

2. Epstein RJ, Smith PJ. Estrogen-induced potentiation of DNA damage and cytotoxicity in human breast cancer cells treated with topoisomerase II-interactive antitumor drugs. *Cancer Res.* 1988;48:297–303.

3. Gregory H. Isolation and structure of urogastrone and its relationship to epidermal growth factor. *Nature* 1975;257:325–7.

4. Niedbala M, Sartorelli A. Regulation by epidermal growth factor of human squamous cell carcinoma plasminogen activator-mediated proteolysis of extracellular matrix. *Cancer Res.* 1989;49:3302–9.

5. Toner G, Geller N, Tan C, Nisselbaum J, Bosl G. Serum tumor marker half-life during chemotherapy allows early prediction of complete response and survival in nonseminomatous germ cell tumors. *Cancer Res.* 1990;50:5904–10.

6. Benchimoi S, Fuks A, Jothy S *et al*. Carcinoembryonic antigen, a human tumor marker, functions as an intercellular adhesion molecule. *Cell* 1989;57:327–34.

7. Epstein RJ. The clinical biology of hormone-responsive breast cancer. *Cancer Treat. Rev.* 1988;15:33–51.

8. Green S, Walter P, Kumar V *et al*. Human oestrogen receptor cDNA: sequence, expression and homology to v-erbA. *Nature* 1986;320:136–9.

9. Sainsbury J, Sherbet G, Farndon J, Harris A. Epidermal growth factor receptors and oestrogen receptors in human breast cancer. *Lancet* 1985;i:364–6.

10. Garcia M, Derocq D, Freiss G, Rochefort H. Activation of estrogen receptor transfected into a receptor-negative breast cancer cell line decreases the metastatic and invasive potential of the cells. *Proc. Natl Acad. Sci. USA* 1992;89:11538–42.

11. Epstein RJ. Drug-induced DNA damage and tumor chemo-sensitivity. *J. Clin. Oncol.* 1990;8:2062–84.

12. Epstein RJ, Smith PJ, Watson JV, Bleehen NM. Estrogen potentiates topoisomerase-II-mediated cytotoxicity in an activated subpopulation of human breast cancer cells: implications for cytotoxic drug resistance in solid tumors. *Int. J. Cancer* 1989;44:501–5.

13. Stern D, Hare D, Cecchini M, Weinberg R. Construction of a novel oncogene based on synthetic sequence encoding epidermal growth factor. *Science* 1987;235:321–4.

14. Sandgren E, Luetteke N, Palmiter R, Brinster R, Lee D. Overexpression of TGF$_\alpha$ in transgenic mice: induction of epithelial hyperplasia, pancreatic metaplasia, and carcinoma of the breast. *Cell* 1990;61:1121–35.

15. Graves D, Jiang Y, Williamson M, Valente A. Identification of monocyte chemotactic activity produced by malignant cells. *Science* 1989;245:1490–2.

16. Keating M, Williams L. Autocrine stimulation of intracellular PDGF receptors in v-sis-transformed cells. *Science* 1988;239:914–16.

17. Peres R, Betsholtz C, Westermark B, Heldin C. Frequent expression of growth factors for mesenchymal cells in human mammary carcinoma cell lines. *Cancer Res.* 1987;47:3425–9.

18. Bejcek B, Li D, Deuel T. Transformation by v-sis occurs by an internal autoactivation mechanism. *Science* 1989;245:1496–8.

19. Wells A, Welsh J, Lazar C *et al*. Ligand-induced transformation by a noninternalizing epidermal growth factor receptor. *Science* 1990;247:962–4.

20. Sacca R, Stanley E, Sherr C, Rettenmeier C. Specific binding of the mononuclear phagocyte colony stimulating factor, CSF-1, to the product of the v-*fms* oncogene. *Proc. Natl Acad. Sci. USA* 1986;83:3331–5.

21. Libermann T, Nussbaum H, Razon N *et al*. Amplification, enhanced expression and possible rearrangement of the EGF-receptor gene in primary human brain tumors of glial origin. *Nature* 1985;313:144–7.

22. Slamon D. Human breast cancer: correlation of relapse and survival with amplification of the HER-2/*neu* oncogene. *Science* 1987;235:177–81.

23. Gusterson B, Machin L, Gullick W *et al*. Immunohistochemical distribution of c-*erb*B-2 in infiltrating and *in situ* breast cancer. *Int. J. Cancer* 1988;42:842–5.

24. D'Emilia J, Bulovas K, D'Ercole K *et al*. Expression of the c-erbB-2 gene product (p185) at different stages of neoplastic progression in the colon. *Oncogene* 1989;4:1233–9.

25. Knabbe C, Lippman M, Wakefield L *et al*. Evidence that trans-forming growth factor-beta is a hormonally regulated negative growth factor in human breast cancer cells. *Cell* 1987;48:417–28.

26. Sieweke M, Thompson N, Sporn M, Bissell M. Mediation of wound-related Rous sarcoma virus tumorigenesis by TGF-β. *Science* 1990;248:1656–8.

27. Epstein RJ, Druker BJ, Roberts TM, Stiles CD. Modulation of a M$_r$ 175,000 c-*neu* receptor isoform in G8/DHFR cells by serum starvation. *J. Biol Chem.* 1990;265:10746–51.

28. Peles E, Bacus SS, Koski RA *et al*. Isolation of the neu/HER-2 stimulatory ligand: a 44 kd glycoprotein that induces differentiation of mammary tumor cells. *Cell* 1992;69:205–16.

29. Gorden P, Hendricks C, Kahn C *et al*. Hypoglycemia associated with non-islet cell tumor and insulin-like growth factors. *N. Engl. J. Med.* 1981;305:1452–5.

30. Thiede M, Strewler G, Nissenson R, Rosenblatt M, Rodan G. Human renal carcinoma expresses two messages encoding a parathyroid hormone-like peptide: evidence for the alternative splicing of a single-copy gene. *Proc. Natl Acad. Sci. USA* 1988;85:4605–9.

31. Mangin M, Ikeda K, Dreyer B, Broadus A. Isolation and characterization of the human parathyroid hormone-like peptide gene. *Proc. Natl Acad. Sci. USA* 1989;86:2408–12.

32. Horiuchi N, Caulfield M, Fisher J *et al*. Similarity of synthetic peptide from human tumor to parathyroid hormone in vivo and in vitro. *Science* 1987;238:1566–8.

33. Mangin M, Webb A, Dreyer B *et al*. Identification of a cDNA encoding a parathyroid hormone-like peptide from a human tumor associated with humoral hypercalcemia of malignancy. *Proc. Natl Acad. Sci. USA* 1988;85:597–601.

34. Epstein RJ. Is your initiator really necessary? *J. Theor. Biol.* 1986;122:359–74.

35. Chackal-Roy M, Niemeyer C, Moore M, Zetter B. Stimulation of human prostatic carcinoma cell growth by factors present in human bone marrow. *J. Clin. Invest.* 1989;84:43–50.

36. Mills G, May C, Hill M *et al*. Ascitic fluid from human ovarian cancer patients contains growth factors necessary for intraperitoneal growth of human ovarian adenocarcinoma cells. *J. Clin. Invest.* 1990;86:851–5.

37. Sargent N, Oestreicher M, Haidvogel H, Madnick H, Burger M. Growth regulation of cancer metastases by their host organ. *Proc.*

Natl Acad. Sci. USA 1988;**85**:7251–5.

38. Guirguis R, Margulies I, Taraboletti G *et al*. Cytokine-induced pseudopodial protrusion is coupled to tumour cell migration. *Nature* 1987;**329**:261–3.

39. Lund-Johansen M, Bjerkvig R, Humphrey P *et al*. Effect of epidermal growth factor on glioma cell growth, migration, and invasion in vitro. *Cancer Res.* 1990;**50**:6039–44.

40. Zabrenetzky V, Kohn E, Roberts D. Suramin inhibits laminin- and thrombospondin-mediated melanoma cell adhesion and migration and binding of these adhesive proteins to sulfatide. *Cancer Res.* 1990;**50**:5937–42.

41. Garin-Chesa P, Old L, Rettig W. Cell surface glycoprotein of reactive stromal fibroblasts as a potential antibody target in human epithelial cancers. *Proc. Natl Acad. Sci. USA* 1990;**87**:7235–9.

5

Angiogenesis, Invasion and Metastasis

ROY BICKNELL

Introduction

It remains true that the majority of cancer patients die as a result of metastatic disease. The metastatic process is a complex one involving many steps and is frequently referred to as the metastatic cascade (Fig. 5.1). The steps involved in metastasis include invasion and entry of tumour cells into the vasculature, dissemination around the body within the vasculature, exit from the vasculature (either by adhesion to the vascular endothelium followed by extravasation or possibly by occlusion of tumour cell/platelet clumps within the microvasculature) and finally the establishment of secondaries. It is now appreciated that angiogenesis (growth of new blood vessels) is not only essential for growth of primary tumours beyond a size of 2–3 mm^3 (the diffusion limit of growth) but is also a prerequisite for metastatic spread, in that the latter occurs primarily through the newly formed tumour vessels. These new tumour vessels are characteristically leaky and ill-formed.

Clinical relevance of tumour angiogenesis

Recent studies have shown that the vascular density of several primary human tumours (including, amongst others, breast, lung, brain, bladder, cervix, melanoma and head and neck cancer) shows a strong correlation with metastasis and survival. In the case of, for example, breast tumours, this is one of very few tumour properties to be identified that correlate with lymph node metastasis. Proteolytic activity is also a component of metastasis and it is noteworthy that the protease urokinase plasminogen activator has also been shown to correlate with lymph node metastasis in breast tumours. Expression of no single angiogenic factor in any solid tumour type has yet been shown to correlate with metastasis. Nevertheless it is now becoming clearer which factors are likely to be key players in tumour angiogenesis. These include soluble extracellular polypeptides that are direct growth factors for endo-thelial cells such as vascular endothelial growth factor (VEGF) as well as more indirect factors, such as thymidine phosphorylase, for which the precise mechanism of the induction of angiogenesis has yet to be elucidated.

Angiogenesis: an essential component of solid tumour development

Several angiogenic factor transfection experiments have confirmed that expression of an angiogenic factor confers a growth advantage on solid tumours. These include experiments in which the angiogenic polypeptide VEGF has been transfected into chinese hamster ovary (CHO) and MCF-7 (Michigan Cancer Foundation breast isolate number) human breast carcinoma cells. In the former case, expression of active VEGF conferred the ability not shown by wild-type cells to form tumours when xenografted into nude mice. MCF-7 cells were chosen for transfection because they form slow growing, poorly vascularized tumours that are hormone (oestrogen) dependent, tamoxifen sensitive and that do not metastasize. It follows that the effect of the transfection on each of these parameters could be examined. Expression of VEGF conferred a growth advantage *in vivo* but not *in vitro*, confirming that the growth of MCF-7 tumours is limited by angiogenesis. The tumours formed by the transfectants were more vascular than those formed by controls showing areas of high vascular density or hot spots (Fig. 5.2, and see below). Transfection had no effect, however, on hormone dependence, tamoxifen sensitivity or metastasis.

Two other elegant experiments that support the tenet that growth of solid tumours is angiogenesis dependent have been reported. First, systemic administration of anti-VEGF monoclonal antibodies blocked growth of three different xenografted tumours. The second experiment involved implantation of cells expressing infective retrovirus that encoded a gene for a dominant negative VEGF receptor (that is a mutant receptor that blocks VEGF

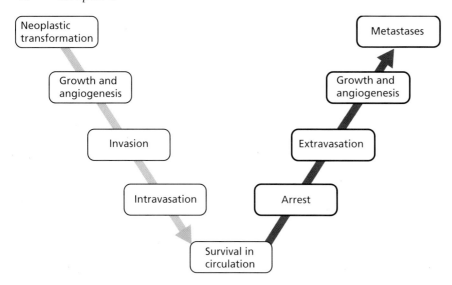

Fig. 5.1 The metastatic cascade.

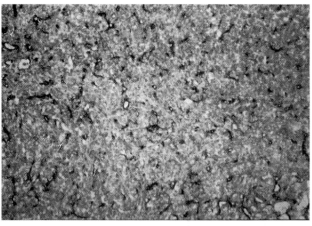

(a)

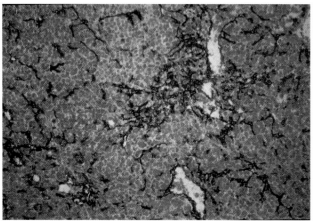

(b)

Fig. 5.2 Vascular density of tumours formed from (a) wild-type MCF-7 breast carcinoma cells, and (b) those transfected and expressing active vascular endothelial growth factor (121 amino acid form). Note the vascular hotspots in (b). It is these that in primary human tumours correlate with metastasis.

signal transduction in cells in which it is expressed) with tumour (glioblastoma) cells. Virus produced by the transfected cells infected the developing tumour endothelium and blocked: (i) signal transduction by tumour produced VEGF; (ii) tumour angiogenesis; and (iii) tumour growth.

Identified angiogenic stimulators and inhibitors

A substantial number of angiogenic stimulators and inhibitors have now been identified (Table 5.1) [1,2].

Angiogenesis and metastatic patterns in cancer patients

Recently two novel and naturally occurring polypeptide inhibitors of angiogenesis have been identified. These are both fragments of larger molecules that have biological activities that are well characterized and quite distinct from that of the inhibition of angiogenesis, namely, thrombospondin and plasminogen. The story of the plasminogen fragment is a particularly interesting one. Folkman and colleagues [3] noticed that removal of primary Lewis lung carcinomas from mice resulted in rapid (within 15 days) development of lung metastases. Metastases were rarely seen in the mice that retained the primary tumour. These workers postulated that the primary tumour was possibly releasing an inhibitor that systemically blocked development of metastases. They went on to show that this was indeed the case and identified the inhibitor as a fragment of plasminogen, which they named angiostatin. Further work then showed that angiostatin is anti-angiogenic and a specific inhibitor of endothelial cells. Thus, it blocked endothelial cell proliferation in response to the potent

Table 5.1 Some identified angiogenic factors

Polypeptide
Basic fibroblast growth factor
Acidic fibroblast growth factor
Angiogenin
Epidermal growth factor
Transforming growth factor-α
Transforming growth factor-β
Tumour necrosis factor-α
Platelet-derived endothelial cell growth factor
(Thymidine phosphorylase)
Vascular endothelial growth factor
Interleukin-1α
Fibrinogen
Fibrin
Laminin

Peptide
Angiotensin II
Substance P
Calcitonin gene-related peptide
Bradykinin

Lipid
Prostaglandins E1 and E2
Platelet-activating factors
Erucamide

Other compounds
Endothelial-stimulating angiogenesis factor
Heparin
Hyaluronic acid fragments
Adenosine
Nicotinamide
Histamine
Spermidine

Table 5.2 Metastatic patterns found at first diagnosis in cancer patients as classified by Folkman [2]

Group	Primary tumour	Metastases	Recurrence of metastases
I	+	0	Months
II	+	+	–
III	0	+	–
IV	+	0	Years

+, cases; 0, no cases.

phenotype is thought to occur. The secondaries then become vascularized and show increased growth. Support for this has come from transgenic mice that express basic fibroblast growth factor (bFGF) in their pancreas. When hyperplastic islands of beta cells start expressing bFGF they become vascularized and the growth rate shows a marked increase. Nevertheless, as discussed above for angiostatin, loss of negative regulators of angiogenesis may also be a significant factor in the development of disseminated tumours.

Adhesion molecules and metastasis

Cell adhesion, either cell-to-cell or cell-to-extracellular matrix, has been extensively researched by those interested in metastasis (see, for example, chapter by Saini in [4]). This is not really surprising in that adhesion clearly plays a critical role in metastatic spread. However, all is not simple in that loss or gain of cell adhesion could each be advantageous for metastasis depending on which step of the metastatic cascade is considered. Thus, loss of cell-to-cell adhesion could aid invasion and escape from the primary, whereas increased adhesion to endothelium might be expected to be advantageous for escape from the vasculature to the secondary site.

As there is much literature concerning the role of adhesion molecules in metastasis, three examples will be chosen for discussion here. Of particular recent interest is the cell-surface glycoprotein CD44. Experiments have shown that CD44 isoforms are generated by differential splicing of the messenger RNA (mRNA). It is possible for 10 out of the 20 exons in the CD44 gene to be removed or expressed in different combinations in the mRNA. Overexpression of certain isoforms of the rat CD44 in a non-metastatic pancreatic carcinoma cell line gave rise to cells that were spontaneously metastatic from a subcutaneous injection site to lymph nodes and the lungs. More significantly an antibody that recognized the sixth exon of CD44 blocked the metastatic spread.

The second and third groups of adhesion molecules to be discussed are the integrins and the cadherins.

angiogenic peptides, basic fibroblast growth factor and VEGF.

The mechanism of this inhibition is at present unknown. Neither has the source of the plasminogen that is proteolytically cleaved to angiostatin been definitively identified. It could come from the primary tumour, but it is is more likely that it is produced as plasminogen in the liver and then cleaved to angiostatin by tumour-produced proteases such as elastase. It is noteworthy that angiostatin disappears from the circulation of the mice 5 days after removal of the primary tumour. This event was followed by an immediate burst of angiogenesis in the disseminated tumours and subsequently rapid tumour growth.

Folkman has classified the metastatic patterns seen in cancer patients as shown in Table 5.2. These groupings have been extensively discussed with regard to angiogenesis and its role in metastasis [2]. Of relevance here is the first of these groups where metastases are not detected when the patient appears with the primary; a switch in the metastasized cells to the angiogenic

Integrins are heterodimeric cell-surface glycoproteins that are composed of two subunits called α and β. A number of different α and β subunits exist, each of which may combine to give a functional heterodimer whose ligand depends on the particular α–β combination. Most integrins interact with components of the extracellular matrix but some are also involved in cell-to-cell interactions. Expression of integrins has been shown to increase the rate of proliferation of carcinoma cells in some cases. However, in terms of metastasis the major role of the integrins is thought to be in the mediation of carcinoma migration on an extracellular matrix and in invasion through the basement membrane. Specific examples where overexpression of integrins leads to an increase in metastasis are the αvβ3 vitronectin receptor in melanoma cells and the α2β1 receptor in rhabdomyosarcoma cells. However, in neither case is the mechanism of the enhanced metastasis known.

The cadherins are also a family of structurally related cell-surface glycoproteins. Cadherins are classified into three groups: E-cadherins (epithelial cadherins), P-cadherins (placental cadherin) and N-cadherin (neural cadherin). Amongst these there exists much evidence that loss of E-cadherin-mediated adhesion leads to increased invasion and metastasis in several tumour types. Thus, in transfection experiments, expression of mouse E-cadherin in human breast carcinoma MDA-435S cells reduced the invasive capacity of the cells. Treatment of the transfected cells with a dissociating E-cadherin antibody restored invasiveness. It is noteworthy that in human tumours, loss of E-cadherin expression (determined immunohistochemically) is a common feature of many tumour types (e.g. breast and colon carcinomas).

Conclusion

In this chapter an attempt is made to show that tumour metastasis is a complex multi-step process that always involves both angiogenesis and invasion. Modern biology now provides the tools with which to determine the mechanisms of these processes at the molecular level. While much progress has been made in recent years, for example, in the identification of angiogenic polypeptides and adhesion molecules, in many cases a full assessment of the role that these individual factors play (if any) in the metastatic process is still to be proven. An observation concerning endocrine tumours is that they are usually adenomas and rarely invade and metastasize. It would be interesting to determine the molecular basis of this behaviour.

References

1. Auerbach W, Auerbach R. Angiogenesis inhibition: a review. *Pharmacol. Ther.* 1994;**63**:265–311.
2. Folkman J. Angiogenesis in cancer, vascular, rheumatoid and other diseases. *Nature Med.* 1995;**1**:27–31.
3. O'Reilly MS, Holmgren L, Shing Y *et al.* Angiostatin: a novel angiogenesis inhibitor that mediates the suppression of metastases by a Lewis lung carcinoma. *Cell* 1994;**79**:315–28.
4. Vile RG. (ed.) *Cancer Metastasis: From Mechanisms to Therapies.* Molecular Medical Science Series. Chichester: John Wiley, 1995.

6

Prospects for Gene Therapy of Endocrine Malignancies

JONATHAN D. HARRIS AND NICK R. LEMOINE

Introduction

Gene therapy may be simply defined as the insertion of exogenous genetic material into somatic cells in order to correct a genetic abnormality or to provide those cells with a new function. This is achieved by the transfer of the new genetic material into the host cell through physical or virus-mediated methods. Two possibilities may therefore occur: a new gene may be introduced in addition to a defective gene (addition therapy), or the new gene may replace the defective one during integration (homologous recombination). Since the gene transfer process is targeted to somatic cells, the genetic information will not be passed to the progeny of the subject. This contrasts with germline gene therapy in which genes would be deliberately introduced into the germ cells (sperm or ova), and therefore passed on to successive generations.

Genetic intervention for endocrine cancer predisposition

The identification of the genetic basis of multiple endocrine neoplasia type 2a, type 2b (MEN-2a, MEN-2b) and familial medullary thyroid carcinoma (FMTC) as inherited mutations in the *ret* growth factor receptor oncogene allows the development of screening tests for carriage of the defective gene in affected families. If an individual has inherited a MEN-2a/FMTC-type *ret* mutation, then biochemical screening would be appropriate as well as genetic screening of any progeny of the mutation carrier.

For some cancer predisposition syndromes, for instance familial adenomatous polyposis caused by knockout of the adenomatous polyposis coli (APC) tumour-suppressor gene and Li Fraumeni syndrome caused by inactivation of the *p53* tumour-suppressor gene, it might be possible to reverse the disease phenotype by addition of a normal copy of the gene into all cells at risk of cancer development. This, in principle, could be done by germline therapy (introducing the gene into ova, or even sperm, before fertilization) but this approach has been deemed ethically unacceptable by all societies that have debated the issue. It might be possible to introduce the gene by somatic gene therapy into the stem cells of organs at risk of neoplasia due to the genetic defect and while this is being explored experimentally it remains a remote possibility at present due to the difficulties of gene transfer into human cells *in vivo*.

The question of genetic intervention for MEN-2 and FMTC is further complicated by the fact that the *ret* mutations are predicted to activate the gene product and so these cancer predisposition syndromes do not conform to the classic tumour-suppressor paradigm. Hence the possibility of restoring function by gene addition therapy is probably inappropriate until we understand more of gene function. The possibility of gene therapy for MEN-1 must await the identification of the gene responsible.

An alternative to genetic intervention, which is already in practice for the prevention of inherited disease, is preimplantation genetic diagnosis after *in-vitro* fertilization and it is possible that this might be extended to inherited predisposition to endocrine cancers [1]. While the technical aspects of this approach have become almost routine in specialist centres, the ethical issues are extremely complicated and will have to be carefully considered before couples can be offered such treatment for cancer predisposition.

Somatic gene therapy for established cancer

There are a number of strategies currently under development that may be considered for gene therapy as shown in Fig. 6.1.

if targeted to tumour cells by a specific monoclonal antibody, may increase the scope of targeted therapy. As yet, clinical applications of these therapies have been limited to small numbers of subjects in phase I and II trials but data, so far, for the treatment of lymphomas are promising.

Medium

The following host factors play a role in preventing antibody from reaching the target: non-specific binding to antigens on normal tissues; sequestration by circulating antigen; clearance from the circulation and interstitium; and metabolic degradation. If murine monoclonal antibodies are used, human anti-mouse antibody (HAMA) responses will develop in approximately 90% of patients after three doses, which precludes the use of fractionated doses. Recombinant-chimeric human or humanized antibody may circumvent this problem but an immune response to the chelator, enzyme or toxin may be elicited.

Access of the antibody to its target may be reduced by variable tumour blood supply, impaired transport across the microvascular wall and reduced interstitial transport [5]. The tumour vasculature is disorganized structurally and functionally with perfusion varying in different areas and over short periods of time. Tumour blood flow may be reduced compared with normal tissues, and may be lower in large compared to small tumours. Transport of macromolecules across the microvascular wall is reduced by raised tumour interstitial pressure and this effect may be magnified with increasing tumour size. The expanded interstitial space and centrifugal fluid flux in tumour deposits further limit access of antibody to its targets.

Target cell

Having reached the target cell, a number of factors may prevent effective cytotoxicity. High concentrations of tight junctions may prevent antibody penetration between cells and limit access to antigens. Antigen-poor cells or cells that shed antigen after antibody binding may escape destruction. Alternatively, cells with high concentrations of antigen may bind excess antibody, reducing binding at more distant sites or in antigen-poor cells. The optimal situation requires homogeneous antigen expression throughout the tumour leading to high levels of direct and crossfire irradiation. This ideal situation is unlikely to occur *in vivo*, fuelling attempts to modulate tumour cell antigen expression with various cytokines.

Tumour cell radiosensitivity and radiation dose rate are important determinants of efficacy. Radioimmuno-therapy dose rates (0.1–0.2 Gy/h) are lower than for either external beam radiotherapy (0.25–1.0 Gy/min) or brachytherapy (0.4–0.5 Gy/h). The dose rate also varies due to antibody flux within the tumour and radioisotope decay. Low and declining dose rates have less biological effect than higher dose rates and at present are unlikely to control macroscopic disease. It has been calculated that a radiolabelled antibody with a dose rate of 0.15 Gy/h and an effective half-life of 4 days could deliver only 21 Gy to a tumour deposit, considerably below the threshold for control of macroscopic disease [6]. Improvements in both the initial dose rate and the effective half-life are required if the goal of effective primary radical radioimmunotherapy is to be achieved. It is likely that similar constraints will apply to immunotoxin and antibody-directed drug therapy.

Clinical data

The clinical application of targeted therapy has been largely restricted to the sphere of radioimmunotherapy and has been assessed in a diverse range of tumours [7]. Phase I to II studies have been conducted in patients with ovarian, gastrointestinal, lung and bladder cancers, melanoma, glioma and haematological tumours. Ovarian carcinoma and lymphoma have been most extensively investigated and serve as useful models. The use of radio-iodinated octreotide to localize phaeochromocytomas, pituitary, pancreatic and carcinoid tumours has been reported, with the suggestion that this method might provide a new therapeutic avenue in the treatment of somatostatin receptor positive endocrine cancers. Identification of specific markers of endocrine tissues and the generation of specific antibodies against them should be the next step forward in the process of applying tumour targeting to the treatment of endocrine tumours.

The presence of lineage-specific surface markers on malignant lymphocytes and their sensitivity to low total doses and low dose rates of radiotherapy have made them suitable candidates for targeted therapy. The application of radioimmunotherapy to the treatment of lymphoma was initially reported for ^{131}I-labelled polyclonal antiferritin antibodies in Hodgkin's disease with overall response rates of 40.5–62%. Non-Hodgkin's lymphoma has been treated with radiolabelled antibodies to surface antigens such as CD37 or CD20. Both low- and high-dose (with autologous bone marrow rescue) protocols have been used with encouraging results in patients with disease refractory to standard treatment [7]. The precise role of targeted therapy in patients with lymphoma remains to be determined. The encouraging responses in patients with end-stage disease suggests that its incorporation into first-

or second-line treatment protocols might yield improved results.

In the treatment of ovarian cancer, tumour and normal organ ablation by hysterectomy and bilateral salpingo-oophorectomy is a standard part of therapy. This is in contrast to marrow stem cell ablation in the treatment of lymphoma, which is an unwanted adverse effect. Therefore, in targeted therapy of ovarian cancer, organ-rather than tumour-specific antibodies can be employed. Intraperitoneal localization until late in the natural history of the disease means that intracavitary targeted therapy offers a chance to improve the therapeutic index by avoiding systemic administration. Most studies deal with intraperitoneal therapy of heavily pretreated patients with macroscopic disease at relapse. Palliation of malignant ascites and pleural effusions has been reported, as have responses in patients with residual or recurrent disease. The results of treatment for microscopic or minimal residual (< 2 cm) disease are better than for bulky disease (> 2 cm). Adjuvant intraperitoneal ^{90}Y-anti-human milk fat globulin 1 (HMFG1) antibody treatment of patients in complete remission after standard surgery and chemotherapy has been shown to produce a significant reduction in the rate of recurrence compared to a historical control group [8]. A follow-up randomized phase III study should define more clearly the role of adjuvant-targeted therapy in ovarian cancer.

Conclusion

With the advent of monoclonal antibody techniques there has been renewed interest in targeted therapy for many tumour types. As yet, clinical applications of this therapy have been limited mainly to phase I and II studies of radioimmunotherapy with the prospect of radical treatment remaining a research goal. Until larger total doses are delivered at higher initial dose rates specifically to tumour deposits it is likely that the role of radioim-munotherapy will be restricted to delivering a moderate (10–20 Gy) tumour boost or as an adjuvant treatment in patients with minimal residual disease after definitive primary treatment. This approach is supported by a recent randomized trial of unlabelled monoclonal antibody in the adjuvant treatment of resected Duke's C colorectal carcinoma, which detected a significant reduction in both overall death rate and recurrence rate [9].

As yet, this form of treatment for endocrine tumours has not been investigated. The presence of cell-specific markers in endocrine tissues and the experience gained from both laboratory and clinical application of the available techniques suggests that tumour targeting of endocrine neoplasms will provide a fruitful avenue of future research.

References

1. Kohler G, Milstein C. Continuous culture of fused cells secreting antibodies of predefined specificity. *Nature* 1975;**256**:495–7.
2. Harrington KJ, Epenetos AA. Recent developments in radio-immunotherapy. *Clin. Oncol.* 1994;**6**:391–8.
3. Wessels B, Rogus RD. radionuclide selection and model absorbed dose calculations for radiolabeled tumour associated antibodies. *Med. Phys.* 1984;**11**:638–75.
4. Bagshawe KD. Antibody directed enzymes revive anti-cancer prodrugs concept. *Br. J. Cancer* 1987;**56**:531–2.
5. Jain RK. Physiological barriers to delivery of monoclonal antibodies and other macromolecules in tumours. *Cancer Res.* 1990;(Suppl.)**50**:814–19.
6. Fowler JF. Radiobiological aspects of low dose rates in radio-immunotherapy. *Int. J. Radiat. Oncol. Biol. Phys.* 1990;**18**:1261–9.
7. Bast RC. Progress in radioimmunotherapy. *N. Engl. J. Med.* 1993;**329**:1266–8.
8. Hird V, Maraveyas A, Snook D *et al.* Adjuvant therapy of ovarian cancer with radioactive monoclonal antibody. *Br. J. Cancer* 1993;**68**:403–6.
9. Riethmuller G, Schneider-Gadicke E, Schlimok G *et al.* Randomised trial of monoclonal antibody for adjuvant therapy of resected Duke's C colorectal carcinoma. *Lancet* 1994;**343**:1177–83.

8

Chemotherapy and Endocrine Manipulation

TIMOTHY J. IVESON AND TREVOR J. POWLES

Introduction

Chemotherapy has been used in the treatment of endocrine tumours although the response rate to cytotoxic chemotherapy is often low. Cancer chemotherapy started in the 1940s when it was found that nitrogen mustard was active against Hodgkin's disease and since then many new cytotoxic agents have been introduced (Table 8.1). More recently biological therapies have also been used in the treatment of endocrine tumours. Some solid non-endocrine tumours have been shown to be dependent on hormones for their growth and treatments either preventing the synthesis of these hormones, or preventing their action can be successful against these tumours.

Theories of chemotherapeutic action

Before discussing individual cytotoxic agents it is first necessary to discuss both the theories of chemotherapeutic treatment and the modes of action of these drugs. One of the initial theories about chemotherapy was Skipper's law, which assumed that all cancer cells were actively dividing and each course of chemotherapy killed a percentage of cells, thus allowing calculation of the number of courses of treatment needed to eradicate a tumour [1]. It was then realized that not all cells are dividing and therefore exponential growth does not occur, rather a Gompertzian growth curve occurs which is sigmoid in shape. More recently the Goldie–Coldman hypothesis proposed that spontaneous mutations occur in tumours, resulting in the emergence of drug-resistant clones even in the absence of chemotherapy, and this has led to the use of combination chemotherapy [2].

Mode of action

Cytotoxic drugs are active against dividing cells, killing them and thus resulting in a reduction in tumour size.

They are also active against normal cells that are rapidly dividing, such as haematopoietic cells and cells lining the gastrointestinal tract, thus explaining some of the common toxicities of nearly all cytotoxic drugs, namely myelosuppression and mucositis.

All dividing cells divide to produce two daughter cells identical to the original cell. At any one time dividing cells are found in one of four phases of a well-ordered process called the cell cycle or in a resting phase. The five phases in which a cell can be found are:
1 G0, a resting phase out of the cell cycle;
2 G1, an initial resting phase in the cell cycle;
3 S, the synthetic phase when the amount of DNA is doubled;
4 G2, a second resting phase (pre-mitotic phase);
5 M, period of mitosis.
DNA consists of two chains of polynucleotides arranged in a double helix fashion which in turn is then supercoiled to allow it to fit into as small a space as possible. The nucleotides are either a purine derivative (adenine or guanine) or a pyrimidine derivative (cytosine or thymine) both of which have to be synthesized *de novo* by cells. Antimetabolites are a class of drugs that act by interfering with purine and pyrimidine synthesis, the basic building blocks of both DNA and RNA. Two of the enzymes that are inhibited by antimetabolites are dihydrofolate reductase and thymidylate synthetase.

Prior to cell division DNA needs to replicate and each strand of DNA acts as a template for production of a complementary strand using the enzyme DNA polymerase. As DNA exists as a double helix it has to be unwound into two parallel strands to allow DNA polymerase to act and this is achieved by the enzyme topoisomerase II. Cell division may be prevented by drugs that cause cross-links between the two DNA chains, such as alkylating agents or inhibitors of topoisomerase II.

During mitosis the chromosomes line up along the middle of the cell and spindles develop from two opposite

58

Table 8.1 The historical development of cytotoxic agents

Decade	Agent
1940s	Nitrogen mustard
1950s	Methotrexate Busulphan Mitomycin C 5-fluorouracil (5-FU) Cyclophosphamide
1960s	Vinca alkaloids Adriamycin Bleomycin
1970s	Cisplatin Streptozotocin
1980s	Etoposide Epirubicin Mitoxantrone Carboplatin
1990s	Taxol

poles of the cell and pull the chromosomes apart before the cell divides into two giving rise to two daughter cells each with identical DNA content. Drugs interfering with spindle formation such as the vinca alkaloids and taxanes also inhibit cell division.

Classes of cytotoxic drugs

Alkylating agents

An alkylating agent contains an alkyl group which is able to form a covalent bond with DNA. The most susceptible area for alkylation is the nitrogen atom in the N7 position on the purine base guanine. Most of the commonly used alkylating agents are so called 'bifunctional' alkylating agents, in that they possess two alkylating groups enabling them to bind to two nitrogen atoms and form both inter- and intra-strand DNA links, preventing normal DNA replication, repair and transcription. Alkylating agents may all cause sterility. This is more likely to occur in males than females, although in females the risk increases the closer they are to their natural menopause. Alkylating agents are also potentially carcinogenic and may therefore give rise to second tumours following treatment.

Cyclophosphamide

Cyclophosphamide itself is inactive and needs to be metabolized by mixed function oxidases in the liver which gives rise to two active agents, phosphoramide mustard and acrolein. Phosphoramide mustard is thought to be the major cytotoxic derivative while acrolein is responsible for the bladder toxicity seen with cyclophosphamide.

Administration

Cyclophosphamide may be administered orally but is usually given intravenously at a dose of 500–1000 mg/m² every 3 weeks or as high-dose therapy at doses up to 7 g/m².

Clinical use

Cyclophosphamide is active against ovarian cancer.

Toxicity

Cyclophosphamide causes bone marrow suppression and, when given intravenously, causes alopecia. At high doses it is moderately emetogenic and can cause cardiac toxicity. Haemorrhagic cystitis occurs due to the production of acrolein and can be prevented by intravenous hydration and the use of Mesna which binds to acrolein.

Busulphan

Busulphan is an orally active alkylating agent which shows activity against germ-cell tumours. Its major toxicity is pulmonary toxicity.

Streptozotocin

Streptozotocin is a naturally occurring drug produced by fermentation of *Streptomyces achromogenes*, which belongs to a class of drugs called the nitrosoureas and acts as a monofunctional alkylating agent. Its active metabolites are formed both by spontaneous dissociation and by metabolism by hepatic mixed-function oxidases.

Administration

Streptozotocin is given intravenously.

Clinical use

Streptozotocin has been reported to be active against pancreatic endocrine tumours and carcinoid tumours.

Toxicity

The major dose-limiting toxicity of streptozotocin is myelosuppression. It is moderately emetogenic and can cause both renal tubular damage and pulmonary toxicity.

Antibiotics

Doxorubicin (Adriamycin)

Cytotoxic antibiotics were discovered by chance as products of the fungal species *Streptomyces*. The first two to be discovered were daunorubicin and doxorubicin. Both belong to the class of agents known as anthracyclines and Adriamycin is one of the most active known single-agent cytotoxic agents. The antitumour antibiotics have several actions including intercalation with DNA and inhibition of topoisomerase II covalent binding to DNA and free radical formation. Because of the planar nature of the Adriamycin molecule it is able to fit in between DNA strands, a process called intercalation and so interfere with DNA replication. Adriamycin allows the topoisomerase to cause strand breaks but then inhibits repair leading to DNA double-strand breaks preventing DNA replication. It is thought that the main cytotoxic mode of action is intercalation and topoisomerase II inhibition, while free-radical formation is responsible for much of the cardiac toxicity seen with this class of drug.

Administration

Adriamycin is given intravenously often as a bolus, although there is now evidence that giving Adriamycin as an infusion over several days reduces the cardiac toxicity of the drug without impairing its therapeutic efficacy.

Adriamycin is a vesicant, that is if it extravasates from the vein then it causes pain and erythema which can progress to necrosis. When administering vesicant cytotoxic agents, prevention of extravasation is of paramount importance and they should be administered by experienced personnel. When given as a bolus they should be given into a fast-flowing drip, and if being given as an intravenous infusion, they must be given into a central line.

Adriamycin is metabolized by the liver, therefore the dose should be reduced if there is hepatic impairment, as may occur with hepatic metastases.

Clinical use

Adriamycin shows activity against ovarian tumours, medullary cell carcinoma of the thyroid, anaplastic carcinoma of the thyroid and carcinoid tumours.

Toxicity

The major short-term, dose-limiting toxicities of the anthracyclines are myelosuppression and mucositis. The anthracyclines are moderately emetogenic and also cause alopecia which may be prevented, or a least reduced, by scalp-cooling.

The most serious long-term toxicity of the anthracyclines is cardiac toxicity. This is usually cumulative and although no dose of Adriamycin is completely safe, the incidence of cardiomyopathy rises steeply after cumulative doses of greater than 550 mg/m^2 of Adriamycin.

Epirubicin

Epirubicin is a structural analogue of Adriamycin developed to try to improve the therapeutic index, especially to achieve a reduction in cardiac toxicity. It is active against a similar range of solid tumours as doxorubicin.

Mitoxantrone

Mitoxantrone is a synthetic DNA intercalator based on the anthracenedione ring structure. It acts as an intercalator and topoisomerase II inhibitor and has reduced cardiac toxicity compared to doxorubicin.

Mitomycin

Mitomycin is an antibiotic the main mode of action of which is as a bifunctional alkylating agent following enzymatic reduction. Recently a toxic interaction between mitomycin and tamoxifen causing haemolytic uraemic syndrome has been reported and so the combination of these two drugs should be avoided [3].

Bleomycin

Bleomycin is an antitumour antibiotic isolated from *Streptomyces verticullus* that causes single-strand and double-strand DNA breaks. Bleomycin is not myelosuppressive but its use is associated with the development of pulmonary fibrosis. It is active against germ-cell tumours. It can also be installed into the pleural cavity once an effusion has been drained to dryness to prevent recurrence of pleural effusions.

Platinum compounds

The discovery of platinum compounds as cytotoxic agents followed the chance observation of the effect of electric current through platinum electrodes on cell culture. Platinum compounds bind to DNA forming 'DNA adducts'. This results in intrastrand DNA links inhibiting DNA replication.

Cisplatin

Administration

Cisplatin is administered intravenously. It is 90% renally excreted and the creatinine clearance should be shown to be at least 60 ml/min before giving cisplatin. In order to decrease renal toxicity, cisplatin has to be given as an in-patient procedure with intravenous pre- and post-hydration together with a forced diuresis. Cisplatin may also be given intraperitoneally.

Clinical use

Cisplatin has been shown to have considerable activity against germ-cell tumours and ovarian carcinoma. Activity has also been reported against adrenal cortical carcinomas and carcinoid tumours.

Toxicity

Cisplatin is highly emetogenic and this is its major short-term toxicity, although since the introduction of the 5HT3 antagonists emesis is much better controlled. Cisplatin is not particularly myelosuppressive so the major dose-limiting toxicities are renal failure, peripheral neuropathy in a glove and stocking distribution and ototoxicity. The major long-term problems with cisplatin are renal toxicity and ototoxicity.

Carboplatin

Carboplatin is an analogue of cisplatin developed to retain the potent cytotoxic effects with fewer side-effects: that is with decreased renal toxicity and emetogenicity. Carboplatin is more myelosuppressive than cisplatin especially causing thrombocytopenia. Like cisplatin, carboplatin is given intravenously and excreted renally. Its excretion from the body has been shown to correlate with renal function and the dose should therefor be calculated according to a chosen AUC (area under curve) of a plot of serum concentration versus time which is dependent on the creatinine clearance rather than surface area [4].

Plant products

Taxanes

Taxanes are a new class of compound, of which Taxol is the lead compound. Taxol is extracted from the bark of the Pacific yew (*Taxus brevifolia*). The mode of action is by promoting microtubule assembly resulting in long microtubules which become entangled with themselves so preventing normal tubule function and cell division. The major toxicities of the taxanes are neutropenia, neurotoxicity, alopecia, anaphylaxis and nausea and vomiting. In initial testing the taxanes have shown activity against ovarian cancer. Because of the scarcity of Pacific yew trees other analogues are being developed, the first of these is Taxotere which is extracted from yew tree needles. The major toxicities from these drugs appear to be myelosuppression and peripheral neuropathy [5].

Vinca alkaloids

Vinca alkaloids are natural products obtained from the periwinkle plant (*Catharanthus roseus*) which prevent tubule formation. The most commonly used vinca alkaloids are vincristine and vinblastine. Both show activity against germ-cell tumours. Their major toxicity is a peripheral neuropathy.

Epiphyllotoxins

Epiphyllotoxins are extracts of the mandrake plant. The major compound used clinically is etoposide (VP16), a glycoside derivative of the parent compound podophyllotoxin. Initially the epipodophyllotoxins were thought to act by inhibiting microtubule formation but now their major mode of action is known to be inhibition of topoisomerase II. Etoposide is active by both the oral and intravenous routes and as it exerts its cytotoxic effect on actively dividing cells the schedule of administration is important. The major toxicities are myelosuppression and alopecia. It is active against germ-cell tumours.

Antimetabolites

The two most commonly used antimetabolites are methotrexate and 5-FU. Methotrexate inhibits both dihydrofolate reductase and thymidylate synthetase while 5-FU inhibits thymidylate synthetase. Both are active intravenously and 5-FU has been reported to have some activity against adrenal cortical carcinomas and pancreatic endocrine tumours. Recently, infusional 5-FU plus α-interferon has been reported as having a 47% response rate in malignant neuroendocrine tumours [6].

Chemotherapy administration and toxicity

As the major side-effect of nearly all cytotoxic drugs is

myelosuppression the dose of drug has to be tailored to the individual patient. Therefore instead of giving a standard dose of a drug, the surface area is calculated from the patient's height and weight and the dose of the drug given is per square metre of surface area. If a patient becomes neutropenic following chemotherapy, they need immediate hospital admission and treatment with broad-spectrum antibiotics, especially covering Gram-negative organisms.

As discussed previously, the Goldie–Coldman hypothesis proposes that once a tumour is large enough to be clinically detectable it is likely to have drug-resistant clones. If a single cytotoxic agent is used against this tumour, some of the tumour cells may be resistant to this drug therefore the tumour will not be eradicated and the patient will not be cured. It is less likely that there will be a clone of cells resistant to two cytotoxic agents, therefore if two cytotoxic drugs are used in combination the chance of resistance is reduced and so the chance of cure is increased. In practice often three or more drugs are given in combination. When choosing drugs to be used in combination chemotherapy, the drugs should ideally have different modes of action and different toxicities enabling each one to be given at a dose close to the maximum tolerated dose without unmanageable toxicity.

While normal tissues must be allowed to recover in between courses of chemotherapy, the concept of the dose intensity of a regimen (the dose of drug administered per unit time) has been developed and this may be an important predictor of response [7]. It is therefore very important to try and deliver cytotoxic drugs on time and at the intended dose in order to gain the maximum therapeutic benefit.

Biological therapies and haematopoietic growth factors

In recent years, due to recombinant DNA technology, various biologically active peptides, most notably interleukins and interferons, have become available for the treatment of many conditions. They have been used in the treatment of some tumours including endocrine tumours.

Interferons have antiproliferative effects, antitumour effects, can induce differentiation and are capable of potentiating the immune system. Interferons are usually given by subcutaneous injection and their side-effects include pyrexia, malaise, rigors, nausea, vomiting and diarrhoea. To date the most widely used biological therapy against endocrine tumours has been α-interferon, which has shown activity against carcinoid tumours and has been combined with infusional 5-FU in the treatment of neuroendocrine tumours [6].

Haematopoietic growth factors such as granulocyte colony-stimulating factor (G-CSF) have been developed, which can decrease both the severity and duration of neutropenia following cytotoxic chemotherapy. This is useful to enable chemotherapy to be given on time and at the desired dose intensity. However, these aims are only important if chemotherapy is curative in intent and therefore currently they are not of use in the chemotherapeutic treatment of endocrine tumours.

Endocrine therapy

The two common tumour types that can be treated by hormone therapy are breast cancer and prostatic cancer, as some of these tumours require oestrogens and androgens, respectively, for their growth. The development of endocrine treatments for breast cancer is shown in Table 8.2.

Breast cancer

Endocrine treatment of breast cancer aims either to decrease the production of oestrogen or to block the actions of oestrogen. Tamoxifen and progestins block the action of oestrogen on breast cancers and therefore are effective in both premenopausal and postmenopausal women. In premenopausal women oestrogens are produced mainly from the ovaries therefore the luteinizing-hormone-releasing hormone (LHRH) analogues, which cause a medical oophorectomy, will cause a significant fall in oestrogen concentration. In postmenopausal women oestrogens are mainly formed by the peripheral aromatization of androgens, therefore inhibition of the

Table 8.2 The historical development of endocrine treatment of breast cancer

Year/decade	Treatment
1896	Oophorectomy
1953	Adrenalectomy
1956	Hypophysectomy
1950s	Oestrogens
	Androgens
	Progestins
1970s	Tamoxifen
	Aminoglutethimide
1980s	LHRH analogues
	More potent aromatase inhibitors
1990s	Pure anti-oestrogens
	Anti-progestins

LHRH, luteinizing-hormone-releasing hormone.

aromatase enzyme causes a significant fall in circulating oestrogen levels. In patients with breast cancer the most important determinant of whether they will respond to hormone therapy is their oestrogen receptor status, although other biological parameters such as progesterone receptor and PS2 may give further prognostic information. If a tumour is oestrogen-receptor-positive, then there is a 60% chance that it will respond to hormone therapy, while if the tumour is oestrogen-receptor-negative, then this likelihood falls to only 10%. Overall, about 60% of breast cancers are oestrogen-receptor-positive, therefore overall approximately one-third of breast tumours will respond to hormone therapy.

Anti-oestrogens

The most commonly prescribed hormone therapy is tamoxifen which acts as an anti-oestrogen against breast cancer cells although on other tissues it acts as a weak oestrogen. Tamoxifen has a low incidence of side-effects, is effective in both pre- and postmenopausal women and can be used as treatment for metastatic disease and as adjuvant therapy. Pure anti-oestrogens are now being developed.

Progestins

Progestins, such as medroxyprogesterone acetate or megestrol acetate are effective in both pre- and postmenopausal women and are used as second-line hormone therapy. They are effective in approximately 50% of patients who have previously responded to endocrine therapy. Antiprogestins such as onapristone have also shown activity against breast cancer and are currently under development.

Aromatase inhibitors

Aromatase inhibitors, such as aminoglutethimide and formestane, are effective against breast cancer in postmenopausal women and are often used as second-line therapy. Newer, more potent aromatase inhibitors are currently under development.

LHRH analogues

LHRH analogues, such as leuprorelin or goserelin, induce an early menopause and are effective treatments in premenopausal women.

Endocrine therapy for breast cancer can be used for patients with metastatic disease, but recently it has been shown that adjuvant tamoxifen therapy following initial diagnosis of breast cancer can prolong both time to relapse and overall survival in both pre- and postmenopausal women [8].

Prostatic cancer

The most common hormone therapies used against prostatic cancer are the LHRH analogues, which cause androgen concentrations to fall to castrate levels and result in response rates of approximately 30%. There are also anti-androgens, such as cyproterone acetate and flutamide, which show activity against prostatic cancer and there is current interest in whether combination therapy or sequential therapy results in longer remission rates in prostatic cancer. Currently endocrine therapy for prostatic cancer is used for metastatic disease and a role for adjuvant therapy has not been established.

References

1. Skipper HE. Historic milestones in cancer biology: a few that are important to cancer treatment (revisited). *Semin. Oncol.* 1979;**6**:506–14.
2. Goldie JH, Coldman AJ. A mathematical model for relating the drug sensitivity of tumours to their spontaneous mutation rate. *Cancer Treat. Rep.* 1979;**63**:1727–33.
3. Montes A, Powles TJ, O'Brien MER *et al.* A toxic interaction between Mitomycin C and tamoxifen causing the haemolytic uraemic syndrome. *Eur. J. Cancer* 1993;**29A**:1854–7.
4. Calvert AH, Newall DR, Gumbrell LA *et al.* Carboplatin dosage: prospective evaluation of a single formula based on renal function. *J. Clin. Oncol.* 1989;**7**:1748–56.
5. Verweij J, Clavel M, Chevalier B. Palitaxel (Taxol™) and docetaxel (Taxotere™): not simply two of a kind. *Ann. Oncol.* 1994;**5**:495–505.
6. Andreyev HJN, Scott-Mackie P, Cunningham D *et al.* A Phase II study of continuous infusion of fluorouracil and interferon alfa 2b in the palliation of malignant neuroendocrine tumors. *J. Clin. Oncol.* 1995;**13**(6):1486–92.
7. Hryniuk W, Bush H. The importance of dose intensity in chemotherapy of metastatic breast cancer. *J. Clin. Oncol.* 1984;**2**:1281–8.
8. Early Breast Cancer Trialists' Group. Systemic treatment of early breast cancer by hormonal, cytotoxic, or immune therapy. *Lancet* 1992;**339**:1–15, 71–85.

Techniques in Radiation Medicine

P. NICHOLAS PLOWMAN

External beam radiotherapy

External beam radiotherapy is the backbone of modern radiotherapy. One or more skin entry portals are used for the beam(s) of X-rays or gamma-ray photons, emitted from a source (tungsten target of a linear accelerator or high specific activity cobalt-60 source, respectively) standing off 75–100 cm from the patient. The advantage of multiple fields (skin entry portals) is that this allows the radiation dose to be concentrated on the premapped tumour which is thereby 'cross-fired'. With a single portal/field, the dose at (or just below) the skin will be higher than at the tumour's depth beneath the skin; with multiple portals/fields, a concentration of radiation is achieved on the tumour with sparing of surrounding normal tissues.

The radiation damage by such external beam treatment occurs instantly and the patient is not radioactive on leaving the treatment room.

The unit of radiation dose is the Gray; 1 Gy represents 1 J of ionizing radiation energy absorbed per kilogram of tissue (i.e. the units of radiation are energy deposited per unit mass of absorbing substance).

Modern linear accelerators provide the most sophisticated method of delivering external beam radiotherapy. These machines generate megavoltage X-ray beams that are more penetrating than previous orthovoltage (deep X-ray) or even cobalt beams; that is, they give a higher dose of radiation at tumour depth per unit dose delivered on the body surface (entry portal). Furthermore, the beams are skin sparing (deliver maximum dose below rather than at the skin surface) and they are better collimated beams (i.e. less penumbra and side scatter). These characteristics alone make the linear accelerator the external beam machine of choice. However, advances in technology have allowed greater potential to be realized. Linear accelerators are isocentrically mounted such that it is routine to position the tumour volume at the centre of the arc of rotation of the linear accelerator, which may then rotate to effect the multiple portals described above (isocentric technology).

Previously, linear accelerator portal/field shaping was effected by defining 'jaws' (collimators) working in perpendicular planes to create square or rectangular portals from the X-ray emissions emanating from the tungsten target (beam flattening filters produced a fairly ±2% flat beam across the portal). Corners or segments of the treatment fields could be obliterated by extra lead blocks placed manually in the beam by radiographers/technologists. Thus a square portal treating the mediastinum could have its left inferolateral corner shielded/screened to reduce the dose received by the heart. Nowadays, linear accelerators have multileaf collimation, whereby the 'jaws' are replaced by 40–52 finger-like lead processes, which can project into the beam by any predetermined extent to effect much more sophisticated beam shaping than hitherto possible. Furthermore, the technique of portal imaging ('beam's eye view') allows verification of treatment set up (i.e. reproducibility of simulated field set-ups) with greater immediacy than the old technique of beam filming. This is critical if beam shaping by multileaf collimation is screening tissues adjacent to tumours with more crucial accuracy than previously obtainable.

The simulator is an X-ray imaging machine that assists mapping by X-ray screening and filming capabilities. Using a simulation table identical to the linear accelerator treatment couch, identical 'set-up' positions for treatment may be planned and marked on the patient's skin or individually made in mobilization mask. CT simulation allows skin portal entry planning in conjunction with CT images. The simulator is nowadays networked with the linear accelerators and a planning computer accepts planning information to optimize the isodosimetry of multiple fields plans.

'Conventionally fractionated' radiotherapy has evolved over decades, following the original observations that small daily doses of external beam radiation led to a cumulative effect on the tumour but allowed relative sparing of normal tissues. 'Conventional' fractionation for adults comprises 200 cGy daily fractions, whereas for children this is usually 160–180 cGy each day. In multiple portal techniques, each portal is treated daily and the minimum tumour isodose is usually chosen for the pre-scription from computer-planning-generated isodosimetric plan; this is the lowest isodose that completely encom-passes the tumour volume. In a good plan, the gradient across the tumour volume should be less than 5%, there should be no 'hot spots' outside the tumour volume and the isodoses should 'fall-off' sharply at the edge of the tumour volume.

Developments of technology have allowed the stereo-tactic mapping of intracranial lesions and the delivery of focal/focused radiation to extremely discrete targets within the head. Unlike most radical radiotherapy treat-ments to the brain, where conventional fraction sizes are used to spare toxicity to the nervous system, these fo-cal radiation techniques allow much larger doses to be delivered as the normal brain surrounding the tumour/target volume receives such a small fraction of the dose. Indeed, this can be used to advantage where some tumours will only respond to high-dose fractions (that previously could not safely be given for fear of radiation morbidity to surrounding normal brain). The two most common forms of focal stereotactic radiotherapy are the cobalt-gamma knife method and the more versatile linear accelerator stereotactic multiple arc radiation therapy (SMART) method.

Another capability of modern linear accelerators is the generation of megavoltage electron beams of vary-ing energies. This allows the clinician the potential of irradiating more superficial tumours with a beam that delivers ionizing radiation fairly homogeneously to a depth (determined by the previously chosen electron energy) and then 'falls off' sharply. The advantages of such a beam can be enormous: for example, a loin tumour can be irradiated to radical dosage without giving this high dose to an underlying kidney.

An adaptation of electron beam therapy is intra-operative radiotherapy. In this case, electron beams of preselected energy are used to deliver radiotherapy through a sterile-tipped cone placed through an operation wound onto a resected/or unresectable tumour bed.

Radioisotope therapy

Tumour-specific radiopharmaceuticals delivering radiation therapy specifically to tumour cells theoretically meet Ehrlich's objective of 'magic bullets' for cancer. Such treat-ment is systemic, non-invasive and should cause few immediate or long-term side-effects. Interestingly, long-term follow-up of patients treated with radioisotope therapy has shown a lower oncogenic potential than for chemotherapy or external beam radiation; is this due to high linear energy transfer (LET) radiation (see below)?

An avid and selective uptake of radioisotope by tumour cells and a lengthy retention of the isotope by these cells is the requirement for successful therapy. The absorbed radiation dose (DB) in Grays delivered by a β-emitting radionuclide can be calculated by the slightly rough and ready equation:

$$DB = 19.9 \times c \times E \times T_{eff}$$

where: c is the concentration of isotope measured in megaBecquerels per gram (MBq/g) tissue; E is the average β energy in MeV; and T_{eff} is the effective half-life in days (a composite of physical and biological half-lives).

The activity concentration (or specific activity) within target tissue requires volumetric assessment of the tumour (from palpation or imaging). The effective half-life of the isotope in the tumour and whole body can be determined by several serial quantitative scans.

It must be realized that the requirements of the imaging nuclear medicine physician and the radiation oncologist differ when it comes to selecting radioisotope-labelled pharmaceuticals or monoclonal antibodies. The former requires good quality imaging and is in favour of deliver-ing a relatively high specific activity of a short half-life isotope which is rapidly taken up by the target tissue and, during its short physical half-life, emits a high signal of gamma-photons of ideal energy for detection by a gamma camera. The radiation oncologist wants an isotope with a high emission of short path length β particles delivering high LET/cytocidal radiation to the tumour cell in which the atom resides plus its neighbours; the gamma emission is undesirable. It is for these reasons that in both meta-iodobenzylguanidine (MIBG) and monoclonal antibody radioisotope labelling work ^{123}I is used for imaging and ^{131}I for therapy. The only conflict that arises is when, to establish the effective half-life of the labelled substance in the tumour (required to obtain an estimate of absorbed dose), the radiation oncologist needs 48–72 hour data points (difficult for ^{123}I with a physical $T_{1/2}$ of 13.2 hours) in the initial diagnostic/imaging scan. This can be undertaken retrospectively after administration of the therapy by subsequent serial imaging.

Radio-iodine (^{131}I)

The ^{131}I isotope has a physical half-life of 8 days and at disintegration emits β rays (average energy of 0.55 MeV with penetration of approximately 1 mm in soft tissue) and photons (average energy 0.37 MeV).

Between 50 and 80% of differentiated thyroid cancer concentrates radio-iodine. Although Pochin [1] found papillary and follicular cancers equally likely to be iodine avid, other workers found a lower fraction of papillary cancers as compared to follicular cancers to concentrate iodine [2]. Paediatric cancer was more likely (89%) than adult cases (64%) to concentrate ^{131}I in the Villejuif experience, despite a higher percentage of papillary cases in children (M.Tubiana, personal communication 1985). As the avidity of thyroid cancer for iodine is usually less than that of normal thyroid tissue, a policy of normal thyroid ablation (surgery and ^{131}I) is employed prior to therapy.

Administered activities of 7.4 GBq (200 mCi) are usually prescribed for treatment of metastatic, iodine-avid, differentiated thyroid cancer. Halnan [3] demonstrated that if a tumour concentrated 0.1% activity/g with an effective half-life of 3 days, it would receive an absorbed dose of 6200 cGy from a 7.4 GBq, whilst at the same time the whole body dose would be below 1% of this; indeed the marrow dose is usually of the order of 0.1 mGy/MBq (0.5 cGy/mCi). If there is a significantly larger uptake and retention in either a normal thyroid remnant or bulky metastatic cancer, the whole body/bone marrow dose is increased up to 4- to 10-fold. Renal impairment, leading to reduced iodine excretion and hence increased effective half-life, also increases the whole body dose. Of the complications of repeated therapy dose of ^{131}I, marrow depression and pneumonitis are best documented; the latter being most important in patients presenting with 'miliary' lung metastases. Radiation nephritis is a rare risk. Gonadal damage leading to infertility is unusual and Edmonds and Smith [4] could not find evidence to support the concept of reduced fertility, although the calculated dose to the gonads, particularly in some males, is in the range known to cause oligospermia, at least temporarily. Similarly, genetic damage in offspring was not detectable [5]. With regard to late oncogenesis, Edmonds and Smith [4] found a slight excess of acute leukaemia (risk one in 100 000 patient-Gray-years) and bladder cancer (risk five in 10 000 patient-Gray-years).

With regard to lower doses of ^{131}I used as therapy for thyrotoxicosis, say 185–370 MBq (5–10 mCi) administered activities, the imperceptible risks with regard to carcinogenesis, leukaemogenesis, genetic and fetal damage from huge analyses of more than 100 000 patients, are well reviewed by Halnan [6].

Metaiodobenzylguanidine

MIBG, a guanethidine analogue, was developed as a radio-iodinated pharmaceutical by Sisson et al. [7] and since then has established itself as an important agent in the imaging and treatment of neural crest tumours. Hoefnagel [8] estimates that 88% of phaeochromocytomas, 91% of neuroblastomas, 70% of carcinoid and 35% of thyroid medullary carcinomas concentrate MIBG. In this author's experience the therapeutically useful avidity percentages are lower, certainly for neuroblastomas and carcinoid carcinomas.

In an analysis of the dosimetry of 25 children with advanced neuroblastoma treated by therapeutically prescribed activities of 3.7–7.4 GBq (100–200 mCi) of ^{131}I-MIBG following induction chemotherapy, Fielding et al. [9] found red marrow and whole body absorbed doses of the region of 0.1–0.7 mGy/MBq with a mean of approximately 0.35 mGy/MBq (approximately 1 rad/mCi). Obviously, where bone marrow infiltration by neuroblastoma has resisted induction chemotherapy, the bone marrow dose will be higher, as the path length of β rays from ^{131}I is approximately 1 mm in soft tissues.

The mean dose to the bladder in non-catheterized patients was 27 Gy, the dose per unit activity varying from 2.5 to 5.3 mGy/MBq. The liver doses were 1.6–11.3 Gy (0.3–1.9 mGy/MBq). The tumour doses varied widely from 2 to 53 Gy (0.2–16.6 mGy/MBq). Repeated administration of 8 GBq (150–200 mCi) activities have been delivered with cumulative beneficial effect to malignant phaeochromocytoma and neuroblastoma patients, although the optimal scheduling of ^{131}I-MIBG into neuroblastoma therapy is still to be decided. The innovative use is as first-line treatment to shrink tumours and render them operable [8]. In other tumours, such as metastatic carcinoid and paraganglioma, this author has also observed cumulative tumour response with successive ^{131}I-MIBG doses.

A scheme that has been proposed is the use of ^{125}I-MIBG therapy, utilizing the Auger electrons from ^{125}I disintegrations as therapy. These have path lengths of the order of 10 nM only, which is sufficient since the cytoplasm in neuroblastoma is thin and MIBG in cellular storage vesicles (its point of sequestration in MIBG-avid cells) is sufficiently close to target DNA for useful cytocidal action. ^{131}I-MIBG has been shown by Shapiro [10] to be as successful in the therapy of neuroblastoma as ^{125}I-MIBG.

Radiolabelled monoclonal antibodies

Diagnostic radioimmunoscintigraphy (RIS) is now a highly developed technique and because tumour deposits show up so well on these static scan pictures, the unwary person is beguiled into thinking that radioimmunotherapy (RIT) should be currently useful for many situations in oncology.

Monoclonal antibodies for both RIS and RIT are gammaglobulin molecules comprising paired heavy and light chains from which, for RIS, antigen-specific Fab fragments are cleaved and may reach tumour cells more easily than the whole antibody molecules; however, the whole antibody molecule often has a greater binding affinity for tumour, which is more important for RIT. Also relevant is that for RIS, the rapid uptake of a high specific activity but short half-life isotope allows a high signal from the tumour (which swamps the background 'noise') to give a good imaging scan. This does not necessarily imply good potential for RIT, which is more dependent on a sustained, preferential uptake and retention of the monoclonal antibody by the tumour cells, and preferably all the tumour cells, with retention for days.

Monoclonal antibodies have been tagged as immuno-toxins or immunoconjugated with chemotherapy drugs, but radioisotopes have the theoretical advantage in that the complex does not have to be internalized after binding to a cell-surface receptor and there is the real possibility of cell-to-cell crossfire, not applicable to toxins or chemotherapy.

Intravenous administration of monoclonal-antibody-directed therapy has to date not been successful. However, such therapy directed towards recurrent cancer, particularly growing in fluid phase or monolayer/bilayers in confined spaces (peritoneum, pleural space, cerebrospinal fluid (CSF)/leptomeninges or intratumour), has generated more interest and appears to hold more potential. However, even this last statement appears optimistic from the data available. Britton *et al.* [11] reviewed the data on RIT with the, then available, ^{131}I-monoclonal antibodies intraperitoneally for stage III ovarian cancer, reduced to small bulk by prior surgery and chemotherapy. The overall response rate was 18% but these responses were not durable. In the CSF, some slightly better evidence of response exists: using a range of monoclonal antibodies directed at neurectodermal surface antigens and radio-iodinated with ^{131}I, Lashford *et al.* [12] found a response rate of 11 from 16 patients with leptomeningeal disease from neuroectodermal primaries, but again mainly poorly sustained. The conclusion so far is that single-stage RIT has yet to fulfil its exciting theoretical potential. A two- or three-stage approach using a bifunctional antibody may be more useful in the future.

Intracystic therapy for craniopharyngioma

Recurrent cystic craniopharyngioma represents another area in which unsealed source radioisotope therapy has shown promise. Craniopharyngiomas are difficult to resect completely and often cystic relapse occurs. These cysts may be problematic in that they fill, causing pressure symptoms and, even if treated by a tube drainage (usually to a subcutaneous reservoir), they may require multiple aspirations. The secreted fluid comes from the thin secreting epithelium of the cyst; this has proved sensitive to high-dose β radiation. Baklund described fourteen consecutive patients with cystic craniopharyngioma treated with intracystic instillation of yttrium (^{90}Y). Following diagnostic and volumetric estimation of the cyst (usually by puncture of the cyst and injection of radio-opaque medium prior to X-ray) the cyst was re-punctured to inject ^{90}Y. In the fourteen originally reported cases, activity of 7.4–118 MBq (0.2–3.2 mCi, average 1.4 mCi) was injected into the cyst, although in one case 289 MBq (7.8 mCi) was injected into a large volume cyst of 45 ml. The activity was calculated (from the volumetric exercise) to deliver a dose of 20 000 rad (200 Gy) to the secretory epithelium of the cyst. Due to the short path length of the β rays, the surrounding brain was spared. Retreatment was safe, if needed. The vast majority of the cysts responded by reducing in size and secretion rate and without complication [13,14].

Although other isotopes have been used (e.g. ^{32}P), ^{90}Y is preferred; it has a half-life of 2.67 days (64.1 hours), it is a pure β emitter (maximum energy 2.3 MeV) with a maximum range in biological tissue of 11 mm.

References

1. Pochin EE. Prospects from the treatment of thyroid carcinoma with radioiodine. *Clin. Radiol.* 1967;**18**:113–35.
2. Simpson EJ, Panzarella T, Carruthers JS, Gospodarowicj HK, Sutcliffe SB. Papillary and follicular thyroid cancer. Impact of treatment in 1578 patients. *Int. J. Radiat. Oncol. Biol. Phys.* 1988;**14**:1063–75.
3. Halnan KE. The treatment of thyroid cancer. *Ann. Radiol.* 1977;**20**:826–30.
4. Edmonds CJ, Smith T. The long term hazards of the treatment of thyroid cancer with radioiodine. *Br. J. Radiol.* 1986;**59**:49–51.
5. Sarkar SD, Beierwattes EH, Gill SP, Cowley BJ. Subsequent fertility and birth histories of children and adolescents treated with ^{131}I for thyroid cancer. *J. Nucl. Med.* 1976;**18**:460–4.
6. Halnan KE. Risks from radioiodine treatment of thyrotoxicosis. *Br. Med. J.* 1983;**287**:1821–2.
7. Sisson JC, Frager MS, Valk TW *et al.* Scintigraphic localisation of phaeochromocytoma. *N. Engl. J. Med.* 1981;**305**:12–17.

8. Hoefnagel CA. Radionuclide therapy revisited. *Eur. J. Nucl. Med.* 1991;**18**:408–431.

9. Fielding J, Lashford LS, Lewis I. Dosimetry of [131]Iodine metaiodo-benzylguanidine for the treatment of resistant neuroblastoma: results of a UK study. *Eur. J. Nucl. Med.* 1991;**18**:308–16.

10. Shapiro B. '*Quo Vadis* MIBG'. Paper presented to the International Nuclear Medicine Symposium, Westerland, Germany, 1994.

11. Britton KE, Mather SJ, Granowska M. Radiolabelled monoclonal antibodies in oncology III radioimmunotherapy. *Nucl. Med. Comm.* 1991;**12**:333–47.

12. Lashford LS, Davies AG, Richardson RB *et al*. A pilot study of ^{131}I-monoclonal antibodies in the therapy of leptomeningeal tumours. *Cancer* 1988;**61**:199–209.

13. Baklund EO. Studies on craniopharyngioma. III Stereotactic treatment with intracystic yttrium-96. *Acta Chir. Scand.* 1973;**139**:237–47.

14. Baklund EO, Axelsson B, Bergstrand CG *et al*. Treatment of craniopharyngiomas—the stereotactic approach in a ten to twenty three years perspective. *Acta Neurochir. (Wien)* 1989;**99**:11–19.

10

Interventional Radiology

JAMES E. JACKSON

Introduction

Interventional radiological procedures are useful for both the *localization* and *treatment* of endocrine tumours. *Localization* techniques are employed when tumours are too small to be visualized by more conventional imaging or when they have not been localized at initial exploratory surgery; for example, procedures such as selective angiography or venous sampling may be useful in the detection of neuroendocrine tumours of the pancreas and functioning parathyroid adenomas. These techniques are dealt with elsewhere in this book and will not be discussed further.

Interventional radiological techniques which may be useful in the *treatment* of patients with endocrine tumours can be broadly categorized into those that involve vessel occlusion, embolization, and those that involve recanalization. The indications for these forms of treatment are listed in Table 10.1. Hepatic arterial embolization for metastatic liver disease is the most common therapeutic procedure performed in this group of neoplasms and has been shown to be of proven benefit and this chapter will therefore concentrate upon this technique. The other indications listed in Table 10.1 will also be discussed.

Chemotherapeutic agents may be administered directly into the liver via an arterial or portal catheter. Such a catheter is usually placed surgically and this form of therapy will, therefore, not be discussed in this chapter. The role of chemotherapy in the treatment of endocrine tumours is discussed in Chapter 8.

Embolization

Hepatic arterial embolization

Transcatheter hepatic arterial embolization is the deliberate occlusion of part or all of the arterial supply to the liver via an intravascular catheter. The basic principle underlying hepatic arterial occlusion in the treatment of primary and secondary malignant liver tumours is that the principal blood supply to the tumour(s) is arterial with little or no supply from the portal vein. Should the hepatic artery be occluded, then the tumour, being deprived of its blood supply, undergoes necrosis, whilst the normal liver, still being supplied by the portal vein, does not.

Tumours that are likely to respond best to embolization, therefore, are those that are highly vascular and that derive most of their supply from the hepatic artery. Hepatic metastases from islet cell (neuroendocrine) tumours meet these criteria and in the West it is for the treatment of these deposits that hepatic embolization is most commonly indicated. Worldwide, irresectable hepatocellular carcinoma is the most common indication for embolization.

Indications

Patients with neuroendocrine tumour metastases exhibit a wide variety of severe symptoms, which will vary depending upon the hormonal production by the tumour. There is usually extensive liver involvement at presentation but the tumours are relatively slow-growing and survival for several years can often be expected. Curative hepatic resection is not usually possible because both lobes are commonly involved by the disease.

The distressing symptoms caused by these hepatic metastases are often well palliated with medical therapy, and certainly the number of patients at this author's institution with such hepatic metastases requiring embolization has decreased quite significantly with the increased availability of somatostatin analogues. Embolization remains, however, a successful form of therapy in those patients who remain symptomatic despite medical treatment. The cost of long-term medical treatment should also be taken into consideration, and in some instances hepatic arterial embolization may prove to be cheaper, while being equally effective. Rarely, patients may have a single large hepatic metastasis which is irresectable because of its

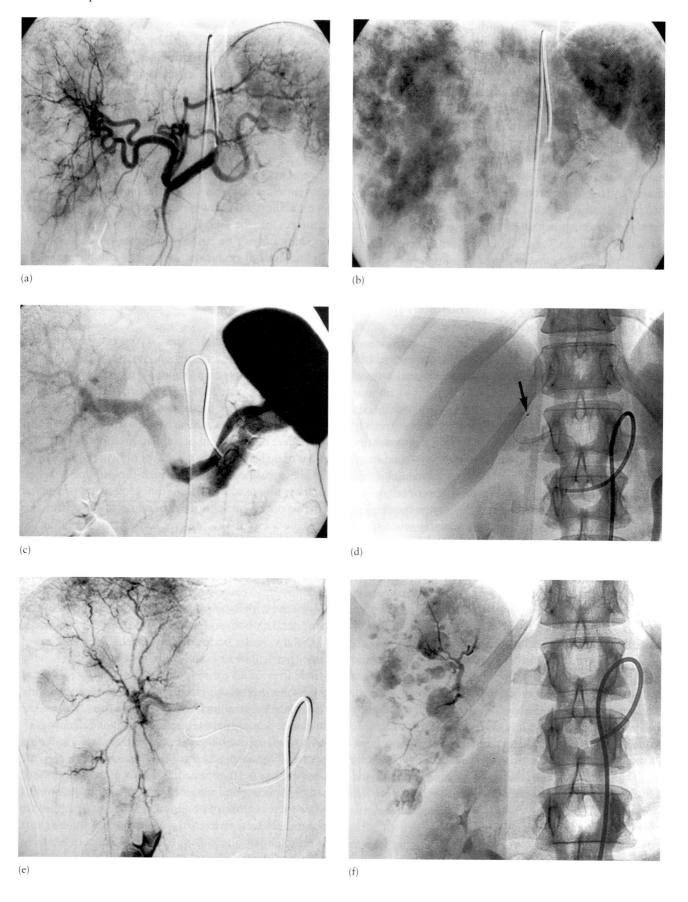

(a)

(b)

(c)

(d)

(e)

(f)

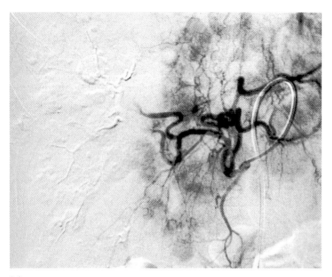

(g)

Fig. 10.1 Embolization of the right lobe of liver in a patient with carcinoid syndrome. (*Facing page*) (a) Coeliac axis arteriogram, arterial phase. There is hypertrophy of the common hepatic artery and its branches. Extensive neovascularity is seen in both lobes of the liver. (b) Coeliac axis arteriogram, capillary phase. Numerous tumour blushes are seen throughout an enlarged liver. (c) Indirect splenoportogram. The main portal vein and its branches are patent. Despite the extensive tumour bulk in the right lobe of the liver, the intrahepatic portal venous branches are well opacified. (d) A 3 French co-axial catheter has been introduced into the right posterior segmental artery (arrow) prior to embolization. (e) An angiogram prior to embolization confirms satisfactory position of the co-axial catheter. (f) Control film of the abdomen after embolization of both the right anterior and posterior segmental hepatic arteries shows contrast stasis within these vessels and within the tumour deposits. (*Above*) (g) Postembolization arteriogram confirms complete occlusion of the right hepatic artery with preservation of the arterial supply to the left lobe of the liver.

depend, to some extent, upon the indication for the procedure. The ideal particle size is that which will produce an arterial occlusion that is sufficiently distal to prevent the rapid development of collaterals, yet will leave normal sinusoidal perfusion by the portal vein uninterrupted. There is a fine dividing line when attempting peripheral hepatic arterial embolization between that particle size which will produce liver infarction and that which will not. Absorbable gelatin sponge and polyvinyl alcohol are the two most commonly used agents for hepatic embolization. The latter agent is preferred by this author because of its availability in a variety of different sizes and its ease of use.

As previously mentioned most patients will have disease in both lobes of the liver at presentation and the total tumour bulk may be massive. It is often prudent, therefore, to perform embolization of one lobe of the liver only during a single procedure (see Fig. 10.1). The patient can then return a few months later for embolization of the other lobe if his/her symptoms are not sufficiently palliated. Embolization is usually performed of that lobe that is most severely affected and this will often, by itself, provide excellent palliation for several months or even years. Patients who have undergone unilobar embolization may show improvement in terms of reduction in size of tumour deposits within the lobe which has not been embolized together with normalization of 5-hydroxy indole acetic acid (5-HIAA) levels. The reasons for this finding are unknown; some authors have suggested that systemic effects other than tumour ischaemia may play a role in tumour response following embolization.

Complications

Serious complications are fortunately uncommon provided the above-mentioned contraindications are heeded and the procedure is performed with a meticulous technique. Good postprocedural care is equally important in reducing morbidity and mortality. The most common complications may be divided into immediate and delayed.

Immediate complications

Complications occasionally associated with any angiographic procedure may of course occur, for example groin haematoma, contrast medium reaction or arterial dissection.

Immediate complications specifically related to hepatic arterial embolization include pain, nausea and vomiting, a hormonal crisis associated with the sudden release of massive amounts of vasoactive substances from the embolized tumour mass and the inadvertent embolization of an adjacent or distant normal vascular territory such as the spleen, stomach, duodenum, pancreas or small bowel. The latter is fortunately uncommon provided a meticulous technique is employed during the embolization procedure.

Delayed complications

Death. Death within a few weeks of the procedure is usually related to hepatorenal failure in patients with severe pre-existing liver function impairment and serious consideration should be given as to whether embolization should be carried out in such patients.

Postembolization syndrome (PES). This consists of a combination of nausea, pain, pyrexia and a leucocytosis; it occurs in the majority of patients who have undergone a major embolization procedure which has resulted in significant tissue necrosis. It may be difficult to differentiate this syndrome from a septicaemic illness, which, although uncommon in patients who have undergone hepatic arterial embolization, may be life threatening. Regular blood cultures are, therefore, very important if a pyrexia persists.

Hepatic abscess formation. This rarely occurs but when it does it may require percutaneous or surgical drainage. It is common, however, to note intrahepatic gas following embolization without signs of infection. This may be due to the production of carbon dioxide by anaerobic reticulocyte metabolism or may represent oxygen released from oxyhaemoglobin trapped in blood cells in embolized vessels.

Extrahepatic infarction. Although presumably occurring at the time of embolization, extrahepatic infarction may not manifest itself until several days following the procedure. The cystic artery is that vessel most susceptible to embolization, despite good technique, but even when this does occur gall bladder infarction is thankfully rare, presumably because the organ continues to receive an adequate blood supply from collateral sources such as its partial peritoneal investment and the gastroduodenal artery.

Derangement in the hepatic enzyme levels. This is almost invariable to some extent but is rarely clinically significant. Most enzyme measurements will have returned to near normal within two weeks of the procedure.

Percutaneous alcohol injection

Inoperable liver tumours may also be treated by the direct injection of absolute alcohol into their substance via a fine needle. The alcohol causes cellular dehydration and protein denaturation with subsequent coagulative necrosis. The procedure is usually performed under ultrasound control and multiple treatment sessions are often required.

This form of therapy has been used predominantly in the treatment of patients with irresectable hepatocellular carcinomas (HCC). In this group of patients the best results are obtained in those who have three or fewer lesions that are 3 cm or less in diameter. Serious complications of the procedure are rare and include: infarction of normal liver due to an intravascular injection of alcohol; haemorrhage, which may be intrahepatic, subcapsular or intraperitoneal; and hepatic decompensation.

It is unlikely that the encouraging results obtained using this technique in patients with small HCC will be equally applicable to patients with liver metastases from other primary tumours. Many of these patients, and particularly those with metastatic lesions from a neuroendocrine tumour, will have multiple hepatic deposits and percutaneous therapy of all of these would be impracticable. Occasionally, however, this form of therapy may prove useful in those patients whose hepatic artery has been occluded either surgically or by embolization or in those in whom hepatic artery embolization is contraindicated due to portal vein occlusion.

Results

Of patients with neuroendocrine tumours, those with carcinoid syndrome represent by far the largest subset and it is not surprising, therefore, that much of the literature regarding embolization of hepatic metastases concerns this group. Unfortunately there are no prospective, randomized, controlled trials comparing this form of therapy with medical treatment and one has to rely upon retrospective, non-randomized studies to try and determine the efficacy of this form of therapy.

In contrast to patients with metastases from other primary tumours, patients with neuroendocrine hepatic metastases frequently survive for a long time, sometimes years after presentation, though often with severe symptoms related to hormonal secretion by the tumour and hepatomegaly; for example, patients with carcinoid syndrome have a median survival of 38 months from the time of their first flush. This is reduced to 14 months if urinary 5-HIAA levels are more than 150 mg/24 h and is reduced still further to 11 months if there is clinical evidence of carcinoid heart disease. The primary aim of any form of therapy in this group of patients is the amelioration of symptoms rather than the modification of some objective parameter such as tumour bulk or serum hormone levels and there is no doubt that hepatic arterial embolization achieves this in a large proportion of these patients, thus vastly improving their quality of life.

The efficacy of this form of treatment in terms of improved survival is more difficult to assess because of the usually prolonged course of the disease but a significant prolongation of life has not been demonstrated. This is perhaps best illustrated in a paper by Coupe *et al.* [1], who retrospectively analysed 63 patients with carcinoid syndrome treated over a 10-year period. Thirty of these patients were referred for hepatic arterial embolization because of severe systemic symptoms poorly controlled by pharmacological treatment or because of marked local pain. Six of these patients did not undergo hepatic arterial embolization for a variety of reasons, including the presence of portal vein occlusion and inadequate arterial access. The mean survival in those patients followed to death was 58.7 ± 9.7 months in those undergoing hepatic artery embolization ($n = 18$) and 44.5 ± 9.6 months in those treated medically ($n = 11$). This result is not significant. A more accurate comparison can be drawn, however, between those patients successfully embolized and those in whom the procedure was unsuccessful. There was no significant survival difference between these two groups. The mean survival from the angiographic procedure was 18 ± 3.26 months in those undergoing hepatic artery embolization ($n = 18$) and 19.6 ± 6.5 months in those six patients in whom embolization was intended but not performed. The conclusion that can be drawn from this paper is that hepatic artery embolization does not prolong survival, although it is undoubtedly very useful for the relief of symptoms.

It is useful also to look at the findings of a second, more recent, retrospective study, in which Wängberg *et al.* [2] reviewed their results of treatment of 48 patients with carcinoid syndrome over 5 years. They treated all their patients aggressively with surgical excision of the primary tumour together with regional lymph node metastases. A cholecystectomy was also performed in all patients to reduce complications due to subsequent embolization or octreotide therapy.

Patients with unilobar hepatic disease underwent hepatic resection at a second operation, whilst those with bilobar disease ($n = 27$) underwent embolization of both lobes of their liver at separate sessions performed 1–2 months apart. The authors reported 11 'cures' of whom six had undergone hepatic resection and five (without liver metastases) had undergone extensive lymph node resection. The mean follow-up of this group of patients was 42 ± 7 months. Ten patients underwent surgery and octreotide therapy, of whom eight died during a mean follow-up of 19 ± 3 months. Twenty-seven patients underwent surgery and hepatic artery embolization. These patients were divided into 13 'responders' (no visible hepatic tumours or more than 50% tumour regression on follow-up), and 14 'non-responders' (less than 50% regression or progression). The authors noted that the reduction in 5-HIAA levels postembolization was much more pronounced in the responders group and these patients had long-lasting biochemical and radiological improvement without the need for further embolization over a mean follow-up period of 26 ± 5 months. There were no deaths in this group during the follow-up period. In contrast there were six deaths in the non-responders group, with a mean follow-up of 37 ± 4 months. The authors concluded that the initial biochemical response to embolization with marked decrease of 5-HIAA levels, in combination with tumour regression may serve as an indicator of a good prognosis. There may, therefore, be a group of patients in whom embolization will produce symptom relief and some prolongation of life.

Treatment of other endocrine tumours

The treatment of other endocrine tumours by radiological means is much less frequently performed than hepatic artery embolization, although it is useful to review some of these techniques which may prove to be helpful in certain individuals.

Primary tumours

Parathyroid adenoma

Percutaneous alcohol injection

Ablation of functioning parathyroid adenomas may be achieved by direct percutaneous injection of absolute alcohol, which is usually performed under ultrasound guidance. The results using this technique are, however, variable and subsequent surgery, should ablation not be achieved, is reported as being more difficult because of the presence of surrounding fibrosis which is presumably induced by extravasation of alcohol during the original injection. As a result of this, and because of the fact that the majority of parathyroid adenomas are easily found and removed by a competent surgeon, the technique has not been widely used.

Transarterial embolization

Parathyroid adenomas may respond well to transarterial embolization. The feeding vessel to the adenoma is selectively catheterized and embolization is then performed with absolute alcohol.

This technique, once again, has not been widely used and long-term results of the procedure are not known. For the same reasons as for percutaneous alcohol injection above, this form of therapy is unlikely to gain much popularity. Both techniques should perhaps be reserved for patients who are poor surgical candidates or those who have undergone several previous negative surgical explorations. Parathyroid adenomas within the mediastinum may be amenable to transarterial embolization, particularly if they have a single feeding vessel arriving from the inferior thyroid or internal mammary to activity; in patients with hyperplasia aldosterone levels rise during the day, whilst in patients with adenomas, levels tend to remain static or even fall. In adrenal adenomas there is a functional deficiency of corticosterone methyl oxidase 2 and, as a result, unlike patients with adrenal hyperplasia, a very raised 18-hydroxycorticosterone level. These two tests give a 90% accuracy rate and are particularly useful when scanning measures are equivocal, avoiding surgery, which in the case of bilateral adrenal hyperplasia is inappropriate.

The diagnosis of phaeochromocytoma mainly depends on the high index of clinical suspicion, coupled with evidence of excessive catecholamine secretion in the form of adrenaline, noradrenaline or dopamine or their metabolites. A considerable number of patients present with hypertension and symptoms suggestive of phaeochromocytoma with borderline elevation of both plasma catecholamines and urinary metabolites.

The diagnosis of insulinoma presents very special problems. The diagnosis is made by persistent hypoglycaemia and an inappropriate elevation of plasma insulin. This may need a prolonged (72 hours) fast. The C-peptide level must be measured because it will be elevated in patients with tumours or in nesidioblastosis and will allow exclusion of patients with fictitious hypoglycaemia due to self-administration of insulin. Urinary measurement of glibenclamide levels is essential in doubtful cases since fictitious hypoglycaemia with a raised serum insulin as well as raised C-peptide levels will occur due to the self-administration of the drug.

The multiple endocrine neoplasia (MEN) types 1 and 2 present formidable diagnostic and therapeutic problems for the surgeon. The MEN-1 syndrome usually results from a mutation of a gene on the long arm (band q12–13) of chromosome 11. The disorder is a distinctive syndrome of neoplasia in parathyroid, gastrointestinal endocrine cells, anterior pituitary and other tissues. Until the MEN-1 gene has been cloned and sequenced it is not possible to make a clear distinction between MEN-1 and the sporadic form. It is essential that an aggressive endocrine approach is made to all possible involved organs so that an appropriate assessment can be made of each of them. The high instance of somatostatin receptors in the various organs involved with tumours in MEN-1 allow the use of somatostatin receptor scanning with radionuclear-labelled somatostatin analogues.

MEN-2, which is subdivided into Sipple's syndrome (MEN-2a) and the rarer MEN-2b with its mucosal neuromas, marfanoid features and absence of hyperparathyroidism are both caused by mutations in a cell surface tyrosine receptor, *ret*. In the past, screening of relatives of patients with known MEN-2 syndrome had relied on either basal or stimulated calcitonin levels and surgical interference was based on these results. In the future, it is hoped that the absence of the genetic abnormality will allow patients to be discharged and, conversely, patients shown to have the genetic defect will need to be subjected to early surgery, long before calcitonin levels are detected. Such an aggressive policy based on genetic information will allow patients to be cured of the medullary thyroid carcinoma aspect of their disease. To date not all the genetic abnormalities have been identified and this approach remains for the future.

Very rarely, a raised calcitonin may exist in the absence of either C-cell hyperplasia or medullary thyroid carcinoma. The absence of a genetic abnormality in such patients will allow these patients to be reassured and not subjected to unnecessary thyroidectomy. Patients with medullary carcinoma must be reviewed regularly since phaeochromocytomas may appear subsequently and are regularly bilateral and associated with adrenal medullary hyperplasia.

Making the patient safe

The second principle of endocrine surgery is the ability to render the patient safe for their surgical procedure. In hyperparathyroidism, adequate hydration coupled with the use of loop diuretics will lower the calcium to satisfactory levels in the majority of cases. In severe primary hyperparathyroidism the administration of isotonic saline, coupled with intravenous diphosphonate or occasionally mithramycin will control the situation and allow urgent parathyroidectomy to be performed. Intravenous phosphate is completely contraindicated, since it may produce intravascular precipitation of calcium phosphate salts and cause pulmonary insufficiency, vascular calcification, hypertension and even, on occasions, death. There is little role for the use of steroids, calcitonin and other agents which are less effective than the diphosphonates.

In patients with Conn's syndrome the replacement of potassium, either orally or intravenously, together with spironolactone 200–400 mg/day will result in the patient having a normal potassium prior to surgery.

The exploration of a patient with an uncontrolled phaeochromocytoma can be a surgical disaster. Treatment has been revolutionized by the preoperative use of the α-blocker phenoxybenzamine. This drug causes postural hypotension and is started in a dose of 10 mg orally, and increased if necessary to 120–140 mg/day. Management of such patients should be on an in-patient basis since an adequate blockade is indicated by symptomatic postural hypotension. Beta-blockers should not be given prior to α blockade and should be added particularly if there is a cardiac arrhythmia or a persistent tachycardia over 100 beats/min. Some patients are resistant to α blockade and when this happens, α-methyl-P-tyrosine may be used. This drug acts by blocking tyrosine hydroxylase and inhibits noradrenaline synthesis. Preoperative blood transfusion may be necessary because of associated vasodilatation and haemodilution. Nitroprusside may be necessary at operation to avoid excessive rises in blood pressure.

Patients with insulinomas vary in the severity of their hypoglycaemia. They should be rendered safe by the use of diazoxide, a thiazide which raises blood glucose, coupled with intravenous glucose perioperatively.

Localization of the tumour

Once an endocrine diagnosis has been made it is important to ascertain whether there is single or multiple gland disease. It also must be emphasized that it is important to ascertain whether the disease is benign or malignant. Malignancy may be very difficult to diagnose preoperatively, unless there are obvious metastases.

In the patient with primary hyperparathyroidism who has not previously been operated on, localization procedures are rarely necessary. A good endocrine surgeon will find 85% of tumours. In patients who have had previous surgery, a large number of tests may be used. These include ultrasound, CT, MRI, venous sampling and parathyroid subtraction scans. These tests when used singly usually have an accuracy of no more than 50% but when used in conjunction with each other the accuracy of the localization is increased to 75–80%.

The small size of Conn's tumours of the adrenal make preoperative localizing essential. Ultrasound is rarely of use since the tumours are usually less than 2 cm in diameter. Spiral CT has a diagnostic rate of about 80% but will miss some lesions less than 1 cm in diameter. Venous sampling may aid lateralization.

Scanning of the adrenal with radioactive labelled cholesterol is helpful in distinguishing a hot adrenal from one with bilateral uptake. In the USA, iodocholesterol is the only available agent, while in the UK, selenocholesterol, which has a longer half-life and allows labelled cholesterol to be cleared from the liver is considered a better agent. The addition of high dose dexamethasone to suppress the adrenocorticotrophic hormone (ACTH)-dependent layers of the adrenal improves the accuracy of the technique.

The localization of phaeochromocytomas has been revolutionized by the advent of MIBG. ^{123}I-MIBG is the agent of choice. It produces clear images, has a short half-life and is about 95% accurate. CT is also of great value, since most phaeochromocytomas are larger than 2 cm and it allows the surgeon to have a clear idea of the relationship of the adrenal tumour to surrounding structures. Ultrasound is extremely important in evaluation of right-sided adrenal tumours which may grow into the inferior vena cava.

The small size of insulinomas presents difficult diagnostic problems and renders abdominal ultrasound unreliable, except as an intra-operative procedure. A combination of high quality CT and selective angiography will demonstrate the tumours in approximately 90% of cases. Recently, the use of a selective calcium infusion into the feeding vessels of the pancreas with simultaneous measurement of insulin and C peptide allows the successful excision of minute insulinomas undetectable by other methods. A similar technique has been used for gastrinomas. Glucagonomas on the whole are large and tend not to present difficulty with localization. Trans-splenic portal venous sampling is rarely used in patients with pancreatic tumours since it has been superseded by the other methods described.

The need to operate

Not all patients with endocrine tumours need surgery. This is true in some cases of asymptomatic primary hyperparathyroidism. Patients over 50 years of age with mildly elevated calcium, normal bone density and no complications (e.g. nephrocalcinosis) may be safely watched. However, watching such patients involves effort and expense. They should have regular serum calcium measurements every 6 months, together with annual checks of renal function, calcium excretion and bone density. This complicated regimen of management must be balanced against the fact that parathyroid surgery usually takes less than 40 minutes and is successful in 98% of cases.

In patients with Conn's syndrome and mild disease, long-term treatment with spironolactone may be satisfactory. Conn's tumours are virtually never malignant and if control is lost on spironolactone therapy they can still be operated upon. Treatment of the adrenal adenoma, almost uniformly unilateral, results in a 90% cure of hypokalaemia and a 70% cure of hypertension. Clearly the treatment of idiopathic bilateral adrenal hyperplasia causing aldosteronism is medical and surgery is not justified.

Patients with phaeochromocytoma always require operation. When phaeochromocytomas occur in association with Sipple's syndrome, the phaeochromocytomas should be dealt with prior to thyroid surgery.

The management of medullary carcinoma is total thyroidectomy. Relatives with a proven genetic abnormality should now be subjected to thyroidectomy, even though their calcitonin levels and scans are normal. This aggressive approach should result in reduced mortality of this difficult group of patients.

Surgical tactics

The primary surgical aim is to return the patient to a normal endocrine state. This principle may or may not always be possible. In primary hyperparathyroidism due to a single adenoma, removal of the adenoma and biopsy of the normal parathyroid will usually result in cure of the patient.

The situation is much more difficult in hyperplasia of all four glands where three options exist.

1 Removal of all the parathyroid tissue and placement of the patient on vitamin D and calcium supplements. This approach, although not elegant, has the advantage that the patient is cured of disease, although dependent on supplements lifelong.

2 Performance of a sub-total parathyroidectomy, leaving approximately 100 mg of parathyroid tissue in the neck. This will result in about 50% of patients remaining normocalcaemic but the remaining 50% may develop recurrent hypercalcaemia and thus need difficult re-exploration of the neck with all its hazards.

3 Performance of a total parathyroidectomy with parathyroid transplantation in the forearm. The results of this vary from centre to centre, but if practised carefully and coupled with cryopreservation, patients with hyperplasia can be maintained normocalcaemic and, if enough parathyroid tissue has not been transplanted, cryopreserved parathyroid tissue can be further transplanted at a later date into the forearm. Conversely, if the patient becomes hypercalcaemic, small amounts of parathyroid tissue can be removed from the forearm under local anaesthetic.

Patients with the rare entity of parathyroid carcinoma are difficult to treat and it is absolutely essential that as far as possible all parathyroid tissue is removed. Great care should be taken not to break into the capsule of the tumour and usually the local lymph nodes and ipsilateral lobe of the thyroid need to be removed together with the tumour.

In Conn's syndrome, unilateral adrenalectomy is the treatment of choice. With the recent advances in technology this can now be performed as a laparoscopic procedure in experienced hands. Although total adrenalectomy in

the past has been advocated it is now possible to perform a meticulous excision of the tumour alone, enucleating it from the surrounding adrenal tissue. This technique is not associated with a high incidence of recurrence of symptoms. Patients with phaeochromocytoma should undergo total adrenalectomy with meticulous preservation of the tumour capsule since disruption of the tumour may result in implantation of tissue in the adrenal bed and late recurrence of symptoms. This may occur even though the tumour is non-malignant. In the MEN-2 syndrome where tumours are often bilateral, total adrenalectomy should be performed, usually on both sides, although on occasion a sub-total adrenalectomy with preservation of some adrenal tissue may be justified. In patients who are being operated on for pituitary-dependent Cushing's syndrome it is absolutely essential when removing the adrenals that all the surrounding area is examined meticulously for possible ectopic adrenal tissue.

Patients with insulinoma usually respond to simple enucleation of the tumour. Rarely, a distal pancreatectomy or a Whipple's procedure may be necessary. When exploring patients with the MEN-1 syndrome the pancreas should be meticulously examined, as well as the duodenum, where small tumours the size of millet seeds may be found in the submucosal layers. Gastrinomas and vipomas should be dealt with on their merits but usually need a major resection of the pancreas.

When exploring a pancreas with a huge tumour bulk and possibly associated tumour in the liver, the extent of the resection has to be balanced against morbidity and the role of pharmacological agents to control symptoms; for example, it may be better to treat a relatively static metastatic insulinoma with diazoxide and do a limited debulking procedure, rather than an attempted curative resection which will be associated with a high morbidity and mortality.

The delicate balance of the use of drugs and surgery emphasizes the importance of a team approach. The team should consist of an endocrinologist, a specialist endocrine surgeon and endocrine pathologist, a radiotherapist experienced in endocrine problems and an oncologist. Such a team approach will result, in the future, in a better understanding of these fascinating cases and also better results.

Reference

Lynn J, Bloom S (eds). *Surgical Endocrinology*. Oxford: Butterworth Heinemann, 1993.

General Management of Cancer Patients

MARCIA HALL

Introduction

This chapter summarizes the guiding principles in the active management of the cancer patient, in particular the management of endocrine-related tumours, although most issues discussed are fundamental to all cancer patients. There are two main sections; the first deals with problems common to the cancer patient irrespective of therapy undertaken and the second discusses the complications of specific therapies. Specific metabolic and endocrine complications are covered in separate chapters.

The diagnosis of cancer is often a complicated, prolonged process requiring extensive and unpleasant investigations. Great patience is occasionally required to await a difficult pathological diagnosis, particularly in the case of many endocrine-related tumours. Diagnostic and staging information should clarify whether treatment should be aimed at cure or palliation. Treatment can usually be tailored to minimize most of the complications of disease, although the therapy itself may cause other problems. Good communication with the patient and their family at this stage is vital to ensure that the aims and limitations of any therapeutic strategy are understood. Distinguishing between cure and palliation is essential to avoid misleading patients and their families, resulting in understandable distress. Finally, regular review, which should include documenting the history, current symptoms, diagnostic results, therapy and the content of discussions with the patient and their family, is essential for quality care of the cancer patient.

Complications of disease

Pain

Pain is the most feared consequence of cancer. It occurs in approximately one-third of patients (15% with non-metastatic disease and 60–90% with advanced disease). There are two main types of cancer pain.

1 *Acute*: clearly defined temporal onset usually associated with objective physical signs together with signs of increased autonomic nervous system activity. This type of pain is usually self-limiting and readily treatable.

2 *Chronic*: poorly defined onset, usually present for greater than three months, with no associated objective clinical signs. This type of pain often results in changes in personality, lifestyle and functioning.

Of cancer pain 70–80% is thought to be due to direct tumour involvement (bone, 50%; nerve, 25%; hollow viscus, 15%). Twenty to 30% is related to cancer therapy and 3–10% to unrelated previous disease processes, for example rheumatoid arthritis.

Pain symptoms should be clearly identified and documented: somatic (e.g. bony), visceral (e.g. liver metastases), or deafferent (injury to peripheral or central nervous system); assessment must include the degree of functional impairment. Psychosocial factors may be influential and should also be addressed. Verification of the history by another family member may help to prioritize the management of multiple complaints. Painful benign conditions may coexist in patients with cancer and should not be overlooked.

Adequate pain relief usually involves two or more different classes of analgesics (Table 12.1). No additional therapeutic effect exists beyond the maximum tolerated dose of most non-steroidal drugs and each one in this category has a different anti-inflammatory to analgesic ratio. H_2-blockers such as ranitidine given prophylactically have *not* been shown to prevent gastrointestinal adverse effects from non-steroidal drugs. However there is some evidence that misoprostol may help prevent gastric ulceration in those receiving non-steroidal anti-inflammatory drugs (NSAIDs).

As with non-steroidal drugs, a similar pragmatic approach with different opiate doses and preparations

Table 12.1 Pharmacological treatment options for pain

Class	Drugs	Indications	Dose/route	Contraindications	Side-effects	Interactions
Non-steroidals	Voltarol	Mild/moderate pain especially if inflammatory component present	50 mg tds oral/rectal or 100 mg SR bd	Active peptic ulcer Proctitis Aspirin allergy	Gastrointestinal Haematological Headache, oedema	Steroids Anticoagulants Digoxin Quinolones
Narcotics Partial agonists Weak opioids	Buprenorphine Dihydrocodeine Codeine phosphate Distalgesic	Not recommended Moderate/severe pain	60–120 mg qds 30–90 mg qds 2 tablets qds (8 max.)	Respiratory depression/COAD	Nausea, vertigo tolerance, constipation, drowsiness	CNS depressants MAOIs
Opioids	Diamorphine Morphine sulphate Morphine sulphate (slow release) Fentanyl	Severe pain	Start 5 mg sc Start 10–30 mg 4 hourly Start 20–30 mg 12 hourly Available as patches	Respiratory depression Hepatic failure	Sedation, nausea constipation (see text)	CNS depressants MAOIs
Tricyclics	Amitriptyline	Dysaesthetic pain	25–50 mg max. nocte Ten-day trial	Ischaemic heart disease	Sedation, dry mouth constipation	Cimetidine Anticoagulants
Anticonvulsants	Carbamazepine	Shooting/stinging pain	100 mg bd increasing slowly (100 mg every 3–4 days) 200 mg tds max.	AV conduction abnormalities, porphyria, agranulocytosis	Dizziness, nausea, hyponatraemia, blood dyscrasias, severe skin rash	Anticoagulants Oral contraceptive MAOIs, cimetidine
Antiarrhythmics	Flecainide	Refractory neuropathic pain	50–150 mg bd	Ischaemic heart disease	Nausea, photosensitivity, ataxia, deranged liver enzymes	Cardiac depressants Digoxin
Steroids	Dexamethasone	Pain associated with tumour pressure or oedema	12–16 mg (high dose) for 5 days then reduce by 2 mg every 2–3 days; maintain 2–4 mg daily	Infections, recent surgery, active peptic ulcer	Gastrointestinal, hyperglycaemia, mood changes, proximal myopathy	Anticoagulants NSAIDs
Bisphosphonates	Pamidronate Clodronate	Pain from bony metastases	30–60 mg iv in 500 ml N/saline over 4 h 300 mg iv daily for 5 days 1600–3200 mg oral daily (very poor GI absorbance hence poor efficacy by this route)		Renal failure if given as a bolus	

AV, arterioventricular; CNS, central nervous system; COAD, chronic obstructive airway disease; GI, gastrointestinal; MAOIs, monoamine oxidase inhibitors; NSAIDs, non-steroidal anti-inflammatory drugs; SR, slow release.

produces the best result. Sedation may be a problem initially but usually lessens with continuing therapy. Nevertheless it is prudent to reduce or stop any concomitant sedative drugs and avoid drugs (such as cimetidine) whose metabolism affects morphine metabolism, by increasing its half-life. Nausea and vomiting may occur with the first doses of morphine but tolerance usually develops rapidly (i.e. within 48–72 hours). Constipation however remains a difficult persisting problem; tolerance develops also, but much more slowly. The use of laxatives with narcotics minimizes constipation but higher than routine recommended doses may be required. A combination of laxatives with different modes of action (e.g. senna and sodium docusate) is frequently useful. Dietary advice and increased fluid intake are also helpful.

Total pain, as first described by Cicely Saunders, is recognized as pain comprising physical, psychological, emotional and spiritual elements and this underlines the importance of a multidisciplinary approach to its control. The non-drug treatment of pain includes the use of nerve-stimulating (transelectrical nerve stimulation (TENS)) and nerve-blocking techniques for neuropathic pains as well as a range of psychological interventions, including relaxation techniques and the teaching of cognitive coping strategies.

Infection

Infections occur commonly in cancer patients, either as a consequence of the underlying malignancy or as a complication of therapy. They may be life threatening. In treating cancer it is important to recognize risk factors contributing to infection and to have a good knowledge of available therapies.

Host defence mechanisms may be compromised by virtue of the malignant disease itself; for example, impaired antibody production in multiple myeloma, altered cellular immunity in lymphomas. The cancer patient is also rendered more vulnerable by cancer treatment. Cytotoxic chemotherapy and radiotherapy deplete granulocyte numbers and produce defects of neutrophil function; corticosteroids diminish phagocytosis and neutrophil migration. As if to add injury to insult, therapy may also break down some of the physical barriers to pathogenic invasion, such as mucosal and skin reactions. Antibiotic therapy, active or empiric, may induce secondary colonization of these 'chinks' in the armour, resulting in systemic invasion. Malnutrition exacerbates any or all of the above, adding to the cancer patient's susceptibility.

The febrile response is often significantly diminished in cancer patients, particularly when neutropenic, and fevers may be masked by concomitant steroid or NSAID

treatment. If undetected and untreated, infections may be rapidly fatal. Fifty-five to 70% of febrile episodes in this population have an infective aetiology. This incidence is higher in neutropenic patients, where 85–90% are bacterial in origin (Table 12.2), although only 30–50% will be positively identified.

Empirical therapy should be considered in non-neutropenic patients after two or three temperature readings greater than 38°C (Fig. 12.1). Antibiotics must be commenced in neutropenic (absolute neutrophil count $< 1 \times 10^9/mm^3$) patients after a single temperature reading of $> 37.5°C$. This reduces mortality from 80% to 10–30%. Bactericidal antibiotics covering Gram-negative bacteria are essential therapy. Single-agent, third-generation cephalosporins, such as ceftazidime 1 g tds have recently been shown to be as successful as combination therapy. If the response is slow or if organisms are isolated that are not covered, early modifications will be required. Standard empirical antibiotics should be tailored for each institution taking into account local microbial isolates, antibiotic resistance patterns and cost. Prophylactic antibiotics should be considered for patients undergoing intensive therapy involving long periods of neutropenia, for example autologous bone marrow transplantation (ABMT), as the major source (85%) of infection is from endogenous flora, (50% from the hospital environment via a human vector). Complete gut decontamination is not recommended as resistant strains emerge and the antibiotics involved are unpalatable and poorly tolerated. Selective gut decontamination (cotrimoxazole, 2 tablets bd) preserves the anaerobic gastrointestinal flora, preventing colonization, and is more tolerable. The benefits are still not entirely clear despite a few enthusiastic reports. Acyclovir 200 mg

Table 12.2 Common infective agents in cancer patients

Form of infection	Organism
Gram-positive	e.g. *Staphylococcus aureus*, *Corynebacterium*
Gram-negative	e.g. *Escherichia coli*, *Klebsiella*
Multiply resistant	e.g. *Enterobacter* spp., *Citrobacter* spp., *Acinetobacter* spp., *Serratia marcescens*, multiresistant *Staphylococcus aureus*
Anaerobes	5%, often associated with anal and oral lesions
Fungi	Candida, aspergillosis
Viral	Herpes zoster, herpes simplex, CMV, toxoplasmosis
Parasites	*Pneumocystis carini*

CMV, cytomegalovirus.

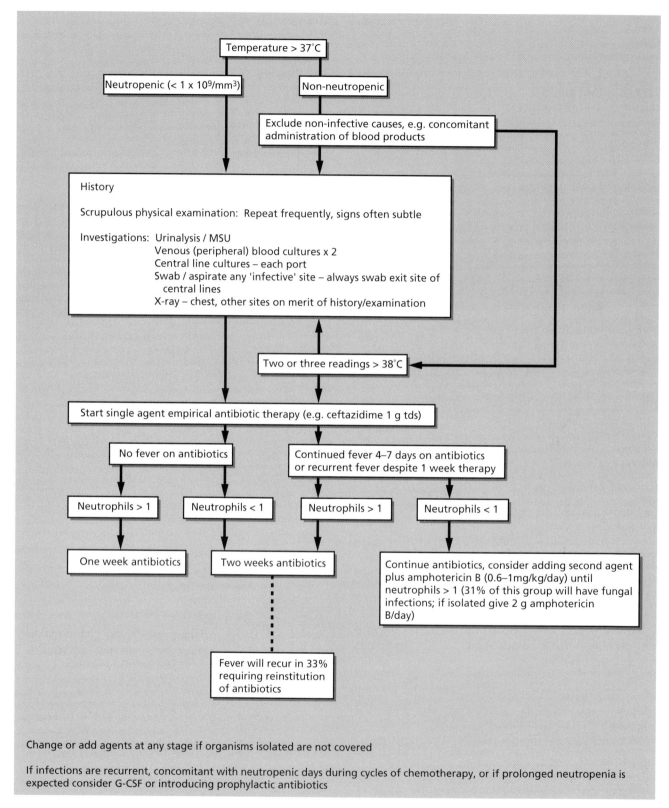

Fig. 12.1 Management of pyrexia of unknown origin in cancer patients.
G-CSF, granulocyte colony-stimulating factor; MSU, midstream urine.

twice daily for a year after ABMT prevents recurrent herpes simplex virus (HSV) infections. Cytomegalovirus (CMV)-seronegative blood products should always be used in CMV-seronegative patients. The recent introduction of recombination granulocyte colony-stimulating factor (G-CSF) promises to be a useful adjunct to reducing the chances of infection, by limiting the period of neutropenia.

Anorexia–cachexia syndrome

Malnutrition is frequently a serious problem in patients with cancer, contributing substantially to the morbidity and mortality from the disease. Approximately one-quarter of cancer patients have lost 10% or more of their pre-morbid body weight and one-third require some form of nutritional support [1]. Clearly certain tumour types, such as those affecting the gastrointestinal tract, are more commonly associated with significant weight loss and malnutrition. There is often no correlation, however, between tumour extent and weight loss, suggesting influences from many other factors. A complex cytokine cascade, triggered in the host by the tumour, is believed to result in the progressive weight loss, lethargy, weakness and anorexia that characterizes cachexia. This chronic abnormal metabolic state may be exacerbated by other tumour-related phenomena such as ectopic hormone production and infective episodes causing hypermetabolism. Abnormalities of taste and smell are common amongst cancer patients, frequently exacerbated by cancer therapy.

The anorexia–cachexia syndrome is notoriously difficult to treat without regression of the underlying cancer. Nevertheless there are numerous therapeutic strategies that can be tried (Table 12.3). Although corticosteroids (prednisolone 20 mg daily) have been shown to improve both quality of life and appetite, this adjunct to therapy rarely results in non-fluid weight gain. Progestogens (medroxyprogesterone acetate 10 mg tds) have been shown to have a dose-related effect on appetite and weight, which is neither secondary to fluid retention nor to tumour response. Enteral feeding can be useful but parenteral feeding should not be undertaken except as a short-term option in the severely malnourished patient expected to respond well to active cancer treatment.

Psychological morbidity

Studies of psychiatric disorders in cancer patients have estimated a prevalence rate of 20–47%. The majority

Table 12.3 Feeding strategies

Oral diet	
Education	High calorie foods
	Small meals frequently
	Add supplements, e.g. Hical, Ensure
	Specific diets may help, e.g. low fibre/ low fat/lactose for short bowel and radiation enteritis
Location/presentation	Eat away from bed
	Small portions
	Tastefully presented
Drugs	
Appetite stimulants	Corticosteroids: prednisolone 20 mg mane, reduce to lower maintenance dose as soon as possible
	Progestogens: medroxyprogesterone acetate 10–20 mg tds
Adequate anti-emetics	5-HT$_3$ antagonists: ondansetron 8 mg bd
	Metoclopramide: 10–20 mg qds as necessary, trial of high dose with procyclidin may be considered
	Cannaboids: nabilone 1–2 mg bd
Enteral feeding	
Nasogastric	Short-term use
Gastrostomy ⎫	Suitable for long-term feeding
Jejunostomy ⎭	Percutaneous placement via endoscopy
	Possible under local anaesthetic
Parenteral feeding	Durable and reliable central venous access required
	Metabolic monitoring and individual TPN prescriptions

5-HT$_3$, 5-hydroxytryptamine 3; TPN total parental nutrition.

suffer from anxiety and depressive disorders, although other problems include anticipatory nausea and vomiting, marital and sexual dysfunction. The spectrum of severity is considerable and ranges from mild, transient 'adjustment reactions' to severe and disabling anxiety and mood disorders. No matter how 'understandable' patients' distress, thorough assessment including a collateral history and appropriate physical investigations should be undertaken if appropriate treatment strategies, both psychological and pharmacological, are to be provided. Many patients will benefit from counselling of a supportive/educational approach, although more specific cognitive behavioural techniques may be needed in severe, persistent disorders [2]. Antidepressant medication is generally underprescribed in cancer patients and with the advent of newer agents with fewer side-effects (e.g. selective serotonin reuptake inhibitors (SSRIs)) this should be considered if symptoms of anxiety and depression are either of a severe degree or

Table 12.4 Commonly used antidepressants

Class	Drug	Indications	Dose/route	Contraindications	Side-effects	Interactions
Tricyclics	Lofepramine	Non-sedating	70 mg bd tds	Heart block, acute MI, severe liver disease	Anticholinergic, e.g. dry mouth, constipation	CNS depressants, anticonvulsants, cimetidine
	Trimipramine	If anxiety and sleep disturbance prominent	50–150 mg nocte	Heart block, acute MI, severe liver disease	Anticholinergic, e.g. dry mouth, constipation	CNS depressants, anticonvulsants, cimetidine
SSRIs	Sertraline	Depression and anxiety	50–100 mg mane	Hepatic insufficiency insomnia, dizziness	Nausea, dry mouth e.g. sumatriptan	MAOIs, serotinergic drugs
	Fluoxetine	Depression especially if somnolent	20–40 mg mane (available as syrup)	Severe renal failure unstable epilepsy	Nausea, insomnia anxiety, headache	MAOIs, anticonvulsants flecainide, vinblastine
Atypical	Trazodone	Useful if sleep disturbance prominent	50–300 mg nocte	Epilepsy, severe renal or hepatic failure	Drowsiness, headache, postural hypotension, priapism, blood dyscrasias	CNS depressants, volatile anaesthetics, MAOIs, digoxin

MAOIs, monoamine oxidase inhibitors; MI, myocardial infarction; SSRIs, selective serotonin reuptake inhibitors.

are non-responsive to psychological treatments (Table 12.4).

Complications of therapy

Cytotoxic therapy

Cytotoxic agents are renowned for their toxic and plentiful adverse effects. These are often closely related to their very action, killing cells. Malignant cells are targeted by these drugs because, in general, they undergo mitosis faster than normal cells. Clearly this crude warfare will inevitably have some action on other normally dividing cells. One very common and underestimated side-effect is lethargy. A patient may feel lethargic as part of their underlying disease but the addition of cytotoxic therapy will invariably exacerbate the situation. The lethargy is particularly profound during episodes of neutropenia. There is no effective remedy for this debilitating condition except to reassure patients that improvements occur with the resolution of neutropenia. Table 12.5 lists adverse effects common to many cytotoxic treatments and mentions a few problems specific to individual agents, noted in parentheses. Strategies to overcome some of these problems are suggested.

Biological agents

Although conventional cytotoxic and radiotherapeutic strategies retain the pivotal role in the treatment of cancer,

biological therapies are emerging fast as a powerful adjunct, or sole therapy, for some tumour types [3]. Those currently used in the management of endocrine-related tumours include somatostatin analogues and α-interferon; monoclonal antibodies are increasingly being used for radioimmunodiagnosis and when conjugated with therapeutic doses of appropriate radionuclides are also beginning to be used as treatment. Recombinant G-CSF, as mentioned earlier in this chapter, is also proving to be an extremely useful agent in allaying prolonged neutropenia. Interleukins remain experimental and will not be discussed here. It must be emphasized that, with the exception of somatostatin which appears to be relatively non-toxic, biological therapy has the potential to cause severe and serious adverse effects (Table 12.6).

Quality of life

'The good physician knows his patient through and through and his knowledge is bought dearly. Time, sympathy and understanding must be lavishly dispensed but the reward is to be found in that personal bond which forms the greatest satisfaction of the practice of medicine. One of the essential qualities of the clinician is interest in humanity, for '*the secret of the care of the patient is in caring for the patient.*' Peabody, 1927 [4].

The general management of the cancer patient requires a multidisciplinary team approach, which is concerned as much with the quality of life as its duration. The modern

Table 12.5 Management of common adverse effects of cytotoxic agents

System	Adverse effect	Management
Local	Phlebitis	Inject/infuse drugs more slowly; resite cannula if persistent. NB Phlebitic drugs, e.g. anthracyclines, should *always* be administered as an infusion or via running saline
	Local tissue necrosis	Irrigate/cold compress/infiltrate with hydrocortisone

Gastrointestinal	Nausea and vomiting	*Emetogenic potential of agents*
		Low
		  e.g. 5-FU/chlorambucil
		  domperidone 30 mg qds prn
		  prochlorperazine 10 mg tds prn
		Medium
		  e.g. cyclophosphamide, methotrexate, Adriamycin
		  dexamethasone 8 mg iv with chemotherapy
		  plus 2 mg tds for 2–3 days
		High
		  e.g. platinum
		  dexamethasone 8 mg iv
		  ondansetron 8 mg iv plus
		  2 mg dexamethasone tds orally
		  (and ondansetron 8 mg bd,
		  if required) for 2–3 days
		NB Rectal preparations of domperidone and prochlorperazine can be useful

	Stomatitis	Mouthwash 2–4 hourly, e.g. Corsodyl or Difflam (latter contains local anaesthetic)
	Diarrhoea	Rarely life-threatening: admit to rehydrate. Usually use loperamide or codeine phosphate (occasionally require excessive doses, e.g: 90–120 mg qds). Try somatostatin analogues if neuroendocrine-related. Try cyproheptadine or parachlorophenylalanine for carcinoid
Haematological	Leucopenia	Dose reduction or G-CSF support if severe. Consider prophylactic antibiotics if infections are recurrent during cycles of chemotherapy
	Thrombocytopenia	Platelet transfusions if bleeding or $< 20{\times}10^3/\text{mm}^3$
	Anaemia	Transfuse packed cells, if necessary
Renal	Hyperuricaemic nephropathy	Allopurinol 100–200 mg tds for 5 days prior to treatment thought to provoke massive lysis of malignant cells. Treatment should also be accompanied by high rate of urine flow, oral or parenteral fluid plus alkalinization by administering sodium bicarbonate 600–1200 mg qds until urine pH > 8.0
	Acute tubular necrosis	Cisplatin induced: check creatinine clearance prior to first dose. If using carboplatin, adjust dose using creatinine clearance. Always prehydrate prior to cisplatin and post hydrate with magnesium afterwards. Monitor plasma creatinine (± clearance) to adjust subsequent doses
Neurological	Ototoxicity (platinum)	Check hearing prior to first dose and between repeated high doses
	Peripheral neuropathy (vinca alkaloids, platinum)	Mostly reversible, although may worsen prior to improving. Stop drugs immediately if significant
Miscellaneous	Haemorrhagic cystitis (cyclophosphamide, ifosphamide)	Forced diuresis: orally if low/medium dose cyclophosphamide Forced diuresis: plus mesna qds with high doses of ifosphamide

continued over page

Table 12.5 (*Continued*)

System	Adverse effect	Management
Miscellaneous (*Continued*)	Alopecia (Adriamycin, 5-FU, cyclophosphamide)	Cold cap may reduce hair loss initially: only suitable with bolus injections
	Hand–foot syndrome (5-FU)	Pyridoxine 50 mg tds, reduce dose of 5-FU if necessary
	Cardiotoxicity (Adriamycin)	Perfusion imaging and ECG prior to commencing large doses in elderly and those with history of ischaemic heart disease. Reconsider agent if ejection fraction poor
	Sterility	Consider sperm banking if appropriate. Semen may be poor quality when unwell. Chances of banking suitable sperm may decrease after first cycle of treatment

ECG, electrocardiogram; 5-FU, 5-fluorouracil; G-CSF, granulocyte colony-stimulating factor.

Table 12.6 Common adverse effects with biological agents

Agent	Adverse effect	Observation
Interferons	Fever and chills	Prophylactic paracetamol 1 g tds, tolerance develops in 48–72 hours
	Fatigue	Dose-dependent
	Mood changes	Often subtle, frequently dose limiting
	Mild–moderate alopecia	Occurs in 20%, reversible
	Anorexia/weight loss	In 17%, dose-dependent
	Autoimmune disorders	Occurs in 19%, 13% thyroid-related
	Leucopenia	Rare if dose < 6 Mu daily
Monoclonal antibodies	Fever, chills, pruritis, rash, arthralgia, myalgia, dyspnoea	Related to speed of antibody infusion
	HAMA response	?Reduces antitumour response: awaiting sufficient production of human antibodies in mice
Radionuclide antibody conjugates	^{131}I: neutropenia 25–30 days post-treatment ^{90}Y: marrow toxicity	Dose-dependent, chelating agents may limit effect
Granulocyte colony–stimulating factor	Mild musculoskeletal pain	Occurs in 10%, severe in 3%, if necessary use prophylactic NSAIDs
	Mildly deranged liver function tests	Dose-dependent, reversible
Somatostatin analogues	May worsen hypoglycaemia	Suppression of counter-regulatory glucagon and growth hormone

HAMA, human antimouse antibody; NSAIDs, non-steroidal anti-inflammatory drugs.

approach to clinical oncology must include quality of life assessments, increasingly important with the advent of more aggressive, often toxic therapies. Quality of life assessment by doctors is notoriously poor and should always be supplemented by self-reported questionnaires, which patients can complete in a few minutes. Until now the most commonly used questionnaires in cancer patients have been the Rotterdam Symptom Checklist and the Hospital Anxiety and Depression Scale. The European Organization for Research and Treatment in Cancer (EORTC) has developed a new questionnaire which is easy to score and measures dimensions such as symptoms of disease, side-effects of treatments, physical functioning, psychological distress, social interaction, sexuality, body image and satisfaction with medical care. It also has modules to make it specifically applicable to individual cancers.

Clearly, improving quality of life is not solely a result of enhanced symptom control; good psychosocial care invariably reduces the need for hospital admission. A multidisciplinary team approach involving nurses, doctors, psychologists and social workers is most successful with 'professional' psychiatric assistance when required. The value of peer support, often informally or as self-help groups, should not be underestimated. Cognitive and behavioural psychotherapy, supportive counselling and psychotropic medication need to become an integral part of 'orthodox' cancer therapy. It must be emphasized that psychosocial oncology is an area of skilled practice, requiring knowledge of and application of researched, available treatment strategies. It is no longer acceptable simply to delegate to a 'sympathetic ear'.

References

1. Shike M, Brennan M. Nutritional support. In Devita V, Hellman S, Rosenberg SA (eds). *Cancer Principles and Practice of Oncology*, 3rd edn. Pennsylvania: Lippincott Company, 1989:2029–42.
2. Watson M. (ed.) *Cancer Patient Care: Psychosocial Treatment Methods*. Cambridge: BPS Books, 1991.
3. Oberg K. Chemotherapy and biotherapy in neuroendocrine tumours. *Curr. Opin. Oncol.* 1993;5(1):110–20.
4. Peabody SW. The care of the patient. *JAMA* 1927;88:877–82.

2

THYROID AND PARATHYROID TUMOURS

Assessment of Thyroid Neoplasia

NEIL J.L. GITTOES AND MICHAEL C. SHEPPARD

Introduction

Thyroid carcinomas are by far the most common endocrine gland malignancies, although clinically apparent thyroid cancer is rare, accounting for less than 0.5% of all new malignancies and less than 0.5% of all cancer deaths in the UK. In contrast the prevalence of thyroid nodules is considerable. The diagnostic challenge faced by the clinician is to identify those few patients with malignant change within the thyroid nodule.

Clinically apparent thyroid swellings have been reported in up to 10% of the population in the UK, affecting females four times more frequently than males. Autopsy studies, however, suggest that the true prevalence is higher, with up to 50% of the population having either single or multiple thyroid nodules. Ultrasound scan assessment of thyroid glands of patients over 50 years of age has confirmed this very high figure.

The risk of malignancy is lower in multinodular goitres than solitary nodules. Rather surprisingly, results from post-mortem studies have shown small foci of 'occult' carcinoma in up to 5% of thyroid glands that were deemed normal on clinical assessment. Most of these tumours were only a few millimetres in diameter and the substantial prevalence of occult cancer in patients who have died from unrelated causes suggests that it has little clinical significance. In contrast, of those patients with thyroid nodules selected for surgery on clinical grounds alone, only approximately 10% show malignant change.

Clinical assessment of thyroid neoplasia

Most patients with thyroid enlargement have no symptoms other than a coincidental finding of a mass in the neck, often noticed by others. A short history of an enlarging thyroid should increase the suspicion of a potentially malignant goitre (Table 13.1). In general a positive family history of thyroid dysfunction or goitre is indicative of a benign lesion. The exceptions are medullary carcinoma of the thyroid, either alone or as part of the multiple endocrine neoplasia (MEN) syndrome. There also appears to be a familial relationship between colon adenocarcinoma and papillary thyroid carcinoma. This is observed in defined genetic syndromes such as Gardener's syndrome and Cowden's disease but is also seen in families with more than one case of papillary thyroid carcinoma. Whether patients with family histories of thyroid cancer or colonic neoplasia have an increased risk of carcinoma per thyroid nodule or simply have more nodules remains to be determined.

The age of a patient has great bearing on the likelihood of an ongoing malignant process. There is a greater risk of malignancy in nodules developing in those over the age of 60 years. Conversely, thyroid dysfunction and nodule formation are rare in childhood and should be regarded with great suspicion. The incidence of carcinoma within thyroid nodules in children has been shown to be as high as 40%. This figure may be related to external irradiation formerly used to treat a wide range of benign conditions during childhood including thymic enlargement, tonsilitis and adenoiditis, enlargement of cervical lymph nodes, haemangiomas, tinea capitis and acne. Several studies have established a clear dose-relationship between radiation and thyroid nodules and thyroid cancers (see Chapter 83).

Although the presence of local mechanical symptoms, such as dysphagia, difficulty breathing or a hoarse voice, may suggest local invasion from an aggressive malignant tumour, all of the aforementioned may be associated with a large benign goitre, especially if multinodular. The reported incidence of carcinoma in the presence of mechanical obstructive symptoms is approximately 10%, although less than 5% of patients with thyroid carcinoma suffer local symptoms. The degree of upper airway obstruction, as assessed by flow volume loop analysis, appears to bear no relationship to the histological

Table 13.1 Clinical features suggesting the possibility of a benign or malignant cause of thyroid enlargement

Benign	Malignant
Age between 18 and 60 years	Age < 18 years or > 60 years
Long history	Short history
Family history of thyroid disease excluding rare cases of medullary carcinoma of the thyroid as part of multiple endocrine neoplasia syndrome	No family history of thyroid disease
	Exposure to radiation
	Dysphagia/SOB/stridor
	Lymphadenopathy
	Distant metastases

SOB, shortness of breath.

diagnosis of the obstructive thyroid lesion. Compression or deviation of the trachea, as seen on thoracic inlet X-rays, may be caused by both benign and malignant neoplasms. The presence on X-ray of stippled calcification of the thyroid is highly suggestive of papillary neoplasia.

The physical characteristics of a thyroid swelling are, on the whole, poor indicators of malignant potential. The only exceptions to this are the presence of lymphadenopathy and local fixation to adjacent structures. Patients occasionally present with evidence of distant metastases in the lungs, bone or liver in association with clinically inapparent thyroid pathology.

A well-differentiated follicular carcinoma may, rarely, present with features of thyrotoxicosis. Often in this instance there is evidence of metastatic disease.

Laboratory investigations

There is no laboratory investigation that can distinguish benign from malignant thyroid tumours. Nonetheless, it is important to assess thyroid function in all patients presenting with thyroid enlargement. The presence of hyperthyroidism makes the diagnosis of malignancy extremely unlikely. A clinically 'firm' goitre, initially raising the suspicion of a carcinoma, may be explained on the basis of biochemical hypothyroidism as a manifestation of Hashimoto's thyroiditis. The presence of positive autoantibodies in this situation would also help to confirm this diagnosis. There is, however, an increased risk of lymphoma in association with Hashimoto's thyroiditis.

Serum thyroglobulin levels are often elevated in the presence of well-differentiated thyroid cancer, although this is seen in a variety of other thyroid conditions including endemic goitre, multinodular goitre, benign adenoma, Graves' disease and Hashimoto's thyroiditis. Serum thyroglobulin therefore has no role in the initial differential diagnosis of thyroid carcinoma. It does, however, serve

an important role as 'tumour marker' in the follow-up of patients with treated differentiated thyroid cancer.

Radionucleotide scanning

The rationale for the use of radionucleotide imaging in the differential diagnosis of thyroid nodules is based on the assumption that malignant tumours do not incorporate iodine; thus scanning with ^{131}I or ^{99m}Tc-pertechnetate (which is trapped like iodine) should indicate poor uptake (a 'cold' spot) in the region of a malignant tumour (Fig. 13.1).

Technetium (99m-pertechnetate) is currently the most widely used thyroid imaging agent. Although technetium is concentrated within the thyroid, it is not incorporated into thyroglobulin, unlike iodide. The uptake of technetium provides a map of the trapping function of thyroid tissue and normally there is uniform tracer uptake throughout both lobes. A solitary thyroid nodule can be characterized by its tracer uptake compared with that of the surrounding normal thyroid tissue. A hypofunctioning (cold) nodule is characterized by decreased tracer uptake within the nodule compared with the surrounding tissue.

Iodine radioisotopes permit tracer studies of the en-

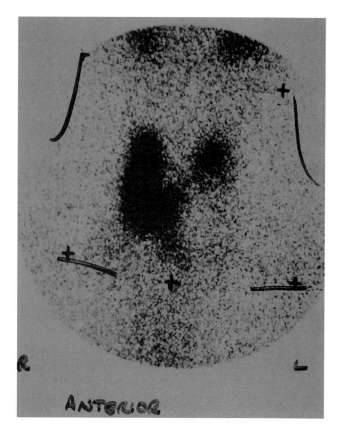

Fig. 13.1 ^{99m}Tc-pertechnetate scan of the thyroid gland. A 'cold' nodule is identified.

tire metabolic pathway of iodine. This includes trapping, organification, coupling, hormone storage and secretion. In practice only two radioisotopes, ^{131}I and ^{123}I, are clinically useful. Radioiodine is administered as sodium iodide by the oral route. Imaging is usually performed 18–24 hours after administration, at which time the majority of radioactivity within the thyroid is present as radiotyrosine residues on thyroglobulin, reflecting hormonogenesis. The imaging patterns for radioiodine scanning of the thyroid are similar to those of technetium. The disadvantages of iodine scanning are the expense of the isotope and the inconvenience of the necessity of two visits. There are few advantages of using radioiodine over technetium scanning.

The resolution of radionucleotide scanning is limited especially for lesions at the periphery of the gland, at the isthmus or if the nodule overlies normal tissue. The technique has also rather poor sensitivity and specificity in the diagnosis of malignancy. A review of a series of patients who underwent surgery regardless of the findings of radionucleotide scanning showed 84% of the nodules were 'cold', 10.5% 'warm' and 5.5% 'hot' [1]. At surgery, malignancy was found in 16% of 'cold', 9% of 'warm' and 4% of 'hot' nodules. Therefore, a 'cold' nodule has the greatest probability of being malignant, but the majority are benign, and the finding of a 'hot' nodule does not exclude malignancy. A radionuclide scan result must therefore be interpreted in the light of physical examination findings.

In most centres the role of radionucleotide scanning in the diagnosis of nodular thyroid disease has been supplanted by the successful use of fine needle aspiration cytology (FNAC).

Ultrasound scanning

Like radionucleotide scanning, ultrasonography does not allow differentiation between benign and malignant thyroid swellings and has been superseded by the use of FNAC. This mode of imaging is most useful for assessing thyroid size and consistency. High-resolution scanning can detect nodules as small as 1 mm in diameter. Ultrasound scanning may detect these coincidental, subclinical nodules in patients deemed to have a solitary nodule on palpation. Although solitary nodules pose greater risk for malignancy than multiple nodules, the finding of additional nodules does not eliminate the possibility of malignancy or the need for further evaluation.

Ultrasonography is very reliable at classifying nodules into solid, cystic or mixed solid and cystic with an accuracy of 90%. True cysts tend to be benign although most large nodules contain cystic areas. Carcinomas may also

undergo infarction causing degenerative cystic change within their substance. In a review of a series of ultrasound scans of thyroid swellings, 69% of nodules were solid, 19% cystic and 12% mixed [1]. Of those cases proceeding to surgery, 21% of the solid lesions were found to be malignant, compared with 12% of the mixed lesions and 7% of the cystic lesions. A solid nodule is therefore most likely to contain malignant cells, conversely most solid lesions are benign, and the presence of a cystic lesion does not exclude malignancy. With the ready availability of FNAC, ultrasonographic assessment of a thyroid nodule has nothing in addition to offer.

Fine needle aspiration cytology

FNAC is the first line investigative tool in nodular thyroid disease. The procedure (described elsewhere [2]) can be performed in an out-patient setting (Fig. 13.2); is quick to execute; has had no significant side-effects associated with its use and in the hands of an experienced cytopathologist a 97% diagnostic accuracy can be obtained. Other than those patients with suspicious or frankly malignant cytology on first examination (who will be immediately referred for surgery), repeat FNAC should be performed in all patients 6–12 months after initial aspiration as this reduces the proportion of false-negative results. One large series revealed changed cytology after repeat FNAC in 13 of 196 (7%) patients, 10 of whom underwent surgery leading to the diagnosis of an additional four carcinomas [3].

Solitary thyroid nodules harbour the majority of thyroid carcinomas, although there is an identifiable risk of malignancy in all types of thyroid swelling. Characterization of thyroid swellings by clinical means is also notoriously

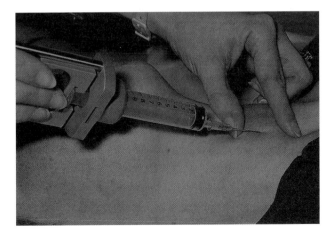

Fig. 13.2 Demonstration of the technique of fine needle aspiration of the thyroid gland.

unreliable, hence we advocate FNAC of all types of thyroid enlargement, whether this is due to a solitary nodule or a diffuse or multinodular goitre. Multiple samples are often necessary from large goitres, and in the case of multinodular goitres there is usually a dominant nodule which should be the preferred site for aspiration.

Inaccurate results are usually due to sampling error, especially if the lesion is small (< 1 cm), illustrating the importance of multiple sampling. If non-diagnostic samples are repeatedly obtained, then ultrasound-guided FNAC may be performed to attain a conclusive cytological diagnosis. It remains to be seen whether new techniques such as polymerase chain reaction (PCR) DNA amplification combined with gene analysis, flow cytometry with chromosome ploidy analysis, or cell cycle analysis can be combined with traditional cytology to improve diagnostic accuracy.

An important limitation of the test is the inability reliably to distinguish benign from malignant follicular neoplasms on the basis of cytological features. Surgical excision of all such lesions is therefore required to provide an accurate histological diagnosis.

The ability to make a preoperative cytological diagnosis allows speedy referral for surgery, planning of the extent of the operative procedure and also facilitates early counselling of the patient. Introduction of FNAC has resulted in a 50% decrease in thyroid surgical procedures, while the total number of thyroid carcinomas diagnosed has remained stable.

Investigation strategy

Patients presenting with a thyroid swelling should have FNAC performed as the first line investigation (Fig. 13.3). Scintigraphy and ultrasound examination have now largely been superseded and have no role in the initial assessment of thyroid neoplasia. Patients with a benign cytological diagnosis should have a repeat FNAC performed after a period of 6–12 months to confirm the benign nature. Those with suspicious or frankly malignant cytology should immediately proceed to surgery. Patients with a non-diagnostic aspirate should be repeatedly subjected to FNAC with or without ultrasound guidance until a cytological diagnosis can be made.

In addition to the obvious advantage of saving patients with benign thyroid disease from surgery, the estimated financial saving of using FNAC in the USA is $400–750 per patient evaluated, or more than $15 million annually.

Conclusion

Thyroid enlargement is common but malignant thyroid swellings are rare. Detecting the minority that fall into the latter category should employ the use of an investigative tool which is highly specific and sensitive; involves little risk or inconvenience to the patient, and is cost effective. FNAC fulfils all these criteria and should therefore be the sole investigation required prior to elective surgery in all patients with suspicious or malignant cytology.

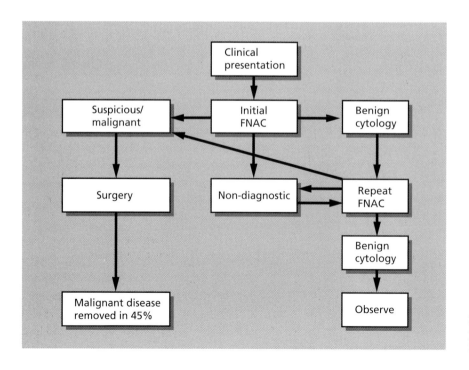

Fig. 13.3 Protocol for dealing with a patient presenting with euthyroid goitre. FNAC, fine needle aspiration cytology.

References

1. Ashcraft MW, Van Herle AJ. Management of thyroid nodules. II. Scanning techniques, thyroid suppressive therapy and fine needle aspiration. *Head Neck Surg.* 1981;**3**:297–322.

2. Solomon D. Fine needle aspiration of the thyroid: an update. *Thyroid Today* 1993;**16**(3):1–10.

3. Dwarkanathan AA, Staren ED, D'Amore MJ *et al.* Importance of repeat fine needle aspiration biopsy in the management of thyroid nodules. *Am. J. Surg.* 1993;**166**(4):350–2.

thyroglobulin measurement is the most appropriate technique to detect recurrence. Successful ^{131}I uptake by the tumour tissue requires induction of endogenous TSH to stimulate ^{131}I uptake, which is achieved by discontinuation of T3 for 2 weeks prior to scanning [13]. Exogenous TSH may also be used. Occasionally, where the scan is equivocal in the presence of an elevated serum thyroglobulin level, ^{201}Tl whole body imaging may be useful, since this is very sensitive for tumour tissue, but not specific (Fig. 14.7) [13].

Following the removal of medullary carcinoma, serum calcitonin levels are used to detect recurrence, and a persistently elevated level is the best indicator of residual or recurrent tumour. In such cases ^{99m}Tc-pentavalent dimercaptosuccinic acid ((v) DMSA) (see Plate 14.1, opposite p. 272), ^{201}Tl, ^{123}I-metaiodobenzylguanidine (MIBG), and ^{111}In-pentetreotide (a radioactive compound related to the analogue of somatostatin octreotide) scanning techniques have all been used. These agents show increased uptake at the site of primary and secondary sites. One postulate is that pentavalent DMSA resembles the phosphate ion, and is therefore taken up by tumours that tend to calcify, particularly medullary carcinoma of the thyroid. Uptake has also been noted in other frequently calcifying tumours: osteosarcoma, prostatic carcinoma and soft-tissue sarcoma [13]. Nevertheless, neither [99m]Tc-(v) DMSA nor ^{123}I-MIBG have been shown to be reliable in the detection of primary or recurrent medullary carcinoma of the thyroid.

Computed tomography

CT is seldom used in the detection and evaluation of thyroid tumours, but has specific roles in demonstrating the extent of local invasion, the presence of retrosternal and retrotracheal extension, regional lymph nodes and in detecting local recurrence. CT may also provide proof that an anterior mediastinal mass is thyroid in origin (Fig. 14.8). The thyroid gland is of higher attenuation than surrounding muscles and vessels before intravenous contrast medium due to the iodine content of the gland. A malignant nodule will most frequently show as a mass of lower density then normal thyroid. After intravenous contrast injection, the tumour enhances less than the intensely enhancing normal gland.

CT may alter the surgical planning of thyroid malignancy by detecting intrathoracic extension. This applies particularly to patients with anaplastic carcinoma where CT may show a large mass of low attenuation accompanied by dense calcification, frequently with central necrosis. Infiltration of adjacent structures such as the carotid artery, internal jugular vein, trachea, larynx, oesophagus and mediastinum is readily evaluated.

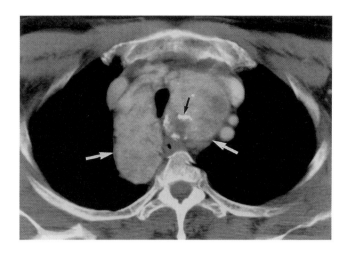

Fig. 14.8 Retrosternal multinodular thyroid goitre. Contrast-enhanced CT through the superior mediastinum. The enlarged thyroid gland (white arrows) is surrounding and compressing the trachea, and displacing the major vessels laterally. Some large foci of calcification are present (black arrow).

A specific role for CT has been suggested in the detection of *medullary carcinoma* of the thyroid in patients with multiple endocrine neoplasia type 2 (MEN-2). Here, pretreatment with oral potassium iodate (total iodine dose 500 mg) has been recommended as this causes increased attenuation of the thyroid gland on CT scanning, improving the rate of detection of small nodules of medullary carcinoma which appear as regions of reduced attenuation. Masses as small as 1–2 mm can be detected by this method, and results have been shown to correlate well with pathological specimens [14]. This scanning technique is particularly useful in confirming an abnormality when stimulated calcitonin levels are equivocal, and in the detection of small or multicentric tumours. When such a tumour is detected, CT forms part of the staging procedure as carcinomas less than 5 mm in diameter are usually treated by thyroidectomy alone, whereas patients with a mass greater than 5 mm also receive a cervical lymph node dissection. Where lymph node metastases are present, a modified neck dissection is performed [14].

The usual mode of spread of thyroid carcinomas is by direct invasion of adjacent structures, involvement of regional lymph nodes and haematogenous dissemination to lungs, bone and other organs. A rare but recognized phenomenon in *follicular* and *anaplastic carcinomas* is direct extension into the great veins and right atrium. As elsewhere, detection of lymph node infiltration from thyroid malignancy relies on demonstrating enlargement. Lymph nodes in the neck are regarded as pathological when the short axis of the node exceeds 1 cm.

CT is extremely sensitive in the detection of calcified lesions. Calcification is found in 30% of the involved lymph nodes and liver metastases from medullary carcinoma.

Magnetic resonance imaging

Thyroid imaging is best performed using a neck coil and preferably in a high field-strength magnet. The normal gland is typically homogeneous in appearance, being of similar or slightly higher signal intensity than adjacent muscle on T_1 weighting, and significantly higher signal intensity on T_2 weighting.

As experience with MRI imaging of the thyroid has grown, it has become apparent that there are no distinctive features on various imaging sequences reliably to distinguish carcinoma from adenomas and multinodular goitre. Lymphoma of the thyroid gland also has similar appearances. On T_1 images, malignant tumours have been shown to have slightly raised, lowered or a similar signal to normal thyroid tissue. Parts of the tumour may have high signal on T_1, usually due to focal haemorrhage. This does not help in the diagnosis, since benign masses can bleed, and a diffusely raised signal on T_1 is seen in colloid cysts. Carcinomas are usually hyperintense on T_2 sequences, as is lymphoma affecting the thyroid. Diffusely raised signal on both T_1 and T_2 sequences is a feature of Graves' disease [15].

As with CT, MRI becomes more useful in staging of a known malignant tumour, showing local invasion and regional lymph nodes. Again, MRI cannot distinguish between benign and malignant lymph nodes, as lymph node size criteria are the only means of detecting pathology. Some information can be gained regarding the 'pseudocapsule' around a tumour, and whether this has been invaded, but clearly, microscopic invasion cannot be detected. Magnetic resonance may be very helpful in determining whether or not there is recurrence of a tumour following thyroidectomy, offering a distinct advantage over ultrasound and CT. A positive predictive value of 82%, and a negative predictive value of 86% has been achieved using MRI in the detection of recurrent disease in the neck. Recurrent tumour is of low signal intensity on T_1-weighted images, and high signal on T_2-weighted images, whereas scar tends to be of low signal intensity on both sequences. False-positive results can be caused by inflammatory lymphatic hyperplasia and granulation tissue.

Parathyroid gland imaging

Modalities available for assessing the parathyroid gland are ultrasound, scintigraphy, selective venous sampling, CT and MRI.

Normal parathyroid glands cannot reliably be imaged by any radiological technique at present, but if visualized on ultrasound, normal glands are small, with the same echotexture as thyroid parenchyma. Only enlarged glands become reliably detectable [2]. When a parathyroid adenoma weighs less than 250 mg, the sensitivity of any imaging modality falls below 50% [16]. Both the number and location of the parathyroid glands are variable. There are more than four glands in 15% of patients, and less than four glands in 5% [6]. About 80% of abnormal parathyroid glands are situated adjacent to the thyroid. Ectopic glands may be found anywhere from the level of the third pharyngeal pouch, just behind the angle of the mandible at the level of the hyoid bone (undescended), down to the aortic root inferiorly. They may lie within or outside the carotid sheath, and from anterior to the thyroid gland anteriorly to behind the oesophagus or pharynx, including intrathyroidal. The inferior gland shares its origin from the third pharyngeal pouch with the thymus explaining the incidence of perithymic or intrathymic location. Up to 5% may lie in the posterior mediastinum [6,17,18]. No single imaging procedure can reliably locate an abnormal gland. These factors combine to make parathyroid imaging a complex issue.

Investigation of parathyroid gland abnormalities

Except in exceptional circumstances preoperative localization of parathyroid tumours is not indicated for patients undergoing initial neck exploration. All authors, however, advocate the use of localization studies before re-operation, when surgical cure rate without localization is 30–40% lower than in the first-time operation patients [19]. The remaining glands are more difficult to find operatively with scarring and loss of normal tissue planes. Even though an increased proportion of pathological glands will lie in an ectopic site, the pathological gland is still most likely to be located in the neck. Levin analysed the causes for failure of first parathyroid operations in 81 patients, finding 62% to be due to multiple abnormal glands, 49% due to ectopic gland location and 21% due to supernumerary glands. Surgeon and histopathologist error, and metastatic parathyroid carcinoma, were responsible for the remainder [20]. In these patients, radiology improves surgical results, especially by demonstrating the size of the parathyroid tumour.

Parathyroid localization techniques

Ultrasonography

Ultrasonography has notable benefits, namely that it is quick to perform, inexpensive, and does not involve ionizing radiation or physical risk to the patient. However, scanning for abnormal parathyroid glands is technically difficult, and only an experienced ultrasonographer will achieve the sensitivity and specificity rates often published in the literature [18].

Typically, parathyroid adenomas appear as oval, well-defined, anechoic or hypoechoic masses, posterior to the thyroid gland and anterior to the longus colli muscle (Fig. 14.9). They tend to be of the order of 10 mm in diameter, but can grow to very large sizes (4–5 cm) [6]. As glands become larger, they are more likely to be multilobulated and to contain areas of increased echogenicity, cystic areas and calcifications.

There are several problems inherent in ultrasound localization of parathyroid adenomas. Retro-oesophageal, retropharyngeal and mediastinal glands, which account for 5–15% of all glands, will be inaccessible by ultrasound. Intrathyroidal parathyroid adenomas account for approximately 1% of the total, and are difficult to detect since they look indistinguishable from thyroid nodules (Fig. 14.10), particularly if the patient has concurrent, occult, thyroid nodules. Occasionally, in primary hyperplasia one gland may predominate, leading the radiologist, erroneously, to the conclusion that there is a solitary adenoma [6]. Ultrasound can produce false-positive results by virtue of thyroid nodules on the periphery of the gland, hyperplastic lymph nodes, longus colli muscle and sympathetic ganglia.

There have been numerous studies giving the sensitivity and specificity of ultrasound in the localization of parathyroid abnormalities, before both first operation and re-operation for primary hyperparathyroidism. Most of the studies involve between 27 and 100 patients each. When considering only those studies where appropriate equipment was used (7.5 or 10 MHz high-resolution probes), and studies where correct localization rather than just the correct side was considered a true positive, the range of sensitivity for ultrasound before first operation is between 52 and 82%. The specificities are high, as with most modalities in parathyroid imaging, ranging from 78 to 100% [16,19,21–24]. Several studies show that the sensitivity increases when more than one modality

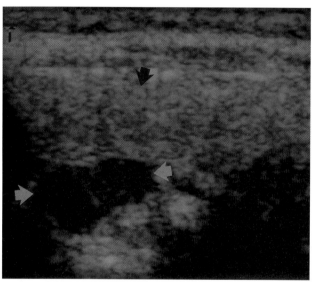

(a)

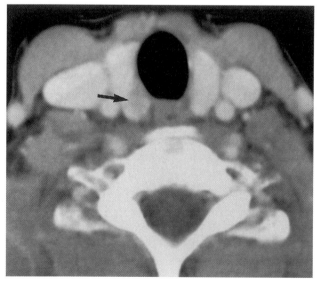

(b)

Fig. 14.9 Parathyroid adenoma. (a) Longitudinal ultrasound scan showing an ovoid hypoechoic mass (white arrows) posterior to the thyroid gland (black arrow). (b) Contrast-enhanced CT scan in the same patient showing the right-sided adenoma (arrow) which enhances less than the adjacent thyroid tissue.

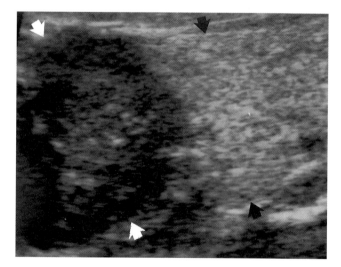

Fig. 14.10 Intrathyroid parathyroid adenoma. Longitudinal ultrasound scan showing hypoechoic mass (white arrows) within the thyroid gland (black arrows).

is used, rising from 53% using ultrasound alone to 85% when combined with scintigraphy [16], and 86% when combined with MRI [25]. In the group of patients that have already had an operation, and in common with all imaging modalities, the sensitivity of ultrasound falls to between 36 and 63%.

Examination of the thyroid gland before parathyroid operation may reveal thyroid nodules that require investigation. Thyroid cancer has been reported to be present in between 6 and 11% of patients with hyperparathyroidism. Thyroid nodules tend to be of increased vascularity when greater than 1 cm in diameter, whereas parathyroid nodules are relatively avascular until they reach 2 cm. Colour Doppler may therefore be of some interest, but cannot categorically distinguish between thyroid and parathyroid lesions. In fact, colour Doppler does not increase the sensitivity of ultrasound for parathyroid adenomas. Parathyroid cysts are a rare phenomenon, but 15% are functioning.

Intra-operative ultrasound has been shown to be of value during re-operation for primary hyperparathyroidism, assisting the surgeon in the localization of the abnormal glands, and reducing operating time. This facility is likely to become increasingly available.

Fine needle aspiration

Using ultrasound guidance, a 22 gauge needle can be directed into a suspected parathyroid nodule and cells aspirated. This technique will usually provide enough cellular material for cytological analysis. This may be particularly useful in patients with hyperparathyroidism where ultrasound reveals an equivocal mass in the neck which cannot be confidently related to the parathyroid glands, or in patients investigated prior to re-operation. Radioimmunoassay of the aspirate for parathyroid hormone is also of value, especially if trying to confirm the nature of a mainly cystic mass.

Alcohol ablation of parathyroid adenomas

A parathyroid adenoma may be ablated by injection of 96% alcohol under ultrasound guidance. Where practised, this technique is reserved for patients where surgery is contraindicated or refused. Normocalcaemia and good clinical results have been achieved in most patients in small series. Permanent vocal cord paralysis has been reported, however.

Computed tomography

Detection of abnormal parathyroid glands on CT depends on careful attention to detail, both in the technique of scanning and in the interpretation. Normal parathyroid glands are not visualized on CT. Rapid 'spiral' scanning achieves excellent resolution, reduces artefacts, and provides the best chance of detecting a subtle abnormality. The patient should be scanned from the hyoid bone (the level of the third pharyngeal arch) to the carina, before and after intravenous injection of contrast medium, depending on what is seen on the non-contrasted scans [16,26].

Most parathyroid adenomas have an attenuation equal to that of muscle before contrast, and homogeneous enhancement after intravenous injection of contrast medium (Fig. 14.11). Unfortunately, these characteristics do not distinguish adenomas from lymph nodes and this can lead to false-positive interpretations. On occasions, the adenoma may enhance non-uniformly due to cystic degeneration or haemorrhage and rarely, an adenoma may calcify [26]. The presence of calcification should, however, raise the possibility of a parathyroid carcinoma. It is possible to use CT as the guidance technique for FNAC of a suspected parathyroid lesion.

CT does not have any advantage over ultrasound when an adenoma is situated in a normal parathyroid site, but it is very useful for detecting abnormalities lying in sites inaccessible to ultrasound, such as behind the trachea. It may also demonstrate an adenoma in an undescended inferior parathyroid gland lying in the carotid sheath. This is a common site to be missed at the initial neck exploration, since extensive dissection is necessary to expose the gland behind the internal jugular vein. CT is no better than ultrasound at distinguishing parathyroid from thyroid masses. The strength of CT lies in its ability

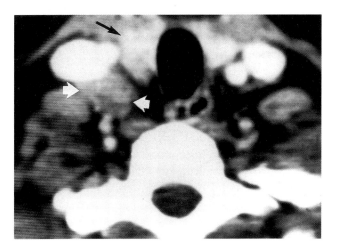

Fig. 14.11 Parathyroid adenoma. Contrast-enhanced CT showing the mass (white arrows) posterior to the right lobe of the thyroid (black arrow).

to detect lesions in the mediastinum, and is essential in localization before re-operation for primary hyperparathyroidism. The sensitivities for CT range from 68 to 81% with specificities from 92 to 95% [16,21,24,26], and after failed exploration of the neck, a sensitivity of 44 to 50% can be expected.

Magnetic resonance imaging

Using high field strength and a small surface coil, excellent images of the neck are obtainable, and results appear at least comparable to the other imaging modalities available for localization of parathyroid abnormalities. MRI has certain advantages over CT in the neck. The hard bone artefact across the root of the neck arising from the shoulders on CT scans is avoided with MRI. The vascular structures of the neck are visualized without intravenous contrast injection due to the effect of flowing blood on MRI, allowing easy distinction from lymph nodes and small masses. Even so, ghost artefacts from respiratory motion and flow within neck vessels can degrade the images and lead to false results [21]. These artefacts, and those from swallowing, may be reduced by the use of a presaturation pulse [27]. Ectopic thymus tissue in the lower neck can lead to a false-positive result.

Uncomplicated parathyroid adenomas typically show medium signal intensity on T_1-weighted images, equivalent to muscle, and high signal on T_2-weighted images [21,28]. This pattern does not apply in all instances. Haemorrhage within the gland will alter the appearance by causing a high signal intensity on both T_1- and T_2-weighted images, whereas fibrosis will lower the signal intensity on T_2 weighting. Calcification shows no signal on all MRI sequences and will not be detected.

The sensitivities and specificities quoted in the literature are similar or slightly better than those found for ultrasound and CT. Sensitivities range from 57 to 82%, and specificities from 78 to 97% [16,21,22,24,25,28]. Attie and colleagues found MRI to be more sensitive than either ultrasonography or subtraction scintigraphy (82% versus 73% and 59% respectively) [22]. Auffermann and co-workers also found MRI more sensitive than scintigraphy or ultrasonography, MRI being equally successful in the neck and mediastinum [25]. As with ultrasound and CT, thyroid nodules lead to false-positive diagnoses. Cervical ganglia also show low signal on T_1-weighted and high signal on T_2-weighted images, and may mimic parathyroid pathology [27].

MRI, like CT, is particularly valuable in evaluating the mediastinum, and is likely to replace CT in the preoperative localization following previous surgery.

Radionucleotide imaging

Imaging of the parathyroid glands is best achieved by the double-tracer technique [29]. This has superseded selenium 75 imaging, which produced poor results. The double-tracer technique involves imaging with ^{201}Tl, which is taken up by both parathyroid and thyroid tissue, and subtracting the image acquired after injection of ^{99m}TcO$_4$, which is taken up by the thyroid only. Success has been achieved with a double-tracer technique using ^{99m}Tc-MIBI instead of ^{201}Tl (see Plate 14.2, opposite p. 272).

If only searching for mediastinal parathyroid glands, the ^{99m}TcO$_4$ image is not necessary, and single photon emission computed tomography (SPECT) of the thorax can be performed [10]. When glands are small or situated in a deep ectopic site, there is a higher chance of a false-negative result. False-positives are most commonly generated by patient movement between image acquisitions. Other false-positives may be produced by thyroid pathologies such as benign and malignant thyroid nodules, multinodular goitre or thyroid metastases, and malignant lymph nodes from other distant pathology. Further limitations include an inability to define the depth of an abnormality, and its relationship to adjacent structures.

The success of double-tracer radionucleotide imaging in the detection of parathyroid adenomas varies between studies, the overall sensitivity ranging from 27 to 95%, over 50% in the majority of studies. Specificities are high, from 91 to 98% [16,21–25,30]. These are similar figures to those given for ultrasound, CT and MRI, but as mentioned before, the sensitivities increase if the modalities are used in combination. As with all imaging modalities, sensitivity in four-gland hyperplasia falls to around 40% [10].

In a controlled trial comparing the ^{99m}Tc-MIBI/^{99m}TcO$_4$ method to the ^{201}Tl/^{99m}TcO$_4$ method in 57 patients, the detection of adenomas by ^{99m}Tc-MIBI/^{99m}TcO$_4$ was 98% compared with 90% with ^{201}Tl, and for hyperplasia the detection rate was 55% compared to 47.5% [31]. Taking into account the dosimetric and practical advantages, the ^{99m}Tc-MIBI/^{99m}TcO$_4$ double-tracer technique has become the radionucleotide investigation of choice for the parathyroid glands [30].

Parathyroid venous sampling

The goal of venous sampling is to obtain specimens from veins in the neck and mediastinum for parathyroid hormone assay in order to localize a parathyroid adenoma. The technique involves direction of a transfemoral catheter into selected veins. Some radiologists perform arteriography with venous phase imaging first in order to provide a venous 'road-map'. The normal drainage route for both the superior and inferior parathyroid glands is via the right and left inferior thyroid veins. Samples are also obtained from the superior thyroid, middle thyroid, vertebral, jugular, subclavian, innominate, thymic and internal mammary veins when feasible in order to detect adenomas in ectopic positions. Midline samples are not helpful, but middle thyroid veins provide very useful results. Unfortunately, these vessels are frequently tied-off in postoperative cases. When most of the thyroid veins have been ligated, venous drainage may be entirely into the vertebral veins bilaterally [32]. The sites from which samples are taken are recorded on a map to aid interpretation of results. Simultaneous samples are taken from a peripheral vein to establish the background levels. A gradient of twice the background venous level of parathyroid hormone is considered a significant result. An adenoma is usually associated with a background level of hormone on the contralateral side due to suppression of normal glands [33]. Raised levels at several sites within the neck indicate multiple adenomas or hyperplasia.

The venous drainage of the thyroid gland, however, forms a latticework of small veins, and crossover of blood can occur, giving false localization results. The most common inferior thyroid variant is a lateral accessory vein from the right or left lobe, and, when present, will often carry the venous blood from an adenoma. Anastomoses between inferior thyroid and thymic veins are very common, but occasionally, inferior thyroid drainage is entirely into the thymic system, especially in a postoperative case. If this evidence is relied upon, the surgeon may be led into performing an unnecessary sternal split [18]. Many mediastinal glands drain cranially into the inferior thyroid veins, especially when the arterial supply is inferior thyroidal, so elevated levels in the neck cannot exclude a mediastinal adenoma. In practice venous sampling is only performed after a failed operation, and normal venous anatomy is rarely present as surgeons ligate neck veins during the search for enlarged glands. Venous sampling results, therefore, cannot be relied upon in isolation.

Selective venous sampling has its main value where other imaging techniques have failed to localize masses. Before reoperation, sensitivities of 69–80% have been recorded, exceeding ultrasound and CT, and achieving a higher level of accuracy when used in combination with ultrasound and CT.

Arteriography

Selective angiography with digital subtraction can identify up to 85% of adenomas, but there is a risk of vascular injury to the spinal cord. As a diagnostic procedure, arteriography is largely outmoded, and is reserved for cases where less invasive techniques have not been successful [32]. Venous phase imaging does produce a venous map, however, which is useful during venous sampling procedures.

Angiographic ablation of mediastinal adenomas is possible by selective intra-arterial injection of ionic contrast material to avoid a sternotomy. A clinical success rate of 83% at 1 month, and 71% at 5 and 9 years has been achieved. This is not a widely practised technique.

References

1. Mettler FA, Williamson MR, Royal HD *et al*. Thyroid nodules in the population living around Chernobyl. *JAMA* 1992;**268**:616–19.
2. Solbiati L, Cioffi V, Ballaratti E. Ultrasonography of the neck. *Radiol. Clin. North Am.* 1992;**30**(5):941–54.
3. Solbiati L, Volterrani L, Rizzato G *et al*. The thyroid gland with low-uptake lesions: evaluation by ultrasound. *Radiology* 1985;**155**:187–91.
4. De los Santos ET, Keyhani-Rofagha S, Cunningham JJ, Mazzaferri EL. Cystic thyroid nodules. *Arch. Intern. Med.* 1990;**150**:1422– 7.
5. Clark OH, Duh Q-Y. Thyroid cancer. *Med. Clin. North Am.* 1991;**75**(1):211–34.
6. Gooding G. Sonography of the thyroid and parathyroid. *Radiol. Clin. North Am.* 1993;**31**(5):967–89.
7. Hajek PC, Salomonowitz E, Turk R *et al*. Lymph nodes of the neck: evaluation with US. *Radiology* 1986;**158**:739–42.
8. Samaan NA, Schultz PN, Ordonez NG, Hickey RC, Johnston DA. A comparison of thyroid carcinoma in those who have and have not had head and neck irradiation in childhood. *J. Clin. Endocrinol. Metab.* 1987;**64**:219–23.
9. Hancock SL, Cox RS, McDougall IR. Thyroid masses after treatment of Hodgkin's disease. *N. Engl. J. Med.* 1991;**325**:599–605.
10. Price D. Radioisotopic evaluation of the thyroid and the parathyroids. *Radiol. Clin. North Am.* 1993;**31**(5):991–1015.
11. Ramanna L, Waxman A, Baunstein G. Thallium-201 scintigraphy in differentiated thyroid cancer. Comparison with radioiodine scintigraphy and serum thyroglobulin determinations. *J. Nucl. Med.* 1991;**32**:441–6.
12. Al-Sayer HM, Krukowski ZH, Williams VMM, Matheson NA. Fine needle aspiration cytology in isolated thyroid swellings: a prospective two year evaluation. *Br. Med. J.* 1985;**290**:1490–2.
13. Sandler MP, Delbeke D. Radionuclides in endocrine imaging. *Radiol. Clin. North Am.* 1993;**31**(4):909–21.
14. Vette JK. Computed tomography of the thyroid gland. *Acta Endocrinol. [Suppl.] (Copenh.)* 1985;**268**:1–82.
15. Gefter WB, Spritzer CE, Eisenberg B *et al*. Thyroid imaging with high-field-strength surface coil MR. *Radiology* 1987;**164**:483–90.
16. Krubsack AJ, Wilson SD, Lawson TL *et al*. Prospective comparison of radionuclide, computed tomographic, sonographic, and magnetic resonance localization of parathyroid tumors. *Surgery* 1989;**106**:639–44.
17. Higgins CB, Auffermann W. MR imaging of thyroid and parathyroid glands: a review of current status. *Am. J. Roentgenol.* 1988;**151**:1095–106.

18. Lloyd MNH, Lees WR, Milroy EJG. Pre-operative localisation in primary hyperparathyroidism. *Clin. Radiol.* 1990;**41**:239–43.

19. Reading CC, Charboneau JW, James EM *et al*. High-resolution parathyroid sonography. *Am. J. Roentgenol.* 1982;**139**:539–46.

20. Levin KE, Clark OH. The reasons for failure in parathyroid operations. *Arch. Surg.* 1989;**124**:911–15.

21. Kneeland JB, Krubsack AJ, Lawson TL *et al*. Enlarged parathyroid glands: high-resolution local coil MR imaging. *Radiology* 1987;**162**:143–6.

22. Attie JN, Khan A, Rumancik WM *et al*. Preoperative localization of parathyroid adenomas. *Am. J. Surg.* 1988;**156**:323–6.

23. Summers GW, Dodge DL, Kammer H. Accuracy and cost-effectiveness of preoperative isotope and ultrasound imaging in primary hyperparathyroidism. *Otolaryngol. Head Neck Surg.* 1989;**100**:210–17.

24. Kohri K, Ishikawa Y, Kodama M *et al*. Comparison of imaging methods for localization of parathyroid tumors. *Am. J. Surg.* 1992;**164**:140–5.

25. Auffermann W, Gooding GAW, Okerlund MD *et al*. Diagnosis of recurrent hyperparathyroidism: Comparison of MR imaging and other imaging techniques. *Am. J. Roentgenol.* 1988;**150**:1027–33.

26. Cates JD, Thorsen MK, Lawson TL *et al*. CT evaluation of parathyroid adenomas: Diagnostic criteria and pitfalls. *J. Comput. Assist. Tomogr.* 1988;**12**:626–9.

27. Higgins CB. Role of magnetic resonance imaging in hyperparathyroidism. *Radiol. Clin. North Am.* 1993;**31**(5):1017–28.

28. Spritzer CE, Gefter WB, Hamilton R *et al*. Abnormal parathyroid glands: high-resolution MR imaging. *Radiology* 1987;**162**:487–91.

29. Young AE, Gaunt JI, Croft DN *et al*. Location of parathyroid adenomas by thallium-201 and technetium-99m subtraction scanning. *Br. Med. J.* 1983;**286**:1384–6.

30. Geatti O, Shapiro B, Orsolon PG *et al*. Localization of parathyroid enlargement: experience with technetium-99m methoxyisobutyl-isonitrile and thallium-201 scintigraphy, ultrasonography and computed tomography. *Eur. J. Nucl. Med.* 1994;**21**:17–22.

31. O'Doherty MJ, Kettle AG, Wells P, Collins REC, Coakley AJ. Parathyroid imaging with technetium-99m-sestamibi: preoperative localization and tissue uptake studies. *J. Nucl. Med.* 1992;**33**:313–18.

32. Miller DL. Endocrine angiography and venous sampling. *Radiol. Clin. North Am.* 1993;**31**(5):1051–67.

33. Doppman JL. Parathyroid localization. Arteriography and venous sampling. *Radiol. Clin. North Am.* 1976;**14**:163–88.

15

Pathogenesis of Thyroid Carcinoma

DAVID WYNFORD-THOMAS

Introduction

Tumours of the thyroid follicular epithelium represent a good example of human tumour induction by ionizing radiation and of tumour promotion by trophic hormone stimulation [1]. More recently they have proven an extremely instructive model for understanding the molecular pathogenesis of epithelial neoplasia. The molecular mechanisms underlying thyroid tumorigenesis are reviewed in this chapter.

Control of thyroid follicular cell proliferation

In common with most mammalian cells, follicular cell proliferation is regulated by stimulatory and inhibitory extracellular growth factors, each acting through a cascade of intracellular signals, the 'balance' of which determines the rate of cell cycling (Fig. 15.1). In the normal adult thyroid, the 'set-point' of this system is such that proliferation is negligible (although the gland retains a capacity for rapid growth following an increase in stimulation, as seen for example in the hyperplasia of Graves' disease). In principle, the inappropriate proliferation seen in neoplasia could result from any irreversible disturbance in this equilibrium, due to an increase in activity of the stimulatory signal pathways, or conversely to loss of inhibitory signals. In practice, however, it seems that only a small subset of signalling molecules are susceptible to such abnormal function (Fig. 15.1). Presumably, many potential oncogenic changes can be effectively compensated by built-in feedback loops. Thus far, analysis of thyroid tumour samples has revealed five critical targets for mutation in the stimulatory pathways: thyroid-stimulating hormone (TSH) receptor, its transducer protein $G_s\alpha$ (gsp), two other growth factor receptors, ret and trk, and a second G protein transducer, ras. In contrast, only a single inhibitor, the tumour-suppressor protein p53, has so far been implicated. It is

important to note that many more genes show abnormally elevated expression in thyroid tumours (notably the hepatocyte growth factor (HGF) receptor coded for by the met gene) but in the absence of any demonstrable genetic abnormality, these are potentially secondary consequences, rather than primary causes, of neoplasia and will not be considered further here.

Overactive stimulatory signals: activation of oncogenes

Irreversible (constitutive) activation of mitogenic signalling proteins can be the result of either a structural mutation, which increases the activity of the protein (qualitative activation) or of overexpression of an otherwise normal protein resulting from amplification of the gene or alteration in its regulatory region (quantitative activation).

Activation of the TSH-induced signal pathway

Although constitutive activation of this pathway might seem the most predictable means of inducing follicular cell proliferation, this appears to be surprisingly rarer than other less obvious targets. Activation was first demonstrated at the level of the transducing protein $G_s\alpha$, and only very recently at the TSH receptor itself.

$G_s\alpha$ (Table 15.1)

The heterotrimeric G_s transducer protein, which normally relays the TSH signal from its receptor to adenyl cyclase, is activated constitutively by mutation of the α subunit (coded by the gsp gene) at one of two critical codons, 201 or 227 [2], the effect of which is to 'lock' the protein in its active signal transducing conformation independent of the presence of TSH. Predictably, such an event can activate both thyrocyte function as well as growth, and

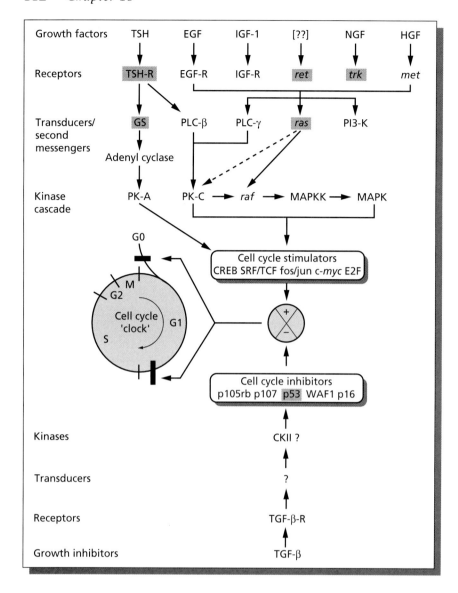

Fig. 15.1 Signal pathways regulating normal and neoplastic follicular cell proliferation. A complex intracellular cascade, largely involving sequential protein phosphorylations, relays signals from stimulatory and inhibitory extracellular growth factors to the nucleus. The 'balance' of such signals determines the entry into (G0 → G1), and progress through the cell division cycle (G1 → S). Autonomous (neoplastic) proliferation can result from constitutive activation of stimulatory signals or inactivation of inhibitors, due to mutations in the corresponding genes. The six known targets that can be mutated in thyroid tumours are highlighted (shaded boxes). (Note that precise connections are not shown for pathways, such as those downstream of *ras*, which are still uncertain in the follicular cell.) CREB, cAMP response element-binding protein; EGF, epidermal growth factor; HGF, hepatocyte growth factor; IGF, insulin-like growth factor; MAPK(K), mitogen-activated protein kinase; NGF, nerve growth factor; PK, protein kinase; PLC, phospholipase C; R, receptor; SRF, serum response factor; TCF, tertiary complex factor; TSH, thyroid-stimulating hormone.

Table 15.1 *gsp* oncogene in thyroid neoplasia, prevalence of point mutation (%, with numbers of cases in parentheses)

Follicular adenoma	Follicular adenoma (toxic)*	Papillary carcinoma	Follicular carcinoma	Anaplastic carcinoma	Reference
0 (0/2)	25 (1/4)	0 (0/4)	0 (0/4)	0 (0/1)	[2]
–	–	8† (1/13)	13† (2/15)	–	[3]
0 (0/16)	38 (5/13)	0 (0/5)	0 (0/3)	–	[4]
3 (1/37)	–	0 (0/23)	0 (0/9)	0 (0/2)	[5]
7 (2/30)	33 (4/12)	8 (3/35)	10 (2/20)	0 (0/1)	H. Suarez (Villejuif) (personal communication)

* Hyperfunctioning adenoma ('hot' nodule).
† All with high basal adenylate cyclase.

it is not surprising therefore that the highest incidence of *gsp* mutation is found in the relatively rare subgroup of hyperfunctioning thyroid tumours, the so-called 'hot' nodule or toxic adenoma (Table 15.1). *gsp* mutation has, however, been observed at lower frequency in tumours (including papillary cancer), in which there is no evidence of thyroid hormone production [3]. Presumably in such cases mutations in other genes have already abolished the ability of the neoplastic follicular cell to respond functionally to cyclic adenosine monophosphate (AMP) stimulation, while leaving the growth response intact.

TSH receptor (Table 15.2)

Although an obvious candidate, the initial search for activating mutations of the TSH-receptor gene was negative [5], although these authors did not specifically analyse known 'hot' nodules. Later studies focusing on the latter have, however, unequivocally demonstrated point mutation at sites (mainly the third intracellular loop) known to result in constitutive signalling in the absence of bound ligand [6].

One unexplained paradox raised by these findings is that sustained activation of this pathway by *extracellular* TSH results in a much more limited proliferation of follicular cells (as seen for example in goitrogen-treated rats) [7].

Activation of other growth factor pathways: *ret* and *trk* (Table 15.3)

Contrary to prediction, activation of receptors for other well-known thyroid mitogens, such as epidermal growth factor (EGF) and insulin-like growth factor 1 (IGF-1), does not seem to occur. Instead, two quite unexpected receptors are activated. These are *trk*, the receptor for nerve growth factor (NGF), and *ret*, the ligand for which remains unknown (but from its pattern of tissue expression would also appear to be associated with neuro-ectodermal differentiation).

In contrast to the TSH-receptor and *gsp*, these two genes are activated not by point mutation but by a chromosomal rearrangement (either translocation or inversion). This produces a hybrid gene in which the signal-generating (tyrosine kinase) domain of *ret* or *trk* becomes fused to a new upstream region derived from a variety of non-oncogenic genes, which are highly

Table 15.3 *ret* oncogene in thyroid neoplasia, prevalence of rearrangement (%, with numbers of cases in parentheses)

Follicular adenoma	Papillary carcinoma	Follicular carcinoma	Anaplastic carcinoma	Reference
–	25 (5/20)	–	–	[8]
–	25 (4/16)	–	–	[9]
0 (0/16)	33 (14/42)	0 (0/13)	0 (0/8)	[10]*
–	17 (11/65)	0 (0/7)	0 (0/2)	[10]†
0 (0/18)	11 (8/70)	0 (0/13)	0 (0/5)	[10]‡
0 (0/26)	8 (3/38)	0 (0/9)	0 (0/4)	P. Soares *et al.* (unpublished data)§
0 (0/8)	11 (4/36)	0 (0/3)	–	[11]

* Milan and Naples samples.
† Minnesota samples.
‡ Lyon samples.
§ Cardiff plus Barcelona plus Porto samples.

expressed in the normal follicular cell [10]. The net effect is to switch on expression of the active portion of *ret* or *trk*, which are not normally expressed in the follicular cell.

The fascinating question is as to why these genes are selected so specifically in thyroid cancer and, within that, the papillary subtype [10,12], since such a mechanism of activation could, in theory, work equally well in a wide range of cell types. The answer may lie in the embryological relationship of follicular cells to the C cell component of the thyroid. It has been postulated that a subpopulation of such cells may share a common origin from an ultimobranchial progenitor. *ret* is normally expressed in the C cell (as in many neuro-ectodermal derivatives) and indeed can be activated (although in this case by point mutation) in C cell tumours. Ultimobranchial-derived follicular cells, if they retain expression of the signal pathway to which *ret* normally communicates, but have lost expression of the receptor itself, may be uniquely sensitive to activation of *ret* expression.

The specific association of *ret* with the papillary subtype of thyroid cancer suggests that it may be responsible for

Table 15.2 Thyroid-stimulating hormone receptor in thyroid neoplasia, prevalence of point mutation (%, with numbers of cases in parentheses)

Follicular adenoma	Follicular adenoma (toxic)*	Papillary carcinoma	Follicular carcinoma	Anaplastic carcinoma	Reference
0 (0/37)	?	0 (0/23)	0 (0/9)	0 (0/2)	[5]
–	27 (3/11)	–	–	–	[6]
–	8 (3/37)	–	–	–	H. Suarez (Villejuif) (personal communication)

* Hyperfunctioning adenoma ('hot' nodule).

Table 15.4 *ras* oncogenes in thyroid neoplasia, % prevalence of point mutation (all three *ras* genes; numbers of cases in parentheses)

Follicular adenoma	Papillary carcinoma	Follicular carcinoma	Anaplastic carcinoma	References
33 (8/24)	18 (3/17)	53 (8/15)	60 (6/10)	[14]; [15]
46 (6/13)	62 (8/13)	100 (1/1)	100 (1/1)	[16]
–	0 (0/20)	–	–	[8]
–	13 (2/16)	–	–	[9]
25* (6/24)	21 (3/14)	0 (0/3)	–	[17]
85 (11/13)	0 (0/12)	50 (3/6)	–	[18]†
17 (2/12)	0 (0/10)	10 (1/10)	–	[18]‡
0 (0/9)	7 (1/15)	14 (2/14)	–	[19]

* Also 21% (4/19) of multinodular goitre nodules.
† Iodine-deficient area (Hungary).
‡ Iodine-sufficient area (Newfoundland).

Table 15.5 Tumour-suppressor gene *p53* in thyroid neoplasia, prevalence of point mutation (%, with numbers of cases in parentheses)

Follicular adenoma	Papillary carcinoma	Follicular carcinoma	Anaplastic carcinoma	Reference
–	0 (0/11)	0 (0/5)	0 (0/4)	[22]
–	0 (0/20)	0 (0/13)	33 (11/33)	[23]*
–	0 (0/33)	0 (0/4)	46 (6/13)	[24]
–	0 (0/10)	–	86 (6/7)	[25]
0 (0/31)	0 (0/37)	9 (1/11)	83 (5/6)	[26]
–	–	–	22 (2/9)†	[27]

* Immunocytochemical analysis only.
† Mutation not present in coexisting papillary cancer.

determining the pattern of tumour development. Indeed, gene transfer experiments in cell culture have shown that introduction of an activated *ret* gene into normal follicular cells results in the growth of colonies whose morphology and behaviour show many features consistent with an *in vitro* analogue of occult papillary cancer [13].

Activation of the signal transducer, *ras* (Table 15.4)

The *ras* oncogene family (H,K and N-*ras*) encode small monomeric G proteins which, like $G_s\alpha$, transduce mitogenic signals from growth factor receptors. Despite the general importance of *ras* as the most commonly mutated oncogene in human cancer, it is only recently that the upstream and downstream components of its signal pathway have been defined, and even now it is not at all certain which growth factors signal through *ras* in specialized cell types such as thyroid.

Whatever its physiological role may be, however, there is no doubt that constitutive activation of *ras* protein (at codons 12, 13 or 61) results in a potent mitogenic signal. Such mutations are found in approximately 50% of all stages of follicular tumour as well as in anaplastic cancer (Table 15.4). In thyroid (as opposed to colon), *ras* mutations appear in the earliest lesions available for analysis, suggesting that it is an initiating event. This conclusion is greatly strengthened by *in vitro* gene transfer experiments, which have demonstrated a dramatic stimulation of proliferation when a mutant *ras* gene is introduced into normal follicular cells in tissue culture [13].

Failure of growth inhibition: inactivation of tumour-suppressor genes

By analogy with other epithelial tumour types, multi-

stage thyroid tumorigenesis would be expected to involve loss of growth inhibitory genes as well as activation of oncogenes. Unfortunately, progress has been rather slow in this area, due in part to the lack of material suitable for cytogenetic analysis. Several candidate tumour-suppressor genes (TSGs) appear not to be involved, notably the retinoblastoma susceptibility gene *RB* and the *APC* gene responsible for familial polyposis coli [20]. (The latter was suggested by the increased frequency of thyroid cancer in Gardner's syndrome.) One of the few studies of allele loss in thyroid cancer points to an important potential locus on chromosome 3p, which may be a key step in malignant conversion [21]. The nature of this gene however is currently unknown.

p53 (Table 15.5)

The only TSG to be unequivocally associated with thyroid cancer is *p53*, which is currently the gene most commonly mutated in human cancer in general. The normal p53 protein appears to inhibit cell proliferation in response to genomic damage and hence acts as a 'brake' on the development of genomic instability in cancers. Consequently inactivation of *p53* by mutation is associated not with malignant conversion *per se*, but with the further progression to high-grade neoplasia. In accord with this idea, in thyroid such mutations are virtually confined to poorly or undifferentiated cancers (Table 15.5).

Conclusion: genetic basis of thyroid tumour behaviour

The above observations permit a tentative assignment of cancer gene mutations to particular subtypes and stages of human follicular cell neoplasia as outlined in Fig. 15.2. The relationship with stage is particularly clearcut, with the five oncogenes, *gsp*, TSH-R, *ras*, *ret* and *trk*, localizing to the earliest stages available for analysis, in contrast to

Fig. 15.2 Multistep tumorigenesis in the thyroid follicular cell. The diagram summarizes the most clearcut associations observed to date between somatic genetic lesions and specific thyroid tumour subtypes. Note that the model is neither totally specific nor exhaustive; for example, *gsp* mutation may also be found in non-toxic adenomas and in papillary cancers (and *ras* mutation in some papillary cancers), and many adenomas contain neither *ras*, *gsp*, *ret* nor *trk* mutations. Likewise, the strictly linear relationship between follicular adenoma and carcinoma (and between occult and clinical papillary cancer) has not been formally proven.

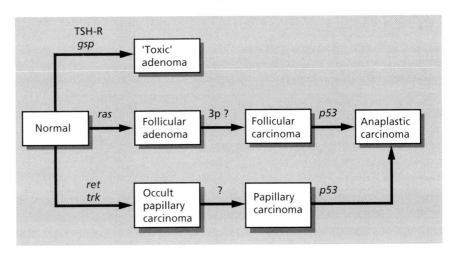

the TSG, *p53*, which is involved only in the most advanced cancers.

There is also an emerging pattern with regard to histological subtypes. *ret* and *trk* are specific for the papillary 'branch,' *gsp* and TSH receptor are predominantly found in toxic adenomas and, while less specific, *ras* mutation is chiefly associated with 'classical' follicular tumours. This observational data is greatly strengthened by the results of *in vitro* gene transfer experiments in which activated *ras* or *ret* genes, when introduced into normal follicular cells, are sufficient alone to generate 'lesions' consistent with an early follicular adenoma or occult papillary cancer respectively [13]. Taken together, these data suggest a model in which the pattern of tumour development is determined by the nature of the initiating oncogene, for example *ras*, *ret*, *trk*, *gsp* or TSH receptor.

Clearly a major remaining question concerns the additional genes that must cooperate with these initiating events to generate clinically apparent cancers. The finding of *ras* or *gsp* mutations in some papillary cancers might suggest that cooperation could occur between the different members of the known set of oncogenes; for example a tumour initiated by *ret* may progress as a result of an additional *ras* mutation. However, in a large series of tumours in which the *same* samples were analysed for all five genes, in nearly all cases only *one* gene was found to be mutated in any given case, indicating that the oncogenes identified to date are alternative rather than complementary in action [28].

The nature of the genes, most likely TSGs, involved in progression to malignancy remains unknown, although at the time of writing the *p16* gene, which appears to be mutated at a frequency rivalling *p53* in many human cancers [29], must be regarded as a strong candidate. Definition of the genetic basis of this step is, of course, of more than academic interest since, of all stages, it is the transition from follicular adenoma to follicular carcinoma that poses the greatest diagnostic problem in thyroid pathology. Unfortunately the quality of DNA preservation in routinely fixed, wax-embedded tumour material is often so low as to permit only a limited range of polymerase chain reaction (PCR)-based studies. Careful collection of representative tumour samples (with, where possible, matched normal tissue) by rapid freezing in liquid nitrogen should therefore be encouraged to provide a bank of specimens suitable for future genetic analysis.

References

1. Franceschi S, Boyle P, La Vecchia C *et al*. The epidemiology of thyroid carcinoma. *Crit. Rev. Oncogenesis* 1993;**4**:25–52.
2. Lyons J, Landis CA, Harsh G *et al*. Two G protein oncogenes in human endocrine tumours. *Science* 1990;**249**:655–9.
3. Suarez HG, du Villard JA, Caillou B *et al*. *gsp* mutations in human thyroid tumours. *Oncogene* 1991;**6**:677–9.
4. O'Sullivan C, Barton CM, Staddon SL, Brown CL, Lemoine NR. Activating point mutations of the gsp oncogene in human thyroid adenomas. *Mol. Carcinogen.* 1991;**4**:345–9.
5. Matsuo K, Friedman E, Gejman PV, Fagin JA. The thyrotropin receptor (TSH-R) is not an oncogene for thyroid tumours: structural studies of the TSH-R and the alpha-subunit of Gs in human thyroid neoplasms. *J. Clin. Endocrinol. Metab.* 1993;**76**:1446–51.
6. Parma J, Duprez L, Van Sande J *et al*. Somatic mutations in the thyrotropin receptor gene cause hyperfunctioning thyroid adenomas. *Nature* 1993;**365**:649–51.
7. Wynford-Thomas D, Stringer BMJ, Williams ED. Dissociation of growth and function in the rat thyroid during prolonged goitrogen administration. *Acta Endocrinol. (Copenh.)* 1982;**101**:210–16.
8. Fusco A, Grieco M, Santoro M *et al*. A new oncogene in human papillary carcinomas and their lymph-nodal metastases. *Nature* 1987;**328**:170–2.

9. Bongarzone I, Pierotti MA, Monzini N *et al*. High frequency of activation of tyrosine kinase oncogenes in human papillary thyroid carcinoma. *Oncogene* 1989;4:1457–62.

10. Santoro M, Carlomagno F, Hay ID *et al*. Ret oncogene activation in human thyroid neoplasms is restricted to the papillary cancer sub-type. *J. Clin. Invest*. 1992;89:1517–22.

11. Jhiang SM, Caruso DR, Gilmore E *et al*. Detection of the PTC/*ret*TPC oncogene in human thyroid cancers. *Oncogene* 1992;7:1331–7.

12. Santoro M, Sabino N, Ishizaka Y *et al*. Involvement of ret oncogene in human tumours: specificity of ret activation to thyroid tumours. *Br. J. Cancer* 1993;68:460–4.

13. Bond JA, Wyllie FS, Rowson J, Radulescu A, Wynford-Thomas D. *In vitro* reconstruction of tumour initiation in a human epithelium. *Oncogene* 1994;9:281–90.

14. Lemoine NR, Mayall ES, Wyllie FS *et al*. High frequency of *ras* oncogene activation in all stages of human thyroid tumorigenesis. *Oncogene* 1989;4:159–64.

15. Wright PA, Lemoine NR, Mayall ES *et al*. Papillary and follicular thyroid carcinomas show a different pattern of *ras* oncogene mutation. *Br. J. Cancer* 1989;60:576–7.

16. Suarez HG, du Villard JA, Severino M *et al*. Presence of mutations of all three *ras* genes in human thyroid tumours. *Oncogene* 1990;5:565–70.

17. Namba H, Rubin SA, Fagin JA. Point mutations of ras oncogenes are an early event in thyroid tumorigenesis. *Mol. Endocrinol*. 1990;4:1474–9.

18. Shi Y, Zou M, Schmidt H *et al*. High rates of *ras*-codon 61 mutation in thyroid tumors in an iodide-deficient area. *Cancer Research* 1991;51:2690–3.

19. Karga H, Lee J-K, Vickery AL *et al*. *Ras* oncogene mutations in benign and malignant thyroid neoplasms. *J. Clin. Endocrinol.*

20. Curtis L, Wyllie AH, Shaw JJ *et al*. Evidence against involvement of APC mutation in papillary thyroid carcinoma. *Eur. J. Cancer* 1994;30A:984–9.

21. Hermann MA, Hay ID, Bartelt JDH *et al*. Cytogenic and molecular genetic studies of follicular and papillary thyroid cancers. *J. Clin. Invest*. 1991;88:1596–604.

22. Wright PA, Lemoine NR, Goretzki P *et al*. Mutation of the p53 gene in a differentiated human thyroid carcinoma cell line, but not in primary thyroid tumours. *Oncogene* 1991;6:1693–7.

23. Wright PA, Jasani B, Newman GR, Schmid KW, Wynford-Thomas D. p53 immunopositivity is a late event in human thyroid carcinoma development. *J. Pathol*. 1993;169S:230.

24. Donghi R, Longoni A, Pilotti S *et al*. Gene p53 mutations are restricted to poorly differentiated and undifferentiated carcinomas of the thyroid gland. *J. Clin. Invest*. 1993;91:1753–60.

25. Ito T, Seyama T, Mizuno T *et al*. Unique association of p53 mutations with undifferentiated but not with differentiated carcinomas of the thyroid gland. *Cancer Res*. 1992;52:1369–71.

26. Fagin JA, Matsuo K, Karmakar A *et al*. High prevalence of mutations of the p53 gene in poorly differentiated human thyroid carcinomas. *J. Clin. Invest*. 1993;91:179–84.

27. Nakamura T, Yana I, Kobayashi T *et al*. p53 gene mutations associated with anaplastic transformation of human thyroid carcinomas. *J.J. Cancer Res*. 1992;83:1293–98.

28. Said S, Schlumberger M, Suarez HG. Oncogenes and anti-oncogenes in human epithelial thyroid tumors. *J. Endocrinol. Invest*. 1994;17:371–9.

29. Kamb A, Gruis NA, Weaver-Feldhaus J *et al*. A cell cycle regulator potentially involved in genesis of many tumour types. *Science* 1994;264:436–40.

Metab. 1991;73:832–6.

16

Papillary Thyroid Carcinoma

IAN D. HAY

Pathological classification

Papillary thyroid carcinoma (PTC) has been defined as 'a malignant epithelial tumor showing evidence of follicular cell differentiation and characterized by the formation of papillae and/or a set of distinctive nuclear changes' [1]. PTC is the most common thyroid malignancy and constitutes worldwide 50–90% of differentiated follicular cell-derived thyroid cancers [2]. Papillary thyroid microcarcinoma (PTM) is defined by the World Health Organization (WHO) as a PTC 1.0 cm or less in diameter [3]. These microcarcinomas are common in population-based autopsy studies, and as incidental findings in carefully examined resected thyroid glands. The incidence rates for clinically diagnosed PTC in the USA approximate 5/100 000 for tumours more than 1 cm in diameter and around 1/100 000 for PTM. By contrast, the reported incidence of PTM in autopsy material from various continents has ranged from 4 to 36% [1].

The nuclei of PTC cells have a distinctive appearance, which in recent years has acquired a diagnostic significance comparable to that of the papillae (Figs 16.1, 16.2). Often the preoperative diagnosis of PTC can be made solely on the basis of the characteristic nuclear changes seen in fine needle aspiration (FNA) cytology material (as described in Chapter 19). In its most typical form, PTC shows a predominance of papillary structures within the tumour. However, the papillae are usually admixed with neoplastic follicles having similar nuclear features. When the lining cells of the neoplastic follicles have the same nuclear features as those seen in typical PTC, and the follicular predominance over the papillae is complete, the tumour is considered a 'follicular variant' of PTC [1].

Another subtype of PTC recognized by the WHO is the diffuse sclerosing variant characterized by widespread lymphatic permeation, prominent fibrosis and diffuse involvement of one or both thyroid lobes. The tall-cell variant is characterized by well-formed papillae covered by cells that are twice as tall as they are wide. The columnar cell variant differs from other forms of PTC because of the presence of prominent nuclear stratification. The tall and columnar cell variants are considered more aggressive [1]. However, controversy exists regarding outcome in the diffuse sclerosing variant.

Presenting features

Although PTC can occur at any age, most diagnoses are made in patients aged between 30 and 50 years (mean age 44 years). Women are more frequently affected (female predominance 60–80%). The majority of primary tumours are 1–4 cm in maximum size, the average approximately 2–3 cm in greatest diameter [2,4]. Of PTC tumours 95% are classified as histological grade 1 (of 4); 80% of primary PTC tumours are DNA diploid by flow cytometry [2]. Extrathyroid invasion of adjacent soft tissues by PTC is reported in about 15% (range 5–34%) at primary surgery. At presentation, about one-third of PTC patients have clinically evident lymphadenopathy [4]. Microscopic examination of excised neck nodes typically reveals 35–50% involvement, but in children < 17 years old nodal involvement may occur in up to 90% [5]. The primary disease is confined to the neck in about 93–99% of PTC patients at diagnosis [2,5]. Spread to superior mediastinal nodes is usually associated with extensive neck nodal involvement. Only 1–7% of PTC patients have distant metastases diagnosed before or within 30 days of primary treatment [2].

The TNM classification represents an internationally accepted system for tumour staging [6]. Postoperative stage assessment in PTC is dependent not only on TNM categories, but also on whether the patient is under 45 years old or is aged 45 years or older [2,6]. In our experience, the majority of PTC patients present as stage I (60%) or stage II (22%). Patients aged 45 years or older

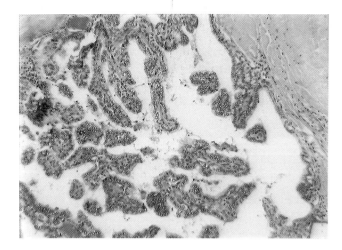

Fig. 16.1 Papillary carcinoma of the thyroid. The typical 'orphan Annie' nuclei are apparent.

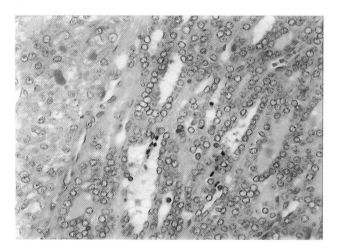

Fig. 16.2 Follicular variant of papillary carcinoma of the thyroid. There is crowding of nuclei in the neoplastic follicles and 'orphan Annie' nucleus formation.

with either nodal metastases or extrathyroid extension (stage III) account for less than 20% of cases [2]. Only about 1–2% of PTC patients present with distant metastases and fulfil the criteria for stage IV disease (aged ≥ 45 years with any T, any N, M1).

Recurrence and mortality

Three types of tumour recurrence may occur with PTC. These are, in order of frequency: (i) postoperative nodal metastases (NM); (ii) local recurrences (LR); and (iii) postoperative distant metastases (DM). An LR may be defined as 'histologically confirmed tumour occurring in the resected thyroid bed, thyroid remnant, or other adjacent tissues of the neck (excluding lymph nodes)' at any time after complete surgical removal of the primary tumour [7]. We have considered nodal or distant spread to be postoperative if the metastases were discovered within 180 days or 30 days, respectively [2]. We have also chosen to consider tumour recurrence only as it occurs to patients without initial DM, who had complete surgical resection of their primary tumours. Figure 16.3 illustrates PTC recurrence at local, nodal and distant sites and compares these rates with those of non-papillary thyroid cancers treated at our institution during the period 1940–90. After 25 years of follow-up, postoperative NM had been discovered in 9%, while LR and DM occurred in 6 and 5%, respectively. When compared to follicular thyroid cancer, there were with PTC fewer LR and DM. Moreover, postoperative NM were significantly more often discovered.

Cause-specific survival rates for differentiated thyroid cancer are shown in Fig. 16.4. Survival rates for PTC were 98% at 5 years, 96% at 10 years, and 95% at 20

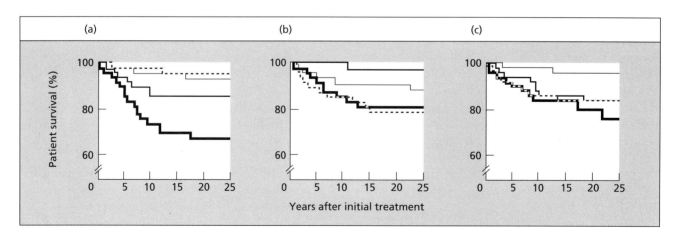

Fig. 16.3 Patient survival of (a) local recurrences, (b) nodal metastases and (c) distant metastases in 2106 patients with differentiated thyroid cancer (DTC) treated at the Mayo Clinic during the period 1940–90. Histological subtypes: —, papillary (1739, 83%);

—, follicular (124, 6%); ▬, Hürthle cell (84, 4%); ----, medullary (159, 7%). The numbers in parentheses represent the numbers or percentages of DTC patients who had complete resection of disease in the neck and had no initial distant spread.

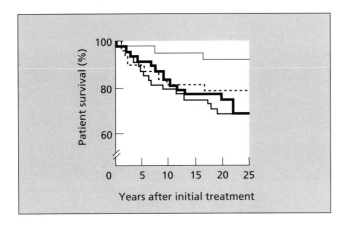

Fig. 16.4 Cause-specific mortality in 2278 patients with differentiated thyroid cancer treated at the Mayo Clinic during the period 1940–90. Histological subtypes as in Fig. 16.3.

years. Of those with lethal PTC, approximately 20% died in the first year after diagnosis. By 10 years, 80% of the deaths from PTC had occurred. It is noteworthy that the 25-year cause-specific survival rate for PTC of 94% greatly exceeded the 79% rate seen with medullary thyroid cancer, and the 71% rates found with both follicular and Hürthle cell cancers.

Outcome prediction

Close scrutiny of the observed rates of recurrence and mortality in PTC reveals that only a small minority (about 15%) of patients are liable to relapse of disease, and even fewer (around 5%) experience a lethal outcome. Those exceptional patients, who pursue an aggressive course, tend to relapse early, and the rare fatalities usually occur within 5–10 years of diagnosis [2–5]. During the past decade many USA centres have used multivariate analyses to identify presenting variables predictive of cause-specific mortality [8–11]. Increasing patient age and presence of extrathyroid invasion have been independent prognostic factors in all these studies [8–11]. The presence of initial DM and increasing size of the primary tumour have also been significant variables in most studies [8,10,11]. We [2,8], and others [9], have found that histopathological grade (degree of differentiation) is an independent variable. The completeness of initial tumour resection (postoperative status) has also been relevant in predicting those at risk of death from PTC [2,10,12]. When analysed by the presence or absence of extrathyroid invasion, the presence of initial neck NM, although very relevant to future nodal recurrence, did not significantly influence cause-specific mortality [2,4,12].

In 1987, we devised a simple scoring system to assign patients to prognostic risk groups [8]. The prognostic index was named the AGES score after the five independent variables of patient's *a*ge, tumour *g*rade, tumour *e*xtent (local invasion, distant metastasis) and tumour *s*ize. Using such a scoring system, the 'minimal risk' group (AGES score < 4) represented 86% of cases, and they experienced a 20-year cause-specific mortality rate of only 1% [2]. By contrast, the minority (14%) of patients with AGES scores of 4+ (high-risk) had a 20-year cause-specific mortality of 40%. The development of such a prognostic scoring system was intended to permit more accurate counselling of patients and to aid in the planning of individualized postoperative management programmes in PTC [8,12].

Although the AGES scheme had the potential for universal application, some academic centres could not include the differentiation (G) variable because their surgical pathologists did not recognize higher grade PTC tumours [13]. Accordingly, we resolved to define a reliable prognostic scoring system for predicting PTC mortality rates using 15 candidate variables that included, for the first time, completeness of primary tumour resection, but excluded histological grade and nuclear DNA ploidy [12]. Cox model analysis and stepwise variable selection led to a final prognostic model that included five variables abbreviated by *m*etastasis, *a*ge, *c*ompleteness of resection, *i*nvasion and *s*ize (MACIS).

The final prognostic score was defined as MACIS = 3.1 (if aged ≤ 39 years) or 0.08 × age (if aged ≥ 40 years), +0.3 × tumour size (in centimetres), +1 (if incompletely resected, +1 (if locally invasive), +3 (if distant metastases present). As illustrated by Fig. 16.5, the MACIS scoring system permitted identification of patient groups with a broad range of risk of death from PTC. Twenty-year cause-specific survival rates for patients with MACIS scores less than 6, 6 to 6.99, 7 to 7.99, and 8+ were 99%, 89%, 56% and 24%, respectively ($P < 0.0001$). The minimal-risk group (MACIS < 6.0) comprised 84% of the patients and had a 20-year PTC mortality of 0.9 ± 0.3% [12]. When cumulative mortality from all causes of death was considered, the approximately 85% of PTC patients, represented by low-risk scores of AGES < 4 or MACIS < 6, experienced no excess mortality over those all-causes rates predicted for appropriate control subjects [8,12].

It should be emphasized that the five variables needed for MACIS scoring are readily available after primary operation, and such a prognostic system has the potential for application in any clinical setting with access to conventional chest and skeletal radiography and accurate surgical pathology reporting. The MACIS scoring system can also provide the attending clinician with an accurate tool for counselling the individual PTC patient and can help guide decision-making on the intensity of postoperative tumour surveillance and the appropriateness of adjunctive radioiodine therapy. Since the CIS variables

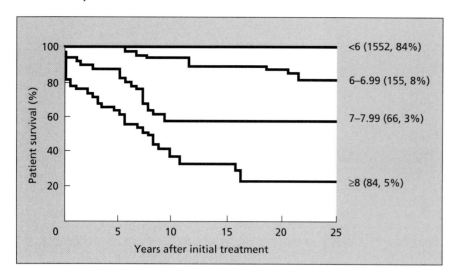

Fig. 16.5 Cause-specific survival plotted by MACIS prognostic risk groups in a cohort of 1851 patients with PTC treated at the Mayo Clinic during the period 1940–90.

need to be verified postoperatively, the scoring system should not be used to decide on the extent of primary thyroid surgery [13].

Impact of surgery

The accepted initial treatment of PTC is adequate surgical excision of the primary tumour. However, the extent of thyroid resection remains controversial, with the choice of definitive therapy ranging from unilateral lobectomy through bilateral, subtotal, lobar resection to near-total or total thyroidectomy [2,7,8,10]. Unfortunately, in many surgical reports where two procedures are compared, only scant attempt is made to match the patient groups with respect to relevant prognostic variables. Accordingly, differences between groups may prove to be primarily due to imbalances in the prognostic factors, rather than to the specific surgical procedure [2].

In an attempt to clarify this issue, we used the AGES scoring system as an adjustment variable in analysing the role of different surgical treatments in PTC [7,8]. In low-risk patients (AGES scores < 4) no improvement in cause-specific survival was demonstrable when patients underwent more than ipsilateral lobectomy. By contrast, in high-risk patients (AGES scores > 4) survival after bilateral resection was much higher than after lobectomy alone [8]. In neither group was survival up to 25 years significantly improved by the performance of a total thyroidectomy. More recently, we used the same approach to assess the impact of surgical resection on subsequent LR [7]. In low-risk patients (AGES < 4) the risk at 30 years of developing LR was 14% after lobectomy and 4% after bilobar resection. In high-risk patients (AGES > 4) the comparable rates were 59% after lobectomy and 20% after bilateral resection. In neither risk group was

there a significant difference in LR frequency between patients undergoing total thyroidectomy and those who had bilateral sub-total or near-total thyroidectomy [7].

Recently we have extended those studies, and used the newer MACIS scoring system to adjust for severity of disease at presentation [14]. The study group consisted of 1848 PTC patients operated on 'with curative intent' for disease confined to the neck and followed up to 53 postoperative years (mean 17 years). As in the AGES studies, we found that extension of the primary resection to include the contralateral lobe led to fewer LR in low-risk (MACIS < 6) patients, and to lower LR and cause-specific mortality (CSM) rates in high-risk (MACIS > 6) cases. Neither LR nor CSM rates after bilateral sub-total or near-total thyroidectomy were significantly different from those seen after total thyroidectomy [14]. In our experience, total thyroidectomy was accompanied by a ten times greater risk of permanent postoperative hypoparathyroidism. We therefore concluded that the performance of a 'total' thyroidectomy seems rarely justifiable in typical PTC. When recurrent laryngeal nerves and parathyroid glands are assuredly preserved, however, total thyroidectomy may be a reasonable, but not necessarily a superior, alternative procedure in the treatment of patients with high-risk (MACIS > 6) PTC [2,7].

'Benefits' of ablation

In the past 5 years there has been a dramatic upsurge in the number of radioiodine remnant ablations (RRA) being performed worldwide for PTC [2]. This has occurred primarily because of optimistic reports showing decreased recurrence rates after apparently successful RRA [10,13] and, more recently, also describing significant reduction in cancer mortality 'following ^{131}I therapy, regardless of the reason for its use' [15]. Of 138 PTC patients without evident postoperative residual disease treated with RRA by Mazzaferri [15], nine (7%) developed cancer recurrence and none to date have died of thyroid cancer. Consequently, Mazzaferri [15] now advises near-total thyroidectomy and routine RRA for all patients with PTC, except those with solitary intrathyroid tumours less than 1.5 cm diameter, not involving cervical nodes. Similar conclusions have been drawn from a University of Chicago study by DeGroot [10,13], who now recommends near-total thyroidectomy and postoperative RRA for all patients with PTC, except those 'individuals with lesions less than 1 cm in size who are under age 30, unless they have a history of X-ray exposure'.

If these recommendations were to be followed, between 87% [15] and approximately 95% [13] of PTC patients would be exposed to RRA and subsequent whole body radioiodine scanning. Since, for the reasons cited in the preceding section on outcome prediction, the majority (95%) of PTC patients are not at risk of developing a life-threatening iodophilic DM, it would seem probably more logical to restrict the use of RRA to those patients who, because of poor prognostic factors, are at heightened risk of cause-specific mortality. In contrast to the recommendations of DeGroot and Mazzaferri, Simpson and his colleagues from Toronto advise the restriction of RRA to that minority (approximately 15%) of PTC patients, whose tumours show extrathyroid invasion, and thus are more likely to have evidence of microscopic residual disease [9]. An alternative approach, which we favour, would be to select for postoperative RRA only those PTC patients considered at 'high-risk' for DM and CSM on the basis of either an AGES score > 4 or a MACIS score > 6.

Practice guidelines

It would be the general expectation that most patients with PTC will be treated initially with bilateral lobar resection, usually near-total thyroidectomy. Nodal metastases would typically be excised and, at most, a modified radical neck dissection would be performed. After the surgical pathology report is available, a MACIS score can be calculated, and the patient assigned to a low- or high-risk category. The majority (probably 80–85%) of patients would be deemed low-risk (MACIS scores < 6), and would be dismissed postoperatively on thyroxine (T_4) therapy, aimed at TSH suppression within a range of 0.1–0.5 mu/l. The serum TSH and thyroglobulin (Tg) would be checked after a minimum of 6–8 weeks. If the Tg level was > 5 ng/ml, the T_4 therapy would be adjusted to permit TSH levels in the 0.01–0.1 mu/l range. If the Tg level

was ≤ 5 ng/ml on adequate T_4 suppressive therapy, the patient would then be followed-up annually by neck palpation, chest X-ray and measurements of serum TSH and Tg. However, if, despite adequate TSH suppression, the serum Tg level was persistently above 5 ng/ml, we would recommend that a high-resolution ultrasound examination of the neck be performed. If a suspicious thyroid bed or nodal lesion were detected, we would recommend an ultrasound-guided FNA biopsy. If recurrent disease was found on biopsy, the patient would be treated as a high-risk patient. A negative ultrasound and a serum Tg level ≤ 5 ng/ml would usually lead to continuing annual surveillance with ultrasound examination, chest X-ray, and measurements of serum TSH and Tg.

The minority (probably 15–20%) of PTC patients, who would be deemed high-risk (MACIS score > 6), would be dismissed from hospital on triiodothyronine therapy, with a view to performing whole body ^{131}I scanning at 6–8 postoperative weeks, after T_3 has been discontinued for 2 weeks. If on scan only remnant uptake is demonstrable, the patient would usually receive an outpatient 29.9 mCi (1100 MBq) [131]I dose for remnant ablation. If, however, ^{131}I uptake was found in a distant metastasis or known residual neck disease, the patient would be considered for an in-patient dose of 100–300 mCi (3700–11 100 MBq) [131]I. Whole body scans and ^{131}I therapy would be repeated at 3–6 month intervals until the iodophilic foci have been eliminated, or evidence for bone marrow toxicity appears. After the whole body ^{131}I scan is negative, the search for potential recurrent or metastatic disease would be based on screening serum Tg levels and, where indicated, confirmatory images of neck, chest or bony skeleton with ultrasound examinations, computed tomography (CT) or magnetic resonance imaging (MRI), or diphosphonate bone scans, respectively. When recurrent disease cannot be treated with ^{131}I, consideration should be given to surgical re-exploration, or, if surgery is contraindicated, external beam irradiation, brachytherapy, or percutaneous ultrasound guided alcohol ablation. At this time, chemotherapy has only exceptionally a role to play in the treatment of widespread, otherwise unmanageable, PTC.

References

1. Rosai J. Papillary carcinoma. *Monogr. Pathol.* 1993;**35**:138–65.
2. Hay ID. Papillary thyroid carcinoma. *Endocrinol. Metab. Clin. North. Am.* 1990;**19**:545–76.
3. Hay ID, Grant CS, van Heerden JA *et al.* Papillary thyroid microcarcinoma: a study of 535 cases observed in a 50-year period. *Surgery* 1992;**112**:1139–47.
4. McConahey WM, Hay ID, Woolner LB *et al.* Papillary thyroid

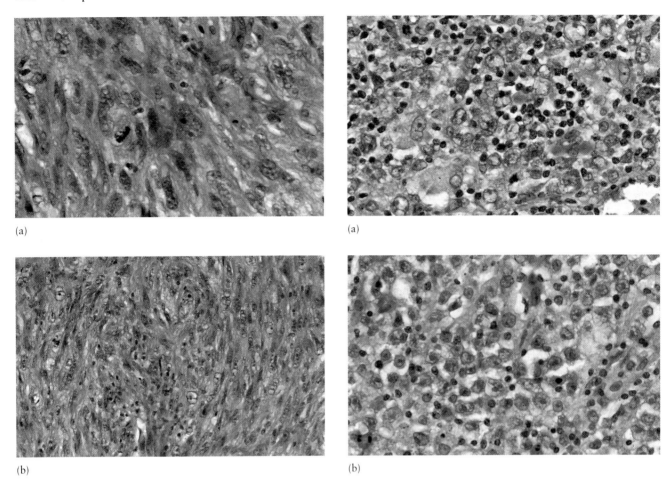

(a)

(b)

Fig. 18.1 Spindle-cell anaplastic carcinoma of the thyroid: (a) low power view; (b) high power view.

(a)

(b)

Fig. 18.2 High grade lymphoma of the thyroid: (a) low power view; (b) high power view.

are diagnosed at weekends, leading to an awkward situation with regard to immediate management. In some circumstances, when symptoms are severe, an emergency tracheostomy may need to be performed to relieve symptoms. Otherwise the dilemma is whether to commence urgent radiation treatment to relieve compression. One useful maneouvre that this author has found helpful is to give a trial dose of high-dose steroids, usually dexamethasone 8–16 mg/day in divided doses. Lymphomas generally melt away very dramatically with such therapy, whereas anaplastic tumours remain refractory. This then allows a little time for consideration of the definitive management.

Surgery

The role of the surgeon in anaplastic thyroid cancer is rather varied and will depend upon his or her own understanding of the literature. There are certainly conflicting reports between the benefits of a more aggressive surgical approach and that of the minimalist approach, where the surgeon's role is merely to obtain enough tissue to establish a diagnosis histologically. There are, however, more reports in the literature that indicate that an aggressive surgical approach is recommended [3–7]. Clearly, when possible, near-total thyroidectomy is the preferred treatment of choice, particularly in the younger, fitter patient. Of course these patients are self selecting in that they are more likely to have tumours amenable to resection; nevertheless in the remaining patients an attempt should be made at debulking surgery even if total tumour resection cannot be achieved. Obviously decompressive surgery, whether radical or debulking, is going to relieve the acute compressive symptoms and permit more careful planning of the next phase of treatment.

Reviewing the largest published series in the literature it is clear from the experience at the MD Anderson Hospital, with a series of 121 patients [3], and from the Mayo Clinic, where 82 patients were treated over a 25-year-period [5], that those patients who have more radical surgery have a better prognosis. It is this definition of radicality that remains a little unclear. It would seem that a super-radical operation, attempting total thyroidectomy with or without lymph node dissection, does not confer any advantage but that, where appropriate, lobectomy, isthmusectomy and sub-total thyroidectomy should be attempted. Clearly, in all these reports the number of patients who were eligible for a more radical approach is small and it is impossible to obtain any meaningful statistical analysis. It may well be a self-fulfilling prophesy that those patients with larger and more aggressive tumours are less likely to be suitable for radical surgery, whereas patients with smaller tumours will be more amenable to a more radical surgical approach. Certainly in our own series of 91 patients from the Beatson Oncology Centre, Glasgow [1], only one-third were able to undergo a partial thyroidectomy and 5% a total thyroidectomy and there was a clear survival advantage to those who underwent partial and total thyroidectomy, especially when they did not have dyspnoea at presentation, but it may well be that this is purely a reflection of a smaller volume of disease.

Radiation therapy

Whether or not patients are able to undergo surgery, most series report the use of radiation therapy [1,8–13], but clearly again there is a wide variation of radiation doses that have been used. The Mayo Clinic experience suggests that there is no consistent trend in survival with increasing dose of radiation, although many patients seem to receive relatively low doses of radiation. Only 18 received in excess of 50 Gy. At the MD Anderson Hospital it was noted that patient survival was longer if they received total or sub-total thyroidectomy and radiation therapy, chemotherapy or both, although this did not reach statistical significance.

It would seem reasonable to suggest that if the patient is fit enough, then a minimum target absorbed dose of 50 Gy in 5 weeks should be prescribed, generally using parallel opposed radiation fields. Depending upon the response it may then be appropriate to give a boost to the residual tumour to take this up to 60 Gy in 6 weeks. Unfortunately the response rates to this would seem to suggest there is no great survival advantage. Nevertheless this would be the optimal conventional treatment.

A number of studies, albeit with small numbers of patients, have looked at unorthodox fractionation schedules including hyperfractionated accelerated treatment. Certainly, on theoretical grounds, such rapidly growing tumours might well respond better to novel radiation techniques but at this point in time such approaches to treatment should be considered to be unproven and

should only be looked at in the context of clinical studies.

Chemotherapy

With such a high incidence of metastatic disease and such a high rate of local failure in spite of initial local control, it is not surprising that approaches have been made to use systemic treatment, either alone or in combination with radiation treatment. From the literature it would seem that Adriamycin (doxorubicin) has been the most active single agent when used as first-line treatment. Gottlieb and colleagues [14] reported a response in 10 out of 28 patients (a response rate of 36%). However the median duration of response tended to be between 4 and 6 months. Small numbers of patients have been treated with other anthracycline analogues such as aclarubicin and mitoxantrone [15,16].

There is also single-agent experience of cisplatin giving around a 20% response rate, and etoposide (no responders). Attempts have been made to use combination chemotherapy particularly with Adriamycin and cisplatin [17] and in the only randomized study reported by Shimaoka and colleagues [18] they compared Adriamycin 60 mg/m^2 with the same drug plus cisplatin 40 mg/m^2 given every 3 weeks. Whilst the response rate was the same, the only two complete responders were both in the combined modality arm.

In conclusion, it is this author's view that the benefits of chemotherapy remain very much unproven. Perhaps we have as yet to find the optimal combination but again one has to feel that any chemotherapy given for undifferentiated anaplastic thyroid cancer should really be within the context of a clinical study or protocol.

Combined modality

There is obviously a major handicap in that there is a dearth of randomized clinical studies for the management of anaplastic thyroid cancer and that most large centres are only able to report on anecdotal numbers of patients treated with chemotherapy alone or combined modality.

Many patients tend to be over the age of 70 years and have relatively poor performance status and therefore are not good candidates for aggressive chemotherapy regimens containing cisplatin. There is however an impression that, for the younger, fitter patient, who is able to undergo radical debulking surgery, follow-up chemotherapy and radiation treatment may have a role to play. There is a desperate need for even the larger centres to cooperate and carry out national studies or even multinational studies in an attempt to resolve whether combined modality therapy does confer an advantage.

Conclusion

Anaplastic carcinoma of the thyroid remains a fascinating and yet frustrating cancer to treat. Patient numbers are very small and therefore most endocrinologists and oncologists will have limited experience in their management. There seems to be some evidence to suggest that surgical debulking with at least a partial thyroidectomy leads to an improved survival rate. Small numbers of patients treated with more aggressive surgery together with a multimodality approach of radiation therapy and chemotherapy for smaller volume disease may lead to improved survival.

Clearly the future direction should be to try to identify those patients for whom there may be a better prognosis and to target them with such aggressive approaches. However these patients should optimally be treated in centres with greater experience in the management of anaplastic carcinoma and there is a great need for multicentre if not multinational studies to be produced to learn more about the optimal management of this rare tumour.

References

1. Junor EJ, Paul J, Reed NS. Anaplastic thyroid carcinoma: 91 patients treated by surgery and radiotherapy. *Eur. J. Surg. Oncol.* 1992;**18**:83–8.
2. Shvero J, Gal R, Avidor I, Hadar T, Kessler E. Anaplastic thyroid carcinoma: a clinical, histologic and immunohistochemical study. *Cancer* 1988;**62**:319–25.
3. Venkatesh YSS, Ordonez NG, Schultz PN *et al.* Anaplastic carcinoma of thyroid: a clinicopathologic study of 121 cases. *Cancer* 1990;**66**:321–30.
4. Starnes HF, Brooks DC, Pinkus GS, Brooks JR. Surgery for thyroid carcinoma. *Cancer* 1985;**55**:1376–81.
5. Nel CJC, van Heerden JA, Goellner JR *et al.* Anaplastic carcinoma of thyroid: a clinical pathologic study of 82 cases. *Mayo Clinic Proc.* 1985;**60**:51–8.
6. Thomas CG, Buckwalter JA. Poorly differentiated neoplasms of thyroid gland. *Ann. Surg.* 1973;**177**:632–42.
7. Rossi R, Cady B, Meissner WA, Sedgwick CE, Werber J. Prognosis of undifferentiated carcinoma and lymphoma of thyroid. *Am. J. Surg.* 1978;**135**:589–95.
8. Kyriakides G, Sosin H. Anaplastic carcinoma of thyroid. *Ann. Surg.* 1974;**179**:295–9.
9. Rafla S. Anaplastic tumours of thyroid. *Cancer* 1969;**23**;668–77.
10. Tubiana M, Haddad E, Schlumberger M *et al.* External radiotherapy in thyroid cancers. *Cancer* 1985;**55**:2062–71.
11. Smedal M, Meissner WA. The results of X-ray treatment in undifferentiated carcinoma of thyroid. *Radiology* 1961;**76**:927–35.
12. Jereb B, Stjernsward J, Lowhagen T. Anaplastic giant cell carcinoma of thyroid. *Cancer* 1975;**35**:1293–5.
13. Rogers JD, Lindberg RD, Hill CS, Gehan E. Spindle and giant cell carcinoma of thyroid: a different therapeutic approach. *Cancer* 1974;**34**:1328–32.
14. Gottleib JA, Hill CS. Adriamycin therapy in thyroid cancer. *Cancer Chemother. Rep.* 1975;**6**:283–96.
15. Samonigg H, Hossfeld DK, Spehn J, Fill H, Leb G. Aclarubicin in advanced thyroid cancer: a phase II study. *Eur. J. Cancer Clin. Oncol.* 1988;**21**:1271–5.
16. Schlumberger M, Parmentier C. Phase II evaluation of mitoxantrone in advanced non anaplastic thyroid cancer. *Bull. Cancer Paris* 1989;**76**:403–6.
17. Williams SD, Birch R, Einhorn LH. Phase II evaluation of doxorubicin plus cisplatin in advanced thyroid cancer: a southeastern cancer study group trial. *Cancer Treat. Rep.* 1986;**70**:405–7.
18. Shimaoka K, Schoenfeld DA, DeWys WD, Creech RH, De Conti R. A randomised trial of doxorubicin vs doxorubicin plus cisplatin in patients with advanced thyroid carcinoma. *Cancer* 1985;**56**:2155–60.
19. Schlumberger M, Parmentier C, Delisle MJ *et al.* Combination therapy for anaplastic giant cell thyroid carcinoma. *Cancer* 1991;**67**:564–6.

19

Thyroid Lymphoma

CHARLES EDMONDS

Introduction

Although most non-Hodgkin's lymphomas arise in lymph nodes, up to 20% start initially in lymphoid tissue located in other structures. The thyroid is one such site, accounting for about 2–3% of extranodular non-Hodgkin's lymphomas [1]. Hodgkin's disease itself, on the other hand, rarely involves the thyroid. Thyroid cancer is an uncommon disease and the rarity of primary thyroid lymphoma is indicated by its accounting for 5% or less of all thyroid cancers. There is, however, considerable practical importance in recognizing it because the response to treatment of the thyroid alone may, in the early stages, be curative.

Pathology

The thyroid is always enlarged, appearing as a diffuse or nodular goitre with tumour replacing much or all of the gland. Exceptionally there is just a single nodule. The tumour is homogeneous and without a clear boundary [2]. The microscopical appearance is of monomorphic cells occupying much of the gland, often within blood vessels and 'packing out' the follicles. There may be regions of necrosis contrasting with functioning follicles particularly at the edges. Because of the frequent association of lymphoma with lymphocytic thyroiditis, some regions of the gland may contain many normal lymphocytes and this may cause confusion in diagnosis [3]. Surface marker studies have established that thyroid lymphomas are nearly always of B-cell origin. For prognosis, assessing whether the tumour is of high- or low-grade malignancy is important [4]. When the disease spreads beyond the thyroid, it does so to lymph nodes and by infiltration of adjacent tissues. But it may, sometimes quite rapidly, affect more distant sites, the gastrointestinal tract becoming frequently involved.

Primary thyroid lymphoma is strongly associated with chronic lymphocytic thyroiditis (Hashimoto's disease), this being present in up to 80% of cases [5]. Lymphocytic thyroiditis is, however, relatively common so it is fortunate that only 1% or less of affected individuals develop lymphoma. It has been proposed that extranodular lymphomas have their origin in lymphoid cell collections, which may occur (usually associated with autoimmune conditions) in such organs as, for example, thyroid, stomach and salivary glands [3]. The acronym MALT (mucosa-associated lymphoid tissue) lymphomas has been suggested for this concept. Extranodular lymphoid tissue associated with autoimmune disease may be especially at risk for developing lymphoma, but against this notion, at least with regards to the thyroid, is the lack of any established association with Graves' disease. No other definite factors in aetiology have been established. Unlike other forms of thyroid cancer, irradiation does not seem to be significant.

Clinical presentation

Thyroid lymphoma is predominantly a disease of elderly women, which is consistent with its association with lymphocytic thyroiditis. The female to male ratio is about 5 : 1 and the median age of onset is around 60–70 years, but the disease may occur in younger people and most series include individuals aged less than 50 years [5–7]. Up to 30% of patients have a history of goitre and some have established autoimmune thyroiditis and may be taking thyroxine. The presentation is most commonly as an enlarging neck mass occurring over a period of a few weeks or months. Discomfort, sometimes pain, tenderness, hoarseness of the voice and even dysphagia and stridor may develop. On examination a firm to hard thyroid mass is found which moves poorly on swallowing. Occasionally one lobe is affected initially but usually the for dealing with the stones adds weight to the argument that surgery is not necessary merely to prevent renal stones developing in a patient without a previous history of stones.

One of the main concerns about conservative management is the theoretical risk that untreated hyperparathyroidism, especially in elderly women, may cause an increased loss of bone mass, worsen osteoporosis and increase the risk of fractures in old age. Current evidence does not allow a definitive answer to be given to this concern. Cross-sectional studies indicate that patients with untreated hyperparathyroidism usually have bone density values within the normal range for their age and sex. Studies at differing sites suggest that there may be some loss of cortical bone but a sparing of trabecular bone. Recent prospective studies have not shown any obvious long-term loss of bone mass compared with age-matched controls [5] but different patients who underwent successful parathyroid surgery showed a 12% increase in bone mass in the four years following surgery [6]. If clinically important bone disease leading to increased fractures was a significant problem, one might have expected mass biochemical screening to have detected many new cases of hyperparathyroidism presenting with fractures to orthopaedic clinics. This does not appear to be the case. Particularly reassuring is a long-term follow-up of nearly 2000 cases of untreated hyperparathyroidism from Sweden, where, after 19 years of follow-up, there was no increased fracture risk [7].

Other long-term follow-up studies have raised the possibility that there is an increased morbidity in untreated hyperparathyroidism, increased deaths from cardiovascular and malignant disease being noted. However, other studies have not shown that successful surgical treatment eliminates this risk.

Very occasionally severe hypercalcaemia is noted in patients who were previously well. The assumption is that they had mild asymptomatic hyperparathyroidism that suddenly worsened. The deterioration being assumed to be caused by an intercurrent illness, leading to dehydration and worsening of the hypercalcaemia. While this is possible, it must be a very rare event. Despite these anxieties, there are now a number of studies reporting that conservative management is a safe option, which can be offered to patients who are older and asymptomatic.

At present there is no effective medical treatment that successfully controls the hyperparathyroid state. Current treatments that lower serum calcium do not reduce and may increase serum parathyroid hormone concentrations. It is the author's view that there is no current effective medical treatment for hyperparathyroidism and therefore conservative management does not involve drug therapy.

It merely monitors patient well-being and biochemistry. Six to twelve monthly serum creatinines and calciums are measured. Patients are asked to report any change in their condition and advised to maintain a good fluid intake in the presence of intercurrent illness.

Surgical management

Once the diagnosis of hyperparathyroidism has been made and surgical treatment recommended, the most important decision is to identify an experienced parathyroid surgeon. Studies from Denmark have shown that the best results are obtained in centres where at least 20 parathyroidectomies are carried out per year.

Indications for surgery

Definite indications

1 Definite complications of the disease; for example renal stones, parathyroid bone disease, symptomatic proximal muscle disease.
2 Young age, irrespective of symptoms. While conservative management of older patients is being evaluated, it seems prudent to offer surgical treatment to all young patients, that is those below the age of 50 years, provided the diagnosis is correct. With asymptomatic young patients, it is essential to exclude the diagnosis of familial benign hypercalcaemia prior to surgery (see below).
3 Moderate to severe hypercalcaemia. Some groups recommend parathyroidectomy in all patients with a serum calcium above 3.0 mmol/l. This seems a very arbitrary view and some elderly patients with calcium levels as high as 3.4 mmol/l may be completely asymptomatic and wish for conservative management. As a broad generalization, serum calcium levels above 3.0 mmol/l usually have symptoms and are best managed surgically.

Possible indications

As serum calcium measurements are often made without being specifically requested during the investigations of a wide range of disorders, hypercalcaemia may be discovered in association with a variety of physical and psychiatric conditions. In many instances, the association is probably coincidental but it is often difficult to exclude completely a link between the two. Under these circumstances it is advisable to offer standard treatment to the other condition and only when this is difficult to manage, should a parathyroidectomy be considered. Hypertension rarely is improved by parathyroidectomy. Psychiatric symptoms, except in the elderly, are rarely helped unless the hypercalcaemia is severe and justifies treatment on its own merits. In the elderly, a more positive attitude to surgery is indicated, as even mild hypercalcaemia can be associated with signs and symptoms of tiredness, depression and dementia which may improve dramatically after successful parathyroidectomy. A good response to surgery cannot be predicted preoperatively. As a consequence, surgery should be offered to all elderly patients with hyperparathyroidism who have a significantly impaired quality of life, which cannot be explained by any other condition. Patients should be told that improvement after surgery is not guaranteed but occurs frequently.

Preoperative localization

Most experienced parathyroid surgeons do not request preoperative localization in a previously unexplored patient, reserving such techniques for previously failed surgery. The reason for this is that the experienced parathyroid surgeon has much greater success in localizing abnormal parathyroid glands than any of the available techniques. These techniques regularly miss small parathyroid tumours, which are the ones the surgeon finds greatest difficulty in identifying. Localizing techniques if employed *must never* be employed until the diagnosis of hyperparathyroidism has been made and a decision has been taken to recommend surgery. False-positive localization is common with many techniques and can be mistakenly used to make an erroneous diagnosis of hyperparathyroidism.

Techniques for localizing parathyroid tumours

Ultrasound

Ultrasound is a readily available technique, which is very operator-dependent. It is the best technique for identifying intrathyroidal parathyroid glands, which occur in about 2–5% of cases of hyperparathyroidism. It is a poor technique for identifying glands outside the neck.

Thallium/technetium scanning

Thallium is taken up both by thyroid and parathyroid tissue and technetium (Tc) is taken up only by the thyroid. The Tc scan is subtracted from the thallium scan to give a parathyroid scan. The technique is most effective with adenomas located within the neck.

Technetium/sestamibi scanning

Sestamibi is taken up by tissues rich in mitochondria. It is taken up by both thyroid and parathyroid tissue but it persists longer in parathyroid tissue. Recent evidence suggests the Tc/sestamibi scanning is superior to thallium/Tc scanning particularly in locating adenomas outside the neck. It is likely that this technique will replace other forms of scanning [8].

Computerized tomography (CT) and magnetic resonance imaging (MRI)

CT and MRI are occasionally useful for identifying abnormal glands in the tracheo-oesophageal groove and the mediastinum.

All the above non-invasive techniques identify 60–70% of parathyroid tumours and each has a 10–15% false-positive rate.

Invasive localizing techniques are selective venous sampling and arteriography. Venous sampling is not a good localizing technique, whereas arteriography, when positive, gives exact localizing information. Neither technique is ever indicated in a previously unexplored case and should only be performed by radiologists with considerable experience of the technique.

Pre- and postoperative management

It is extremely rare to have to give any specific treatment of the hypercalcaemia prior to surgery. In moderate to severe hypercalcaemia, good rehydration is usually all that is needed. Examination of the vocal cords prior to surgery is advisable.

At surgery, attempts should be made to identify visually all four parathyroid glands, removing any obviously enlarged glands, which must be sent for frozen section. Experience of proving, by biopsy, that all parathyroid glands are normal showed an unacceptable incidence of permanent hypoparathyroidism.

Following successful surgery, the serum calcium would be expected to be within the normal range within 24 hours except when the preoperative value was very high. No significant fall of calcium level within 24 hours means either the wrong diagnosis or incomplete surgery. If the diagnosis of hyperparathyroidism is secure, the possibility of an immediate re-exploration looking for a second adenoma, if one has already been removed, should be considered.

In most cases of hyperparathyroidism the serum calcium either does not fall below normal or transiently falls just below normal on days 2–4 and then rises to normal. Treatment of this is not necessary. Occasionally symptomatic, severe hypocalcaemia develops. This is much more likely in those rare cases where there is severe parathyroid bone disease. Hypocalcaemia is associated with healing of the bone disease and eventually resolves. Permanent hypoparathyroidism occasionally occurs after the removal of a single adenoma, but is much more likely when multiple parathyroid glands have been removed.

Management of postoperative hypocalcaemia

When hypocalcaemia is symptomatic, usually with a serum calcium below 2.0 mmol/l, intravenous calcium gluconate is required. A slow (8 hour) infusion of 100 ml of 10% calcium gluconate in 1 l of saline will control symptoms. If prolonged hypocalcaemia is anticipated because of severe bone disease or suspected hypoparathyroidism, then calcitriol 1–2 µg/day should be given by mouth. As the serum calcium rises towards normal, the calcium infusions can be reduced and eventually stopped. Once normocalcaemia has been maintained for a period of weeks, then the calcitriol can be slowly reduced to see whether the serum calcium falls again, which would indicate permanent hypoparathyroidism.

Management of an unsuccessful neck exploration

Patients who have undergone unsuccessful surgery, should be referred to specialized centres experienced in the management of such cases. The diagnosis of hyperparathyroidism needs to be confirmed. Once this has been done, a decision needs to be made as to whether conservative management can be considered. If surgery is thought to be necessary, then this must be performed by a very experienced parathyroid surgeon. Almost invariably the abnormal parathyroid tissue will be found in the expected areas of the neck for parathyroid glands. Parathyroid adenomas that cannot be reached through a standard neck excision are very rare. They do however occur, justifying the use of localizing techniques in previous failed explorations.

Familial hypercalcaemia

Familial hypercalcaemia occurs in several different settings. Familial hyperparathyroidism can occur either as a specific disorder, dominantly inherited, in which only hyperparathyroidism occurs. It can also be a component of multiple endocrine neoplasia (MEN) type 1 and 2. In MEN-1, hyperparathyroidism is the most common

manifestation and usually the earliest to present. It occurs in around 80–90% of affected family members but rarely manifests before the age of 12 years. Pancreatic and pituitary tumours occur in 20–40% of family members. The hyperparathyroidism is often asymptomatic but may occasionally be associated with renal stones but only very rarely with clinical bone disease.

In MEN-2, medullary thyroid carcinoma is almost invariably present with hyperparathyroidism and phaeochromocytomas (usually bilateral) occurring in less than 50% of cases.

In all these forms of familial hyperparathyroidism, the disease is usually mild and frequently asymptomatic, often found by family screening. Almost invariably multiple parathyroid glands are affected, usually by hyperplasia. The condition is much more difficult to cure surgically. Usually a 3.5 gland parathyroidectomy is performed. Following this there is a high risk of either persistent hypercalcaemia or permanent hypoparathyroidism. Attempts to improve surgical results by transplanting parathyroid tissue to the forearm and removing all parathyroid tissue from the neck, have not necessarily given better results but the transplanted tissue is easily accessible if hypercalcaemia recurs. Because of the poorer results and typically benign course of the disease in most cases, an alternative approach is to follow cases conservatively.

Familial benign hypercalcaemia (FBH) also called familial hypocalciuric hypercalcaemia (FHH) is a condition, as mentioned earlier, which emerged as cases of presumed asymptomatic hypercalcaemia were operated upon [9]. In a number of cases, surgery, often repeated, failed to cure the hypercalcaemia. When such cases were further evaluated, multiple affected family members began to be identified, some being hypercalcaemic at a very young age. Many also had relatively low values of urinary calcium excretion.

FBH is a dominantly inherited condition with high penetrance, in which hypercalcaemia is present in affected individuals from birth. This contrasts with familial hyperparathyroidism where hypercalcaemia is virtually never present in childhood. If the index patient is excluded, there is no convincing evidence that any signs, symptoms or complications of the disease occur more frequently in affected family members compared with unaffected family members, with one exception. Very rarely, affected neonates can have severe hypercalcaemia associated with marked parathyroid bone disease, hypotonia and failure to thrive. Such infants appear to have achieved dramatic improvement after early sub-total parathyroidectomy, although there are a few cases who have improved without surgical intervention.

Other features of the condition are a tendency to hypermagnesaemia and hypocalciuria. However, neither measurement differentiates between FBH and hyperparathyroidism. Serum PTH tends to be within the normal range but can be elevated in a minority of cases. When operated upon, early evaluation suggested an increased parathyroid mass but this may be due to extra fat tissue rather than true parathyroid hyperplasia. The explanation of FBH has recently been ascertained in a number of cases and shown clearly to be a genetic disorder associated with molecular changes in the calcium sensing receptor [10].

The 'calcium sensor' is present in parathyroid tissue, renal tubules and a number of other tissues. As a result of the abnormality of the sensor, serum calcium concentrations are maintained at abnormally high values. However, induced changes in the ionized calcium concentrations influence PTH secretion in the expected manner. Of the cases so far studied, around 75% have been shown to have abnormalities in the gene encoding the 'sensor'. The rare cases of severe neonatal hyperparathyroidism have been shown to be homozygous for the abnormality. Interestingly, some families have recently been recognized who have familial benign *hypo*calcaemia. Abnormalities of the calcium sensor have also been found. It therefore appears that differing abnormalities can alter the setting of the sensor either upwards or downwards.

Identification of familial benign hypercalcaemia

Identification of FBH within a family is easy once the index case is known. The problem occurs in identifying new index cases. The diagnosis should be considered in all cases of asymptomatic cases of presumed hyperparathyroidism, especially if surgery is being contemplated. A young age and normal PTH concentrations should especially bring the possibility of FBH to mind. Unfortunately there is no test in the affected patient which will make a positive diagnosis of FBH. A tendency to relative hypercalcaemia and a high serum magnesium suggest, but do not prove, the diagnosis. Currently new mutations are thought to be unlikely but this may in part be due to the difficulty of making the diagnosis in the absence of affected family members. Therefore, if possible, attempts should be made to measure serum calcium in both parents. Where this is not possible, other first-degree relatives can be screened but negative results cannot exclude the condition. The finding of hypercalcaemic family members can also occur in familial hyperparathyroidism. If children are found to be hypercalcaemic, this makes FBH the almost certain diagnosis.

Management of familial benign hypercalcaemia

The identification of FBH is important so that parathyroidectomy is avoided. FBH, except in neonates, appears to be a benign condition requiring no treatment. Within affected families, pregnancies are uneventful but it would be prudent to advise serum calcium measurements on all neonates of affected parents if the baby is unwell and fails to thrive.

Other causes of hypercalcaemia

Malignancy is a common cause of hypercalcaemia but is typically associated with disseminated malignancy. The hypercalcaemia usually is a complication of a known solid tumour. If not, the malignant process can usually be found rapidly. Such patients are usually ill and have other manifestations of malignancy; for example, anaemia, low serum albumin and deranged liver function tests. Such cases usually do not create diagnostic problems. Serum PTH, if measured, is usually suppressed or low normal.

Occasionally hypercalcaemia can be associated with malignancy which is not clinically obvious and the patient is relatively well. Such cases can be readily differentiated from hyperparathyroidism by a low or low normal serum PTH concentration. In this situation, low-grade haematological malignancies are more likely, such as leukaemias or lymphomas. In such cases the hypercalcaemia frequently responds to steroid therapy, which is unusual in most forms of hypercalcaemic malignancy.

Vitamin D intoxication

Vitamin D intoxication almost always occurs in patients known to be on vitamin D therapy and only rarely in patients surreptitiously taking the vitamin. For this reason, routine measurements of vitamin D are unnecessary in the investigation of hypercalcaemia. The greater use of potent vitamin D metabolites has led to a greater incidence of vitamin D intoxication. Temporary withdrawal of treatment is usually all that is required. When more severe, steroid therapy may be required.

Other causes

Sarcoidosis and thyrotoxicosis are rarer causes of hypercalcaemia, which can usually be suspected from the history or initial investigation of the patient.

References

1. Heath DA. Primary hyperparathyroidism: clinical presentation and factors influencing clinical management. *Endocrinol. Metabol. Clin. North Am.* 1989;**18**:631–46.

2. Mundy GR, Cove DH, Fisken RA, Heath DA, Somers S. Primary hyperparathyroidism: changes in the pattern of clinical presentation. *Lancet* 1980;**1**:1317–20.

3. Ratcliffe WA, Heath DA, Ryan M, Jones SR. Performance and diagnostic application of a two site immunoradiometric assay for parathyrin in serum. *Clin. Chem.* 1989;**35**:1957–61.

4. Heath DA, Heath EM. Conservative management of primary hyperparathyroidism. *J. Bone Miner. Res.* 1991;**6**(suppl. 2):5117–20.

5. Silverberg SJ, Gartenberg F, Jacobs TP *et al.* Longitudinal measurements of bone density and biochemical indices in untreated primary hyperparathyroidism. *J. Clin. Endocrinol. Metab.* 1995;**80**(3):723–8.

6. Silverberg SJ, Gartenberg F, Jacobs TP *et al.* Increased bone mineral density after parathyroidectomy in primary hyperparathyroidism. *J. Clin. Endocrinol. Metab.* 1995;**80**(3):729–34.

7. Larsson K, Ljunghall S, Krusema UB *et al.* The risk of hip fractures in patients with primary hyperparathyroidism; a population based cohort study with a follow up of 19 years. *J. Intern. Med.* 1993;**234**:585–93.

8. Mitchell BK, Kinder BK, Cornelius E, Stewart AF. Primary hyperparathyroidism: preoperative localisation using technetium-sestamibi scanning. *J. Clin. Endocrinol. Metab.* 1995;**80**(1):7–10.

9. Heath DA. Familial hypocalciuric hypercalcemia. In Bilezikian JP, Levine MA, Marcus R (eds). *The Parathyroids.* New York:Raven Press, 1994:699–710.

10. Brown EM, Gamba G, Riccardi D *et al.* Cloning and characterization of an extra-cellular Ca^{2+}-sensing receptor from bovine parathyroid. *Nature* 1993;**366**:575-80.

Parathyroid Carcinoma

HITOSHI MIKI AND LORRAINE A. FITZPATRICK

Introduction

Parathyroid carcinoma is a rare and unusual clinical entity. However, it is important to consider the disease in the differential diagnosis of primary hyperparathyroidism due to the substantial morbidity and mortality, and the fact that the best prognosis is associated with an *en bloc* resection at the time of initial operation. Since the first case description in 1933, about 300 cases of parathyroid carcinoma have been reported [1–4]. In this chapter, clinical manifestations, treatment and outcome of parathyroid carcinoma are reviewed.

Aetiology

The aetiology of parathyroid carcinoma is usually unknown, but in a few patients the possibility of radiation-induced malignant change or adenoma-to-carcinoma transformation has been proposed. Recently, the *PRAD1* or cyclin *D1* gene, a cell-cycle regulator, has been implicated in a subgroup of benign parathyroid tumours. The retinoblastoma tumour-suppressor gene (*RB*) is another cell-cycle regulator with functional links to *PRAD1*. In 88% of nine patients with parathyroid carcinoma, abnormal expression of RB protein was found, suggesting that inactivation of the *RB* gene is common in parathyroid carcinoma and may contribute to its molecular pathogenesis [5].

Incidence

Currently, the incidence of parathyroid carcinoma in all patients with primary hyperparathyroidism is about 1% [3,6], although previously the reported incidence was as high as 5% [2]. The incidence of carcinoma has not increased proportionally in spite of an increase in the incidence of asymptomatic primary hyperparathyroidism due to the introduction of the multichannel analyser and routine measurement of serum calcium concentrations.

Clinical manifestations and diagnosis

Parathyroid carcinoma has a tendency to occur in males and females proportionately, in contradistinction to benign hyperparathyroidism, which is much more common in women. The average age of patients with carcinoma was reported to be 44–54 years, in contrast to the higher age of 57–62 years in patients with benign disease. However, reflections of sex and age are of little help in confirming the diagnosis in the individual patient.

Although a few cases of the non-functioning parathyroid carcinoma were reported [7], most cases of parathyroid carcinoma are functional. Patients with functioning carcinoma frequently have clinically severe hyperparathyroidism due to the effects of excessive secretion of parathyroid hormone (PTH) rather than to invasion of adjacent organs by the tumour. The common symptoms are related to hypercalcaemia and include generalized fatigue, polydipsia, polyuria, myalgias, arthralgias and weight loss. Moreover, patients with carcinoma have a greater incidence of renal and bone disease in comparison with patients with benign hyperparathyroidism. In a recent series of 43 patients with parathyroid carcinoma, the reported prevalence of nephrolithiasis, renal insufficiency and bone involvement was 56, 84 and 91%, respectively. Both stone and bone disease were noted in 53% of patients [3]. In contrast, the incidence of renal involvement, and that of bone involvement accompanied with specific radiological signs in the patients with benign hyperparathyroidism were reported to vary from 4 to 37% and 14 to 20%, respectively. Using more sensitive densitometric techniques, a recent series reported 61% prevalence of reduction of bone mineral density [8]. Concomitant bone and stone disease in the patients with benign primary hyperparathyroidism is rare. Another clinical finding that differentiates parathyroid carcinoma from benign primary hyperparathyroidism is a palpable neck mass detectable in one-fourth to one-half of patients with carcinoma.

In a case of hyperparathyroidism, the diagnosis of parathyroid carcinoma should be considered in patients with severe hypercalcaemia, because most benign parathyroid lesions cause mild hypercalcaemia. The serum calcium concentration of patients with carcinoma is usually much higher, generally > 3.5 mmol/l (> 14 mg/dl). PTH levels are also remarkably higher (three to ten times the upper limit of normal) than those seen in patients with benign parathyroid disease (commonly less than twice normal). Serum alkaline phosphatase level is higher in patients with carcinoma, reflecting the high incidence of bone involvement, as compared to patients with benign hyperparathyroidism. The preoperative diagnosis of parathyroid carcinoma is very difficult to make. However, patients with a palpable neck mass, markedly elevated levels of serum calcium (> 3.5 mmol/l; > 14 mg/dl), PTH and alkaline phosphatase, and combined renal and bone disease should be suspected of having parathyroid carcinoma (Table 21.1).

Non-invasive localization studies such as ultrasonography are considered diagnostic of parathyroid carcinoma preoperatively. The presence of malignancy should be considered when signs of gross invasion of surrounding structures and marked irregularity of the tumour margin are demonstrated by ultrasonography [9]. Fine needle aspiration cytology (FNAC) is not recommended if there is any suspicion of parathyroid carcinoma.

Surgical findings are very important and supportive in confirming the diagnosis of parathyroid malignancy. It is frequently difficult to confirm the diagnosis from examination of frozen sections at the time of operation.

Table 21.1 Predictive findings of parathyroid carcinoma

Clinical findings	Laboratory data	Intraoperative findings
Symptoms of severe hypercalcaemia	Serum calcium (> 3.5mmol/l; > 14 mg/dl)	Greyish-white, lobulated, firm or hard tumour
Concomitant bone and stone disease	Parathyroid hormone > three times above the upper limit of normal	Adhesion to or invasion of surrounding structures
Palpable neck mass or recurrent laryngeal nerve palsy in a patient with hyperparathyroidism	Serum alkaline phosphatase > three times above the upper limit of normal	

Grossly, parathyroid carcinoma is characterized by a greyish-white, lobulated, firm or hard mass, and is frequently accompanied by surrounding dense fibrous reaction. Calcification and necrosis are occasionally present. In contrast, the typical benign lesion is usually reddish-brown, round or oval, and soft. Confirmation of capsular or vascular invasion, increased mitotic figures and the presence of fibrous trabeculae in the specimen can be obtained by examination of permanent pathological sections.

Initial treatment

As soon as the diagnosis of primary hyperparathyroidism is made, surgical removal of the diseased parathyroid gland is recommended. Preoperative management of hypercalcaemia consists of vigorous hydration by infusion of isotonic saline and early consideration of the use of bisphosphonates. Other adjuvant medications used for lowering serum calcium include calcitonin and mithramycin. If the patient manifests severe hypercalcaemia along with renal failure, which is sometimes encountered in the patient with parathyroid carcinoma, haemodialysis may be the primary preoperative mode of management.

Surgery

The sole most effective treatment for parathyroid carcinoma is complete surgical resection of tumour, accomplished best at the first operation, since attempts at resection of a recurrent tumour are less likely to lead to a complete cure. In a neck operation for the patient whose clinical findings are suggestive of parathyroid carcinoma, a large collar incision and a transverse section of the strap muscle are made to provide a wide operative field and an exploration of all four parathyroid glands is usually carried out in order to be prepared for the rare combination of adenoma or hyperplasia and carcinoma. The initial operation should be *en bloc* resection, which is usually accompanied by ipsilateral thyroid lobectomy and excision of paratracheal and upper mediastinal lymph nodes. Although the reported incidence of cervical lymph node metastasis is < 20%, the routine dissection of regional nodes appears to be essential [2]. The recurrent laryngeal nerve may be preserved if it can be separated readily from the tumour. Otherwise, sacrifice of the nerve is necessary.

Successful removal usually brings about a marked fall of the serum calcium level, which is controlled by intravenous or oral administration of calcium salt together with oral administration of calcitriol. Replacement of 10 ml of 10% calcium gluconate i.v. over 10 minutes is

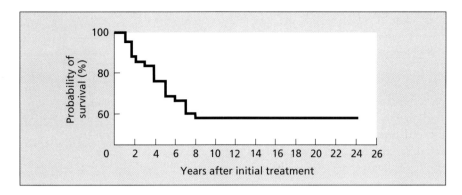

Fig. 21.1 Kaplan–Meier survival analysis of 43 patients with parathyroid carcinoma.

given in an emergency. This can then be followed by 100 ml of 10% calcium gluconate in 1 litre of normal saline over 8 hours. This infusion rate can be adjusted according to results of the serum calcium. When the patient is stable, long term maintenance of the serum calcium can be achieved with oral calcium supplements (1–2 g of elemental calcium/day) and vitamin D supplements (1–4 mg of one alpha/day or 1–2 µg calcitriol) if deficiency is proven.

Serum calcium and PTH levels should be monitored regularly, as the disease may recur after several years.

Outcome

Parathyroid carcinoma carries the risk of local recurrence or distant metastases even after a successful initial *en bloc* resection, and the rate of recurrent disease was recently reported to be 41–67%. Usually patients with recurrent or metastatic parathyroid carcinoma present with recurrent hypercalcaemia from the release of PTH from cancer cells rather than symptoms caused by local tumour growth. The average time between initial surgery and the recurrent disease is approximately 3 years and local recurrence or metastases to the regional lymph nodes or the lung are common.

The management of recurrent or metastatic parathyroid carcinoma is also surgical. Once the tumour has recurred, complete cure is less likely. However, aggressive repeated resection of local recurrent tumours or even distant metastases can provide effective alleviation of recurrent hypercalcaemia and this palliation occasionally prolongs life for several years [10,11]. Parathyroid carcinoma grows slowly and mortality and morbidity are related to the metabolic consequences of hypercalcaemia. When the operation for recurrent disease is impossible or unsuccessful, other non-surgical therapies should be tried. Chemotherapy has only rarely been of benefit in a few patients. Although radiation therapy is frequently ineffective, one case has been in remission 11 years after

receiving radiation therapy [3]. Another therapy is medical treatment, which is directed at inhibiting bone resorption and enhancing urinary calcium excretion, to control the hypercalcaemia. Medical treatment includes a variety of drugs such as oestrogen, calcitonin, mithramycin, gallium nitrate and bisphosphonates. Efficacy is variable and should be evaluated in each case.

Most deaths are usually due to cardiac or renal complications, or uncontrolled hypercalcaemia instead of local invasion by the tumour. Five-year survival rates after initial resection of parathyroid carcinoma are reported to be 40–69% (Fig. 21.1).

References

1. Shane E, Bilezikian JP. Parathyroid carcinoma: a review of 62 patients. *Endocr. Rev.* 1982;**3**:218–26.
2. Obara T, Fujimoto Y. Diagnosis and treatment of patients with parathyroid carcinoma: an update and review. *World J. Surg.* 1991;**15**:738–44.
3. Wynne AG, van Heerden J, Carney JA, Fitzpatrick LA. Parathyroid carcinoma: clinical and pathologic features in 43 patients. *Medicine* 1992;**71**:197–205.
4. Vetto JT, Brennan MF, Woodruf J, Burt M. Parathyroid carcinoma: diagnosis and clinical history. *Surgery* 1993;**114**:882–92.
5. Cryns VL, Thor A, Xu HJ *et al.* Loss of the retinoblastoma tumor-suppressor gene in parathyroid carcinoma. *N. Engl. J. Med.* 1994;**330**:757–61.
6. Shane E. Parathyroid carcinoma. In Bilezikian JP, Levine MA, Marcus R (eds). *The Parathyroids.* New York: Raven Press, 1994:575–81.
7. Klink BK, Karulf RE, Maimon WN, Peoples JB. Nonfunctioning parathyroid carcinoma. *Am. Surg.* 1991;**57**:463–7.
8. Silverberg SJ, Shane E, Jacobs TP *et al.* Nephrolithiasis and bone involvement in primary hyperparathyroidism. *Am. J. Med.* 1990;**89**:327–34.
9. Daly BD, Coofey SL, Behan M. Ultrasonographic appearance of parathyroid carcinoma. *Br. J. Radiol.* 1989;**62**:1017–19.
10. Sandelin K, Thompson NW, Bondeson L. Metastatic parathyroid carcinoma; dilemmas in management. *Surgery* 1991;**110**:978–88.
11. Shortell CK, Andrus CH, Phillips CE Jr, Schwartz SI. Carcinoma of the parathyroid gland: a 30-year experience. *Surgery* 1991;**110**:704–8.

3

PITUITARY AND
HYPOTHALAMIC LESIONS

23

Endocrine Assessment

JOHN NEWELL-PRICE

Introduction

The evaluation of neuroendocrine status requires the integration of information gained in the clinical setting with the appropriate biochemical and imaging investigations. Pituitary hormone levels are assessed basally followed by dynamic tests where indicated. The significance of a borderline low value may be established by a stimulatory test, whilst suppression tests may be needed in conditions of hormonal excess. Symptoms and signs of expanding pituitary fossa masses are predictable from the anatomy of this region. Imaging techniques provide valuable information with respect to the anatomy, allow planning and evaluation of therapeutic intervention, and furthermore often give insights into the underlying aetiology of dysfunction.

Pituitary lesions represent some 10–15% of all intracranial tumours [1]. The prevalence of symptomatic pituitary tumours was 8.9/100 000 in the USA in 1950 [2]. They may present with symptoms of endocrine dysfunction, a mass effect, or both together; there may be either hyposecretion or hypersecretion of pituitary hormones, or both in combination. In addition to primary sellar disease, previous pituitary surgery or irradiation, head injury and parasellar disease may present in a similar fashion, with varying degrees of partial or total hypopituitarism. Anterior pituitary function should be assessed and deficiencies remedied with hormone replacement, prior to the investigation of posterior pituitary function. This chapter deals with the assessment of hypopituitarism associated with pituitary and hypothalamic lesions. The assessment of anterior hormone secretion is the same irrespective of the many causes of hypopituitarism.

Pituitary hormones

The anterior pituitary secretes six major hormones, each with its own target organ and feedback hormone(s). In cases of an expanding lesion within, or impinging upon, the pituitary gland there usually appears a sequential loss of hormone secretion in the following order: growth hormone (GH), luteinizing hormone (LH) and follicle-stimulating hormone (FSH), thyroid-stimulating hormone (TSH) and adrenocorticotrophic hormone (ACTH). Deficiency of prolactin usually represents infarction of the gland. The posterior pituitary secretes oxytocin and vasopressin.

Clinical and biochemical aspects of pituitary hypofunction

Anterior pituitary

Gonadotrophin deficiency

In men, hypogonadism presents with diminishing libido, impotence, infertility, loss of body hair and reduction in shaving frequency. Reduction of muscle bulk, and in long-standing cases, osteopaenia, will supervene. The testes will be diminished in volume, which should be assessed with a Prader orchidometer, and of a softer consistency. A low serum testosterone in conjunction with a low LH confirms a diagnosis of hypogonadotrophic hypogonadism. In women, hot flushes, vaginal dryness, oligomenorrhoea, amenorrhoea, loss of libido and the development of osteopaenia result from the deficiency of oestrogen, and again gonadotrophins will be low. In both sexes a fine, wrinkled skin develops. If occurring in childhood, fusion of long bone epiphyses will be delayed giving rise to a eunachoid appearance, the span being greater than the height. Dynamic testing of gonadotrophin reserve is usually not indicated and is most often performed by a clomiphene stimulation test. Clomiphene 3 mg/kg in divided doses (maximum 200 mg/day) is given for 7 days, and serum LH and FSH is measured on days 0, 4, 7 and 10. A lack of a rise to above the normal range, or a lack of doubling of the basal value suggests gonadotrophin deficiency due to pituitary or hypothalamic disease.

Growth hormone deficiency

Deficiency of GH in adults may be without specific symptoms, but may be disclosed during the evaluation of suspected pituitary disease. By convention, levels of less than 20 mu/l on provocative testing are considered as deficient. GH-deficient adults have a higher proportion of central fat, a lower bone density, an apparent increase in cardiovascular morbidity and mortality, and subjective lack of well-being [3]. Currently, intensive studies are seeking to establish the role of GH replacement in deficient adults. Neonatal GH deficiency may present with hypoglycaemia, older children exhibit decreased growth velocity. GH is secreted in a pulsatile fashion and single random estimations are thus unhelpful. Deficiency is established by the insulin tolerance test (ITT) (Table 23.1, Fig. 23.1) and when this is contraindicated the glucagon stimulation test may be employed. Concern has arisen about the safety of the ITT, especially in children, but when performed in a specialist unit it is a safe procedure [4]. Synthetic GH-releasing hormone (GHRH) analogues such as Hexarelin are undergoing evaluation for this purpose.

Table 23.1 Insulin tolerance test

Indications	Assessment of ACTH/cortisol and GH reserve
Contraindications	Ischaemic heart disease, epilepsy/unexplained blackouts
Precautions	Normal ECG Normal serum T_4 5 and 20% dextrose and hydrocortisone available in intravenous form
Procedure	Fast from midnight Weigh patient, i.v. cannula 08.30 h Soluble human insulin i.v. bolus 09.00 h Usual dose: 0.15 u/kg (0.3 u/kg in acromegaly or Cushing's syndrome) Sample serum for cortisol, GH and glucose at 0, 30, 45, 60, 90 and 120 minutes Observe pulse and look for signs of hypoglycaemia
Normal response	Blood glucose: < 2.2 mmol/l Serum cortisol: rise by more than 170 nmol/l to > 580 nmol/l Growth hormone: rise to > 20 mu/l
Interpretation for cortisol response	Adequate hypoglycaemia must be achieved Normal responders will withstand major surgery, without corticosteroid cover If response just subnormal, corticosteroid cover needed for major surgery or illness — carry steroid card/MedicAlert Other subnormal responders require hydrocortisone replacement

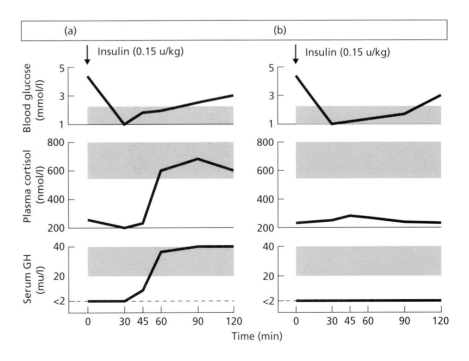

Fig. 23.1 Insulin tolerance test: (a) normal responses; (b) hypopituitary responses.

Thyrotrophin deficiency

Thyrotrophin deficiency is a rare cause of hypothyroidism. Cold insensitivity, weight gain, constipation and skin dryness feature, and in children there is growth retardation. The symptoms are generally less severe than in primary hypothyroidism. A low level of T_4 in conjunction with an inappropriately low TSH confirms the diagnosis. TRH testing does not add further information. The distinction between pituitary and hypothalamic causes is now facilitated by improved neuroradiology.

ACTH deficiency

Isolated ACTH deficiency is extremely rare. Varying degrees of deficiency may occur following pituitary surgery or irradiation, or as part of non-iatrogenic panhypopituitarism. Secondary adrenal insufficiency will result. As the mineralocorticoid axis remains intact, severe crises are less common than in primary adrenal insufficiency caused by destruction of the adrenal glands. Presentation tends to include lethargy, anorexia, malaise, postural hypotension and weight loss. Less commonly, intercurrent illness will unmask the deficiency, causing an adrenal crisis. In contrast to the pigmentation that develops in primary adrenal failure as a result of high levels of circulating pro-opiomelanocortin (POMC) products, the skin becomes pale. The secretion of ACTH, an extremely labile peptide, is pulsatile and follows a circadian rhythm, being highest on waking and falling to undetectable levels at midnight when asleep. It may be assayed by both radioimmunoassay (RIA) and immunoradiometric assay (IRMA) methodologies, but following sampling requires immediate cold centrifugation and subsequent freezing. An 09.00 h serum cortisol of 500 nmol/l or greater means that significant deficiency is unlikely, whilst an undetectable level (< 50 nmol/l) is highly suggestive of ACTH deficiency. Intermediate values require an ITT (see Table 23.1, Fig. 23.1) or glucagon stimulation test to establish the hypothalamus–pituitary–adrenal axis reserve. This is of particular relevance when planning corticosteroid cover for pituitary surgery. The use of the short synacthen test for this purpose is not yet established.

Prolactin

Release of prolactin is under tonic inhibition by dopamine. Factors interfering with this will thus allow serum levels to rise. Excess prolactin causes oligomenorrhoea, amenorrhoea, and galactorrhoea. Levels of this hormone are raised by pregnancy, phenothiazines, all anti-emetics except cyclizine, pituitary tumours, hypothalamic and stalk lesions, primary hypothyroidism, polycystic ovarian syndrome, renal failure, nipple stimulation, stress of phlebotomy and post-ictally. These factors need to be borne in mind when interpreting raised values, which should be tested on at least three occasions. In pituitary tumours a normal serum prolactin, whatever the size of tumour, or in macroadenomas a serum level of less than 2–3000 mu/l, is suggestive of a non-functioning tumour [5]. In these tumours, small doses of D_2 agonists such as bromocriptine reduce prolactin levels to normal but there is no change in the size of the tumour.

Posterior pituitary

Oxytocin is involved in the milk let-down reflex, and will not be considered further. Vasopressin is synthesized in paraventricular and supra-optic nuclei of the hypothalamus. Transport to the posterior pituitary lobe is via neuronal axons. From here release will be stimulated in response to a raised serum osmolality, or less commonly to a reduction in blood volume. Deficiency in synthesis, or interruption of the pituitary stalk will result in cranial diabetes insipidus (DI). This is not usually associated with primary anterior pituitary adenomas, and its presence suggests an alternative diagnosis from anterior pituitary tumour. Features include polyuria and polydipsia, and in severe cases in which access to water is denied, dehydration may result. If suspected, simultaneous plasma (P) and urine (U) osmolalities on rising should be measured. In DI the serum osmolality is usually raised above the normal range of 280–295 mmol/kg, and the urine is inappropriately dilute, the U : P ratio being less than two. When doubt exists a water deprivation test should be performed [6].

Manifestations of pituitary mass effect

The pituitary fossa has bony margins anteroposteriorly, whilst laterally lies the meshwork of the cavernous sinuses containing the internal carotid artery and cranial nerves III, IV, V_1, V_2 and VI. Superiorly the diaphragma sella separates the opic chiasm from this region; inferiorly lies the sphenoid. The effects of mass expansion within this area may thus be predicted, and depend upon size and anatomical position.

Headache is a common presenting feature of pituitary tumours resulting from dural stretching, even in a microadenoma confined to the fossa, particularly if it is locally invasive. The site of pain is often retro-orbital or bitemporal, and may decrease over the course of the day and be relieved by analgesics. A catastrophic headache is associated with pituitary apoplexy, caused by pituitary tumour haemorrhage. A large tumour, such as a germinoma or craniopharingioma, may, rarely, cause obstructive hydrocephalus (Fig. 23.2). Uncommonly (5% of pituitary tumours) lateral extension will impinge upon the cranial nerves resulting in various combinations of opthalmoplegia and peri-orbital pain (Fig. 23.3). In one large series, 42% of cases presented with visual loss and diplopia in less than 1% [7]. Rarely, inferior erosion of the sella turcica may lead to CSF rhinorrhoea (fluid contains glucose), and the potential for meningitis. Very extensive lateral enlargement may, rarely, cause temporal lobe epilepsy. If extensive superior extension impinges upon the hypothalamus, there may result disturbances in temperature regulation, disturbed levels of consciousness, hyperphagia and altered thirst.

Compression of the optic chiasm by suprasellar extension is far more common and will lead to visual field and visual acuity disturbances (Fig. 23.4). The pattern of field loss depends upon the size of tumour and its relative position to the optic chiasm. In 80% of individuals the chiasm lies directly above the pituitary gland; in 15% it lies in an anterior position above the tuberculum sella, a prefixed chiasm; in the remaining 5% the chiasm is post-fixed lying over the dorsum sellae. Assessment of acuity should utilize Snellen charts, although in long-standing compression there may be blindness. Fundoscopy is

(a)

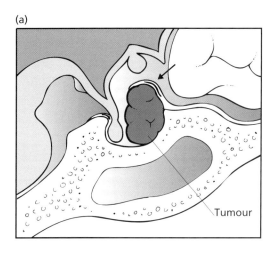

(b)

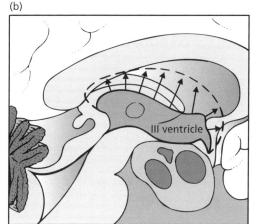

Fig. 23.2 The local effects of a pituitary tumour causing headaches are (a) mainly due to stretching of the dura by the tumour; and (b) rarely, due to hydrocephalus.

(a)

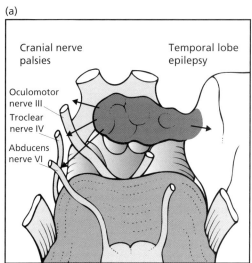

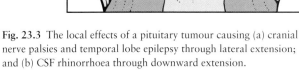

(b)

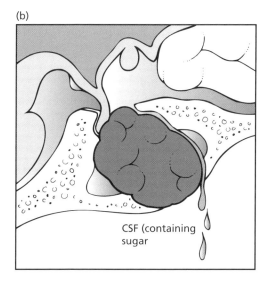

Fig. 23.3 The local effects of a pituitary tumour causing (a) cranial nerve palsies and temporal lobe epilepsy through lateral extension; and (b) CSF rhinorrhoea through downward extension.

(a)

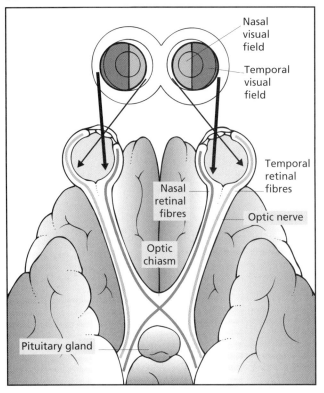

Nasal visual field

Temporal visual field

Temporal retinal fibres

Nasal retinal fibres

Optic nerve

Optic chiasm

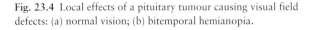

Pituitary gland

(b)

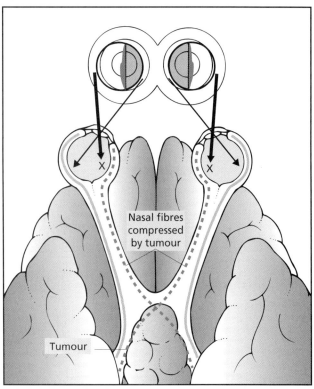

Nasal fibres compressed by tumour

Tumour

Fig. 23.4 Local effects of a pituitary tumour causing visual field defects: (a) normal vision; (b) bitemporal hemianopia.

mandatory in all cases. Visual desaturation to a red pin on confrontational testing may disclose early compression. Perimetry should be performed and the Goldman apparatus remains the standard means of assessment.

Occasionally visual evoked responses may offer additional guidance in the delineation between compressive and demyelinating lesions. Typically, five characteristic field losses occur. Most commonly a bitemporal upper quadrantic defect, with normal acuity, is the result of compression of the inferior nasal fibres from below. Further tumour expansion may cause complete bitemporal hemianopia. Optic neuropathy, with a normal contralateral field will result from anterosuperior tumour expansion and is particularly likely if the chiasm is postfixed. Compression of contralateral inferonasal fibres as they loop forward forming Willibrand's knee, will cause decreased ipsilateral acuity and contralateral upper quadrantic field loss. Posterior chiasmal compression produces bitemporal scotomatous loss, as perimacular fibres are impinged upon, although acuity is preserved. Finally compression of the optic tract by superoposterior extension, or when a prefixed chiasm is present, results

in a homonomous hemianopia. Hypothalamic lesions such as craniopharyngiomas and germinomas will tend to produce these latter two types of visual field loss. It is important to note that changes in visual fields may occur with no great alteration in tumour size on imaging. These techniques thus represent a sensitive means of assessing disease progression, or indeed improvement following therapeutic intervention. Such improvement may occur within hours to days of surgery or the initiation of medical treatment on pituitary lesions (Fig. 23.5).

Pituitary imaging

Imaging of the pituitary fossa region is of vital importance for diagnostic purposes and in the planning of therapeutic intervention and further assessment of its effect. Suprasellar extension may be accurately documented. Magnetic resonance imaging (MRI) is of particular value in this respect as details of internal carotid blood flow may be gained without recourse to invasive angiography, or indeed even intravenous contrast media (see Chapter 24). Postoperative films are required to act as a baseline from which to judge recurrence. Furthermore MRI and computed tomography (CT) provide ideal means of evaluating the response to medical therapy such as in tumour shrinkage of a macroprolactinoma when treated with

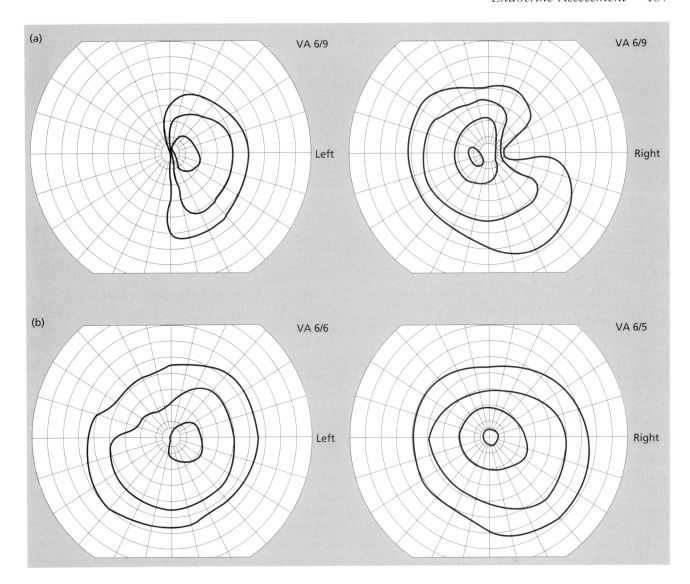

Fig. 23.5 Improvement in visual fields following treatment with bromocriptine of a prolactinoma: (a) before treatment; (b) after treatment.

the dopamine D_2-receptor agonists bromocriptine or carbergoline.

References

1. Kovacs K, Horvath E. Pathology of pituitary tumours. *Endocrinol. Metab. Clin. North Am.* 1987;**16**:585–608.
2. Vance ML. Hypopituitarism. *N. Engl. J. Med.* 1994;**330**:1651–62.
3. Shalet SM, Holmes SI. Growth hormone replacement in adults. *Br. Med. J.* 1994;**308**:1314–15.
4. Jones SL, Trainer PS, Perry L *et al.* An audit of the insulin tolerance test in adult subjects in an acute investigation unit over one year. *Clin. Endocrinol.* 1993;**41**:123–8.
5. Vance ML, Thorner MO. Prolactin: hyperprolactinemic syndromes and management. In DeGroot LY (ed.). *Endocrinology.* Philadelphia: W.B. Saunders, 1989:408–18.
6. Baylis PH, Thompson CJ. Osmoregulation of vasopressin secretion and thirst in health and disease. *Clin. Endocrinol.* 1988;**29**:549–76.
7. Hollenhorst RW, Younge BR. Ocular manifestations produced by adenomas of the pituitary gland: analysis of 1000 cases. In Kohler PO, Ross GT (eds). *Diagnosis and Treatment of Pituitary Tumours.* New York: American Elsevier, 1973:53–64.

Imaging of the Pituitary and Hypothalamus

PETER ARMSTRONG AND MICHAEL CHARLESWORTH

Introduction

Both computed tomography (CT) and magnetic resonance imaging (MRI) provide detailed anatomical information about the pituitary and hypothalamus [1]. With modern equipment, MRI is the optimal imaging technique, although CT can provide almost equivalent information, providing high-quality sections of 1.5 mm or less are available and multiplanar reconstructions are used. The advantages of MRI are that imaging in any desired plane is very simple, it can show higher inherent contrast between tissues and there is no ionizing radiation. It should be noted, however, that MRI is far less sensitive than CT or even plain X-ray film for demonstrating calcification in tumours and other pathological processes. The plain skull film provides very limited information. It can demonstrate calcification in heavily calcified tumours, notably cranio-pharyngiomas, and will show hyperostosis at the base of some meningiomas. The pituitary fossa balloons with large intrasellar tumours and may show pressure deformity with large suprasellar tumours. On rare occasions, the skull X-ray provides the first evidence of a sellar or parasellar tumour, but in the great majority of cases the information provided is subsidiary to the details obtained from MRI or CT and adds little of clinical value. The advantage of plain skull radiographs is that they are relatively inexpensive and easy to obtain. They may, therefore, be useful for follow-up.

With both MRI and CT it is possible to identify the shape and dimensions of the pituitary gland, the pituitary stalk and the hypothalamic region. It is not possible separately to visualize the hypothalamic nuclei, but the boundaries of the hypothalamus (the optic chiasm, third ventricle and mammillary bodies) are clearly visible. The anterior and posterior lobes of the pituitary are separately identifiable by MRI, and the cavernous sinuses can be identified on both MRI and contrast-enhanced CT scans, but the medial walls of the cavernous sinuses (the lateral boundary of the pituitary fossa) are not demonstrable by either modality.

There are two basic methods of CT imaging of the hypothalamo-pituitary region: axial and coronal. Coronal scans provide sections through the pituitary analogous to viewing the region from the front of the patient. They are the optimal imaging plane to show the size of the pituitary gland, in particular any upward bulging, asymmetry, or suprasellar extension (Fig. 24.1), but coronal scans require patients to hold their heads in a markedly extended position. While this position can often be maintained without movement during an individual exposure, it is difficult for a patient to keep still long enough for the multiple sections needed for multiplanar reconstruction. Axial sections with the head in a comfortable position are, therefore, used for top-quality imaging if multiplanar reconstructions are required (Fig. 24.2), but they have the real disadvantage of significant radiation dose to the lens of the eye. The term multiplanar reconstruction refers to the technique of obtaining several adjacent thin sections and then reconstructing the data to display images in alternative planes from the one used to acquire the imaging data. High-quality coronal and sagittal images, for example, can be reconstructed from axial sections provided the axial sections are thin enough, for example 1.0–1.5 mm. The axial sections in themselves are of limited value. Contrast-enhanced images can be obtained quickly, allowing discrimination of enhancing as opposed to non-enhancing tissues. This is particularly useful when demonstrating small pituitary adenomas (Fig. 24.3).

Many different MRI sequences are in use in various centres around the world. The technique used by the authors is to obtain T_1-weighted spin-echo images, with pre- and postcontrast enhanced images, when necessary, supplemented by T_1-weighted gradient echo images taken with three-dimensional Fourier transform (3D FT) techniques which enable display in any desired plane simply by manipulating the data on the console. The

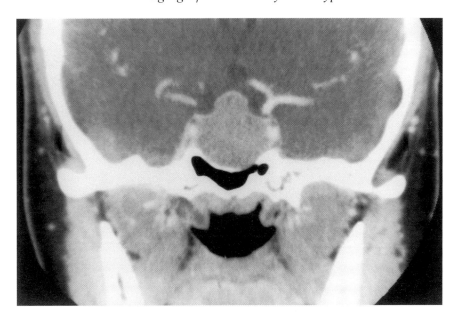

Fig. 24.1 Direct coronal CT scan following intravenous contrast enhancement showing a pituitary adenoma. Note how easy it is to see the suprasellar extension, which in this case was compressing and elevating the optic chiasm.

technical aspects of MRI contrast are complex and well beyond the scope of this chapter. Suffice it to say that on T_1-weighted images cerebrospinal fluid (CSF) appears dark grey, and brain substance, including the optic chiasm, hypothalamus, pituitary and pituitary stalk, appears much whiter than CSF. T_1-weighted images, therefore, show the boundaries of the pituitary and hypothalamic regions exquisitely well (Fig. 24.4a). The posterior pituitary is separately identifiable in 90% of normal patients due to the presence of high signal on T_1-weighted images (Fig. 24.4b), whereas the signal of the anterior lobe is similar to normal white matter. The posterior pituitary high signal is believed to be due to phospholipids in the neurosecretory granules of the posterior lobe.

Intravenously administered contrast media can be used for MRI in a similar manner to contrast-enhancement for CT. The contrast agents are, however, different in chemical composition and produce their contrast in a different manner. Central nervous system MRI contrast agents are currently all gadolinium compounds. Gadolinium, a paramagnetic element, changes the adjacent magnetic field so that signals from regions containing gadolinium are higher on T_1-weighted images than they would be without the contrast agent. Gadolinium is toxic and is therefore administered as a chelate. Gadolinium chelates, like the iodinated media used for CT, do not cross the intact blood–brain barrier. The pituitary and pituitary stalk have no blood–brain barrier and, therefore, enhance brightly on T_1-weighted images. The normal brain substance, including the optic chiasm and hypothalamus, shows no enhancement. Thus, enhancing areas of the pituitary are normal (Fig. 24.5), whereas enhancing

areas in the brain are abnormal. An important point to bear in mind is that in normal individuals the cavernous sinus, the meninges and the mucosa of the paranasal sinuses all show bright enhancement following intravenous gadolinium contrast agents.

Tumours of the pituitary and suprasellar regions

Clinical and endocrinological features play a very important part in diagnosing the nature of tumours in the pituitary and suprasellar regions and often point to a specific diagnosis, particularly if the tumour secretes one or more hormones.

The imaging features of tumours are essentially the demonstration of a mass and displacement of adjacent structures by the mass. Characterizing the nature of a tumour is based on its location, particularly on the presumed site of origin, its shape and size, and on the density/intensity characteristics of the mass.

Pituitary adenomas

Tumours may arise in the anterior lobe of the pituitary; the majority are benign adenomas, though a few are locally invasive and may even metastasize. The size of tumour at presentation varies from 2 mm or even less, in the case of adrenocorticotrophic hormone (ACTH)-producing adenomas, to very large, in the case of non-functioning tumours or those that produce prolactin or growth hormone. Macroadenomas (defined as tumours of greater than 1 cm in diameter) cause recognizable enlargement

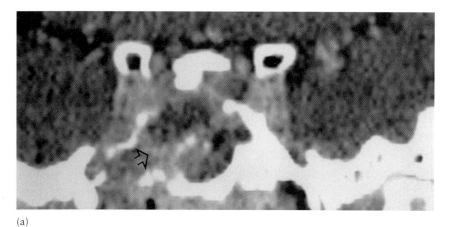

(a)

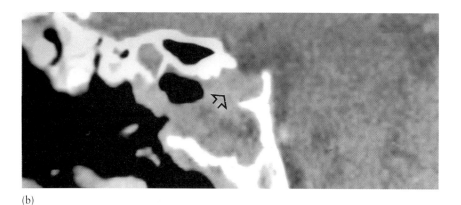

(b)

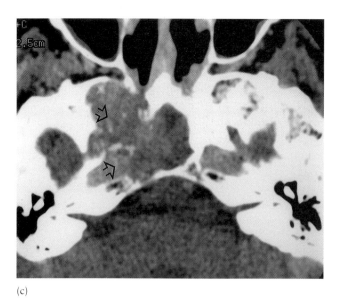

(c)

Fig. 24.2 (a) Coronal and (b) sagittal reconstructions of CT scans in a patient with Nelson's syndrome (pituitary tumour consequent upon adrenalectomy for control of pituitary-dependent Cushing's) showing erosion into the adjacent skull base. (c) One of the axial images used for the reconstructions. The arrows in (a–c) point to the extensive bone destruction by the tumour.

of the gland on CT or MRI, whereas microadenomas may or may not deform the outer contour of the gland.

On T$_1$-weighted MR images pituitary adenomas are of slightly lower signal intensity than the adjacent anterior pituitary tissue (Fig. 24.6), a difference that is markedly accentuated for a short period after contrast enhancement with a gadolinium chelate [2] (see Fig. 24.5). With CT the difference in density between tumours and adjacent tissue is only recognizable after the use of intravenous contrast enhancement (see Fig. 24.3).

Bigger pituitary tumours may show cystic degeneration (Fig. 24.7), calcification (recognizable on CT, but

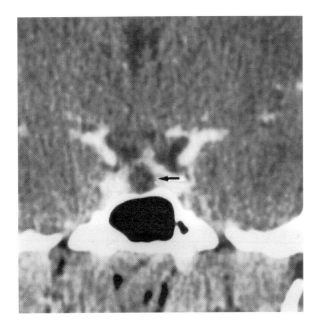

Fig. 24.3 Contrast-enhanced direct coronal CT scan showing the differences in enhancement between the pituitary adenoma (arrow), which does not enhance, and the adjacent normal pituitary gland which enhances substantially.

not usually on MRI), or the features of haemorrhage into the gland. Subacute haemorrhage shows specific signal characteristics at MRI: high signal on T_1- and T_2-weighted

images [3]. Large tumours extend upwards into the suprasellar cistern and may compress the optic chiasm and hypothalamus (Fig. 24.8). Invasive tumours grow into the cavernous sinus, surround the adjacent internal carotid arteries and may even invade the adjacent brain substance (Fig. 24.9). These features are most readily demonstrated with MRI.

Craniopharyngioma

Craniopharyngiomas are benign tumours which develop from cell remnants of Rathke's cleft. They are slow-growing tumours that often have large cystic elements, a feature that is readily demonstrated by imaging. These tumours are most frequently encountered in childhood with a peak incidence between 5 and 10 years of age, although adult cases are reported. They usually arise in a suprasellar location and grow down into the pituitary fossa, the clinical effects being due to compression of adjacent structures, notably the optic chiasm, hypothalamus and pituitary gland. On rare occasions the tumour is confined to the sella, the optic chiasm or hypothalamus.

The imaging features (Fig. 24.10) are essentially those of a mass with cystic or calcified portions. On MRI the solid portions show the typical characteristics of tumours elsewhere in the body; namely, low signal on T_1-weighted images and high signal on T_2-weighted images [4]. The

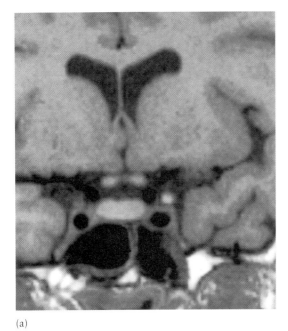

(a)

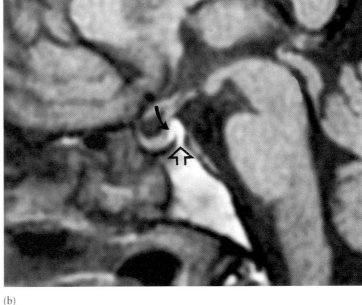

(b)

Fig. 24.4 Normal pituitary on T_1-weighted spin-echo images. (a) Coronal; (b) sagittal. Note that the CSF has low signal (dark), the anterior pituitary gland has intermediate signal (grey) and the posterior pituitary (curved arrow in b) has high signal (white). The posterior high signal is of the same intensity as marrow fat in the posterior clinoid (open arrow in b).

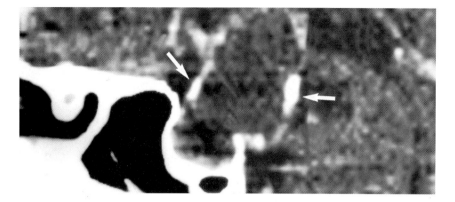

Fig. 24.10 Craniopharyngioma shown by CT (sagittal reconstruction). Note the peripheral contrast enhancement surrounding a low density centre, together with focal calcification (arrow) in the wall.

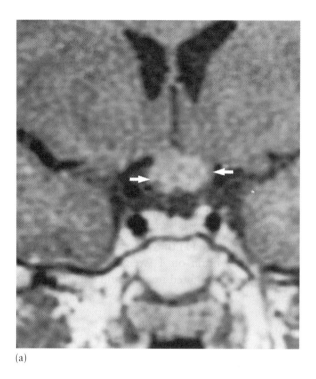

(a)

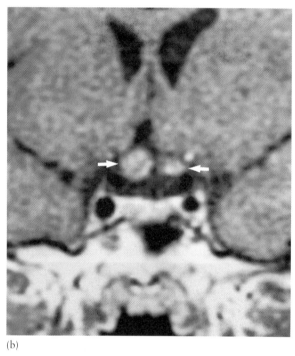

(b)

Fig. 24.11 Optic glioma on coronal T$_1$-weighted images following contrast enhancement. Section (a) is at the level of the optic chiasm and shows considerable enlargement of the chiasm by an enhancing mass (arrows). Section (b) is anterior to the chiasm and shows the mass extending into both optic nerves, with more enlargement of the right than the left (arrows).

is non-specific, resembling other neoplasms. After enhancement with intravenous gadolinium chelate, marked uniform enhancement of the tumour can be seen on T$_1$-weighted images [5]. The combination of shape, namely a well-defined mass based on a portion of the dura, and uniform enhancement after contrast, makes the diagnosis of meningioma highly likely; the presence of adjacent, visible hyperostosis makes it certain.

Similarly, chordomas may occasionally grow into the pituitary fossa (Fig. 24.13).

Metastases

Metastases can occur to any intracranial site including the sella and parasellar areas. The imaging features of the mass are non-specific, but the multiplicity of lesions, particularly a known primary tumour elsewhere in the body, means that the diagnosis is often readily made. Pituitary metastases are found in 1–2% of autopsies in patients with known extracranial primary malignancies: breast and lung carcinoma being the common primary sources. Interestingly, 70% involve the posterior pituitary and diabetes insipidus may ensue. Anterior pituitary hypofunction is uncommon with metastatic involvement of the pituitary. The MRI/CT features are, as expected, those of an enhancing mass in the pituitary, pituitary stalk and/or the hypothalamus [6]. Haemorrhage may be seen within the metastasis.

Hamartoma of the tuber cinereum

Hypothalamic hamartomas are benign non-invasive lesions, which arise from the region of the tuber cinereum or mammillary bodies and project into the adjacent suprasellar and prepontine cisterns. Symptoms and signs, when they occur, are due to compression of adjacent structures. At CT and MRI (Fig. 24.14) they show a characteristic appearance: a sessile or pedunculated mass arising from

the floor of the third ventricle [7]. They show similar signal intensity to normal grey matter both before and after contrast enhancement, that is they do not enhance on T_1-weighted images. Hamartomas do not, for practical purposes, show growth when followed up.

Tumour-like conditions

There are a large range of non-neoplastic lesions that may cause a mass in the hypothalamus or pituitary stalk. On imaging examinations most of these lesions, which include histiocytosis X (Fig. 24.15), dermoid/epidermoid cysts and sarcoidosis may appear indistinguishable from the neoplastic lesions described earlier in this chapter.

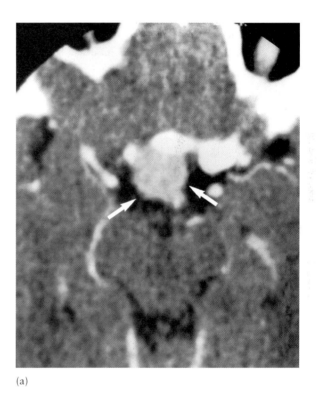

(a)

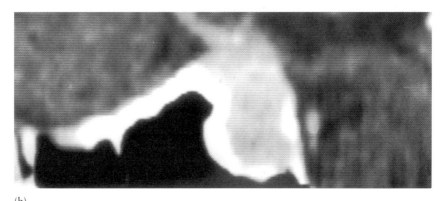

Fig. 24.12 Meningioma of the diaphragma sellae. (a) Axial and (b) sagittal reconstruction of a contrast-enhanced CT scan showing an enhancing mass (arrows) in (a) growing up into the suprasellar cistern and downward into the pituitary fossa. Note the close resemblance in shape and position to a pituitary adenoma.

(b)

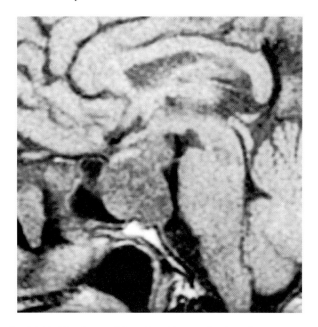

Fig. 24.13 Chordoma of the sphenoid extending into the pituitary fossa, suprasellar cistern and prepontine cistern, closely resembling a pituitary tumour. Sagittal T$_1$-weighted MRI scan prior to contrast enhancement. There was marked, patchy enhancement following intravenous gadolinium.

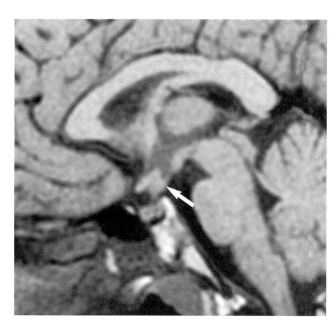

Fig. 24.15 Histiocytosis X in all 11-year-old girl showing a small mass in the region of the infundibulum (arrow). T$_1$-weighted sagittal MRI seen prior to contrast enhancement. The lesion enhanced markedly following intravenous gadolinium.

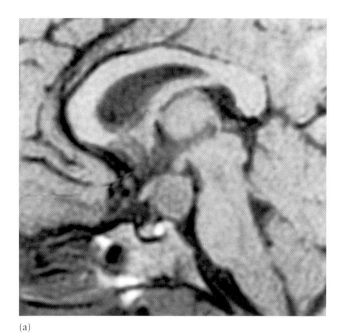

(a)

Fig. 24.14 Hamartoma of the tuber cinereum. Sagittal T$_1$-weighted MRI scans (a) pre- and (b) post-contrast enhancement. Note the non-enhancing mass arising from the floor of the third ventricle.

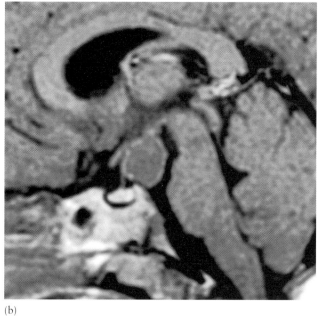

(b)

Note the normal posterior pituitary high signal (a) and the enhancement pattern of the normal anterior pituitary (b).

References

1. Chong BW, Newton TH. Hypothalamic and pituitary pathology. *Radiol. Clin. North Am.* 1993;**31**(5):1147–83.
2. Newton DR, Dillon WP, Norman D, Newton DH, Wilson CB. Gd-DTPA-enhanced MR imaging of pituitary adenomas. *Am. J. Neuroradiol.* 1989;**10**(5):949–54.
3. Bradley WG. MR appearance of hemorrhage in the brain. *Radiology* 1993;**189**:15–26.
4. Karnaze MG, Sartor K, Winthrop JD, Gado MH, Hodges FJ. Suprasellar lesions: Evaluation with MR imaging. *Radiology* 1986;**161**:77–82.
5. Michael AS, Paige ML. MR imaging of intrasellar meningiomas simulating pituitary adenomas. *J. Comp. Assist. Tomogr.* 1988; **12**:944–6.
6. Chaudhuri R, Twelves C, Cox TCS, Bingham JB. MRI in diabetes insipidus due to metastatic breast carcinoma. *Clin. Radiol.* 1992;**46**:184–8.
7. Burton EM, Ball WS Jr, Crone K, Dolan LM. Hamartomas of tuber cinereum: a comparison of MR and CT findings in four cases. *Am. J. Neuroradiol.* 1989;**10**(3):497–501.

Pathology of Tumours of the Pituitary and Related Structures

DAVID LOWE

Introduction

Over the last 25 years the classification of tumours of the anterior pituitary has been refined and simplified by the introduction of immunohistochemical techniques to stain for pituitary hormones. The time-honoured descriptive terms of acidophil, basophil and chromophobe are usually still applied, but adenomas are now classified more specifically. This is done by immunostaining for the hormones contained in the cytoplasmic granules of the tumour cells, and therefore refers to lactotroph, somatotroph, corticotroph, thyrotroph, gonadotroph, mixed and non-staining adenomas [1].

Another classification of pituitary tumours is based on their size and behaviour (judged primarily by imaging techniques rather than histology). This method is useful clinically in the choice of management and correlates with symptoms, signs and prognosis. The classification is into microadenomas or macroadenomas, intrasellar or extrasellar tumours and discrete or invasive tumours (all of which are of course related). Microadenomas are less than 1 cm in diameter. They are a relatively common cause of Cushing's disease and hyperprolactinaemia (79 and 65%, respectively) and a less common cause of acromegaly (30% of cases). Most are not invasive, but occasionally the dura over the sella is infiltrated. Invasive adenomas account for about 7% of all pituitary tumours. Most are macroadenomas, non-functioning and negative on immunostains. A classification of tumours of the pituitary and hypothalamus is given in Table 25.1 (see also [2]).

The 'empty sella' syndrome is a clinical and radiological term that describes the condition that results from an absence of or deficiency in the dura of the sellar diaphragm. The pressure of cerebrospinal fluid (CSF) is transmitted into the sella, and the pituitary is compressed into a rim of tissue at its base and sides. Histologically there are no diagnostic features of this condition: the pituitary appears normal and all cell types are represented. On the rare occasions when a pituitary neoplasm has features of the empty sella syndrome, the histology may be the same as for the more usual pituitary adenomas, or it may be the result of degeneration in the tumour [3].

Histological features of pituitary adenomas

Many of the histological features of pituitary adenomas are common to all types, irrespective of the hormone secreted. The tumour cells are usually polyhedral, and may be of uniform size and shape or may vary considerably. The presence of mitoses is similarly variable and is not a useful indicator of behaviour. The criteria for the diagnosis of aggressive behaviour and malignancy in pituitary tumours are given in Chapter 34.

The neoplastic cells are arranged in diffuse sheets, as cords and papillary structures around sinusoids (Figs 25.1 and 25.2), and rarely in small colloid-containing glands. All of the cells of the anterior pituitary contain cytokeratins, though there are significantly more intermediate filaments in somatotroph and corticotroph cells than the other cell types (see below). Collagen is deposited in some cases, either as hyaline strands dissecting the tumour (Fig. 25.1) or as dense connective tissue containing strands of tumour cells, blood vessels and areas of calcification.

Oncocytic change (Greek *onkisthai* to swell or enlarge) in pituitary adenomas is common; oncocytes may form a small part of a tumour or be the predominant cell type. Oncocytes are large, eosinophilic cells with copious amounts of granular cytoplasm; on electron microscopy the granules can be seen to be very numerous, large, distended mitochondria. They characteristically occur in an older age group of patients than the more usual, non-oncocytic tumours, though exceptions have been described. The metabolism of these cells is thought to be abnormal, with deficient synthesis and export of protein. Oncocytic tumours are almost always non-functioning.

Table 25.1 Histological classification of space-occupying lesions of the pituitary and related structures (after [2])

Pituitary tumours	Hypothalamic tumours

Adenomas that contain demonstrable hormones:
  PRL secreting
  GH secreting
  ACTH secreting
  TSH secreting
  FSH/LH secreting
  mixed tumours
	Tumours apparently derived from developmental abnormalities:
	  craniopharyngioma
	  dysgerminoma
	  hamartoma
	  chordoma
	  haemangioma

Adenomas that do not contain demonstrable hormones	Tumours derived from normal structures of the central nervous system: meningioma
Primary pituitary carcinoma	glioma (including ependymoma)
Primary pituitary sarcoma	sarcoma
Metastatic tumours	Metastatic tumours

ACTH, adrenocorticotrophic hormone; FSH, follicle-stimulating hormone; GH, growth hormone; LH, luteinizing hormone; PRL, prolactin; TSH, thyroid-stimulating hormone.

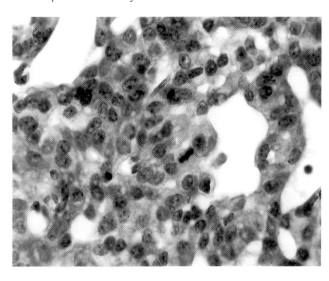

Fig. 25.2 Chromophobe adenoma of pituitary that was shown to be a prolactinoma on immunostains. The tumour cells are polygonal and arranged in trabeculae. Mitotic activity (centre of field) is present, but the tumour behaved in an indolent fashion.

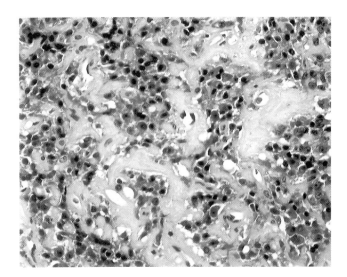

Fig. 25.1 Acidophil adenoma of pituitary that was shown to be a somatotroph adenoma on immunostains. The tumour cells are polygonal and arranged in sheets and cords interspersed with hyaline fibrous tissue.

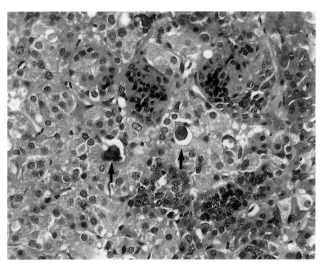

Fig. 25.3 Mixed chromophobe/acidophil adenoma of pituitary that was shown to be a prolactinoma on immunostains. The tumour cells are similar to those in Fig. 25.2. Several psammoma bodies are present (arrows). These are characteristic of prolactinoma but are not pathognomonic.

Psammoma bodies (calcispherites) are formed from concentric deposition of calcium salts in areas susceptible to dystrophic calcification (Fig. 25.3). They may be found in all tumour types but are most common in lactotroph adenomas. The reason for this is unknown. Calcispherites are usually found among tumour cells but also occur in fibrous tissue. They are also found occasionally in the non-neoplastic pituitary, especially in neonates.

Routine histochemical stains will show whether a tumour is acidophil, basophil or chromophobe but this purely descriptive characterization depends on the stain or panel of stains used: for example, a tumour that is chromophobe on haematoxylin and eosin stains may be basophilic with the more sensitive periodic-acid-Schiff orange G stain.

The reticulin stain is very helpful in identifying tumour tissue in sections. The normal anterior pituitary gland is divided into relatively uniform packets or alveoli by reticulin fibres (Fig. 25.4). In the posterior pituitary the reticulin is mainly centred on blood vessels (Fig. 25.5). In adenomas the alveoli of the anterior pituitary are initially expanded and then destroyed by the neoplastic cells, and the difference between tumour reticulin and the normal pattern is usually clear (Fig. 25.6). The reticulin stain is particularly useful when immunostains are difficult to interpret: for example, in the tiny tissue fragments from a trans-sphenoidal hypophysectomy, clusters of acidophil cells can appear to be adenomatous. If they are in fact clusters of normal acidophil cells from

the posterolateral wings of the pituitary, they will have the normal packeted reticulin pattern.

Extension of corticotroph cells into the posterior pituitary occurs normally; this should not be mistaken for infiltration by adenoma (Fig. 25.7). The process begins after puberty and is a common finding, especially in men. In the early stages the corticotrophs move into the junction of the zona intermedia and the pars nervosa. They then progressively migrate posteriorly, in some cases deep into the posterior part of the gland. The cells are immunoreactive for adrenocorticotrophic hormone (ACTH), β-lipotrophic hormone (β-LPH) and endorphins. Despite

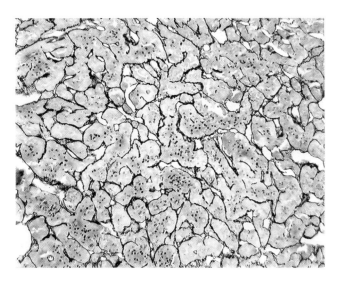

Fig. 25.4 Reticulin pattern of normal anterior pituitary gland. There is relatively uniform packeting of reticulin around small groups of cells.

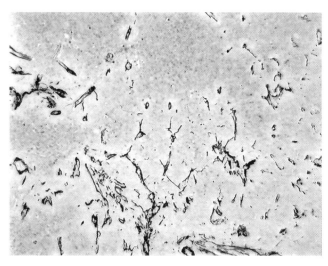

Fig. 25.6 Reticulin pattern of adenoma of pituitary. All adenomas, irrespective of the hormone type, have obliteration of the normal packeting and irregular, sparse deposition of coarse reticulin.

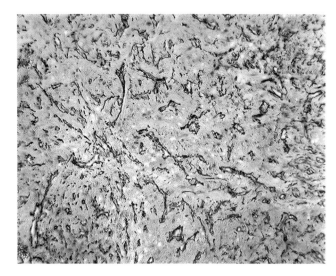

Fig. 25.5 Reticulin pattern of normal posterior pituitary gland. The reticulin is principally perivascular with fine processes between vessels.

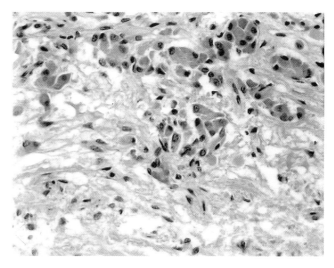

Fig. 25.7 Extension of basophils into the posterior pituitary (centre and lower field), a normal finding that should not be mistaken for tumour invasion.

reports to the contrary, they may occasionally show Crooke's hyaline change in response to hypercortisolaemia, though usually this is less pronounced than in anterior lobe basophils. The significance of basophil migration is unknown.

Occasionally the clinical and imaging features show that there is clearly a pituitary tumour, the patient's condition resolves after trans-sphenoidal surgery, and no pituitary tumour is found in the tissues removed. An obvious reason for this is that the tumour was very small and has not been sectioned; numerous tissue sections may be necessary to demonstrate a tumour. A more subtle reason is that pituitary adenomas have little reticulin or fibrous tissue (see Fig. 25.6) and so tend to be very soft. This is especially so for corticotroph adenomas, which characteristically have very little reticulin. The tumour may be removed inadvertently through the sucker used at operation to remove CSF and blood from the field and so the contents of the sucker sump should be examined histologically. Another putative explanation in such cases may be hypothalamic pathology.

Lactotroph adenomas

Lactotroph adenomas (prolactinomas) are the most common pituitary tumour, and account for about half of all tumours at that site. About two-thirds are micro-adenomas, and these have a female : male ratio of 20 : 1. Most prolactinomas are composed of chromophobe or faintly acidophil tumour cells which are polygonal and arranged as described above. Oncocytic variants are rare.

Calcification, usually as psammoma bodies, is present in about 15% of these tumours (see Fig. 25.3). It begins in mitochondria, especially in papillary areas of the tumour, and grows by concentric accretion. On rare occasions calcification is dense enough to appear on radiographs.

Ultrastructure and amyloid deposition

The secretory granules are distributed uniformly throughout the cytoplasm; most tumours are sparsely granulated. Concentric arrays of rough endoplasmic reticulum ('Nebenkerns') are often seen. Exocytotic vesicles are usually evident on the plasma membrane, and are concentrated at the part of the cell farthest away from the nearest blood vessel (so-called 'misplaced exocytosis'). Prolactin is the only hormone that is discharged by this type of visible granule exocytosis. In sparsely granulated cells the granules are concentrated in the area of the Golgi apparatus.

Tubules and fibrils of amyloid material of endocrine type may be deposited within and around the lactotroph tumour cells. The material is produced in dilated cisterns of the rough endoplasmic reticulum, and appears to be specific to this cell type.

Effects of treatment with bromocriptine

Bromocriptine inhibits prolactin synthesis by slowing transcription of the DNA responsible. The tumour cell cytoplasm becomes smaller, the rough endoplasmic reticulum is reduced and lysosomal activity increases. Shrinkage of the tumour cells does not occur in all patients. Reversal of the changes can occur when bromocriptine is withdrawn but is not inevitable.

Somatotroph adenomas

Somatotroph adenomas are the second most common clinically functioning tumour, accounting for about one-fifth of adenomas of the pituitary. They arise most commonly in the lateral wings of the anterior pituitary. In contrast to prolactin (PRL)-secreting tumours, about two-thirds present as macroadenomas. They are usually more obviously acidophilic than lactotroph adenomas, but may be chromophobe when the content of secretory granules is low. 'Fibrous bodies' may be found (see below and Fig. 25.8) and oncocytic change is also relatively common.

Electron microscopy and fibrous bodies

The granules in somatotroph adenomas vary widely in

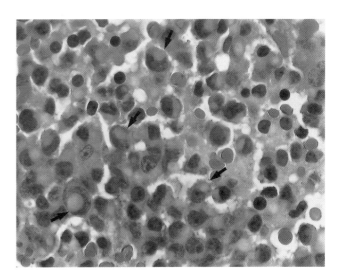

Fig. 25.8 Acidophil adenoma of pituitary that was shown to be a somatotroph adenoma on immunostains. The tumour cells have pale-staining fibrous bodies in their cytoplasm (arrows), characteristic of this adenoma type.

number: some tumours have very many and some very few. In both types, but particularly the latter, fibrous bodies may be found. These are spherical intracytoplasmic collections of microfilaments composed of low molecular weight cytokeratins. They are different from the relatively pure collections of microfilaments found in corticotrophs: in somatotrophs the filaments enclose centrioles, mitochondria and secretory granules. Fibrous bodies are paranuclear and displace the nucleus to one side of the cell. They are characteristic of somatotroph adenomas and are not found in the other types of pituitary tumour.

Effects of treatment with octreotide

Unlike with the effects of bromocriptine on lactotrophs, there are few specific histological changes found in somatotroph adenomas treated with octreotide. In treated and untreated cases, the tumour cells may be large, small, or mixtures of both. Assessment of cell size gives no indication of whether the patient has received octreotide, nor whether the tumour has responded clinically and radiologically by shrinking (shrinkage occurs in about half of treated cases). Some workers found that in treated adenomas the capillaries were sparser, fibrosis greater and necrosis more widespread than in untreated tumours, and these factors rather than reduction in cell size were more likely to be the cause of the tumour shrinkage. Treated adenomas tend to have more growth hormone (GH)-positive cells than untreated tumours on immunostaining.

Corticotroph adenomas

Corticotroph adenomas are the third most common pituitary tumour (5–8% of cases); the majority are microadenomas. They are composed of cells with basophilic or chromophobic cytoplasm that is typically extensive and finely granular [4]. The nuclei are round or ovoid and have prominent single nucleoli. The hormone-containing granules are spread diffusely throughout the cytoplasm when present in large numbers, and condense at the periphery of the cell when there are fewer. Mitoses are not generally a feature. The presence of cellular and nuclear pleomorphism and mitotic activity does not reliably indicate whether aggressive behaviour is likely. Immunostains are positive for ACTH, β-LPH and β-endorphin.

Ultrastructure and Crooke's change

The non-neoplastic corticotrophs show Crooke's hyaline change in many cases. Crooke's change begins as a hyaline band midway between the nucleus and the periphery of the affected corticotroph, with the secretory granules pushed to the periphery or collected as a clump near the nucleus. In severely affected cells the granules are few and are present only as thin rims around the plasma membrane and nucleus. Crooke's change in the pituitary can persist for up to 1 year after hypercortisolaemia has been reversed by adrenalectomy or pituitary adenomectomy.

Corticotroph adenomas are characterized by dense, spherical, secretory granules and microfilaments. The microfilaments are about 7 nm in diameter and are composed of low molecular weight cytokeratins. They are also found in corticotrophs in the normal anterior pituitary, and in the posterior lobe when there is corticotroph extension. The filaments are arranged in perinuclear sheaves; when abundant, the secretory granules are pushed to the periphery of the cell and an appearance similar to Crooke's change in non-neoplastic corticotrophs can result [5].

Similar microfilaments accumulate in the non-neoplastic corticotrophs in Crooke's change. Immunostains for specific low molecular weight cytokeratins show that types 8 and 18 cytokeratins are present in Crooke's change; skin, oesophagus and cornea cytokeratins are absent. The accumulation of microfilaments is the result of hypercortisolaemia.

Gonadotroph and thyrotroph adenomas

Gonadotroph and thyrotroph adenomas are rarely encountered, even in specialized units. Gonadotrophin-containing adenomas account for only about 5% of pituitary tumours, and thyrotroph adenomas for only 1%. Both may be misdiagnosed as non-productive tumours because antisera against gonadotrophins and thyrotrophin are not readily available.

The light microscopical appearances are similar to the more common types of pituitary tumours, though the tumour cells tend to be chromophobe and contain few granules. Perivascular rosette formation is often prominent. Vacuolated tumour cells (called 'castration' cells because they resemble the vacuolated gonadotrophs in the pituitaries of castrated animals) may be evident in functioning gonadotroph adenomas. The nucleus is pushed to the side of the cell by distended vacuoles in the cytoplasm resulting in a signet-ring appearance. Oncocytic change is common.

Electron microscopy

The tumour cells tend to have relatively few granules. Gonadotroph adenomas have larger granules in general than thyrotroph tumours. A sex difference in gonadotroph adenomas has been described: in men the tumour cells have a typical Golgi complex that has the usual unevenly shaped saccules, while women have Golgi complexes composed of collections of perfect spheres of different sizes (the 'honeycomb' Golgi). The granule size tends to be smaller in women than men.

Mixed tumours

Tumours that secrete more than one hormone may be bitypic, polytypic or monotypic in terms of the cells of which it is composed [6]. For example, tumours that secrete both GH and thyroid-stimulating hormone (TSH) have two cell types and so are bitypic; a gonadotroph adenoma that secretes follicle-stimulating hormone (FSH) and luteinizing hormone (LH) does so from one cell type and so is monotypic. Bitypic tumours are relatively common: tumours producing both GH and PRL in different cells are the most common. Tumours with ACTH and GH have been described [7,8], and with ACTH and PRL [9]. These tumours are sometimes called bimorphic, but the cells that contain GH may be indistinguishable in appearance from those making PRL. Monotypic adenomas, in which the same cell makes both GH and PRL, have also been described.

In human beings, monotypic mixed adenomas are rare and are almost always gonadotroph secreting. Vasoactive intestinal peptide is commonly coexpressed by lactotroph, somatotroph and corticotroph adenomas, but the significance of this is uncertain.

Polytypic mixed tumours, composed of more than one cell type, usually secrete GH, PRL and a glycoprotein hormone, the most common being TSH. All mixed tumours tend to be large and infiltrate the surrounding tissues.

Non-functioning adenomas

About half of all pituitary adenomas do not secrete measurable quantities of known hormones. Their clinical effects are of compression of the uninvolved pituitary, the optic chiasm and other structures and are the result of their size. Histologically these tumours are chromophobe or oncocytic; non-oncocytic tumours have the same microscopic features as functioning adenomas and cannot be distinguished from them without immunostains. Sparse secretory granules can be demonstrated in the tumour cells by electron microscopy but not usually by immunostains for hormones on light microscopy. Immunostains for neurosecretory granules, such as chromogranin, are quite often positive, especially in oncocytes.

Craniopharyngiomas and other tumours in the region of the pituitary

Craniopharyngioma is the third most common intracranial tumour after tumours of glial origin and pituitary adenoma, and accounts for about 5%. It is considered to arise from metaplasia of anterior pituitary cells and so to be of Rathke's pouch origin. In relation to this, craniopharyngiomas may occasionally have anterior pituitary cells in their walls, and nasopharyngeal craniopharyngioma has been reported.

Craniopharyngiomas are slow-growing tumours; about 35% are cystic, 25% solid and 40% mixed. The cysts contain granular eosinophilic debris, cholesterol and histiocytes. The cyst wall and septa show squamous epithelium in 26% of cases, epithelium resembling that of the enamel organ in the mouth in 15%, or mixed forms. In the adamantinous or enamel organ type the peripheral cells of the squamous islands are darkly staining and palisaded, and the inner aspects are composed of 'stellate reticulum' cells (Fig. 25.9). Mitoses are quite commonly found. Occasionally glandular tissue with cuboidal or low columnar clear cells may also be present; this is especially so in the 15% of craniopharyngiomas that extend into the sella turcica. Sebaceous differentiation may also be found.

The cyst fluid in a craniopharyngioma may contain human chorionic gonadotrophin (hCG); this can escape into the CSF and so be a useful diagnostic marker. Immunostains for hCG are positive in the squamous epithelium of the tumour.

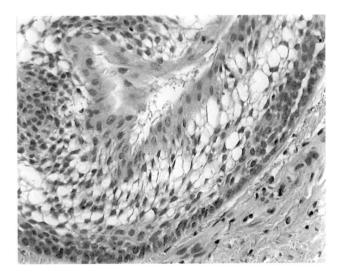

Fig. 25.9 Craniopharyngioma of adamantinous type. The stellate reticulum typical of this type of craniopharyngioma is present in the centre of the epithelium.

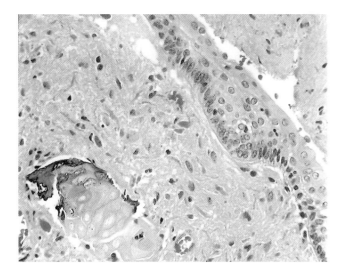

Fig. 25.10 Craniopharyngioma of squamous type. In the upper right part of the field there is squamous epithelium lining a cyst that contains granular necrotic debris. There is calcification occurring in degenerate squamous epithelium in the lower left part of the field.

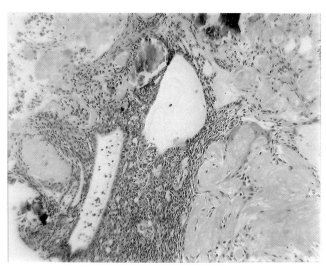

Fig. 25.11 Craniopharyngioma. The tumour is composed of squamous epithelium in which there are small cystic spaces, focal calcification (top centre and lower left) and areas of fibrosis (right).

Granulation tissue may form in the wall as a reaction to escaped cyst contents; in severe cases, cyst rupture can cause sterile fibrosing meningitis. In long-standing tumours, irregular deposition of calcium is common (Fig. 25.10). Fibrosis in the sella and dura around it and gliosis in the compressed or infiltrated cerebral tissue may be extensive. This can lead to histological difficulties in diagnosis because of sampling problems (the excision specimen can sometimes consist of fibrous tissue only) and distortion. In about one-fifth of surgically excised cases there is insufficient material to allow a histological diagnosis to be made. The clinical aspects of craniopharyngioma are discussed in Chapter 35.

Epidermal and dermal cysts

Sellar and suprasellar cysts are considered to be the same type of tumour as craniopharyngioma and to have the same pathogenesis. Craniopharyngioma grows progressively and tends to be multiloculated, while a suprasellar cyst is slower growing, behaves in a more indolent manner and is usually unilocular (Fig. 25.11 and Plate 25.1, between pp. 272 and 273).

Only mature squamous epithelium is found in the walls of epidermoid and dermoid cysts. This has a well-defined granular layer as in the epidermis, and the keratin from the surface forms the cyst contents. Stellate reticulum cells and peripheral palisading are not a feature. Mitoses are rarely found. In dermoid cysts skin appendages, such as hair follicles and sebaceous glands, are present in the squamous epithelium of the wall.

Granular cell tumour of the neurohypophysis

Granular cell tumour of the neurohypophysis is a relatively common tumour of the posterior pituitary and is of glial origin. It was once thought to be a tumour of myoblasts, and so was considered to be a choristoma (a tumour-like malformation of tissues not normally found at the site of occurrence). The granularity is due to the large numbers of lysosomes in the cytoplasm of the tumour cells.

Granular cell tumours are more often found at post mortem than in hypophysectomy specimens and are rarely symptomatic. Glial fibrillary acidic protein can be demonstrated in the tumour cells with immunostains. The differential diagnosis includes oncocytic pituitary adenoma, especially somatotroph adenoma, and metastatic renal cell carcinoma.

Langerhans' cell histiocytosis

Langerhans' cell histiocytosis is a rare condition and is manifest by an apparently uncontrolled proliferation of antigen-presenting, dendritic Langerhans' cells. Secondary to this proliferation and the attendant release of cytokines, these lesions usually have an infiltrate of lymphocytes, fibroblasts, eosinophils and giant cells in varying proportions. Immunostains for certain macrophage markers are positive. Pituitary involvement results eventually in panhypopituitarism; as the posterior pituitary is commonly involved, diabetes insipidus may be the presenting feature (see Chapter 45).

In children there is evidence that the tumour is monoclonal and is a neoplasm, but this has not been established in adults. Disease in the liver, lungs and bone marrow may overshadow the pituitary involvement. Disease in the hypothalamus and brain elsewhere may also occur.

Germ-cell tumours

Germinomas can occur in the pituitary and hypothalamus. The histological features are identical to those of germ-cell tumours of the pineal region, and are very similar to the much more common testicular germ-cell tumours (full differentiation, as is usual in ovarian teratoma, is rare). Primary choriocarcinoma may rarely occur in the pituitary. In most germ-cell tumours of the pituitary hCG is present, and in choriocarcinoma immunostains for β-hCG are characteristically very strongly positive. The CSF and tumour may have demonstrable α subunit and occasionally α fetoprotein.

The tumour cells are pleomorphic and have large, open nuclei with single, prominent, eosinophilic nucleoli. Before the diagnosis of an intracranial, primary germ-cell neoplasm is accepted, metastasis from a gonadal primary must be excluded.

References

1. Herzog T, Schlote W, Lorenz R, Jungmann E, Althoff PH. Pituitary adenomas: serum hormone levels and immunohistochemical staining for ACTH, GH and prolactin. *Clin. Neuropathol.* 1993;**12**:117–20.
2. Faglia G, Ambrosi B. Hypothalamic and pituitary tumours: general principles. In Grossman A (ed.) *Clinical Endocrinology*. Oxford: Blackwell Scientific Publications, 1992:113–22.
3. Robinson DB, Michaels RD. Empty sella syndrome resulting from the spontaneous resolution of a pituitary macroadenoma. *Arch. Intern. Med.* 1992;**152**:1920–3.
4. Kruse A, Klinken L, Holck S, Lindholm J. Pituitary histology in Cushing's disease. *Clin. Endocrinol.* 1992;**37**:254–9.
5. Halliday WC, Asa SL, Kovacs K, Scheithauer BW. Intermediate filaments in the human pituitary gland: an immunohistochemical study. *Can. J. Neurosci.* 1990;**17**:131–6.
6. Kontogeorgos G, Scheithauer BW, Horvath E *et al.* Double adenomas of the pituitary: a clinicopathological study of 11 tumors. *Neurosurgery* 1992;**31**:840–9.
7. Kamijo K, Sato M, Saito T *et al.* An ACTH and FSH producing invasive pituitary adenoma with Crooke's hyalinisation. *Pathol. Res. Pract.* 1991;**187**:637–41.
8. Bugalho MJ, Nunes JF, Sobrinho LG *et al.* Multihormonal response to CRH in a patient with Cushing's syndrome and a pituitary adenoma producing ACTH and GH. *Acta Endocrinol.* 1993;**128**:289–92.
9. Mahler C, Verhelst J, Klaes R, Trouillas J. Cushing's disease and hyperprolactinaemia due to a mixed ACTH and prolactin secreting pituitary macroadenoma. *Pathol. Res. Pract.* 1991;**187**:598–602.

26

Surgery for Pituitary Tumours

JÜRGEN HONEGGER, MICHAEL BUCHFELDER AND RUDOLF FAHLBUSCH

History of pituitary surgery

The evolution of pituitary surgery is one of the most interesting chapters in the history of neurosurgery. In 1889, Horsley undertook the first attempt to expose a pituitary adenoma via a temporal craniotomy. Intra-operatively, he believed that the tumour which compressed the chiasm was inoperable and abandoned tumour removal. Nevertheless, by 1906 he had performed ten operations for pituitary tumours, of which two resulted in death. A (sub)frontal approach was proposed by Krause in 1905, who removed a bullet close to the chiasm. Cushing preferred an approach via a unilateral frontal craniotomy through a smaller osteoplastic flap. Since craniotomy was initially afflicted with unacceptably high morbidity and mortality, surgeons also sought extradural approaches to the sella turcica. In 1907 Schloffer from Innsbruck reported on the first successful trans-sphenoidal operation for a pituitary tumour using a superior nasal approach. He performed a unilateral incision at the nasal circumference and turned the nasal flap aside. His patient was a 30-year-old male who presented with headaches and visual compromise resulting from a massive tumour. The lesion could only be incompletely removed by surgery. However, the patient died 2.5 months later from hydrocephalus due to obstruction of cerebrospinal fluid (CSF) pathways at the level of the foramen of Monro. Illumination of the operative field in the depth and visualization of structures in the sellar region was poor during this procedure and required extensive exposure for the operative approach. Subsequently von Eiselsberg, Hochenegg and Borchert carried out similar procedures. Kocher suggested splitting the nasal bridge. Then, he created a tunnel between the mucous membranes of the nasal septum, which is the principle of today's trans-septal submucosal method. Inferior nasal approaches were soon developed, the principles of which we still use today.

Inferior approaches avoided externally visible skin incisions. One of the pioneers was Hirsch from Vienna, who in 1911 replaced his original endonasal approach by the trans-septal submucosal method. Hirsch who was later working in Boston continued to use the trans-septal approach until 1956. Cushing [1] combined the advantages of various procedures and used an arrangement the basis of which remains contemporary. The surgeon stood behind the patient's head which was slightly reclined from the supine position. He used a sublabial incision and designed a bivalved speculum to maintain retraction of the mucosal tunnel. Despite Hirsch's and Cushing's impressive initial results, most surgeons later abandoned trans-sphenoidal surgery for pituitary tumours because of poor visualization during the procedure, high recurrence rates, and dramatically improved transcranial pituitary surgery. Only a few surgeons continued the use of trans-sphenoidal surgery at this time. However, one advocate of the technique was Cushing's pupil Dott (Edinburgh) who introduced Guiot (France) to the trans-sphenoidal approach. The renaissance of the method started with the improvements added by Guiot and Hardy between 1965 and 1972 [2]. Magnifying glasses were initially used but these were later replaced by the operating microscope. The position of the operative field could be precisely defined by intra-operative radiographs and by televised radiofluoroscopic control. Selective adenomectomy was made possible by the excellent illumination provided by trans-sphenoidal microsurgery. Clear-cut definitions and classifications of pituitary tumours followed and allowed a comparison of different series in respect of their success rate. In the early 1970s an increasing number of neurosurgical centres started to use trans-sphenoidal approaches to pituitary tumours [3].

Preoperative evaluation

Endocrine evaluation of anterior and posterior pituitary

function is an important part of routine preoperative work-up. Insufficiency of the adrenal axis requires perioperative replacement. In selective surgery, hypothyroidism should be corrected preoperatively. Endocrine results are also important for the differential diagnosis; for example, panhypopituitarism and diabetes insipidus are typical findings, even in minute suprasellar germinomas. By contrast, endocrine function is frequently normal in optico-hypothalamic tumours even if they are large in size. Endocrine evaluation detects hypersecretion by pituitary adenomas. If a patient presents with chiasmal syndrome, urgent measurement of prolactin is mandatory for the further management. Generally, non-functioning pituitary adenomas require surgery, while prolactinomas are initially treated medically.

Magnetic resonance imaging (MRI) is the imaging technique of choice. It depicts the precise location of pituitary and hypothalamic lesions and shows their relationship to the adjacent structures. The location of a tumour is the essential criterion for the appropriate surgical approach. MRI demonstrates invasiveness of tumour growth and shows whether the tumour is growing under the diaphragma sellae or above.

Ophthalmological evaluation of visual fields and visual acuity is imperative when dealing with suprasellar tumours. Bitemporal hemianopia is characteristic for tumours that bulge the diaphragm upwards and compress the optic chiasm but other field defects occur.

Medical pretreatment for pituitary adenomas

In *acromegaly*, medical pretreatment with octreotide prior to surgery may be used. The majority of surgeons share the impression that tumour consistency is softer after octreotide pretreatment and tumour removal is facilitated [4]. In our department, octreotide pretreatment in acromegaly is generally performed over a 6–12 week period for large and apparently invasive adenomas. There are as yet no data to suggest that outcome is beneficially affected by this treatment, either in terms of postoperative growth hormone (GH) levels or the frequency of induction of hypopituitarism.

Patients with severe *Cushing's disease* are pretreated for some weeks in order to improve their general condition prior to surgery. Some patients are inoperable at presentation and require pretreatment to reach an operable state. Metyrapone is the most appropriate adrenolytic drug and is suitable for short-term pretreatment.

For non-functioning *pituitary adenomas*, no reliable medical therapy is available and the initial therapy of choice is surgery.

Prolactinomas are primarily treated with dopamine agonists (DA). Surgery is generally indicated in non-responders or hyporesponders to DA therapy and in patients who suffer from severe adverse effects under DA therapy. Other indications for primary surgery are cystic and haemorrhagic prolactinomas.

Trans-sphenoidal surgery

Pituitary adenomas

Trans-sphenoidal surgery outnumbers transcranial approaches for pituitary adenomas. Through a small operative corridor ('keyhole surgery') even large tumours can be removed and the approach can be classified among the minimally invasive surgical techniques.

Special instrumentation is available that is adjusted to the peculiarities of trans-sphenoidal surgery.

Approach

We use a supine positioning of the patient similar to Cushing's original method. A semi-sitting positioning is also common [5]. Usually a small incision is made in the vestibulum oris under the upper lip just above the nasal septum. Alternatively, the incision can be performed in the nasal cavity above the septum, if the patient's nostril is of sufficient size. Then, the cleavage plane between the cartilaginous nasal septum and the perichondrium is exposed. The cartilaginous septum is mobilized and displaced laterally by a bivalved speculum (retractor) that is inserted into the created surgical corridor (Fig. 26.1). Using the microscope, the bony septum is removed in the midline between the bilateral mucosal layers (Fig. 26.2). The sphenoid sinus is widely opened with a punch and a diamond drill. Care must be taken to position the blades of the speculum just below the floor of the sphenoid sinus to avoid fracture of the sphenoid.

The insertion of the vomer at the floor of the sphenoid provides the crucial midline orientation (Fig. 26.2). The sagittal orientation is provided by an X-ray image intensifier. Having removed the mucosa and the bony septum of the sinus, a view can be obtained of the whole sellar floor. If the sphenoid is poorly pneumatized, the sellar floor is exposed by removing sphenoid bone with the drill. It is important to note that a non-pneumatized sphenoid, as found in younger children, is no contraindication for trans-sphenoidal surgery.

The sellar floor, which is usually thinned by pituitary tumours, is removed. The basal dura is opened with microscissors. The width of a normal-sized pituitary fossa is only 12 mm. The exposure is easier in tumours that

Limitations of surgery are firm attachments to perforating arteries, bilateral invasion of the hypothalamus and major calcifications. Under these circumstances, the neurosurgeon should be content with sub-total resection. Craniopharyngiomas tend to grow in different chambers (commonly the intrasellar, suprasellar extraventricular, or third ventricle chamber). For these reasons, combined approaches (i.e. combination of trans-sphenoidal, transcranial basal or transcranial superior approaches) are frequently required [12].

Optico-hypothalamic gliomas are low-grade astrocytomas (grade I or pilocytic astrocytomas) that grow within the optic pathways and the hypothalamus. Surgery is restricted to a biopsy or to resection of exophytic tumour portions. A pterional approach is suitable. *Hypothalamic astrocytomas* are a different entity of gliomas. Both low-grade and high-grade astrocytomas are encountered within the hypothalamus. Hydrocephalus due to foramen Monro occlusion is frequently observed and external CSF drainage or CSF shunting may be required as an emergency measure. The surgical approach depends on the prevailing location. Both superior and basal approaches may be suitable. For these intrinsic brain tumours, removal is generally sub-total and sometimes limited to a biopsy. If neuroradiology suggests diffuse growth within crucial brain tissue, a stereotactic biopsy may be the only feasible procedure and confirms the diagnosis.

Suprasellar germinomas are highly radiosensitive and can be cured by radiotherapy alone. Chemotherapy is also efficient. For these reasons, surgery is restricted to a biopsy. As they most commonly grow above the diaphragm in the area of the pituitary stalk and the basal hypothalamus, a biopsy is obtained by a pterional approach or by a CT-guided stereotactic procedure. β-human chorionic gonadotrophin (β-hCG) may be present in the CSF or serum.

Hypothalamic hamartomas are relatively rare tumours that arise from the tuber cinereum. They are pedunculated or sessile. Clinically, they may cause precocious puberty due to gonadotrophin-releasing hormone (GnRH) release or less frequently gelastic seizures. Surgery is indicated if a symptomatic hamartoma is pedunculated, as it allows total removal. After removal, precocious puberty is likely to be cured. Gelastic seizures may improve after surgery.

Perioperative management

After trans-sphenoidal surgery, the patients are supervised in the recovery room for 2–4 hours. If an intra-operative CSF leak is encountered, a lumbar CSF drainage is inserted in the operating room and 20 ml CSF is withdrawn 3 times daily over a 3–5 day period. It decreases the intracranial pressure and prevents the complication of a postoperative nasal CSF leak.

Following transcranial surgery, the patients are on intensive care for at least 24 hours. In our regimen, perioperative antibiotics and low-dose heparin are given routinely only in patients with Cushing's disease because of a higher risk of infection and hypercoagulability. Patients with adrenal insufficiency receive hydrocortisone cover until the next morning. The dose is then gradually tapered to that required for normal replacement therapy. Fluid intake and output, serum and urine osmolarity and sodium levels are carefully monitored. SIADH with a decrease of sodium levels is usually encountered within 10 days of surgery. It may cause life-threatening hyperhydration and is treated with restriction of fluid intake. Therefore, patients are not sent home until 10 days following surgery. Diabetes insipidus is corrected with deamino-D-arginine vasopressin (DDAVP) injections. One week after trans-sphenoidal surgery, DDAVP can be administered nasally.

Endocrine and ophthalmological reassessment is performed 1 week after surgery, and another re-evaluation after 3 months also includes MRI.

References

1. Cushing H. Surgical experiences with pituitary disorders. *JAMA* 1914;**63**:1515–25.
2. Hardy J. Transsphenoidal microsurgery of the normal and pathological pituitary. *Clin. Neurosurg.* 1969;**16**:185–217.
3. Wilson CB. A decade of pituitary microsurgery. The Herbert Olivecrona Lecture. *J. Neurosurg.* 1984;**61**:814–33.
4. Fahlbusch R, Honegger J, Buchfelder M. Surgical management of acromegaly. *Endocrinol. Metab. Clin. North Am.* 1992;**21**:669–92.
5. Hardy J. *Atlas of Transsphenoidal Microsurgery in Pituitary Tumors.* Tokyo: Igaku-Shoin, 1991.
6. Lüdecke DK. Transnasal microsurgery of Cushing's disease 1990. Overview including personal experiences with 256 patients. *Path. Res. Pract.* 1991;**187**:608–12.
7. Fahlbusch R, Buchfelder M. The transsphenoidal approach to invasive sellar and clival lesions. In Sekhar LN, Janecka IP (eds). *Surgery of Cranial Base Tumors.* New York: Raven Press, 1993:337–49.
8. Laws ER, Kern EB. Complications of trans-sphenoidal surgery. *Clin. Neurosurg.* 1976;**23**:401–16.
9. Nelson AT, Tucker HSG, Becker DP. Residual anterior pituitary function following transsphenoidal resection of pituitary macroadenomas. *J. Neurosurg.* 1984;**61**:577–80.
10. Honegger J, Buchfelder M, Fahlbusch R, Däubler B, Dörr HG. Transsphenoidal microsurgery for craniopharyngioma. *Surg. Neurol.* 1992;**37**:189–96.
11. Apuzzo MLJ, Zee CS, Breeze RE. Anterior and mid-third ventricular lesions: a surgical overview. In Apuzzo MLJ (ed.). *Surgery of the Third Ventricle.* Baltimore: Williams and Wilkins, 1987:495–541.
12. Yasargil MG, Curcic M, Kis M *et al.* Total removal of craniopharyngiomas. Approaches and long-term results in 144 patients. *J. Neurosurg.* 1990;**73**:3–11.

Pituitary Radiotherapy: Techniques and Potential Complications

P. NICHOLAS PLOWMAN

Introduction

Radiotherapy is dramatically effective at controlling pituitary adenomas, converting a very high postoperative relapse rate [1–3] into a very low one [4]. Furthermore it is, if carried out carefully with attention to known sources of possible risk, a very safe form of treatment. In this chapter, we will review current techniques of delivery and current knowledge on possible complications.

Radiotherapy technique

The conventional external beam radiotherapy technique for pituitary tumours requires a head fixation device (usually an individually moulded plastic head shell, made to keep the head absolutely still) with the orbitometal line (Reid's base line) vertical, in a supine patient. Modern radiotherapy simulator facilities together with current-generation computed tomography (CT) scanning (in transaxial, coronal and sagittal planes) allow the fields to be accurately moulded around the tumour volume. The day-to-day reproducibility of the field set-up should be within 2.0 mm.

The volume to be irradiated comprises the boundaries of the tumour as seen on the imaging procedures, plus 0.5 cm in all planes. If the tumour has been resected surgically, the preoperative tumour dimensions are still used to define the volume for radiotherapy as there have been examples of suprasellar recurrences occurring in these circumstances when the treatment volume was confined to the fossa. However, if a tumour has shrunk due to medical therapy (i.e. dopamine agonist-induced prolactinoma shrinkage), the volume for irradiation is accepted as the postmedical therapy volume as the tumour shrinkage is then a total shrinkage, provided dopamine agonist treatment is continued.

Having immobilized the patient and defined the tumour volume (using diagnostic magnetic resonance imaging (MRI)) and field centres, an outline is taken and an isodosimetric plan generated by the planning computer. A three-field (two lateral and one superior-oblique) 6–8 MV X-ray plan is used and, at St Bartholomew's Hospital, a dose of 4500 cGy in 25 fractions over 35 days is delivered (180 cGy per fraction; Fig. 27.1).

There have been differences in the dose prescriptions, but regimens employing 5000 cGy or more have not produced superior control rates to those employing 4000–4500 cGY [3], and the risks of radiation morbidity are greater with higher dose prescriptions.

Recently, there has been considerable interest in focal radiotherapy techniques. Proton beams, cobalt gamma-knife 'radiosurgery' and linear accelerator focal stereotactic technology are all potentially applicable to pituitary adenomas. The conceptual beauty of using focal radiotherapy in this situation is that, being benign, a 'margin of safety' with regard to radiation volume around an adenoma is less necessary than with cancer, and, with so much critical nervous system adjacent to the pituitary, a 'focused' dose would seem highly appropriate with regard to normal tissue sparing. However, the practicalities of focal radiotherapy make the situation not so clear-cut. Due to the labour intensity of all these techniques, it is not feasible to fractionate the radiotherapy over 25 fractions or so; the consequence is that almost all focal radiotherapy techniques use one or 'a few' radiotherapy fractions of, therefore, necessarily large size. This may not be of importance if the optic chiasm is outside the radiation volume but where the target volume abuts the chiasm, or other critically sensitive areas of the nervous system, not even the fast-falling radiation isodoses at the periphery of the radiation volume will spare these structures from high-dose fraction radiotherapy, a major factor in normal tissue morbidity.

For the above reasons, we reserve focal stereotactic radiotherapy for selected cases of pituitary adenoma. Thus

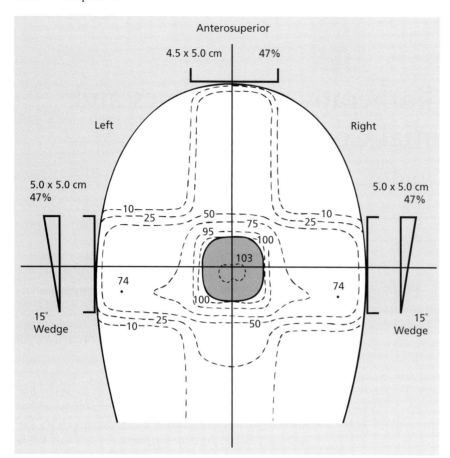

Fig. 27.1 8 MV X-ray isodosimetric plan for pituitary radiotherapy. Three fields are used to restrict the high-dose volume to the target.

a small adenoma placed low in the pituitary fossa would be a good case for focal stereotactic radiotherapy but such cases represent the minority.

Complications of pituitary radiotherapy

With modern radiation methods and techniques, the once-cited risk of brain (especially temporal lobe) necrosis should be close to zero. The three sequelae for consideration are therefore visual impairment, late hypopituitarism and radiation oncogenesis.

Visual impairment

The optic chiasm has long been known to be a particularly radiosensitive structure, and blindness due to chiasmal damage following radiotherapy to tumours in the pituitary region is well documented. However, such a catastrophic event should nowadays be exceedingly rare as the predisposing factors are better understood.

In those cases that have been described, visual deterio-

ration occurs 2–36 months (rarely later) after radiotherapy. It tends to progress over days or weeks. The differential diagnosis includes recurrent tumour, arachnoid adhesions around the chiasm or the empty sella syndrome [5]. MRI has been shown to be the most useful diagnostic investigation, particularly using gadolinium enhancement [6].

The pathological basis of radiation-induced optic chiasmal damage is thought to be vascular damage to the chiasmatic blood supply [7]. It is therefore not surprising that the major factors in the radiation prescription predisposing to such damage are the total dose delivered and the dose per fraction. Whilst employing radiotherapy for pituitary adenoma in a dose range of 4200–5900 cGy in Boston between 1963 and 1973, Harris and Levene [8] found radiation optic neuropathy in four out of the 55 cases, but none in those in whom the daily dose was less than 250 cGy per fraction. Aristizabal and co-workers [9] reviewed 122 patients presenting to their institution over a 20-year period who received pituitary radiotherapy. There were four cases of optic neuropathy; all four occurring within a group of 26 patients who had received more than 4600 cGy total dose, and all four had received more than 200 cGy per fraction. Several other reports exactly mirror these observations, that large daily dose fractions put the optic chiasm at much greater risk [10–13]. Jones [14] reviewed 332 cases of pituitary adenoma receiving megavoltage radiotherapy at St Bartholomew's Hospital, all receiving 4500 cGy in 25–26 fractions over 35 days (i.e. daily fractions of 173–180 cGy). With a minimum follow-up of 10 years for all cases, he found no cases of optic chiasmal damage, although in reviewing the literature from other institutions delivering this prescription he found occasional reports of this complication.

It is clear that the higher the daily dose and total dose, the more the chiasm is risked.

Late hypopituitarism

Anterior pituitary hormone deficiencies have been well documented following radiotherapy to the head and neck when the hypothalamopituitary axis falls within the radiation field. The evidence suggests that the hypothalamus is the site of radiation-induced effects. Studies have demonstrated normal serum growth hormone (GH) responses to bolus doses of GH-releasing hormone (GHRH), but subnormal GH responses to arginine or insulin-induced hypoglycaemia [15]. There have been delayed but present anterior pituitary hormone responses to gonadotrophin-releasing hormone (GnRH) and thyrotrophin-releasing hormone (TRH). The observation of late hyperprolactinaemia following pituitary radiation is interesting, again attributable to a late radiation effect on the hypothalamus [16].

The total absorbed dose to the hypothalamopituitary axis is the major factor in determining the speed of onset, severity and overall incidence of hypopituitarism [17]. Furthermore, the overall incidence of hypopituitarism increases with time after radiation. As expected, the radiation fraction size is another important factor (i.e. the number of treatments in which any total radiation dose is delivered, small numbers of large fractions being proportionately more harmful for any late-responding normal tissue). Thus the Manchester group demonstrated that an increased radiation fraction size, and a short treatment course, was likely to increase the risk of hypopituitarism for any total radiation dose [18].

The GH axis is most sensitive to these effects of radiation. In conventionally fractionated radiotherapy to children, after a total dose of 2700 cGy or more, the serum GH responses to provocative stimuli are blunted. After 2400 cGy the serum GH responses to provocative stimuli are often normal but spontaneous secretion of GH is decreased. After 1800 cGy there is demonstrable and subtle disturbance of the normal pattern of pulsatile GH secretion, in particular a disturbed GH increase at puberty [19].

Prospective studies in irradiated adult pituitary adenoma patients suggest that following GH deficiency, a deficiency of either gonadotrophins or corticotrophin is next most likely to occur, and that the TRH–thyroid-stimulating hormone (TSH) axis is least likely to be affected. Diabetes insipidus is extremely unusual. The reasons for this 'rank order' of radiosensitivity are unknown, but it is interesting that progressive hypopituitarism, often with a non-irradiated pituitary tumour, occurs in the same order.

Lastly, the overall incidence of subsequent hypopituitarism is greater if pituitary function is very abnormal before radiotherapy is delivered, either as a result of the tumour alone or due to both tumour and surgical influences.

All these facts temper the acceptance of exact percentage statistics on the incidence of postradiation hypopituitarism. However, after the application of the St Bartholomew's Hospital radiation prescription to a series of acromegalic patients, 25% of patients required new endocrine replacement therapy by 5 years after radiotherapy, and the incidence rose further in the next 5-year period [20]. Gonadotrophin deficiency occurred before hypoadrenalism, with hypothyroidism being least common. Feek and colleagues [21] reported that by 10 years after radiotherapy, 47% of patients were hypogonadal, 30% hypoadrenal and 16% hypothyroid. These incidences rose to 70, 54 and 38%, respectively, when surgery had preceded radiotherapy.

Radiation oncogenesis

Over the last 40 years, instances of sellar fibrosarcoma, osteogenic sarcoma, meningioma and glioma have been reported as anecdotal case reports, illustrating that second tumours can arise in or around the pituitary fossa in the late follow-up of irradiated pituitary tumours. Jones [22] reviewed the world literature on this subject, also researching the incidence of second intracranial tumours in non-irradiated pituitary tumour patients. In the period from 1959 to 1992 there were 30 case reports of parasellar fibrosarcoma following 2–27 years after irradiation and none reported in non-irradiated cases. There were 16 cases of meningioma reported from 1970 to 1992, with latencies of 8–32 cases (median 20 years), but also noteworthy was the incidence of 19 cases of meningioma in non-irradiated pituitary patients. Similarly, from 1983 to 1992 there were 18 cases of glioma reported in a series of irradiated pituitary patients (with a median latency of 9 years), but nine cases of glioma were reported in non-irradiated pituitary patients [14]. From the above data, there are no figures to suggest the denominator (i.e. the total population of irradiated and non-irradiated patients) for these results, from which the risk/incidence could be calculated.

Jones [22] reviewed a personal series of 332 consecutive, irradiated pituitary adenoma patients 7–27 years (median 11 years) postradiation. No case of fibrosarcoma was encountered. There was one case of glioma, but also one in a parallel non-irradiated pituitary adenoma patient. There was no case of meningioma, although there was one meningioma, synchronous with a pituitary adenoma, occurring in a non-irradiated patient. There was one case of naso-ethmoidal primitive neuro-ectodermal tumour. Statistical advice was that for these small index numbers, comparison with general population statistics would be inappropriate.

Brada and colleagues [4] studied 334 pituitary adenoma patients irradiated in the period 1962–86. They observed five cases of second tumour (two glioma, two meningioma, one meningeal sarcoma) and compared this incidence with the population rates in the South Thames region, and concluded that there was a risk of 1.9% for a second tumour by 20 years after radiotherapy. Whether it is relevant to use normal population rates as a comparison is open to question. Bliss and colleagues [23] reviewed the follow-up of 296 irradiated pituitary adenoma patients from Edinburgh (treated 1962) and found only one malignant brain tumour and one meningioma. They concluded no excess risk.

In conclusion, it is possible that there is a risk of second tumour induction with pituitary irradiation and of parasellar fibrosarcoma with high-dose radiation, but whether the true incidence of this late complication is as high as one in 100 is not yet certain.

References

1. Sheline G, Boldrey EB, Philips TL. Chromophobe adenomas of the pituitary gland. *Am. J. Roentgenol.* 1964;**92**:160–73.
2. Sheline G. Treatment of chromophobe adenomas of the pituitary gland and acromegaly. In Kohler PO, Ross G (eds). *Diagnosis and Treatment of Pituitary Tumours.* Amsterdam: Elsevier, 1973:201–16.
3. Sheline G. Pituitary tumours: radiation therapy. In Beardwell C, Robertson GL (eds). *Clinical endocrinology. I. The Pituitary.* London: Butterworths, 1981:106–39.
4. Brada A, Ford D, Ashley S *et al.* Risk of second brain tumour after conservative surgery and radiotherapy for pituitary adenoma. *Br.*
Med. J. 1992;**304**:1343–6.
5. Kaufman B, Tomsak RL, Kaufman BA *et al.* Herniation of the suprasellar visual system and third ventricle into empty sellae: morphologic and clinical considerations. *Am. J. Neuroradiol.* 1989;**10**:65–76.
6. Guy J, Mancuso A, Beck *et al.* Radiation induced optic neuropathy: a magnetic resonance imaging study. *J. Neurosurg.* 1991;**74**:426–32.
7. Hudgins PA, Newman NJ, Dillon WP *et al.* Radiation-induced optic neuropathy. Characteristic appearances on gadolinium-enhanced MR. *Am. J. Neuroradiol.* 1989;**13**:235–8.
8. Harris JR, Levene MB. Visual complications following irradiation for pituitary adenomas and craniopharyngiomas. *Radiology* 1976;**120**:167–71.
9. Aristizabal S, Caldwell WL, Avila J. The relationship of time-dose fractionation factors to complications in the treatment of pituitary tumours by irradiation. *Int. J. Radiat. Oncol. Biol. Phys.* 1977;**2**:667–73.
10. Atkinson AB, Allen IV, Gordon DS *et al.* Progressive visual failure in acromegaly following external pituitary irradiation. *Clin. Endocrinol.* 1979;**10**:469–79.
11. Sheline GE. Role of conventional radiation therapy in treatment of functional pituitary tumours. In Linfoot JA (ed.). *Recent Advances in the Diagnosis and Treatment of Pituitary Tumours.* New York: Raven Press, 1979:289–313.
12. Hammer HM. Optic chiasmal radionecrosis. *Trans. Ophthalmol. Soc. UK* 1983;**103**:208–11.
13. MacLeod AF, Clark DG, Pambakian H *et al.* Treatment of acromegaly by external irradiation. *Clin. Endocrinol.* 1989;**30**:303–314.
14. Jones A. Complications of radiotherapy for acromegaly. In Wass JAH (ed.). *Treating Acromegaly.* Bristol: Journal of Endocrinology, 1994:115–25.
15. Blacklay A, Grossman A, Savage M *et al.* Cranial irradiation in children with cerebral tumours — evidence for a hypothalamic defect in growth hormone release. *J. Endocrinol.* 1986;**108**:25–9.
16. Ciccarelli E, Corsello SM, Plowman PN *et al.* Long term effects of radiotherapy for acromegaly on circulating prolactin levels. *Acta Endocrinol.* 1989;**121**:827–32.
17. Littley MD, Shalet SM, Beardwell CG *et al.* Radiation induced hypopituitarism is dose dependent. *Clin. Endocrinol.* 1989;**31**:363–73.
18. Littley MD, Shalet SM, Beardwell CG *et al.* Hypopituitarism following external radiotherapy for pituitary tumours in adults. *Q. J. Med.* 1989;**70**:145–60.
19. Shalet SM. Radiation and pituitary dysfunction. *N. Engl. J. Med.* 1993;**328**:131–3.
20. Wass JAH, Plowman PN, Jones AE, Besser GM. The treatment of acromegaly by external pituitary irradiation and drugs. In *International Symposium: Challenges in Hypersecretion: Human Growth Hormone.* New York: Raven Press, 1985.
21. Feek GCM, McLelland J, Seth S *et al.* How effective is external pituitary irradiation for growth hormone secreting pituitary tumours? *Clin. Endocrinol.* 1984;**20**:401–8.
22. Jones A. Radiation oncogenesis in relation to the treatment of pituitary tumours. *Clin. Endocrinol.* 1991;**35**:379–97.
23. Bliss P, Kerr GR, Gregor A. Incidence of second brain tumours after pituitary irradiation in Edinburgh 1962–1990. *Clin. Oncol.* 1994;**6**:361–3.

Prolactinomas

JONATHAN WEBSTER AND MAURICE F. SCANLON

Introduction

Prolactinomas are the most common of the functioning pituitary adenomas, accounting for 25–30% of cases. Most occur sporadically and in isolation, but occasionally the tumour is associated with parathyroid and pancreatic islet cell tumours as part of the multiple endocrine neoplasia (MEN) type 1 syndrome. The prevalence of prolactinomas in post-mortem studies of subjects with no ante-mortem evidence of pituitary diseases is over 10%, with equal sex distribution. However there is a marked female preponderance of clinically apparent tumours, particularly microadenomas (< 10 mm diameter), which are relatively rare in men. A higher proportion of prolactinomas in men than in women are macroadenomas (> 10 mm diameter), which reflects the earlier presentation in women. Mixed growth hormone (GH)- and prolactin (PRL)-secreting tumours are well recognized and give rise to acromegaly in association with hyperprolactinaemia. Most consist of both GH- and PRL-secreting cells (5–7% of pituitary adenomas); others, mammosomatotroph adenomas (1–2% of pituitary adenomas) are monomorphous, secreting GH and PRL from the same cells. Mixed PRL- and adrenocorticotrophic hormone (ACTH)-secreting tumours are recognized, but exceedingly rare [1].

The pathogenesis of prolactinomas remains obscure. Most, if not all, comprise a monoclonal population of cells, implying clonal proliferation from a single abnormal cell in which normal mechanisms of growth control are subverted. The underlying abnormality may be a mutation which results in activation of dominant oncogenes and/ or inactivation of tumour-suppressor genes. The MEN-1 locus represents a tumour-suppressor gene, one copy of which is absent in patients inheriting the syndrome. Subsequent inactivation of the remaining normal copy of the gene by spontaneous mutation is thought to allow tumour development. Chromosome 11 deletions, spanning the MEN-1 site at 11q13, have been demonstrated in approximately 10% of sporadic prolactinomas: loss of both copies of the MEN-1 gene may therefore be important in a minority of these lesions [2]. The mechanism of action of the MEN-1 gene product, and the genetic abnormalities in the remaining 90% of prolactinomas have yet to be defined. Hypothalamic dysregulation may have a role in tumour development, possibly by allowing increased cell turnover and hence a greater probability of a somatic mutation occurring.

Malignant prolactinomas are exceedingly rare. A number of cases have been described, however, of relentless prolactinoma expansion and increasing serum PRL despite aggressive surgery, radiotherapy and dopamine agonist therapy. In a small proportion of such cases, distant metastases have been documented in liver, lungs, lymph nodes and bone [3]. Point mutations in the proto-oncogene H-*ras* have been detected in metastatic prolactinoma deposits, and it has been suggested that such mutations may play a role in initiating or maintaining tumour metastasis [4].

Clinical features

The clinical symptoms and signs of a prolactinoma may be divided into those due to hyperprolactinaemia and, in the case of larger tumours, those related to space occupation. Hyperprolactinaemia has an inhibitory action on hypothalamic gonadotrophin-releasing hormone (GnRH) release, possibly via alterations in hypothalamic opiate or dopaminergic tone. In women, the frequency of luteinizing hormone (LH) secretory pulses is reduced, the positive feedback effect of oestrogens on LH secretion is impaired and the ovulatory surge of gonadotrophins is abolished. Gonadal function may also be disturbed by a direct effect at the ovary to inhibit progesterone

189

and/or radiotherapy were the only effective treatments for prolactinomas. Surgery is usually performed via a trans-sphenoidal approach, craniotomy being reserved for particularly large macroadenomas. Results depend on both the skill of the surgeon and the size of the tumour. Normoprolactinaemia is achieved postoperatively in 60–90% of patients with microprolactinomas in most large centres, the highest rates (exceeding 95% in some series) being for those patients with lesions of 4–9 mm diameter. Macroprolactinoma patients fare less well: PRL levels are restored to normal in less than 75% of patients with lesions > 10 mm. Cure rates also correlate closely (and inversely) with preoperative PRL levels: in our centre normoprolactinaemia was restored in over 80% of patients with PRL values below 5000 mu/l (167 µg/l) and in approximately 60% of those with levels of 5000–10 000 mu/l (167–333 µg/l). None of the seven patients with preoperative levels > 10 000 mu/l (333 µg/l) were cured by surgery [7]. Preoperative dopamine agonist therapy of more than 6 weeks' duration may be associated with a lower surgical cure rate. It has been suggested that irregular tumour shrinkage and dopamine agonist-related fibrosis of prolactinomas may hinder surgical excision. Complications of surgery include anterior hypopituitarism (partial or complete), diabetes insipidus (usually transient), cerebrospinal fluid (CSF) rhinorrhoea and, less frequently, visual loss, cranial nerve palsies, meningitis, vascular injuries and haemorrhage.

Recurrence of hyperprolactinaemia with or without radiological evidence of tumour re-expansion is well recognized. Its incidence varies considerably from centre to centre. Early reports of recurrences in up to 50% and 80% of micro- and macroadenoma patients, respectively, are probably not representative of most neurosurgical centres. In our experience, early recurrence (within 6 weeks) occurred in five out of 65 patients with normal PRL 1–3 days postoperatively and late recurrence was documented (at 26, 48 and 50 months) in only three cases (mean follow-up > 5 years) [7]. Surgery is usually now reserved for patients intolerant of, or resistant to, dopamine agonists and those with a strong preference for surgery (frequently reflecting anxiety over long-term medication or the presence of an 'intracranial tumour').

Radiotherapy

Pituitary irradiation, at a dose of 4500 cGy, administered over 25 fractions using a three-field technique, reduces PRL levels in the majority of prolactinoma patients, but its effects are slow (over a period of years) and complete normalization of PRL is achieved in only a minority of cases. Dopamine agonist therapy may therefore be re-

quired after completion of radiotherapy, the drug being withdrawn from time to time for PRL estimation. A late complication of pituitary radiotherapy is the development of hypopituitarism, which occurs to varying degrees in up to 60% of patients, over a 5–15-year period, necessitating regular assessment of pituitary function during long-term follow-up. Radiotherapy is not therefore used as first-line treatment, but may be used together with dopamine agonists in patients not cured by surgery, especially where there are signs of aggressive tumour expansion or the patient is unfit for surgery. Radiotherapy also has a place in the management of rare cases with dopamine agonist resistance in whom progressive tumour expansion occurs despite maximum tolerated drug doses.

Dopamine agonists

The introduction of dopamine agonists in 1971 revolutionized the treatment of prolactinomas. Bromocriptine, a semi-synthetic ergot alkaloid, was the first such drug and remains the most widely used. A number of other agents including pergolide, lisuride, quinagolide and cabergoline have since been introduced.

These drugs directly activate pituitary D2 dopamine receptors, mimicking the action of endogenous hypothalamic dopamine. In addition to inhibiting PRL secretion, D2 receptor stimulation results in rapid involution of the cellular protein synthetic machinery and thus marked reduction in cell size. This effect, together with an antimitotic action, probably accounts for the rapid and sustained tumour shrinkage observed in the large majority of prolactinomas during dopamine agonist therapy (Fig. 28.1). Reasons for the failure of a minority of tumours to shrink include cystic change within a prolactinoma, incorrect diagnosis (a non-functioning tumour with stalk compression hyperprolactinaemia) and true dopamine agonist resistance, probably related to receptor or intracellular signalling defects.

PRL levels can be suppressed to normal in the majority of prolactinoma patients, allowing restoration of normal gonadal function and cessation of galactorrhoea. Both micro- and macroadenomas typically respond well, although normalization of serum PRL may be incomplete and usually takes longer to achieve in patients with larger tumours. Recovery of impaired anterior pituitary function as a result of tumour shrinkage is variable and patients need to be monitored and treated on an individual basis. Testosterone replacement may be required in up to two-thirds of men with macroprolactinomas as gonadal function is often not adequately restored during dopamine agonist therapy, even in those achieving normoprolactinaemia.

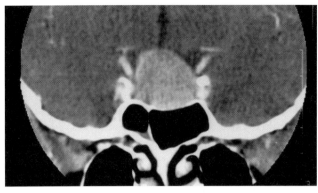

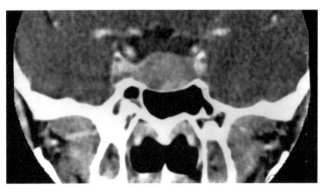

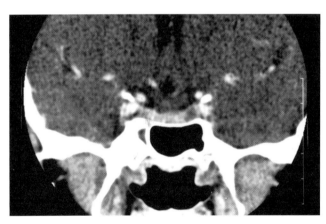

Fig. 28.1 Dopamine agonist-induced prolactinoma shrinkage, as demonstrated by serial CT. (a) The patient, a 26-year-old female, was diagnosed as having a macroprolactinoma (23 × 23 mm) with PRL levels in excess of 15 000 mu/l (500 μg/l). (b) After 3 months' treatment with cabergoline 0.5 mg twice weekly, PRL was suppressed to 800 mu/l (27 μg/l) and the tumour size had decreased (13 × 19 mm). The cabergoline dose was increased to 1.0 mg twice weekly, resulting in suppression of PRL to 300 mu/l (10 μg/l) within 4 months. (c) The scan performed 30 months later shows further reduction in tumour size to 6 × 4 mm. Visual fields were full throughout.

There are isolated reports of patients with disease progression despite dopamine agonist therapy and it is therefore important to monitor all patients clinically, biochemically and, in the case of larger tumours, radiologically. During follow-up, the treatment dose should be titrated according to clinical and biochemical response. In most cases, satisfactory results are obtained with bromocriptine 2.5 mg twice or three times daily, depot bromocriptine or cabergoline 0.5 mg twice weekly. Side-effects are common and include nausea, postural hypotension and headache. These can be minimized by gradual introduction of the drug, starting with 1.25 mg bromocriptine or 0.25 mg cabergoline, taken in the evening, with food and while recumbent, and gradually increasing the dose (in 1.25 mg increments every 3–4 days for bromocriptine, or from 0.25 mg twice weekly to 0.5 mg twice weekly after 2 weeks for cabergoline). Side-effects, if they occur, tend to resolve with continued treatment, but may necessitate a pause in dose escalation or treatment withdrawal, perhaps with subsequent more gradual re-introduction of the drug.

A recent multicentre study comparing bromocriptine and cabergoline in the treatment of hyperprolactinaemia suggested that the latter drug has significant advantages over the reference preparation in terms of clinical efficacy and side-effects. Stable normoprolactinaemia was achieved in 83% of women treated with cabergoline (up to 1 mg twice weekly) and 59% of those receiving bromocriptine (up to 5 mg twice daily) during the 24-week study period [8].

A particular therapeutic problem, not infrequently encountered, is that of a patient with a large pituitary tumour and visual failure. Urgent decompression is indicated, and this can be achieved either by surgery or, if the tumour is a prolactinoma, with dopamine agonists. In such cases serum PRL should be measured urgently before surgery. A PRL level in excess of 5000 mu/l (167 μg/l) in a patient with a macroadenoma is virtually diagnostic of a prolactinoma, and treatment with a dopamine agonist should be instituted, with an excellent chance of significant tumour shrinkage and improvement in vision. A PRL level of 2500–5000 mu/l (83–167 μg/l) provides an area of diagnostic uncertainty, as approximately 50% of such patients will have non-functioning tumours with stalk compression hyperprolactinaemia. The decision as to how to treat such patients will depend on the severity of visual failure, local expertise, clinical judgement and patient preference. A closely supervised trial of dopamine agonist therapy is reasonable, provided surgery is performed in the event of visual deterioration or failure of the lesion to shrink after, at most, 3 months. In cases where vision is severely impaired most would opt for surgery as primary treatment.

Prolactinomas and pregnancy

Hyperprolactinaemic women who present with infertility are frequently treated with dopamine agonists. Fertility is usually restored, sometimes very rapidly, and occasionally patients become pregnant without resuming menstruation. As soon as pregnancy is confirmed, treatment is usually discontinued. The average duration of fetal exposure to dopamine agonists in large studies is 30 days (probably longer in the case of long-acting drug agonists or depot preparations). Bromocriptine does not appear to have any adverse effects on pregnancy and the incidence of spontaneous abortions and congenital abnormalities is comparable to that seen in the normal population. Although experience with newer dopamine agonists is necessarily more limited, there is no evidence to date of any increased incidence of spontaneous abortions or congenital malformations with either cabergoline or quinagolide.

The management of prolactinomas during pregnancy remains controversial. Tumour expansion is a particular concern as the normal pituitary volume has been shown to expand considerably (by approximately 70%) during pregnancy and expansion of a prolactinoma may be expected to occur as a result of oestrogenic stimulation. In practice, clinically significant expansion is not usually a problem in microprolactinoma patients, symptomatic enlargement occurring in 1–2% of cases, and asymptomatic expansion in 5%. Patients with pre-existing macroprolactinomas, however, present a very different problem, as significant tumour enlargement occurs in up to 25% of cases, including 9% with symptoms [9]. Close monitoring for symptoms and signs of tumour enlargement is therefore required. Such expansion can be treated medically, with the reintroduction of a dopamine agonist, surgically, or expectantly, according to the clinical situation.

Because of the significant risk of macroprolactinoma expansion in pregnancy, surgery or radiotherapy prior to conception has been advocated in some centres. This appears to be associated with a considerably reduced incidence of significant tumour expansion during pregnancy. However, after radiotherapy, a dopamine agonist is usually still required to restore normoprolactinaemia and fertility, and both surgery and radiotherapy may be complicated by secondary hypogonadism resulting in subfertility. Such treatments are therefore not widely practised.

References

1. Kovacs K, Horvath E, Ezrin C. Anatomy and histology of the normal and abnormal pituitary gland. In De Groot LJ (ed.). *Endocrinology*, 2nd edn. Philadelphia: W.B. Saunders Co, 1989:264–83.
2. Boggild MD, Jenkinson S, Pistorello M *et al*. Molecular genetic studies of sporadic pituitary adenomas. *J. Clin. Endocrinol. Metab.* 1994;**78**:387–92.
3. Walker JD, Grossman A, Anderson JV *et al*. Malignant prolactinoma with extracranial metastases: a report of three cases. *Clin. Endocrinol.* 1993;**38**:411–19.
4. Pei L, Melmed S, Scheithauer B, Kovacs K, Prager D. H-*ras* mutations in human pituitary carcinoma metastases. *J. Clin. Endocrinol. Metab.* 1994;**78**:842–6.
5. Bevan JS, Webster J, Burke CW, Scanlon MF. Dopamine agonists and pituitary tumor shrinkage. *Endocr. Rev.* 1992;**13**:220–40.
6. Molitch ME. Pathologic hyperprolactinemia. *Endocrinol. Metab. Clin. North Am.* 1992;**21**:877–910.
7. Webster J, Page MD, Bevan JS, Richards SH, Douglas-Jones AG, Scanlon MF. Low recurrence rate after partial hypophysectomy for prolactinoma: the predictive value of dynamic prolactin function tests. *Clin. Endocrinol.* 1992;**36**:35–44.
8. Webster J, Piscitelli G, Polli A *et al*. Cabergoline Comparative Study Group. A comparison of cabergoline and bromocriptine in the treatment of hyperprolactinemic amenorrhea (1994). *N. Engl. J. Med.* 1994;**331**:904–9.
9. Molitch ME. Endocrine emergencies in pregnancy. *Baillières Clin. Endocrinol. Metab.* 1992;**6**:167–91.

Acromegaly

RICHARD SHEAVES AND JOHN A.H. WASS

Introduction

The term acromegaly, introduced by Pierre Marie in 1886, is derived from the Greek, *akron* meaning extremity and *megas* meaning great. The typical clinical signs result from prolonged excess growth hormone (GH) secretion, which in more than 99% of cases is due to a functioning pituitary adenoma [1]. Rarer causes of acromegaly result from excess growth hormone-releasing hormone (GHRH) secretion and may be secondary to the presence of a hypothalamic hamartoma or ganglioneuroma or to ectopic production from carcinoid and other neuroendocrine tumours such as those found in the pancreas, upper gastrointestinal tract or lung.

Recent progress in the understanding of the pathogenesis of pituitary tumours has identified specific gene mutations and chromosome rearrangements [2]. Mutations of the G_s protein (*gsp* oncogene) occur in 30–40% of GH-secreting adenomas [3] and this is the same defect that is found in a variety of pathological tissues of the McCune–Albright syndrome [4]. Rapid development of molecular technology and a greater understanding of tumorigenesis may soon lead to improved diagnosis and treatment for patients with somatotroph adenomas. This chapter describes our current knowledge of the assessment and management of acromegaly.

Epidemiology

Acromegaly is rare, with an estimated prevalence rate of 40–60 cases per million population. Data from the UK suggest an annual incidence rate of four per million [5]. Based on these estimates there would be 240 new cases per year in the UK with a population of approximately 60 million.

There is equal frequency of the disease in both sexes. The majority of patients are diagnosed between the ages of 40 and 60 years, although the insidious nature of the disease often contributes to the considerable time lag between onset and diagnosis [6]. Acromegaly during childhood may be more likely to be diagnosed earlier since it also causes the syndrome of gigantism. Very rarely acromegaly may present as part of a familial endocrine syndrome such as multiple endocrine neoplasia (MEN) type 1 syndrome.

Clinical presentation

The clinical presentation of acromegaly results either from the general metabolic effects of prolonged excess growth hormone and insulin-like growth factor-1 (IGF-1) or from the local effects of an expanding pituitary tumour causing visual loss and hypopituitarism (Table 29.1). In addition, hyperprolactinaemia, resulting either from direct secretion by the adenoma or from pituitary stalk compression, can contribute to the significant number of patients presenting with galactorrhoea, menstrual disturbances and impotence [7].

The coarse acromegalic facial features and enlarged hands and feet remain the most striking of the clinical signs. If the patient is able to produce a series of photographs taken over many years, it may be possible to date the onset of the disease. Occasionally the patient demonstrates an arm span greater than standing height and this suggests the possibility that the disease was manifest during childhood before closure of the epiphyses (Fig. 29.1). In our series of over 400 acromegalic patients at St Bartholomew's Hospital, 2% showed evidence of pituitary gigantism with eunuchoid features.

A typical acromegalic face demonstrates coarse features including deep nasolabial furrows, thick lips, an enlarged nose and frontal bossing. Growth of the mandible causes prognathism and separation of the teeth. Tongue enlargement together with swelling of the nasopharynx and soft

Table 29.1 Clinical symptoms and signs in 60 patients presenting with acromegaly (adapted from [7])

Symptoms and signs at presentation	Overall prevalence (%)
Facial change and acral enlargement	100
Excessive sweating	83
Acroparaesthesiae	68
Tiredness and lethargy	53
Headaches	53
Arthropathy	37
Goitre	35
Ear, nose, throat or dental problems	32
Congestive cardiac failure/arrhythmia	25
Hypertension	23
Visual loss or visual field defects	17

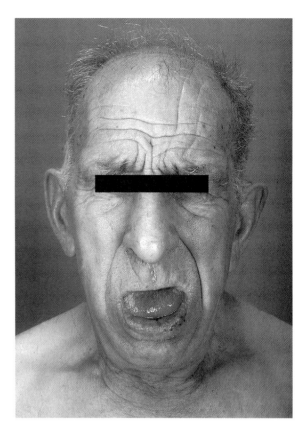

Fig. 29.2 An acromegalic patient with typical coarse features and tongue enlargement who eventually required a resection to allow the tongue to fit into his mouth.

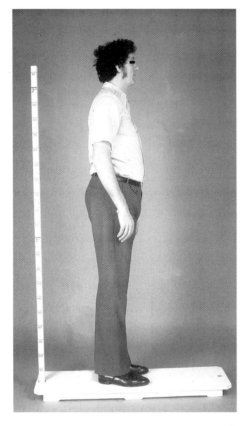

Fig. 29.1 An acromegalic giant (height 228 cm) who was found at St Bartholomew's Hospital, at the age of 27 years, to have a growth hormone-secreting pituitary adenoma, clinical and biochemical evidence of hypogonadotrophic hypogonadism and radiological confirmation of unfused epiphyses.

tissues of the upper airways contributes to respiratory difficulties, with sleep apnoea being prominent amongst the varied list of complications (Fig. 29.2).

The musculoskeletal changes are a cause of significant morbidity in the acromegalic patient. Subtle enlargement of the hands and feet can be recognized by increasing ring and shoe size, whereas more severe changes result in typical spade-like appearances. Degenerative changes in the joints cause osteoarthritis, particularly of the hips and knees. Changes in the stability of the vertebral column results in kyphoscoliosis (Fig. 29.3). In addition, soft tissue swelling may contribute to neuropathies with carpal tunnel syndrome (40% of patients) a frequent finding at presentation. The combination of these pathologies together with a generalized myopathy is probably a major factor contributing to the weakness and lethargy which seem so prominent in this disease.

Chronic excess of GH and IGF-1 is associated with generalized organomegaly. Clinically detectable goitre can be found in 10–70% of patients at presentation. Cardiomegaly, which is well recognized in acromegalic patients, may result directly from GH excess or alternatively be caused by the additional risk factors of hypertension and diabetes mellitus with subsequent ischaemic heart disease. The gastrointestinal tract increases in size, usually without symptoms, although there is a well-recognized increased incidence of colonic polyps. The incidence of colonic carcinoma and premalignant polyps is increased in acromegaly [8]. The physical challenge in providing

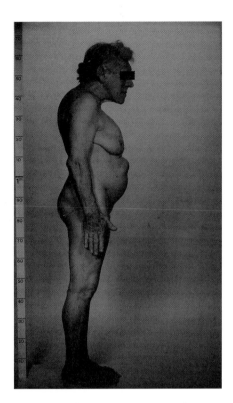

Fig. 29.3 A patient with long-standing acromegaly presenting with symptoms and signs of chronic osteoarthritis and a kyphosis.

routine colonoscopy in patients with a greatly enlarged colon is widely acknowledged.

The local effects of pituitary tumours largely result from expansion within the pituitary fossa, causing hypopituitarism, and from suprasellar extension, causing chiasmal compression with decreased visual acuity, visual field defects and optic atrophy. Exceptionally, these tumours may be large enough to cause hydrocephalus and others which invade the cavernous sinus produce ophthalmoplegia. Headaches are particularly common and are thought to result from dural stretching by the enlarging adenoma. The tumour, by expanding within the fossa, also results in the symptoms and signs of hypogonadism, adrenal insufficiency and hypothyroidism. In a group of 100 patients that we recently studied the prevalence of these conditions at presentation was 28, 8 and 2% respectively. In addition hyperprolactinaemia was found in 30% of these patients.

Diagnostic work-up

Confirmation of acromegaly

The physiological fluctuations of GH secretion in both normal and acromegalic subjects makes a random GH estimation unhelpful as an initial step in the investigation. From a practical point of view the daily GH output can be reasonably assessed by measuring serial plasma samples

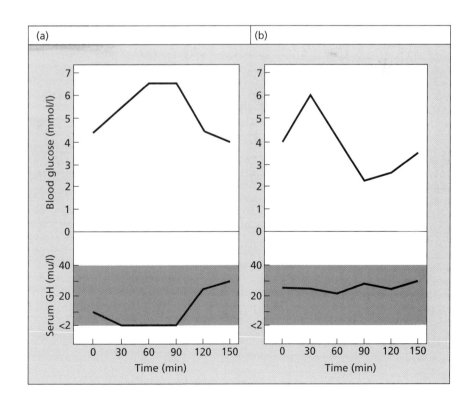

Fig. 29.4 Demonstration of the response of the plasma GH to an oral glucose load of 75 g in a normal and acromegalic subject.

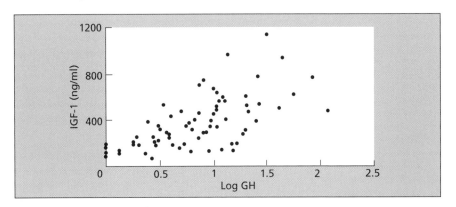

Fig. 29.5 The relationship between the serum IGF-1 level and log mean growth hormone (GH) in 73 acromegalic patients from St Bartholomew's Hospital.

for GH throughout the day. In healthy subjects basal GH levels are below the sensitivity of most assays (less than 0.5 mu/l) for most of the time, whereas in acromegalic patients the levels are usually significantly higher during the day curve. However, the definitive test for acromegaly remains the demonstration of failure to suppress the plasma GH to undetectable levels during an oral glucose load (Fig. 29.4). The oral glucose tolerance test is also useful in identifying the significant number of patients with impaired glucose tolerance (40%) and overt diabetes mellitus (20%).

More recently, the laboratory diagnosis of acromegaly has also been made by measuring a serum IGF-1 level. This reflects the integrated effect of GH on the tissues and has been shown to differentiate between active untreated acromegaly and normal individuals [9]. The long half-life of IGF-1, due mainly to its binding to specific carrier proteins, excludes the necessity for multiple sampling and this may therefore prove to be a precise and cost-effective test during the initial screening for acromegaly (Fig. 29.5).

A further test that may be useful, especially in borderline cases, is the GH response to thyrotrophin-releasing hormone (TRH). About 60% of acromegalic patients show a paradoxical increase of GH levels following intravenous administration of 200 mg of TRH. The routine use of this test is not normally necessary since the clinical assessment, failure of GH to suppress following a glucose load, and the IGF-1 level are usually conclusive for a diagnosis of acromegaly.

Radiological assessment

Despite being so simple a lateral skull X-ray in acromegaly can give useful information very quickly (Fig. 29.6). An enlarged pituitary fossa indicates the presence of a pituitary tumour, whereas enlargement of the frontal sinuses and thickening of the calvarium are well-known features of acromegaly.

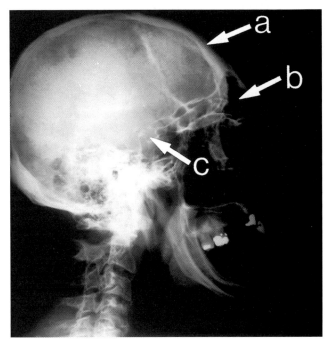

Fig. 29.6 A lateral skull X-ray in an acromegalic patient showing an enlarged pituitary fossa (c), enlarged frontal sinus (b) and a thickened calvarium (a).

Computed tomography (CT) or magnetic resonance imaging (MRI) may be used to assess the pituitary fossa for the presence of an adenoma. Evidence of a pituitary tumour is found in the majority of cases and macroadenomas with extrasellar extension are found in about one-third of cases [7]. Tumours that infiltrate bone and other surrounding structures are well recognized. MRI has been considered particularly helpful by some neurosurgeons in these cases, by delineating which parasellar structures, especially the vascular components, are involved by the tumour (Fig. 29.7). However, tumour invasion is often suggested by MRI, although no such invasion can be demonstrated at operation. The role and accuracy of MRI in determining invasion requires further assessment.

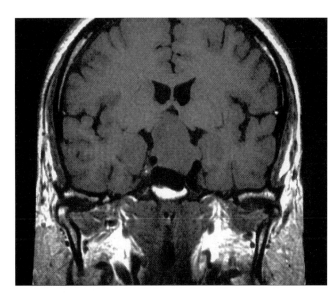

Fig. 29.7 An MRI scan of the pituitary fossa of an acromegalic patient demonstrating a pituitary tumour invading the parasellar structures.

Visual field testing

The visual fields should be tested by confrontation using a red pin during the initial examination. In addition, the visual fields can be formally documented using Goldman perimetry.

Pituitary function tests

Standard basal pituitary function should be assessed by measuring the serum prolactin and by assessing the pituitary–gonadal axis (luteinizing hormone (LH), follicle-stimulating hormone (FSH), oestradiol, testosterone), the pituitary–thyroid axis (T_4, T_3, thyroid-stimulating hormone (TSH)) and the pituitary–adrenal axis (09.00 h serum cortisol). Dynamic testing of the adrenocorticotrophic hormone (ACTH) reserve to stress using the insulin-tolerance test may also be necessary. Paired early morning plasma and urine osmolarity are necessary to investigate for diabetes insipidus, although in our experience, even with very large pituitary tumours, this is extremely rare and its presence is more likely to indicate hypothalamic disease.

Confirmation of the aetiology

Although in more than 99% of patients presenting with acromegaly the cause is due to a GH-secreting pituitary adenoma, occasionally patients are seen in whom excess GHRH can be demonstrated. A variety of neuroendocrine tumours (gut, pancreas, lung) are known to cause the clinical syndrome of acromegaly by secreting GHRH. A routine chest X-ray is mandatory in all patients and may identify chest lesions, but further investigations, including measuring a serum GHRH level, may be indicated if an obvious pituitary adenoma is not demonstrated by CT or MRI scanning. The presence of hypercalcaemia or a family history of endocrine neoplasia may also raise the suspicion of MEN-1.

Aims of treatment and definition of cure

Acromegaly is a chronic disease causing significant morbidity and is associated with a mortality about double the expected rate in healthy, age-matched subjects. Some form of therapy is therefore considered in virtually all patients. The decision on recommending medical therapy, surgery or radiotherapy is influenced by the age and general health of the patient and also whether the pituitary tumour is causing local compressive effects, particularly on the visual pathways. In general, however, the treatment aims are as follows.

1 removal of the pituitary tumour to relieve local mass effects;
2 relief of symptoms and signs of acromegaly;
3 restoration of GH secretion and IGF-1 levels to normal;
4 maintenance of normal pituitary function;
5 prevention of disease recurrence;
6 assessment and treatment of chronic complications.

The most controversial aim and that which has proven difficult to define is the restoration of normal GH secretory dynamics [10]. A precise definition of biochemical cure in acromegaly is impossible to substantiate at the present time. Whereas many published surgical series suggest a single GH level of less than 10 mu/l as confirmation of cure, we consider GH levels < 5 mu/l more in keeping with biochemical cure. Also, in view of the wide fluctuations of GH seen in acromegalic patients, a single random sample is considered by many to be inadequate and the mean GH from a day curve may therefore be used in its place.

We propose that obtaining a mean GH level of < 5 mu/l together with a normal IGF-1 level represents an important biochemical aim in the treatment of acromegaly. The scientific basis for this is that mean GH levels of < 5 mu/l and not < 10 mu/l are associated with restoration of the normal body composition of salt and water [11]. Also, a reduction in mortality similar to that of the general population was reported for patients with the lower mean GH levels of < 5 mu/l but was not demonstrated in those patients whose GH levels remained < 10 mu/l following treatment [12].

Treatment

Trans-sphenoidal surgery is currently the treatment of first choice in most centres for acromegaly. It is associated with a low mortality (< 0.5%) and the most serious of the complications, such as cerebrospinal fluid (CSF) leaks and meningitis, are reported to occur in less than 1% of cases [13]. The prevalence of hypopituitarism at presentation is appreciable and although trans-sphenoidal surgery causes deterioration of pituitary function (Fig. 29.8), hormone replacement therapy is readily available for long-term treatment. In some individual patients tumour removal by trans-sphenoidal surgery may even restore previously documented pituitary failure. Selective removal of a pituitary adenoma via the trans-sphenoidal route limits the development of hypopituitarism and may be guided by MRI images of the sellar region. This allows prediction of tumour localization, as well as identifying sites of invasion. In the case of focal invasion into the cavernous sinus it is now possible to follow the tumour by direct vision and achieve total removal of the adenoma [13].

Serial MRI and CT imaging have also been used to investigate a role for preoperative octreotide treatment. GH-secreting adenomas show shrinkage in approximately 40% of cases after several months of octreotide treatment, although the degree of shrinkage is small. This treatment has not yet been shown to influence the immediate postoperative outcome and no long-term follow-up studies favourably support the use of preoperative octreotide. This is still, however, an area of considerable interest and research.

Publications relating to the use of trans-sphenoidal surgery in the management of acromegaly consistently quote remission rates of 60–90% and low recurrence rates of less than 10% [13–16]. More recently, however, medical therapy with octreotide has been used with considerable success as a first-line treatment. Although many centres still offer surgery to virtually all patients, there are now good arguments to consider chronic octreotide treatment alone for elderly patients [17]. Pituitary radiotherapy may be offered as an alternative or as adjunctive treatment, although one of the main disadvantages is the long time period, often many years, for the effects of radiotherapy to normalize GH levels.

Results of trans-sphenoidal surgery

Published postoperative remission rates vary considerably. One reason for this is the previous lack of consistent remission criteria. Lowering the postoperative basal GH to < 20, < 10, < 5 and < 2 mu/l have all been used in the past, while suppression of GH to < 4 mu/l following a glucose load has also been proposed as an important aim of treatment. Data from Germany [13] and from the USA [15] quote remission rates of 71% and 74% respectively in obtaining postoperative basal GH levels of < 10 mu/l. The Newcastle group [14], however, with an 84% success rate using the same criteria, clearly demonstrated how the outcome of surgery varies according to the remission criteria (Table 29.2). Our currently accepted biochemical treatment aim is for a postoperative GH level of < 5 mu/l and 76% of patients from the Newcastle group achieved this goal.

In a large series of 100 patients from St Bartholomew's Hospital, a postoperative mean GH of < 5 mu/l was achieved by 42% of patients. The lower success rate compared to the Newcastle study might be partly explained by the influence of known adverse prognostic factors. Thus, the likelihood of success was influenced by the preoperative GH level, 65% of patients achieved a 'cure' if this value was < 20 mu/l but only 18% of patients were 'cured' if the preoperative GH level was > 100 mu/l. In addition, tumour size was found to be important, 61% of microadenomas but only 23% of macroadenomas achieved a postoperative mean GH of < 5 mu/l. Tumour

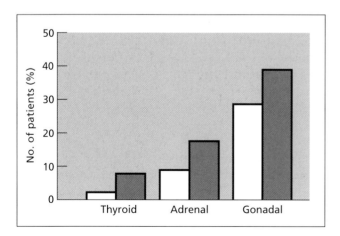

Fig. 29.8 The pre- (▢) and postoperative (▉) incidence of hypopituitarism in 100 acromegalic patients from St Bartholomew's Hospital.

Table 29.2 The outcome of trans-sphenoidal surgery in 76 acromegalic patients as defined by the postoperative growth hormone (GH) level (data from the Newcastle group [14])

	Postoperative GH (mu/l)			
	> 10	< 10	< 5	< 2
Patients (%)	16	84	76	49

invasion is also known adversely to affect the outcome.

Re-emergence of active acromegaly and tumour re-growth following postoperative GH normalization is regarded as a recurrence. The published recurrence rates, as do the remission rates following surgery, vary according to the remission criteria used in the immediate post-operative period. Thus, using a postoperative basal GH level of < 10 mu/l as criterion for remission, the overall long-term (mean 6 years, range 1.5–14.0 years) recurrence rate in 61 patients was found to be 7% [13]. This is similar to other large published series [15]. If a postoperative GH level of < 5 mu/l is used as the criterion for remission then two studies [14,16] showed a zero recurrence rate. Achieving a postoperative GH level of < 5 mu/l is therefore not only associated with an improved overall prognosis [12], but it is also a valuable indicator in predicting that the long-term follow-up will be disease free.

Results of pituitary radiotherapy

Treatment results following the administration of particulate irradiation from supervoltage machines [18] and after implantation of radioisotopes directly into the pituitary fossa [19] can be compared to the more commonly used technique of conventional pituitary irradiation [20]. Particulate irradiation utilizes the Bragg peak phenomenon where a peak of high energy particles are calculated to coincide with the pituitary tumour. Extreme precision is required to avoid damage to adjacent tissues. Although this technique is effective for acromegaly, 77% of patients demonstrating GH levels < 10 mu/l following treatment [18], the limited availability of the expertise and the potentially hazardous complications have limited widespread use. Similarly, the implantation of radioisotopes into the pituitary fossa has not gained wide acceptance. Whilst effective in controlling acromegaly, 87% of patients achieving GH levels < 10 mu/l at 10 years [19], the complication rate is considered high.

Conventional megavoltage radiotherapy has in the past been used either as primary treatment or as an additional alternative following trans-sphenoidal surgery. Comparison of published series are hampered by the varying dose regimens used worldwide. A total dose of 4500 cGy divided into 25 daily fractions of 180 cGy/day is effective in the control of acromegaly and limits the visual complications associated with higher dose schedules. Our series at St Bartholomew's Hospital using this dose schedule as primary treatment for acromegaly demonstrated radiotherapy to be effective after a follow-up period of many years (Table 29.3). The largest fall in serum GH occurs during the first 2 years but the levels of

Table 29.3 Data from the St Bartholomew's Hospital acromegaly series showing the percentage of patients (*n* = 31) achieving a mean growth hormone (GH) of < 10 mu/l following radiotherapy

	Years following radiotherapy			
	0	2	5	7
% patients with GH < 10 mu/l	0	18	40	86

GH continue to fall for many years thereafter. The percentage of patients achieving GH levels of < 10 mu/l is cumulative with time and 7 years post-treatment, 86% of our patients had achieved this target.

Progressive development of hypopituitarism following radiotherapy for acromegaly has been well documented. The prevalence of thyroid, adrenal and gonadal deficiencies 10 years after radiotherapy as sole treatment has been reported in 19, 38 and 55% of patients respectively [20]. Incidence rates are higher for patients who have undergone prior trans-sphenoidal surgery. Hypopituitarism is dose-dependent and favourable results have recently been reported for the treatment of acromegaly using a low radiation dose schedule [21]. Future studies are needed to confirm whether the lower radiation dosages offer effective long-term control of acromegaly.

Results of medical therapy

Dopamine agonists inhibit GH release in some acromegalic patients although the biochemical response is highly variable. Significant clinical improvement has been reported following the administration of bromocriptine, lisuride, pergolide, terguride, quinagolide and, more recently, with the new, long-acting oral dopamine agonist, cabergoline. It has been demonstrated, however, that GH levels can be reduced to < 10 mu/l in only approximately 20% of patients with IGF-1 levels being restored to normal in only 10% [22]. Despite the fact that dopamine agonists are effective in only a minority of patients, their continued use is largely determined by the significant cost savings compared to somatostatin analogues. The current accepted practice is for the patients to be given a trial of bromocriptine, the dose being increased incrementally to 20 mg daily. There are no tests which confidently and consistently predict the bromocriptine responders. If there is no effective GH suppression after 2 weeks of such therapy, then an alternative form of treatment should be considered.

Octreotide, the long-acting octapeptide analogue of somatostatin, is the most effective medical treatment for acromegaly. Subcutaneous administration of octreotide

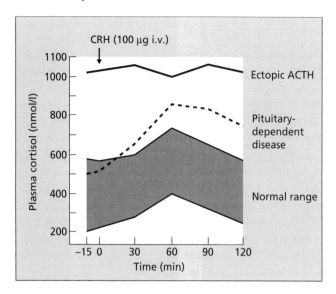

Fig. 30.3 Serum cortisol responses to corticotrophin-releasing hormone (CRH) (100 μg i.v.) in normal subjects, patients with pituitary adrenocorticotrophic hormone (ACTH)-dependent Cushing's disease and patients with the ectopic ACTH syndrome.

A cortisol response to CRH has been defined as an increase in cortisol of four times the coefficient of variation of the mean baseline cortisol. This corresponds to a rise of 20–25% after administration of CRH in normal individuals. Grossman and colleagues [15] reported an exaggerated response to CRH in 16/21 patients (76%) with Cushing's disease. The vast majority of patients with the ectopic ACTH syndrome tested in this way do not respond to CRH, although there have been isolated case reports contradicting this view. One of the main problems with the interpretation of the CRH test is the spontaneous fluctuation of cortisol levels seen in any form of Cushing's syndrome. Thus, the results are usually assessed together with the results of additional tests such as the high-dose DST. Patients showing no response to CRH and failing to suppress with the high-dose DST are highly likely to have the ectopic ACTH syndrome [15].

High-dose DST

The high-dose DST is performed in an identical manner to the low-dose DST, except that 2 mg of dexamethasone is administered 6-hourly in place of 0.5 mg. In Cushing's disease a fall in plasma cortisol of greater than 50% is expected, whereas patients with adrenal tumours or the ectopic ACTH syndrome demonstrate no such suppression. Published results indicate that approximately 90% of patients with Cushing's disease show the expected cortisol suppression, although 10% of patients with the ectopic ACTH syndrome also show this response [13,15].

If the diagnosis is still unclear after both the CRH test and the high-dose DST, then further information may be gained from petrosal sinus sampling. This technique is also used to lateralize the pituitary adenoma prior to surgery in some centres.

Inferior petrosal sinus sampling

Simultaneous bilateral inferior petrosal sinus sampling allows detection of the significant ACTH gradient which exists between the petrosal sinus draining the pituitary gland and peripheral blood in patients with Cushing's disease [16]. Due to the spontaneous variation in ACTH levels, a petrosal to peripheral ratio of > 2 is considered necessary to diagnose Cushing's disease with confidence. Demonstrating a significant ACTH gradient is greatly increased following the administration of CRH (Fig. 30.4). A petrosal to peripheral ACTH ratio of > 3 after CRH was found to give

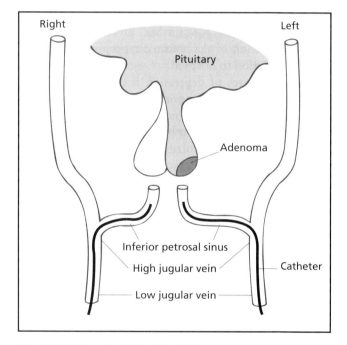

	Plasma ACTH levels (ng/l) after CRH administration			
	0 min	5 min	10 min	15 min
Left inferior petrosal sinus	14	477	280	123
Right inferior petrosal sinus	16	23	28	54
Simultaneous peripheral vein	17	19	25	32

Fig. 30.4 The adrenocorticotrophic hormone (ACTH) response to corticotrophin-releasing hormone (CRH) (100 mg i.v.) in a patient with Cushing's disease during bilateral inferior petrosal sinus sampling.

a 100% accuracy in differentiating pituitary from ectopic sources of Cushing's syndrome [17].

Some consider that lateralization of ACTH-secreting tumours within the pituitary gland is possible from the data obtained during petrosal sinus sampling. In Cushing's disease, accurate preoperative tumour localization is relevant since selective removal of the adenoma by trans-sphenoidal surgery may offer a cure and preserve normal pituitary function. However, a recent analysis of 20 consecutive patients studied with petrosal sinus sampling showed interpretable lateralization data in only 55% [18]. Correct placement of the catheter was unsuccessful in three patients, anatomical variation of the inferior petrosal sinus precluding reliable conclusions was found in five patients and a macroadenoma was present in one further patient. Furthermore, magnetic resonance imaging (MRI) scanning was found to be more successful and identified a pituitary adenoma in 15/20 patients with the correct position of the tumour being confirmed in 14 of the cases (70%) at subsequent trans-sphenoidal surgery. It was therefore concluded from this study that MRI scanning is superior to bilateral inferior petrosal sinus sampling for the lateralization of pituitary microadenomas. A similar recent study, however, concluded that petrosal sinus sampling was far superior to MRI in localizing pituitary adenomas in patients with Cushing's disease [19]. Further data are obviously needed to resolve this issue and this should particularly examine the role of operator dependency.

Pituitary imaging

Most specialized centres report detecting a pituitary adenoma in Cushing's disease by computed tomography (CT) scanning only in a minority of patients. It should be remembered also that a significant number of normal subjects (10%) show subtle pituitary heterogeneity on CT scans and that 20–30% of post-mortem specimens demonstrate the presence of a pituitary adenoma as an incidental finding. MRI scanning has been shown to be superior in the detection and localization of corticotroph adenomas, especially when gadolinium enhancement is used [18]. A sensitivity for the detection of a pituitary adenoma in Cushing's disease has been reported to be 77% for MRI and 47% for CT scanning [20]. With a specificity of only 80–85%, the number of false-positives will be appreciable and pituitary imaging must be interpreted in conjunction with the biochemical data.

Aims of treatment and definition of cure

The prognosis for untreated Cushing's disease is poor

and the condition should be treated even if the biochemistry indicates mild disease. Half the patients are dead within five years with vascular disease and susceptibility to infections strong contributing factors. In addition, in children there may be permanent stunting of growth.

Cushing's disease may be treated by trans-sphenoidal surgery, pituitary radiotherapy, bilateral adrenalectomy or with medical treatment using a variety of drugs including metyrapone, ketoconazole and op'DDD (mitotane). Although the treatment offered will depend on the age and general health of the patient, trans-sphenoidal surgery is regarded as the treatment of first choice in most centres. Selective trans-sphenoidal adenomectomy is now widely practised and is the best available option for control of the hypercortisolaemia and preservation of normal anterior pituitary function.

The primary aim of trans-sphenoidal surgery is to offer the patient the chance of a cure from the disease. Many patients will be improved and will be said to be in remission following surgery, although relapses have been documented to occur in these patients and also those previously said to be cured at the time of surgery. Despite the widespread use of trans-sphenoidal surgery, there has been a lack of consensus in the criteria used to define a successful outcome. Thus, published series quote postoperative cure rates as being defined as the restoration of normal basal cortisol levels, the normalization of urinary-free cortisol and/or cortisol suppression following dexamethasone administration.

There is now good evidence to support the view that a very low or undetectable serum cortisol following trans-sphenoidal surgery defines a successful treatment outcome [21]. In a study of 48 patients who underwent surgery, 25 had undetectable cortisol levels (< 50 mmol/l) postoperatively and the disease had not recurred in any of these patients after a median follow-up time of 40 months. Significantly, three patients in this series, whose postoperative cortisol values had improved (50–300 mmol/l), but were not undetectable, relapsed during the follow-up period.

The above results support the theoretical argument that the high circulating levels of cortisol found in Cushing's disease lead to total suppression of normal corticotrophs. Complete tumour removal should therefore render the patient ACTH-deficient. Persisting cortisol secretion postoperatively, even if subnormal, is not likely to be associated with cure and the possibility of a recurrence at a later date should be considered.

Treatment

Bilateral adrenalectomy was formerly the mainstay of

treatment but is now rarely employed. An appreciable mortality was reported by some centres (5–10%) and significantly, 20–30% of patients developed Nelson's syndrome following this procedure. This complication may be associated with a particularly aggressive and invasive pituitary tumour. Prophylactic pituitary irradiation has been shown to reduce the risk of developing Nelson's syndrome by 50% [22]. The results, however, are not altogether satisfactory since some patients still developed expanding pituitary tumours despite this additional treatment.

Bilateral adrenalectomy still retains a place in the management of patients with the ectopic ACTH syndrome if the primary tumour cannot be removed or treated with radiotherapy or chemotherapy, or medical treatment to lower cortisol levels is inadequate. It may also be useful as primary therapy in Cushing's disease in occasional circumstances. In our department, patients not cured by the initial trans-sphenoidal surgery would be offered a second trans-sphenoidal operation. If the serum cortisol remains detectable following this second operation, pituitary radiotherapy would be considered. Medical treatment with adrenolytic drugs may also be necessary during the interim period before the effects of radiotherapy become apparent. The aim of treatment with these agents is to maintain mean basal cortisol values from a day curve to within 150–300 mmol/l since these levels most closely reflect a cortisol production rate in normal individuals. These levels are also associated with remission of the clinical features of Cushing's disease.

Results of trans-sphenoidal surgery

The variable definitions of postoperative cure of Cushing's disease make a direct comparative appraisal of treatment results from worldwide centres difficult. Remission rates following surgery of 70–90% are however commonly reported. It is important also, and especially since the disease results in such devastating complications, to continue follow-up in the long-term and to assess for recurrence. Of 101 patients reported by Fahlbusch and colleagues [23], 76% were stated as being in remission in the immediate postoperative period. Further assessment of these and additional patients has suggested that a recurrence of Cushing's disease occurred in 11% of patients who appeared to be cured initially [14]. Significantly, recurrences occurred in patients with normal postoperative cortisol levels but not in those shown to have adrenal insufficiency with undetectable ACTH and cortisol levels.

Patients treated at St Bartholomew's Hospital are considered cured if the postoperative cortisol is undetectable (< 50 nmol/l). This was achieved in 42% of patients at

Table 30.4 The postoperative outcome according to the mean serum cortisol levels in 48 consecutive patients undergoing trans-sphenoidal surgery for Cushing's disease at St Bartholomew's Hospital (adapted from [21])

	Postoperative cortisol (< 50 nmol/l)	Postoperative cortisol (50–300 nmol/l)	Postoperative cortisol (> 300 nmol/l)
Clinical outcome	Cured	Controlled	Uncontrolled
Patients (*n* = 48)	20 (42%)	12 (25%)	16 (33%)

first operation, a further 25% being significantly improved by trans-sphenoidal surgery (Table 30.4). Patients not cured at the first attempt were offered a second operation and this resulted in an overall cure rate of 52% with 81% of the total patients achieving a clinical remission with a postoperative cortisol level of < 300 nmol/l [21]. Significantly, Cushing's disease has not recurred in a single patient during the median follow-up period of 40 months in whom the postoperative cortisol was < 50 nmol/l. During this period, normal cortisol secretion had recovered in only 20% of this cured group. Overall, the postoperative incidence of hypopituitarism was appreciable; hypothyroidism was documented in 40% of patients and hypogonadism in 53% of men and 30% of premenopausal women. Diabetes insipidus, persisting for at least 6 months, occurred in 46% of patients.

Pituitary radiotherapy

Pituitary tumours may be treated by proton beam irradiation, implantation of radioisotopes into the pituitary fossa or, more usually, by conventional supervoltage irradiation. Radiotherapy may be offered as primary treatment in those patients unfit or unwilling to have surgery, although in most institutions it is used as secondary therapy in those patients not cured by trans-sphenoidal surgery. The effects of radiotherapy may take months or even many years to be effective and so medical treatment to control the hypercortisolaemia should be offered during this interim period.

Successful treatment of Cushing's disease following both proton beam irradiation and after interstitial implantation of 90-yttrium has been reported. However, the limited availability of these techniques and the potentially serious complications initially reported, have restricted their widespread use. External conventional radiotherapy, using a total dose of 4500 cGy/day divided into 25 daily fractions of 180 cGy/day, has been shown to be effective in the long-term biochemical control of Cushing's disease and also in the management of invasive corticotroph adenomas [24].

Medical therapy

The aim of medical therapy is to achieve mean cortisol values from a day curve of 150–300 nmol/l and so approximate the cortisol production rate in normal individuals. Treatment is normally recommended for patients prior to surgery to prevent postoperative complications such as poor wound healing and susceptibility to infection. Medical therapy would also normally be offered to postoperative patients not cured by surgery. The use of pituitary radiotherapy in these patients is commonplace and drug treatment should be maintained until the successful effects of radiotherapy can be demonstrated.

A number of drugs are available for the management of Cushing's disease. There are no agents that effectively reduce ACTH secretion from corticotroph adenomas, although a small number of patients respond to bromocriptine. Other successes have been reported for cyproheptadine and sodium valproate, although these centrally acting drugs are not indicated for general use. Usually, the hypercortisolaemia of Cushing's disease is controlled using either ketoconazole or metyrapone which block the biosynthesis of cortisol in the adrenal gland. Metyrapone, a blocker of cortisol synthesis, is usually used as initiating therapy and its action starts within a few hours. Doses of 1.5–4.0 g daily may be required [25,26]. Side-effects include nausea and hirsutism. Long-term control is best obtained with ketoconazole. Ketoconazole is often considered the first line in therapy for children since it does not increase the production of adrenal androgens. The dose of ketoconazole needs to be titrated against the mean cortisol level from a day curve but is usually of the order of 200–400 mg three times daily. Gastrointestinal symptoms including nausea, vomiting and diarrhoea comprise the more common side-effects and liver function should be closely monitored since hepatotoxicity is well documented in patients taking ketoconazole.

The adrenolytic agent, op'DDD (mitotane), has a cytotoxic effect on adrenocortical tissue. It is the drug of choice for patients with adrenal carcinoma in order to control the excessive production of adrenal hormones, although the prognosis for this disease remains unaltered. This drug may also be used in patients with Cushing's disease. Gastrointestinal side-effects including nausea and vomiting may occur but are dose dependent. In addition there are also a significant number of patients who develop hypercholesterolaemia on this agent.

Finally, successful treatment of Cushing's disease is associated with adrenal insufficiency. Treatment with prednisolone 5 mg on wakening and 2.5 mg with the evening meal is appropriate replacement therapy to allow endogenous cortisol secretion to be followed. Mineralocorticoid replacement is not required. Assessment of the pituitary–adrenal axis should be performed at regular intervals thereafter to determine recovery of the normal functioning pituitary tissue. For patients treated by bilateral adrenalectomy, hydrocortisone 20 mg on wakening and 10 mg with the evening meal in addition to fludrocortisone 50–100 µg twice daily would be appropriate. All patients should carry a MedicAlert bracelet and a steroid card and be given instructions for intercurrent illness.

Conclusion

Cushing's disease is rare, although it is often suspected in diabetic and hypertensive patients who report weight gain. The most sensitive and specific confirmatory test for Cushing's syndrome is the low-dose DST. The diagnosis of pituitary-dependent Cushing's disease is established by a number of biochemical and radiological investigations. These include suppression of cortisol following the high-dose DST and demonstrating an exaggerated cortisol response during the CRH test. Petrosal sinus sampling and pituitary MRI are also useful confirmatory investigations.

The treatment of first choice in most patients is transsphenoidal surgery. The aim of the treatment is to demonstrate adrenal insufficiency by the finding of an undetectable postoperative serum cortisol. Patients of failing to achieve this treatment aim can be offered a second operation. If the serum cortisol remains high following the second operation, pituitary radiotherapy should be considered. The aim of medical therapy, using ketoconazole or metyrapone, normally given until the successful effects of radiotherapy can be demonstrated, is to maintain a mean serum cortisol value of 150–300 nmol/l and so approximate the cortisol production rate of normal individuals.

The prognosis of treated Cushing's disease is good. Some of the most distressing symptoms such as mood swings, depression and irritability often improve within hours or days of treatment. The Cushingoid facial appearance may also improve dramatically within just a few days. In the majority of patients, diabetes mellitus will resolve, and in many hypertension will also improve. Although osteoporosis may not resolve in the elderly, fresh fractures are prevented. In children, however, osteoporosis tends to resolve well. Within a few weeks, patients often note a marked improvement in muscle strength and this is usually confirmed by the resolution of a previously documented proximal myopathy.

Survival data for patients with treated Cushing's disease are limited, although mortality has been shown to be higher than that expected for the general population [4]. Persistence of diabetes mellitus and hypertension after treatment are positive predictive factors for this increased mortality.

References

1. Krieger DT. *Cushing's Syndrome*. Berlin: Springer Verlag, 1982.
2. Trainer PJ, Grossman A. The diagnosis and differential diagnosis of Cushing's syndrome. *Clin. Endocrinol.* 1991;**34**:317–30.
3. Howlett TA, Price J, Hale AC *et al*. Pituitary ACTH-dependent Cushing's syndrome due to ectopic production of bombesin-like peptide by a medullary carcinoma of the thyroid. *Clin. Endocrinol.* 1985;**22**:91–107.
4. Etxabe J, Vazquez JA. Morbidity and mortality in Cushing's disease: an epidemiological approach. *Clin. Endocrinol.* 1994;**40**:479–84.
5. Aron DC, Findling JW, Tyrrell JB. Cushing's disease. *Endocrinol. Metab. Clin. North Am.* 1987;**16**:705–30.
6. Grua JR, Nelson DH. ACTH-producing pituitary tumours. *Endocrinol. Metab. Clin. North Am.* 1991;**20**:319–62.
7. Levy A, Lightman SL. The pathogenesis of pituitary adenomas. *Clin. Endocrinol.* 1993;**38**:559–70.
8. Ishibashi M, Shimada K, Abe K, Furue H, Yamaji T. Spontaneous remission in Cushing's disease. *Arch. Intern. Med.* 1993;**153**:251–5.
9. Jeffcoate WJ, Silverstone JT, Wass JAH, *et al*. Psychiatric manifestations of Cushing's syndrome: response to initial lowering of plasma cortisol. *Q. J. Med.* 1979;**48**:465–72.
10. Trainer PJ, Besser GM. *The Barts Endocrine Protocols*. Edinburgh: Churchill Livingstone, 1995.
11. Newell-Price J, Trainer P, Perry L *et al*. A single sleeping midnight cortisol has 100% sensitivity for the diagnosis of Cushing's syndrome. *Clin. Endocrinol.* 1995;**43**:545–50.
12. Crapo L. Cushing's syndrome: a review of diagnostic tests. *Metabolism* 1979;**28**:955–77.
13. Howlett TA, Drury PL, Perry L *et al*. Diagnosis and management of ACTH-dependent Cushing's syndrome: comparison of the features in ectopic and pituitary ACTH production. *Clin. Endocrinol.* 1986;**24**:699–713.
14. Von Werder K, Müller OA. Cushing's syndrome. In Grossman AB, (ed.). *Clinical Endocrinology*. Oxford: Blackwell Scientific Publications, 1991:442–56.
15. Grossman AB, Howlett TA, Perry L *et al*. CRF in the differential diagnosis of Cushing's syndrome: a comparison with the dexamethasone suppression test. *Clin. Endocrinol.* 1988;**29**:167–78.
16. Trainer PJ, Besser GM. Differential diagnosis in Cushing's syndrome: the role of inferior petrosal sinus sampling. *Eur. J. Med.* 1993;**2**:261–3.
17. Oldfield EH, Doppman JL, Nieman LK *et al*. Petrosal Sinus sampling with and without corticotrophin-releasing hormone for the differential diagnosis of Cushing's syndrome. *N. Engl. J. Med.* 1991;**325**:897–905.
18. De Herder WW, Uitterlinden P, Pieterman H *et al*. Pituitary tumour localisation in patients with Cushing's disease by magnetic resonance imaging. Is there a place for petrosal sinus sampling? *Clin. Endocrinol.* 1994;**40**:87–92.
19. Landolt AM, Schubiger O, Maurer R, Girard J. The value of inferior petrosal sinus sampling in diagnosis and treatment of Cushing's disease. *Clin. Endocrinol.* 1994;**40**:485–92.
20. Kaye TB, Crapo L. The Cushing's syndrome: an update on diagnostic tests. *Ann. Intern. Med.* 1990;**112**:434–44.
21. Trainer PJ, Lawrie HS, Verhelst J *et al*. Trans-sphenoidal resection in Cushing's disease: undetectable serum cortisol as the definition of successful treatment. *Clin. Endocrinol.* 1993;**38**:73–8.
22. Jenkins PJ, Trainer PJ, Plowman PN *et al*. The long term outcome after adrenalectomy and prophylactic pituitary radiotherapy in adrenocorticotropin-dependent Cushing's syndrome. *J. Clin. Endocrinol. Metab.* 1995;**80**:165–71.
23. Fahlbusch R, Buchfelder M, Muller OA. Transsphenoidal surgery for Cushing's disease. *J. R. Soc. Med.* 1986;**79**:262–9.
24. Howlett TA, Plowman PN, Wass JAH *et al*. Megavoltage pituitary irradiation in the management of Cushing's disease and Nelson's syndrome: long-term follow-up. *Clin. Endocrinol.* 1989;**31**:309–23.
25. Jeffcoate WJ, Rees LH, Tomlin S *et al*. Metyrapone in long-term management of Cushing's disease. *Br. Med. J.* 1977;**2**:215–17.
26. Verhelst JA, Trainer PJ, Howlett TA *et al*. Short and long term responses to metyrapone in the medical management of 91 patients with Cushing's syndrome. *Clin. Endocrinol.* 1991;**35**:169–78.

31

Non-functioning Pituitary Adenomas

GIOVANNI FAGLIA AND BRUNO AMBROSI

Introduction

The term non-functioning pituitary adenoma (NFPA), far from defining a unique biological entity, describes pituitary tumours occurring in patients not presenting with any classical hypersecretory syndromes. These patients rather have pituitary insufficiency of variable degree, due to either compression of the normal pituitary tissue or impingement of the tumour mass on the pituitary stalk and hypothalamus, thus preventing the hypothalamic hormones from reaching the pituitary. This last event may cause slight elevations in serum prolactin. The majority of these tumours are diagnosed at the stage of macro-adenomas because of mass-caused symptoms such as headache, visual field deterioration and/or ocular palsies. NFPAs constitute a clinical problem as they are usually disabling huge pituitary masses, difficult to be totally removed by surgery and, in the absence of any tumour marker, except if the α subunit (α-SU) is high, and prove difficult to be followed-up. Furthermore, up to now there is no established medical treatment.

Epidemiology

NFPAs represent about one-quarter of all pituitary tumours (prevalence 50–60 cases per million; incidence 4.5 per million per year). Twenty-six percent of patients fall between the ages of 40 and 50 and about 70% between 51 and 80 years, without any difference in sex distribution.

Classification

The common characteristic of NFPAs is that they are lacking hypersecretion of any biologically active anterior pituitary hormone up to now identified. Their classification is still a matter of debate as histopathological, immunocytochemical, functional and clinical criteria are unsatisfactory. A classification, based on comprehensive criteria, is proposed in Table 31.1.

Pathology

NFPAs are round-shaped formations of variable size, occupying the pituitary fossa. The largest ones may present with suprasellar expansion up to the foramen of Monro and/or extend laterally towards the cavernous sinuses or downwards in the sphenoid sinus. Some of them may penetrate into the orbital cavity, or even reach the occipital foramen. Staining negatively with acidic, basic or periodic-acid-Schiff dyes, NFPA show no hormone production with immunoperoxidase techniques [1]. However, in about 85% of tumours there is positive immunostaining in scattered cells for at least one glycoprotein hormone or subunit, 8% for pro-opiomelanocortin (POMC) derivatives, and 2.5% for growth hormone (GH). On electron microscopy, most null cell adenomas appear composed of small polyhedral cells with irregular nuclei, poor rough endoplasmic reticulum (RER) and organelles and small mitochondria; the Golgi apparatus may be prominent. The secretory granules are few, round, 100–250 nm in diameter, with a dense core. In some tumours the majority of cells may undergo oncocytic transformation such that the cells appear filled by dense mitochondria. An aneuploid DNA pattern has been shown by flow cytometry in about 50% of NFPAs. Some tumours show a frequency of S-phase cells higher than 10% indicating a certain degree of aggressiveness.

Origin and pathogenesis

Immunocytochemical as well as *in situ* hybridization and *in vitro* secretion studies have documented that most NFPAs contain and release gonadotrophins and/or their common α-SU [2]. Therefore, it has been hypothesized that they derive from gonadotrophs. It has been suggested

Table 31.1 Classification of non-functioning pituitary adenomas

Type	Morphology	Immunoreactivity
Null cell adenomas	Lacking distinctive structural and/or immunocytochemical markers. Small polyhedral chromophobic cells with irregular nuclei. Poorly developed rough endoplasmic reticulum, prominent Golgi. Clusters of ribosomes. Small mitochondria. Sparse small secretory granules (100–250 nm)	Scattered cells staining for FSH, LH, α-SU, LH-β, and occasionally for other hormones
Oncocytomas	Cells filled with 'dark' or 'light' mitochondria, such that intracellular organelles are hidden	Scattered cells staining for FSH, LH, α-SU, LH-β, and occasionally for other hormones
Silent corticotroph adenomas	Heterogeneous (see below)	Staining for ACTH and POMC derivatives
Subtype 1	Basophilic, ultrastructural appearance similar to that of typical ACTH-omas	Most cells staining for ACTH or POMC-der.
Subtype 2	Chromophobic, with sparse PAS-positive basophilic granulation. Secretory granules up to 450 nm	Most cells staining for ACTH or POMC-der.
Subtype 3	Chromophobic or slightly acidophilic. Large cells resembling those of glycoprotein-secreting tumours. Secretory granules up to 250 nm	Few cells staining for ACTH or POMC-der., and occasionally for GH and/or PRL or for glycoprotein hormones

α-SU, α subunit; ACTH, adrenocorticotrophic hormone; der., derivatives; FSH, follicle-stimulating hormone; GH, growth hormone; LH, luteinizing hormone; POMC, pro-opiomelanocortin; PAS, periodic-acid-Schiff; PRL, prolactin.

that the subset of NFPAs known as oncocytomas originate from either pre-existing pituitary oncocytes or intermediate lobe rests, while silent corticotroph adenomas presumably originate from corticotrophs.

Recent studies support the theory that the genesis of pituitary tumours is a multistep process in which somatic mutations of proto-oncogenes or loss of suppressor genes lead to neoplastic transformation (initiation) and then to the growth of the mutated clone. Stimulatory factors either of hypothalamic origin or locally produced by the tumour itself may also sustain clone expansion (promotion). Very recently, in agreement with this theory, it has been demonstrated that NFPAs are monoclonal in origin [3], possess functioning cell membrane receptors for several hypothalamic neurohormones and produce growth factors.

Hormone production

Most NFPAs are able to produce hormones. In fact the secretion of follicle-stimulating hormone (FSH), luteinizing hormone (LH), thyrotrophin (TSH), α-SU, LH-β, FSH-β, or POMC-derivatives has been documented by *in vitro* hormone release from cultured adenomas under both basal conditions and after appropriate stimulation [4], and complementary DNA *in situ* hybridization has shown the expression of mRNA of hormone genes. Evidence of *in vivo* hormone production is much less common. Only a minority of patients with NFPA (about 15–20%) show inappropriately high circulating levels of gonadotrophins and/or their subunits. The release of FSH, LH, α-SU, and LH-β is stimulated by gonadotrophin-releasing hormone (GnRH) and thyrotrophin-releasing hormone (TRH) and inhibited by dopaminergic agents. On the contrary, the *in vivo* release of other anterior pituitary hormones occurs in less than 10% of cases. The discrepancy between the findings of an *in vitro* secretory activity, which often takes place at quite high rates, and the absence of elevations in circulating hormone levels, may be explained by the observation, obtained with the reverse haemolytic plaque assay, that only a few tumour cells have hormone-releasing activity.

Signs and symptoms

In the absence of any hormone hypersecretion causing specific biological effects, there is not a typical presentation of patients with NFPA. As most patients have large tumours, 50–60% of cases present with visual field defects (quadrantanopia or hemianopia, mainly bitemporal) due to compression of the optic chiasma, or diplopia or ophthalmoplegia due to tumour expansion towards the cavernous sinuses. A deep, generally frontal, headache is common (35%), while intracranial hypertension, nausea, vomiting and diabetes insipidus, are less frequent. A dramatic, severe headache accompanied by rapid loss of sight, hypotension and mental confusion is typical of tumour haemorrhagic infarction. NFPAs may also incidentally be discovered in asymptomatic patients undergoing computed tomography (CT) or magnetic resonance imaging (MRI) investigations for other reasons.

Gonadal function defects are the most frequent endocrinological features (40–45% of cases). Galactorrhoea may occur in 10–20% of affected women. About one-third of cases show signs and symptoms of secondary hypothyroidism, or hypoadrenalism. Profound stress may precipitate latent hypoadrenalism into acute adrenal failure. Total anterior hypopituitarism is clinically evident in about 10% of patients.

Diagnosis

On standard radiography of the skull, about 20% of patients show a widely destroyed sella turcica, 40% have diffuse alterations of the bony walls, 35% a sellar enlargement without osseous deformities and only 5% a slight bulging, double floor, or focal alterations. On axial and coronal CT, the tumours are visualized in the sellar and suprasellar region and usually show homogeneous enhancement after the injection of contrast medium. Necrotic or cystic areas are demonstrated by heterogeneous enhancement surrounded by a peripheral ring; calcification may be present too. MRI is equally sensitive and also gives precise three-dimensional information about surrounding structures and the characteristics of tumour expansion.

On ophthalmological study, visual fields defects are the most common alterations (> 70% of cases), although visual acuity may also be impaired. Fundoscopy may reveal optic nerve pallor, atrophy or papilloedema.

As most patients with NFPA lack a specific serum hormone marker, it is difficult to differentiate NFPA from other lesions resembling pituitary adenomas in their clinical, endocrinological and radiological appearance, such as craniopharyngiomas, meningiomas, gliomas, hypophysitis, granulomatous diseases, metastatic tumours and hamartomas. Therefore, the diagnosis largely rests on histological examination of the surgically removed lesion. The recently developed three-step immunoscintigraphy with radiolabelled antichromogranin A (CgA) monoclonal

antibodies [5] offers the possibility of distinguishing between CgA-secreting (as usually NFPAs are) and CgA-non-secreting pituitary masses (Plate 31.1, between pp. 272 and 273). In some cases also the hormonal study may help. In fact, inappropriately high serum levels of FSH, or α-SU, more rarely of LH or LH-β, may facilitate the preoperative diagnosis of NFPA. Serum α-SU levels are frankly high in 12–18% of cases and may constitute a useful marker of the tumour. The finding of elevated circulating levels of gonadotrophins and their subunits in response to TRH (50–70% of cases) and of α-SU greatly enlarge the number of preoperatively diagnosed patients [6]. Postoperative persistence of these abnormal responses implies residual tumour, which may need further treatment. In postmenopausal women bearing a pituitary mass, the lack of gonadotroph desensitization (i.e. the persistent release of gonadotrophins and α-SU after repetitive administration of long-acting GnRH) is of diagnostic value. Subtle alterations of hypothalamic–pituitary–adrenal axis regulation, such as plasma ACTH hyperresponsiveness to corticotrophin-releasing hormone (CRH) or vasopressin, facilitate the preoperative diagnosis of silent corticotroph adenomas. The search for tumour markers other than basal and TRH-stimulated gonadotrophins and their subunits has so far failed. The only promising putative marker, serum CgA concentration measurement, has not yet been extensively investigated.

The majority of patients show pituitary insufficiency involving, in descending order, GH (80–90%), TSH (30–80%), ACTH (25–60%). About 80–90% of patients with NFPA do not increase serum GH levels after insulin tolerance tests (ITT) or growth hormone-releasing hormone (GHRH) tests. Impaired or absent serum cortisol responses to ITT are present in more than 50% of patients, while CRH tests elicit a normal response in most cases. Central hypothyroidism is a common finding. Alterations of TSH response to TRH are frequently found: absent, impaired, sometimes delayed, exaggerated, or prolonged responses may be recorded. Multiple factors, such as inappropriately normal or low gonadotrophin levels, secretion of gonadotrophins with reduced biological activity, or of their bioinactive free subunits, and associated mild hyperprolactinaemia, may contribute to secondary hypogonadism (45–90% of patients). Absent or impaired responsiveness of gonadotrophins after GnRH is found in about half the cases. Mildly elevated serum prolactin (PRL) levels are recorded in more than 50% of patients. Contrary to patients with prolactinomas, the majority of patients with NFPA show serum PRL elevation after TRH administration, while in only a minority of patients does serum PRL increase after dopamine receptor blockers. Diabetes insipidus is a very uncommon finding and its presence suggests hypothalamic-pituitary lesions other than pituitary tumour.

Therapy

Surgical resection of the tumour is the best way to control tumoral expansion and to remove the mass effects (Fig. 31.1). In patients without mass symptoms, particularly if elderly, close follow-up alone is indicated, while a more aggressive approach is advisable in younger patients, as they carry a greater potential risk for tumour progression. Macroadenomas require resection in order to debulk the tumour mass and to have some tissue available for histopathological confirmation of the diagnosis. Transsphenoidal surgery is a valid and safe tool to achieve these goals. This procedure has negligible mortality and morbidity rates (0.4–1.0%) and may result in total tumour excision in patients with intrasellar adenomas, while in those with large tumours and extrasellar expansion it may result in the resolution of symptoms due to mass effects even if the tumour resection is partial. Transcranial surgery is associated with higher mortality and morbidity rates (2–10%). Whatever the surgical approach, pituitary surgery is infrequently curative and tumour remnants may cause recurrence. Contrary to hypersecreting adenomas, there is no helpful hormonal criterion to assess the outcome of operation, except in those patients with high circulating levels of gonadotrophins or their subunits and/or in those with paradoxical response to TRH. In fact, the normalization of the basal levels and/or the disappearance of the paradoxical response is suggestive of successful surgery. However, residual tumour and those

with recurrence should undergo pituitary radiation therapy (4.5 Gy at 1.8 Gy/day, utilizing conventional three-field radiotherapy) [7].

Pituitary function should be carefully assessed. Although in some series hypopituitarism has been reported to improve following tumour ablation, in most patients a deterioration of anterior pituitary function is observed. Patients receiving radiotherapy should have pituitary hormone function carefully monitored, as radiation may result in partial or complete hypopituitarism over several years after radiation. In a recent survey, it has been shown that the 10-year progression-free survival rate was 77% and overall tumour control was achieved in 83% of patients treated by surgery and postoperative radiotherapy, in comparison with about 50–60% estimated in other series after surgery alone. It is worth mentioning that in the aforementioned study the 10-year progression-free survival rate was about 60% and overall tumour control was achieved in more than 70% of patients treated by radiotherapy only.

Contrary to PRL- or GH-secreting pituitary tumours where medical therapy with dopamine agonists or somatostatin, respectively, is able to suppress hormone secretion and to reduce tumour size; medical treatment of NFPAs has remained elusive (Fig. 31.2). In a few patients with FSH or α-SU hypersecretion, bromocriptine has been described to cause hormone levels to fall, but not to cause any significant tumour shrinkage in most patients, although it improves tumour mass and/or visual fields in a minority. Administration of the long-acting somatostatin analogue, octreotide, has been reported to reduce gonadotrophins and their free subunit levels along with a reduction of

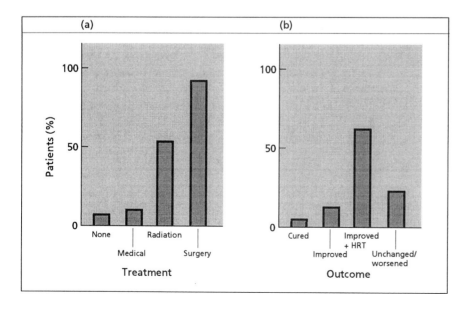

Fig. 31.1 (a) Therapeutical approach and (b) outcome in a series of 286 patients with non-functioning pituitary adenomas (NFPAs) studied over a 20-year period. In this series radiation therapy was given as first therapeutical approach in less than 5% of patients. About 8% of patients had more than one surgical operation. Cured: patients in whom no postoperative residual tumour tissue was detectable and did not need any other adjunctive or hormone replacement treatment. Improved: patients in whom tumour mass-induced disturbances disappeared, and did not need any hormone replacement treatment. Improved + hormone replacement therapy (HRT): as in cured and improved, but needing HRT.

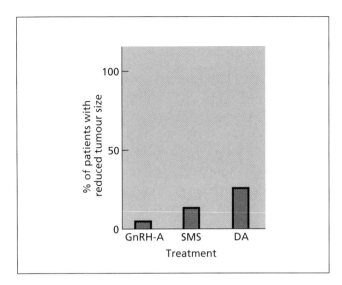

Fig. 31.2 Only few patients with non-functioning pituitary adenomas (NFPAs) benefit from medical treatment. This figure shows the percentage of patients with NFPAs who had a reduced tumour size after medical treatment. GnRH-A, GnRH superagonist analogue ($n = 18$); SMS, somatostatin analogue octreotide ($n = 46$); DA, dopaminergic drugs ($n = 141$). (From available literature.)

tumour size in a small number of patients. The responses of NFPA to octreotide administration have been extremely heterogeneous: most patients show transient improvement in visual field defects, but do not shrink the tumour; a small number of patients (less than 20%) show slightly reduced tumour size, while some demonstrate an increase. These findings probably reflect the fact that somatostatin receptors are found in a limited subset of such tumours, that the improvement of visual fields may be due to a direct action of octreotide on optic pathways or their vascular flow, that the effect of octreotide on tumour size and serum hormone levels may be independent, and that in a subset of NFPA, somatostatin is able to increase in-

tracellular calcium concentration, which might result in paradoxical stimulation of tumour growth. The use of GnRH agonists has been suggested (as they can suppress gonadotrophin secretion from normal pituitary gonadotroph by desensitizing GnRH receptors) but they are not effective since neither gonadotrophin- nor α-SU-secreting adenomas seem to desensitize.

The second aim of therapy of NFPAs is to correct any hormonal deficiencies. The endocrine management of hypopituitary patients mainly consists of hormone replacement therapy according to the widely accepted usual schedules. Overall, hormone therapy is required in about 50–60% of patients. Optimal treatment permits normal activity and a good prognosis for life expectancy. The usefulness of treating GH deficiency in these patients is, at present, under investigation.

References

1. Horvath E, Kovacs K. The adenohypophysis. In Kovacs K, Asa SL (eds). *Functional Endocrine Pathology*, vol. 1. Boston: Blackwell Scientific Publications, 1991:245–80.
2. Katznelson L, Alexander JM, Klibanski A. Clinically nonfunctioning pituitary adenomas. *J. Clin. Endocrinol. Metab.* 1993;**76**:1089–94.
3. Alexander JM, Biller BMK, Bikkal H *et al.* Clinically nonfunctioning pituitary tumors are monoclonal in origin. *J. Clin. Invest.* 1990;**86**:336–40.
4. Spada A, Vallar L, Faglia G. Cellular alterations in pituitary tumors. *Eur. J. Endocrinol.* 1994;**130**:43–52.
5. Colombo P, Paganelli G, Magnani P *et al.* Immunoscintigraphy with anti-chromogranin A antibodies in patients with endocrine/neuroendocrine tumor. *J. Endocrinol. Invest.* 1993;**16**:841–3.
6. Faglia G, Spada A, Beck-Peccoz P *et al.* Clinically nonfunctioning pituitary adenomas: advances and perspectives. *Excerpta Medica Int. Congress Ser.* 1991;**961**:373–82.
7. Hughes MN, Llamas KJ, Yelland ME, Tripcony LB. Pituitary adenoma — long term results for radiotherapy alone and postoperative radiotherapy. *Int. J. Radiat. Oncol. Biol. Phys.* 1994;**27**:1035–43.

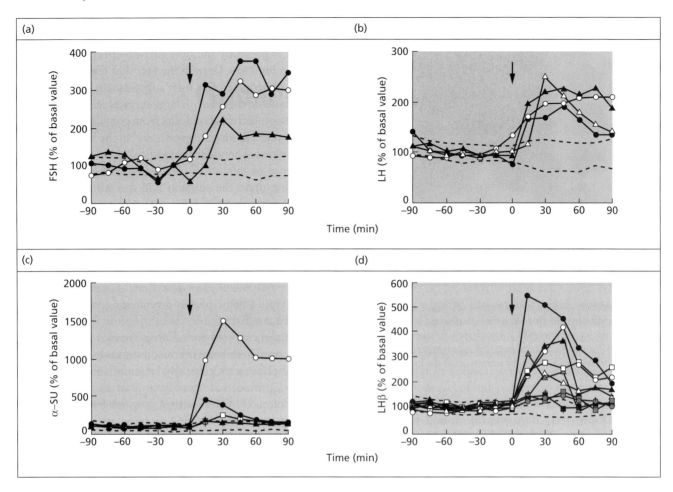

Fig. 32.2 Responses of serum (a) follicle-stimulating hormone (FSH), (b) luteinizing hormone (LH), (c) α subunit (α-SU) and (d) LH-β to the intravenous administration of 400 μg of thyrotrophin-releasing hormone (TRH) in 16 women with non-secreting pituitary adenomas. The values are expressed as a percentage of the mean of seven values determined before the administration of TRH (arrows). The dashed lines represent the mean ±2 sd in 16 healthy age-matched women. The solid lines and various symbols represent individual patients whose responses to TRH increased significantly (by analysis of variance) above basal values and exceeded the range in the healthy age-matched women. Eleven women with non-secreting adenomas had significant LH-β responses to TRH, four had significant LH and α-SU responses, and three had significant FSH responses. (Redrawn from [4] by copyright permission of the Massachusetts Medical Society.)

References

1. Snyder PJ. Clinically non-functioning pituitary adenomas. *Endocrinol. Metab. Clin. North Am.* 1993;**22**:163–75.
2. Jameson JL, Klibanski A, Black PM *et al.* Glycoprotein hormone genes are expressed in clinically nonfunctioning pituitary adenomas. *J. Clin. Invest.* 1987;**80**:1472–8.
3. Demura R, Jibiki K, Kubo O *et al.* The significance of α-subunit as a tumor marker for gonadotropin-producing pituitary adenomas. *J. Clin. Endocrinol. Metab.* 1986;**63**:564–8.
4. Daneshdoost L, Gennarelli TA, Bashey HM *et al.* Recognition of gonadotroph adenomas in women. *N. Engl. J. Med.* 1991;**324**:589–94.
5. Daneshdoost L, Pavlou SN, Molitch ME *et al.* Inhibition of follicle-stimulating hormone secretion from gonadotroph adenomas by repeti-tive administration of a gonadotropin-releasing hormone antagonist. *J. Clin. Endocrinol. Metab.* 1990;**71**:92–7.
6. Katznelson L, Oppenheim DS, Coughlin JF *et al.* Chronic somatostatin analog administration in patients with α-subunit-secreting pituitary tumors. *J. Clin. Endocrinol. Metab.* 1992; **75**:1318–25.

33

Thyrotrophinomas

ROBERT C. SMALLRIDGE

Introduction

Thyrotrophin-secreting tumours (TSHomas) comprise approximately 1% of all pituitary tumours. This review reports on 176 published [1–3] and unpublished cases which have presented since 1970.

Clinical features (Table 33.1)

TSHomas almost always produce hyperthyroid symptoms (often mild), although rarely a patient appears euthyroid. Unlike the female predominance seen in Graves' disease, TSHomas occur with equal frequency in men and women. While most present in the third to sixth decades of life, ages have ranged from 11 to 84 years (Fig. 33.1). Most patients have a goitre. Visual field abnormalities in about half the patients are expected given the high frequency of macroadenomas (90%). Multiple hormone oversecretion is common, with 21% of patients exhibiting clinical acromegaly and half that number having amenorrhoea and/or galactorrhoea.

Autoimmune thyroid disease, as determined by various thyroid antibodies and ophthalmopathy, has been detected in a small percentage of TSHoma patients [1]. Graves' disease and a TSHoma in the same individual, while rare, has occurred. It is noteworthy that tumour invasion of the orbit has produced unilateral proptosis.

Diagnostic evaluation

Measurement of an increased serum T_4 with detectable or increased thyroid-stimulating hormone (TSH) presents an interesting differential diagnosis (Fig. 33.2). Transient causes are identified by history and physical examination, and laboratory studies can characterize abnormal thyroid-binding proteins or antibodies. If these possibilities are excluded, the patient probably has inappropriate TSH secretion. Resistance to thyroid hormone (RTH), when generalized, is usually autosomal dominant; clinically hyperthyroid patients have predominantly pituitary resistance, and are often sporadic cases. In neither instance is a pituitary tumour present [4].

Distinguishing between RTH and a TSHoma requires both laboratory [5] and radiological studies. The single most helpful blood test is an α subunit (α-SU) level, with calculation of an α-SU/TSH molar ratio. This ratio, indicating selective oversecretion of uncombined α-SU to intact TSH, is > 1.0 in 92% of patients with TSH-secreting tumours, but is ≤ 1.0 in RTH cases. It is more meaningful than the absolute α-SU value, which may be in the normal reference range. Serum TSH-β is not elevated.

The TSH response to thyrotrophin-releasing hormone (TRH) also is helpful [1–3]. In RTH, this response is always normal or exaggerated, while a twofold or greater increase occurs in only 20% of TSHomas. Other pharmacological manipulations in tumour patients have not yielded a useful diagnostic test. Baseline levels of other pituitary hormones should be measured (e.g. prolactin, PRL), as they are increased in some tumour patients (see Fig. 33.1).

When a TSH tumour is suspected a pituitary imaging study is mandatory. Most tumours are large and readily visible. Interestingly, several tumours have not been found radiologically. Because of convincing biochemical evidence, selective petrosal sinus sampling has been performed and shown to confirm the presence of a microadenoma in some cases [3].

Therapy (Table 33.2)

Treatment of TSHomas is often unsuccessful, as patients usually have large tumours with suprasellar, sphenoid or cavernous sinus extension. Where size was mentioned, from 1970 to 1987, 57 of 60 (95%) tumours were macroadenomas [1]. The high frequency of such large, unresectable tumours may be due to improper initial diagnosis. Some patients underwent thyroid ablation for suspected Graves'

Table 33.1 Clinical and laboratory features in 176 patients with thyrotrophin-secreting pituitary tumours (1970–94)

Clinical characteristics	Number*	Laboratory results	Number*
Sex:		α/TSH > 1.0	84/91 (92)
Male	88	GH ↑	40
Female	88	PRL ↑	36
Goitre	108/119 (91)	LH/FSH ↑	8
Abnormal visual fields	50/104 (48)	ACTH ↑	1
Ophthalmopathy	6/89 (7)	Thyroid Abs	6/50 (12)
Acromegaly	35 (21)	TSH-R Abs	3/57 (5)
Amenorrhoea/galactorrhoea	19 (11)	TSH ↑ to TRH	26/132 (20)
		Macroadenoma	138/154 (90)

* Numbers in the numerators and denominators indicate the number affected and total number of cases available, respectively. The numbers in parentheses indicate percentages.

↑, elevated; Abs, antibodies; ACTH, adrenocorticotrophic hormone; FSH, follicle-stimulating hormone; GH, growth hormone; LH, luteinizing hormone; PRL, prolactin; TRH, thyrotrophin-releasing hormone; TSH, thyroid-stimulating hormone; TSH-R, TSH-receptor.

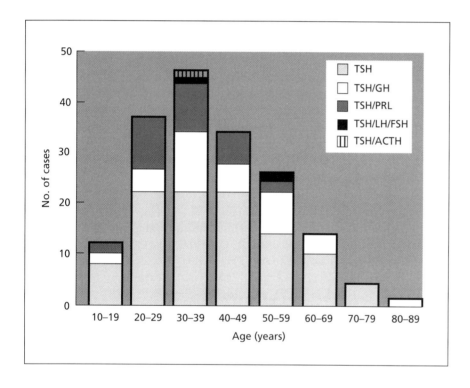

Fig. 33.1 Distribution by decades of patients with thyrotrophin-secreting tumours. ACTH, adrenocorticotrophic hormone; FSH, follicle-stimulating hormone; GH, growth hormone; LH, luteinizing hormone; PRL, prolactin; TSH, thyrotrophin-secreting hormone.

disease. While euthyroidism or hypothyroidism occurred, the pituitary tumour enlarged over years to decades. With sensitive TSH assays and greater appreciation of this disorder microadenomas have been identified more often, with only 81 of 94 (86%) being macroadenomas (1987–94). Unfortunately, the biochemical cure rate with pituitary surgery alone remains unchanged, at less than 40%.

The most exciting advance in management of TSHomas is the use of octreotide administered subcutaneously [3]. In 48 cases reviewed, serum TSH was reduced in all but three. Of the 46 cases with specific values, TSH decreased by 0–25% in six, 26–50% in seven, 51–75% in 11 and

76–100% in 22. Serum T_4 fell in all 32 patients in whom data were available, and hyperthyroid symptoms often improved. Tumour size decreased in 14 of 26, vision improved in six of seven, and goitre shrank in four cases.

Octreotide altered glycosylation of serum TSH in one patient, suggesting a change in biological activity [3]. This might explain the decrease in serum T_4 and clinical improvement in a few patients whose serum TSH was unchanged. Most patients received octreotide injections subcutaneously (100–1500 µg/day in divided doses), but a few received continuous subcutaneous infusions (200–300 µg/day) and four received a slow-release formulation

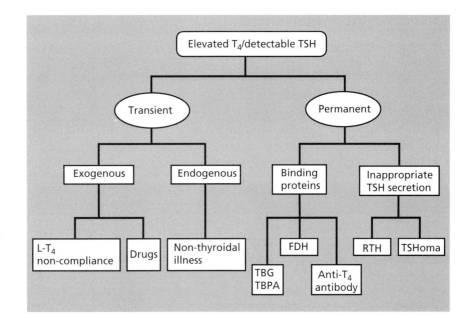

Fig. 33.2 Causes of an elevated serum T$_4$ and a detectable serum thyrotrophin-secreting hormone (TSH) level. TBG, thyroxine-binding globulin; FDH, familial dysalbuminaemic hyperthyroxinaemia; RTH, resistance to thyroid hormone; TBPA, thyroxine-binding prealbumin (transthyretin); TSHoma, thyrotrophin-secreting pituitary tumour.

Table 33.2 Results of various therapies in patients with thyrotrophin-secreting tumours and hyperthyroidism

Therapy	Results		
	Success	Failure	Unknown
Pituitary surgery	43	67	8
Pituitary irradiation (X-ray therapy)	1	8	1
Surgery and X-ray therapy	17	31	8
Thyroidectomy	0	30	0
Radioactive iodine	0	30	1

of the analogue lanreotide two to three times monthly. Side-effects from somatostatin analogues have included abdominal cramps or pain, increased frequency of stools or diarrhoea, nausea, gall stones, steatorrhoea and glucose intolerance.

Long-term results

Long-term follow-up is available in a few patients. In one series of five macroadenoma patients treated with surgery and radiation (X-ray) therapy, all had residual tumour and inappropriate TSH secretion 3.5–6 years later. Two microadenoma patients remained cured 2.5 and 4 years after trans-sphenoidal surgery [2].

At our institution, of six patients treated with trans-sphenoidal surgery and X-ray therapy for macroadenomas, two were cured at 2.5 and 4.5 years. A third was not cured 2 years after therapy, and a fourth, also not cured, has been controlled with octreotide for 8 years.

A fifth patient initially received iodine-131 (^{131}I) for suspected Graves' disease. Twenty-one months after trans-sphenoidal surgery and X-ray therapy she has extensive tumour and active acromegaly; serum T$_4$ and T$_3$ are normal, and TSH is slightly elevated. The sixth patient, treated initially with trans-sphenoidal surgery, received ^{131}I to control her hyperthyroidism, then received X-ray therapy. Nineteen years later, she has no residual tumour on magnetic resonance imaging (MRI). Her acromegaly is cured; T$_4$ and T$_3$ levels have been normal for many years. TSH remains detectable (2.5 mu/l) and minimally responsive to TRH. The α-SU/TSH molar ratio is 2.4 (preoperatively, it was 35.8); LH/FSH are low.

Our approach to follow-up is similar to that of patients with other types of pituitary tumours. We recommend annual testing of pituitary hormonal function. Visual field tests and an MRI are performed every 1–2 years, and patients are advised that they need such re-evaluations indefinitely.

Pathophysiology/pathogenesis

Alterations in glycosylation of tumour and serum TSH have been reported, as has an increase in biological activity of serum TSH. Circadian rhythms of secreted TSH may also be altered. Receptors for TRH and dopamine may be absent. Tumour TSH-β mRNA has been shown to be normal in several patients, and G protein ($G_{s\alpha}$) gene sequence and function normal in one. Whether a molecular defect causes these tumours is unknown.

Conclusion

Much has been learned about these fascinating tumours in the past quarter century. Once their aetiology is known, more effective therapy will be devised.

Acknowledgements

I wish to thank Drs K. Burman, R. Sjoberg, J. Hennessey and A. Warnet for providing information on unpublished cases. The opinions or assertions contained herein are the private views of the authors and are not to be construed as official or reflecting the views of the Department of the Army or the Department of Defense.

References

1. Smallridge RC. Thyrotropin-secreting pituitary tumors. *Endocrinol. Metab. Clin. North Am.* 1987;**16**:765–92.
2. Gesundheit N, Petrick PA, Nissim M *et al.* Thyrotropin-secreting pituitary adenomas: clinical and biochemical heterogeneity. Case reports and follow-up of nine patients. *Ann. Intern. Med.* 1989;**111**:827–35.
3. Smallridge RC. Thyrotropin-secreting tumors. In Mazzaferri EL, Samaan NA (eds) *Endocrine Tumors.* Boston: Blackwell Scientific Publications, 1993:136–51.
4. Refetoff S, Weiss RE, Usala SJ. The syndromes of resistance to thyroid hormone. *Endocr. Rev.* 1993;**14**:348–99.
5. Smallridge RC. Thyroid function tests. In Becker KL (ed.) *Principles and Practice of Endocrinology and Metabolism.* Philadelphia: J.B. Lippincott, 1990:229–306.

34

Pituitary Carcinoma

ISRAEL DONIACH

Introduction

In his Sherrington lecture (1955) [1] the neurosurgeon Sir Geoffrey Jefferson reviewed the findings in 312 surgically treated pituitary adenomas and drew special attention to 14 of them, showing both clinical and microscopic evidence of invasion and infiltration of the structures in the cavernous sinuses. He proposed that these should be called 'invasive adenomas' and restricted the term 'carcinoma' to the extremely rare cases in which there are metastases by implantation along the cerebrospinal axis and/or metastases outside the axis. In a recent review analysing the pathology of 365 surgically treated invasive pituitary adenomas, Scheithauer and colleagues [2] included the incidence of gross invasion of surrounding structures established by direct observation through the dissecting microscope during surgery or by neuroradiology. Their estimated rate of gross invasion by adenomas of all types was approximately 35%. None had metastasized in spite of access of tumour cells to the cerebrospinal fluid (CSF) and venous system. The ability to establish colonies away from the primary tumour indicates new 'malignant' properties of tumour cells as well as possibly lowered or absent immune resistance by the host. The requirement of the presence of metastases for use of the term carcinoma of pituitary, though arbitrary, has been widely, though not completely, accepted. Checking case reports entitled malignant or carcinomatous anterior pituitary tumours, still reveals occasional examples without metastases, in which there is widespread invasion of local structures and/or marked nuclear pleomorphism and abundant mitoses. Malignancy cannot be determined on histology alone. In fact occasional pituitary adenomas, especially in acromegaly, may show marked nuclear pleomorphism and multinucleated tumour cells. Occasional adenomas, especially in Cushing's disease, may show more mitoses than are usually seen. Some of the carcinomas show good differentiation and no gross excess of mitoses.

Morphological analysis of anterior pituitary tumours shows an ascending degree of aggressive behaviour as follows.

1 Microadenomas are discrete non-encapsulated tumours that compress adjacent parenchyma and may show entrapped non-neoplastic cells in their periphery.

2 Macroadenomas may damage adjacent structures including bone by compression only, without infiltration.

3 Invasive adenomas infiltrate adjacent structures, particularly the cavernous sinuses and sphenoid bones and may even present clinically with nasopharyngeal polyps consisting of anterior pituitary tumour cells continuous with the primary tumour.

4 Malignant tumour cells in the CSF may seed the surface of the brain, spinal cord and cauda equina.

5 Intracranial carcinomas may produce deposits within the depth of the brain non-contiguous with the primary tumour. They may possibly arise as a result of reverse venous flow [3].

6 Extracranial deposits indicate the final stage of aggressive behaviour.

The search is in progress in a number of institutes for DNA markers in adenectomy specimens that might indicate the likelihood of future aggressive clinical behaviour [4].

Reported cases

Using the strict criteria of the presence of metastases, Mountcastle and colleagues [5] reported a case of acromegaly due to carcinoma of the anterior pituitary with spinal and lymphatic metastases and reviewed the literature. They found 36* cases of pituitary carcinoma, both functional and inactive, the first case report dated 1904. Further case reports up to 1993 (cited below) bring

* One case is excluded from Table 34.1 since no age or sex or clinical details are given in the original report.

35

Craniopharyngioma

DAVID B. GRANT

Introduction

Craniopharyngiomas are relatively rare tumours, which are derived from remnants of Rathke's pouch and can arise either within or above the pituitary fossa. With an annual incidence of around 1–2 cases per million they account for approximately 5–8% of all intracranial tumours in childhood and about 1% of intracranial tumours in adults. While the tumour can be classified as benign on histological appearance, it frequently infiltrates surrounding structures and the clinical effects are far from benign because of the close proximity of the tumour to the pituitary gland, the optic chiasm and the hypothalamus. In most instances, histology shows adamantinous epithelial pallisades with cyst formation, keratin nodules and calcification. However, in adults about one-third of tumours show a squamous papillary pattern; these latter tumours do not calcify or infiltrate locally and they have a generally better prognosis [1]. This, together with the more rapid growth of craniopharyngiomas that present in early life, largely accounts for the more favourable postoperative outcome that has been noted in adults compared to children.

Clinical presentation

Craniopharyngiomas can declare their presence at any age from the newborn period onward, and in very roughly 50% of cases the first manifestations are during childhood. Most series suggest that the most common age of presentation is between 5 and 12 years of age. In many patients diagnosis is delayed and average duration of symptoms prior to diagnosis of between 7 and 22 months have been reported, with delays of up to 9 years in some cases.

Most cases present with symptoms of: raised intracranial pressure (headache and vomiting) which may be intermittent at first; loss of vision, which is usually of insidious onset but which can sometimes progress rapidly; or endocrine disturbances such as growth failure often associated with obesity in childhood, amenorrhoea and loss of libido in adult life, or with diabetes insipidus at either age. Diencephalic syndrome, precocious puberty and tall stature are less common endocrine manifestations. Other neurological abnormalities such as cranial nerve palsies, ataxia, convulsions, or paresis may be presenting features and clinical examination often reveals the presence of a visual field defect with optic atrophy (or sometimes papilloedema) on ophthalmoscopy.

Diagnosis

Once the possibility of a craniopharyngioma has been entertained in a child or adult with recurrent headaches, visual failure or clinical evidence of hypopituitarism, confirming the diagnosis is usually relatively straightforward. Prior to introduction of computed tomography (CT) and magnetic resonance imaging (MRI), most cases were identified by plain radiographs of the skull and pituitary fossa. These have been reported to be abnormal in up to 94–98% of cases, showing either calcification within the tumour or an abnormal pituitary fossa which may be generally enlarged or may show more subtle changes such as erosion of the sella turcica. Introduction of cranial CT scanning made the diagnosis of craniopharyngioma more straightforward, particularly if the tumour was small or if the skull radiographs appeared normal. However, cranial MRI with gadolinium contrast is probably the most effective method of detecting craniopharyngiomas (Fig. 35.1) and demonstrating the relationship between the tumour and other intracranial structures [2]. Evaluating invasion of bone or sinuses may still require CT scanning.

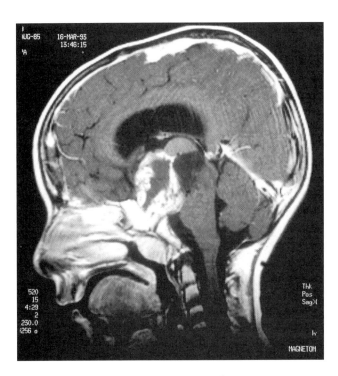

Fig. 35.1 Cranial magnetic resonance image showing a part cyst/part solid craniopharyngioma in an 8-year-old boy who presented with features of intracranial pressure. (Courtesy of Department of Medical Illustration, Great Ormond Street Hospital for Children.)

Surgical treatment

Initial surgical management

The neurosurgical management of craniopharyngioma remains a matter of some controversy. Because of the high risk of tumour recurrence after incomplete removal, some units aim for radical removal of the tumour at the first operation [3]. However, this may carry a relatively high operative mortality and postoperative morbidity, particularly in cases with large tumours. As a result, many neurosurgical units have adopted a much more conservative approach, aiming for radical sub-total removal when complete excision is not possible [4,5]. While such surgery carries a high risk of tumour recurrence, there is now ample evidence that this can be largely prevented by postoperative external irradiation, and sub-total surgical removal followed by radiotherapy is probably the treatment of choice for most cases [6]. Some units have adopted an even more conservative approach with shunting to relieve hydrocephalus (and aspiration if the tumour is largely cystic) followed by external irradiation. Interstitial irradiation, achieved by injecting radioactive isotope (^{90}Yt, ^{198}Au or ^{186}Rh) into tumours which are

cystic, is still used in some centres [7], and intracavitary treatment with methotrexate or bleomycin has also been advocated.

Management of tumour recurrence

In general, most neurosurgical units have reported poorer results with higher mortality after surgery for recurrent craniopharyngioma. In cases that have not been previously given radiotherapy, conservative surgical management followed by external irradiation probably offers the best chance of long-term survival with little or no new neurological handicap. If recurrence occurs after surgery and radiotherapy, further irradiation is likely to lead to problems with vasculitis and brain necrosis or further damage to the optic nerves unless multiple port techniques are used to keep the exposure of normal brain tissue to a minimum.

Endocrine aspects of craniopharyngioma

Like the anterior pituitary, craniopharyngiomas are derived from the foregut but little has been written about their own endocrine activity as opposed to their effects on anterior and posterior pituitary function. However, the presence of immunoreactive human chorionic gonadotrophin (hCG) has been described in fluid from cystic craniopharyngiomas [8] and is invariably present. This immunoreactive material, which appears to have no biological activity, was also present in the cerebrospinal fluid (CSF) of one of nine patients investigated but was not present in the circulation. The presence of hCG in the cyst fluid may therefore be a useful test in the differential diagnosis of a symptomless cyst. In addition, it indicates that the diagnosis of craniopharyngioma must be included with that of germinoma in patients with elevated levels of β-hCG in the CSF.

High levels of insulin-like growth factor-2 (IGF-2) have also been reported in fluid from cystic craniopharyngiomas [9] but the biological significance of this is uncertain. A further intriguing observation is that an immunoreactive form of vasopressin can be found in the circulation soon after subfrontal resection of suprasellar tumours, usually craniopharyngiomas, and that this blocks the antidiuretic effect of vasopressin *in vivo* [10]. Again, the significance of this finding is not known. However, all these results suggest that further studies on the endocrine secretory potential of craniopharyngiomas may be rewarding.

Endocrine management of patients with craniopharyngioma

Preoperative endocrine evaluation

Clinical evidence of endocrine disturbance is relatively common in patients with craniopharyngioma with a reported prevalence of delayed growth in up to 85% of the children in different series. Careful clinical and endocrine assessment is needed to identify features such as diabetes insipidus, growth impairment or hypogonadism, together with an estimation of the adrenocorticotrophic hormone (ACTH) reserve.

Immediate postoperative period

A high proportion of patients develop diabetes insipidus after surgery for craniopharyngioma, particularly when extensive tumour resection has been carried out, and in many patients the diabetes insipidus remains a permanent problem. However, some patients may have a period of inappropriate antidiuretic hormone (ADH) secretion (SIADH) after operation and as a result careful management of fluid balance is essential, together with the use of desmopressin given by injection when appropriate. This is particularly important if the patient has impairment of consciousness or an abnormal/absent sense of thirst and has to rely on others to maintain an appropriate fluid intake. As hypopituitarism is very common after surgery for craniopharyngioma, adequate postoperative steroid replacement therapy with hydrocortisone is almost always indicated.

Long-term endocrine management

Deficits of anterior and posterior pituitary function are very common after surgery for craniopharyngioma and formal endocrine assessment is a very important part of each patient's long-term management. In particular, it is vital to establish whether ACTH deficiency is present, as failure to recognize this and institute appropriate steroid replacement can lead to potentially devastating hypoglycaemia during intercurrent infection [11]. In addition to thyroid replacement when necessary, treatment with growth hormone (GH) to achieve an acceptable adult height will be needed in the majority of children who have had surgery for craniopharyngioma. However, a significant proportion of cases will grow normally for 1–3 years after operation, despite the presence of severe GH deficiency. Such cases often show rapid weight gain associated with high plasma insulin levels during the period of spontaneous growth [12]. The place of GH therapy to maintain muscle and bone mass in adult patients who have had surgery for craniopharyngioma is now under evaluation. Gonadotrophin deficiency is also very common after surgery for craniopharyngioma. Testosterone or oestrogen replacement are required in older children to achieve normal growth and secondary sexual development, and in adults to maintain sexual function.

Hypothalamic disturbances that occur or develop postoperatively can have life-threatening consequences because of problems with fluid balance, hyperphagia and somnolence, despite careful management.

References

1. Adamson TE, Wiestler OD, Kleihues P, Yasargil MG. Correlation of clinical and pathological features in surgically treated craniopharyngiomas. *J. Neurosurg.* 1990;**73**:12–17.
2. Pigeau I, Sigal R, Halimi P, Comoy J, Doyan D. MRI features of craniopharyngioma at 1.5 Tesla: a series of 15 cases. *J. Neuroradiol.* 1988;**15**:276–87.
3. Yasargil MG, Curcic M, Kis M *et al.* Total removal of craniopharyngiomas: Approaches and long-term results in 144 patients. *J. Neurosurg.* 1990;**73**:3–11.
4. Baskin DS, Wilson CB. Surgical management of craniopharyngiomas. *J. Neurosurg.* 1986;**65**:22–7.
5. Graham PH, Gattamaneni R, Birch JM. Paediatric craniopharyngiomas: a regional view. *Br. J. Neurosurg.* 1992;**6**:187–94.
6. Regine WF, Kramer S. Pediatric craniopharyngiomas: long term results of combined treatment with surgery and radiation. *Int. J. Radiat. Oncol. Biol. Phys.* 1992;**24**:611–17.
7. Berge JH, Blaauw G, Breeman WAP, Rahmy A, Wijhgaarde R. Intracavitary brachytherapy of cystic craniopharyngiomas. *J. Neurosurg.* 1992;**77**:545–50.
8. Harris PE, Perry L, Chard T *et al.* Immunoreactive human chorionic gonadotropin from the cyst fluid and CSF of patients with craniopharyngioma. *Clin. Endocrinol.* 1988;**29**:503–8.
9. Zumkeller W, Sääf M, Rähn T, Hall K. Demonstration of insulin-like growth factors I, II and heterogenous insulin-like growth factor binding proteins in the cyst fluid of patients with craniopharyngioma. *Neuroendocrinology* 1991;**54**:196–201.
10. Seckl JR, Dunger DB, Bevan JS *et al.* Vasopressin antagonist in early postoperative diabetes insipidus. *Lancet* 1990;**335**:1353–6.
11. Lyen K, Grant DB. Endocrine function, morbidity and mortality after surgery for craniopharyngioma. *Arch. Dis. Childh.* 1982;**57**:837–41.
12. Stahnke N, Grubel G, Lagenstein I, Willig RP. Long-term follow-up of children with craniopharyngioma. *Eur. J. Pediatr.* 1984;**142**:179–85.

Benign Cysts: Rathke's Cysts, Mucocoeles and Arachnoid Cysts

SHERRY L. TAYLOR AND CHARLES B. WILSON

Introduction

Any sellar, parasellar or suprasellar lesion can produce endocrine dysfunction by compressing adjacent structures, particularly the hypothalamus and the pituitary gland. The most common non-neoplastic lesions in this region are Rathke's cysts, mucocoeles and arachnoid cysts, which can cause headaches and visual manifestations as well as hypopituitarism [1,2]. Table 36.1 gives details of presentation of Rathke's and arachnoid cysts.

Rathke's cleft cysts

Rathke's cysts are lined by epithelial cells and their contents range from a fine, granular, yellowish fluid to a thick mucoid material. They are derived from remnants of Rathke's pouch, which appears between the third and fourth week of gestation.

Although Rathke's cysts have been reported more frequently since the advent of computed tomography (CT) and magnetic resonance imaging (MRI), they are seldom symptomatic and are often found at autopsy, with an incidence of 13 to 23%. Symptomatic cysts may present between adolescence and the seventh decade, but are seen most commonly in young adults, predominantly females. Headache is the most common symptom, followed by amenorrhoea or galactorrhoea. Visual field loss and hypopituitarism, including growth hormone (GH), thyroid and adrenal insufficiency, and, rarely, obstructive hydrocephalus can also be seen. Rathke's cysts can be difficult to diagnose by radiological criteria. Plain skull films may show sellar erosion or enlargement. CT scans typically demonstrate an intrasellar, non-calcified, non-enhancing cystic mass with or without suprasellar extension; however, contrast enhancement, calcification, and an entirely suprasellar location may be seen. T_1-weighted MRI scans show increased signal intensity in about two-thirds of cases and low signal in about one-third (Fig. 36.1). T_2-weighted images showed increased signal in approximately 50%, isointense signal in 25% and low signal in 25%. Administration of gadolinium may produce discrete, intense rim enhancement.

Treatment includes surgical decompression, cyst drainage and partial resection of the cyst wall. The transsphenoidal approach is preferred because postoperative aseptic meningitis is less common than with craniotomy and because there is less operative morbidity. Headache resolved postoperatively in approximately 60% of our patients; visual field impairment was relieved in all and hyperprolactinaemia in all but 12.5%. Panhypopituitarism and diabetes insipidus tend not to improve after cyst drainage. Recurrence in our series was extremely rare and further therapy was rarely needed.

Mucocoeles

Mucocoeles are diffuse expansions from a paranasal sinus with a blocked ostium. Pathologically, they can be indistinguishable from Rathke's cysts and may only be differentiated by radiological evidence of extension from a paranasal sinus. Parasellar mucocoeles originate from the sphenoid, frontal or ethmoid sinus, sometimes producing a painless unilateral exophthalmos without extraocular motor palsy. Mucocoeles of the sphenoid sinus are the least common, representing less than 5% of all paranasal sinus mucocoeles; rarely they may mimic an intrasellar tumour and compress the pituitary gland or optic structures. It is important to differentiate these lesions from intrasellar neoplasms because of the high incidence of severe chemical meningitis if the cyst contents are spilled intracranially. Decompression without attempt at radical removal is the treatment of choice. Recurrence is rare when drainage into the nasal cavity is established.

Table 36.1 Presentation of Rathke's cleft cysts [3] and arachnoid cysts [4,5]

Presentation	Rathke's cleft cysts [3]	Arachnoid cysts	
		Intrasellar [4]	Suprasellar [5]
Mean age (years)	34	42.2	50% < 5, all under 15
Male/female (*n*)	10/33	6/2	15/5
Headache	++++	++	+
Amenorrhoea/galactorrhoea	+++	+	–
Visual field deficits	++	+	++
Hypopituitarism	+	++	+
Precocious puberty	–	–	+
Bobble-head doll syndrome	–	–	+
Incidental finding	–	++	+
Hydrocephalus	–	–	+++*

*Common in infants.
++++, > 75 to 100%; +++, > 50 to ≤ 75%; ++, > 25 to ≤ 50%; +, ≤ 25%.

Arachnoid cysts

Arachnoid cysts are thought to develop from splitting or duplication of the arachnoid. They represent only 1% of all intracranial space-occupying lesions and can arise anywhere in the subarachnoid space along the cerebrospinal axis; the sellar/suprasellar region is the second most common location of intracranial supratentorial arachnoid cysts. These cysts may be either suprasellar or, less commonly, intrasellar.

Most suprasellar arachnoid cysts occur in children; almost half the patients are less than 5 years old. They develop in the chiasmatic cistern and may expand upwards, compressing the hypothalamus, third ventricle and aqueduct of Sylvius, and may encroach on the optic chiasm, optic nerve and pituitary stalk. They usually communicate with the subarachnoid space and on imaging studies may be difficult to differentiate from third ventricular dilatation due to aqueductal stenosis. Hydrocephalus is most common in infants; approximately one-third of cases have visual impairment, spasticity and gait ataxia. Precocious puberty is the most common endocrine presentation; hypopituitarism, including growth retardation and adrenal insufficiency, may also occur. An extremely unusual manifestation is the 'bobble-head doll syndrome', consisting of irregular involuntary head bobbing at a rate of 2–3 times/second that is absent during sleep and can usually be stopped voluntarily for brief periods. Children with this syndrome usually have enlarged heads, growth retardation and delayed developmental milestones. It is twice as common in boys as in girls.

There is no consensus on the treatment for suprasellar arachnoid cysts. The options include shunting of the hydrocephalus alone, fenestration of the cyst membrane into a subarachnoid cistern or adjacent ventricle, cystoperitoneal shunting, or percutaneous ventriculocystostomy. Reoperation is frequently necessary, regardless of the initial approach. In our experience, cystoperitoneal shunting yields the best results.

Intrasellar arachnoid cysts do not occur in infants; the mean age at presentation is 42 years. They are extradural and located outside the pituitary gland, usually at the level of the pars distalis or immediately below the dura. Upwards displacement of the diaphragma sellae and posterior bowing of the sellar contour are common. Even when there is a large suprasellar extension, the diaphragma sellae remains intact; this can be a key finding during radiological evaluation. Approximately 50% of intrasellar arachnoid cysts are found incidentally on radiological evaluation. Symptomatic cysts tend to cause headache; hypopituitarism, decreased visual acuity and bitemporal field deficits may also be present. The preferred treatment is trans-sphenoidal drainage followed by packing of the residual cavity with fat, fascia or muscle and reconstruction of the sella turcica. Headache and visual difficulties can improve with treatment, but the endocrine dysfunction usually does not.

Conclusion

Because of their parasellar location, Rathke's cysts, mucocoeles and arachnoid cysts may cause endocrine dysfunction, including amenorrhoea, galactorrhoea, panhypopituitarism and diabetes insipidus. Headache, visual disturbances and symptoms of hyperprolactinaemia frequently improve after surgical treatment, but panhypopituitarism usually does not.

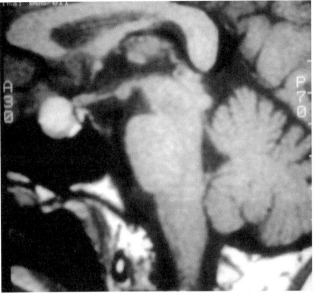

(a)

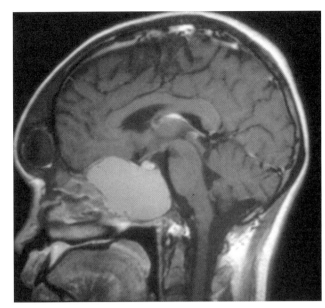

(b)

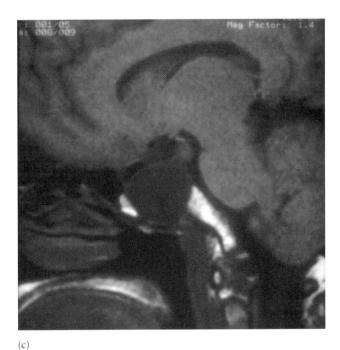

(c)

Fig. 36.1 Sagittal T$_1$-weighted magnetic resonance images showing (a) a Rathke's cleft cyst, (b) a mucocoele, and (c) an intrasellar arachnoid cyst. The high signal intensity of the Rathke's cyst and the mucocoele on T$_1$ imaging reflects the high protein content of the cyst. The low signal intensity of the arachnoid cyst on T$_1$ imaging indicates that the cyst contents have the same density as cerebrospinal fluid. Note compression of the normal pituitary by the mucocoele in (b).

References

1. Rengachary SS. Intracranial arachnoid and ependymal cysts. In Wilkins RH, Rengachary SS (eds). *Neurosurgery*, Vol. 3. New York: McGraw-Hill, 1985:2160–72.

2. Tindall GT, Barrow DL. Tumors of the sellar and parasellar area in adults. In Youmans JR (ed.). *Neurological Surgery*. Philadelphia: W.B. Saunders, 1990:3447–98.3.

3. Ross DA, Norman D, Wilson CB. Radiologic characteristics and results of surgical management of Rathke's cysts in 43 patients. *Neurosurgery* 1992;**30**:173–9.

4. Baskin DS, Wilson CB. Transsphenoidal treatment of non-neoplastic intrasellar cysts. A report of 38 cases. *J. Neurosurg.* 1984;**60**:8–13.

5. Pierre-Kahn A, Capelle L, Brauner R *et al*. Presentation and management of suprasellar arachnoid cysts. Review of 20 cases. *J. Neurosurg.* 1990;**73**:355–9.

37

Epidermoid and Dermoid Cysts

PETER J. HAMLYN

Introduction

The earliest references to epidermoid and dermoid tumours is thought to have been by Verattus in 1745 and Pinson in 1807, respectively. Since then these unusual, non-neuroepithelial tumours or cysts have been subject to considerably confused terminology [1].

Both may occur throughout the cranium and spine though the emphasis here will rest around the sellar region.

Epidermoids

Incidence

Certainly comprising less than 1% of intracranial tumours in adults, fewer than 0.02% of infant brain tumours are epidermoids. Half present during the second and third decade of life though the peak incidence arises during the forties. There is no gender predilection and no confirmed geographical orientation [1,2].

Site

Ninety percent of cranial epidermoids are intradural, associated with the basal subarachnoid spaces. Almost half arise within the cerebellopontine angle where, after acoustic tumours and meningiomas, they are the most common lesion. Approximately 15% arise around the supra and parasellar regions. Isolated reports of intrasellar lesions exist [1–3].

Intra-axial examples are rare, with the fourth ventricle being the most frequent site and only occasional reports of hemisphere, pineal and brain stem lesions occurring. Ten percent of cranial epidermoids are extradural, intra-diploic tumours affecting, in decreasing frequency, the frontal, parietal, occipital and sphenoid bones. Rare and most usually iatrogenic spinal lesions occur.

However, the most common site, when they arise in conjunction with chronic otitis media, is the middle ear from where they may erode the petrous bone.

Pathology

Well delineated they have a smooth, nodular and 'pearly white' surface of thin, translucent, occasionally calcified, simple stratified squamous epithelium. This capsule gradually expands with the build up of desquamated keratin in soft, white and waxy concentric lamellae. Escape of the material may provoke a surrounding granulomatous meningeal reaction. Rarely the contents are thick, brown and viscid; a result perhaps of haemorrhage [2].

They insinuate along cerebrospinal fluid (CSF) pathways to envelop vessels and cranial nerves, distort the adjacent brain and excavate the skull base. Their growth rate is determined by the speed of desquamation which being linear is slow compared to the exponential pattern of solid tumours. Consequently they may acquire great size, the largest recorded having a volume of 3.2 litres. Rarely carcinomatous change occurs when the outcome is rapidly fatal. In common with other parasellar lesions up to 2% have been associated with cerebral aneurysms though this is comparable with the incidental frequency [1].

Clinical features

Many cases have had symptoms for more than ten years prior to diagnosis. No specific symptoms aid clinical diagnosis.

They may cause compression of adjacent neural structures, occlusion of cerebral vessels, obstruction of CSF pathways and erosion of bone. Thus presenting symptoms have included: painless lump, discharging sinus, cognitive impairment, seizures (50% of cases), pressure headache, coma, irritative cranial nerve symptoms such as trigeminal neuralgia and hemifacial spasm, paretic cranial nerve

234

lesions affecting in decreasing frequency the VII, VIII, VI, II, V, IV, III and IX, X, XI, XII nerves, transient ischaemic attacks, stroke and gradually progressive focal deficits of cerebral, brain stem and cerebellar function. Rarely they may rupture to cause a meningitis, or present with proptosis, subarachnoid haemorrhage or prolonged coma following minor head injury. Incidental lesions are found [1,3].

With 15% arising around the pituitary fossa they may cause a variety of hypopituitary and hypothalamic states in association with cavernous sinus involvement and consequent cranial nerve defects principally affecting ocular function. Amenorrhoea and loss of libido have been the most frequent pituitary symptoms. During treatment others may progress to develop pituitary and perhaps hypothalamic dysfunction [3].

Imaging

Skull X-ray may show bone erosion and calcification. Typically they are hypodense, well demarcated, uniform lesions on computed tomography (CT) which do not enhance with contrast (Fig. 37.1). The Hounsfield unit values (5–15 HU) are those of CSF or below. Calcification within the capsule is seen in 15–25% where slight enhancement may also be seen. Reports of central enhancement have been misquoted. Erosion and adjacent sclerosis of bone is seen. Occasionally they may appear hyperdense or patchy which is thought to result from previous haemorrhage or saponification. On magnetic resonance imaging (MRI) they are usually hyperintense on T_1 reflecting the high lipid content, though 'black' epidermoids with long T_1 values, from lower fat content, do arise. Rarely are they mixed. MRI most clearly demonstrates their extra-axial nature. They are avascular on angiography, though arteries, veins and sinuses may be critically occluded by envelopment. Other than with dermoids doubt rarely remains. Colloid cysts, arachnoid cysts, cystic astrocytoma, tuberculoma, hydatid and craniopharyngiomas have to be considered [4].

Treatment

Growth is slow and not all require treatment. Accounts of more than 10 years' conservative treatment testify to this. However, for the majority this is not appropriate

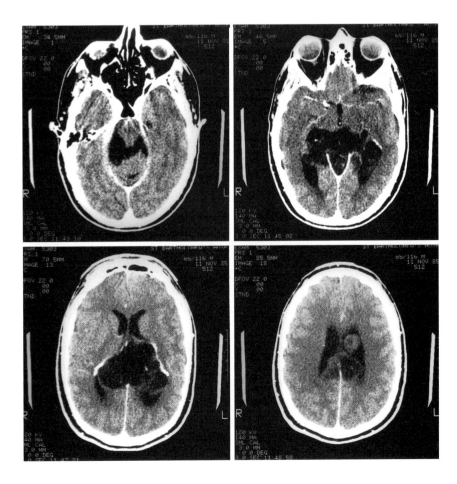

Fig. 37.1 CT scan of an extensive epidermoid tumour. A large epidermoid tumour is seen extending from the lateral ventricles through the third ventricle to encircle the upper brain stem. This 65-year-old male patient presented with headache and cognitive failure. Transventricular and subsequent posterior fossa surgery provided lasting relief.

and here transcranial surgery remains the sole option as radiotherapy and chemotherapy are not effective.

In many instances a complete excision is achieved without additional deficit. Failure arises when adhesions to nervous and vascular structures preclude further dissection. Even then the soft consistency of its contents and the 'dissection' afforded by its slow growth, allows for radical clearances though it is often wise to leave an adherent capsule. Lesions that have extensively crossed the midline may require bilateral approaches and a flexible neuroendoscope may assist in the removal of spread within the ventricles.

A typical operative mortality from the 1930s and 1940s of 70% may now be compared with rates of 5–10% reported in the last two decades. Over 80% may expect to be greatly improved and in some series 70% have returned to the employment held before symptoms developed [1]. Immediate postoperative deficit relates to neural or vascular injury. Disruption of the fine perforating vessels encountered when operating in the para- and suprasellar region may result in hemiplegia or a vegetative state. Postoperatively a crippling chemical meningitis may develop if an extensive keratin-covered capsule is left. With steroids it will eventually settle but may result in hydrocephalus.

Prognosis

Even when excision of the capsule has been incomplete, the outlook is excellent. Follow-up reports have shown that several decades may pass uneventfully in the presence of significant capsular remnants [1]. Surgical caution and on occasions a staged procedure is therefore all the more essential if lifelong deficit is to be avoided.

Dermoids

Incidence

Dermoids are less common in adults than epidermoids although relatively more common in children, where dermal lesions around the fontanelle, occiput and spine account for the majority. They comprise between 0.04 and 0.6% of adult primary brain tumours [1]. The majority of intracranial dermoids present before the fourth decade of life. In general they are probably more common in males and show no geographical pattern. However, the fontanelle lesions may be more common amongst Negro females [2].

Site

Again they centre around the midline. A third of all cases arise in the posterior fossa where they occupy the vermis or fourth ventricle and may communicate with a sinus or dimple on the skin. Parasellar and frontobasal lesions form a significant group. More rarely they arise in the pineal region. Overall the lumbosacral spine is the most frequent neurological site.

Pathology

The capsule consists of dermal appendages as well as epithelium. It is these follicles, hair, sweat, sebaceous and occasional apocrine glands, which differentiate them from the classical epidermoid [2]. Surrounded by dense fibrosis the capsule fills with buttery, thick, brown fluid, the result of desquamation and glandular secretion. Calcification may occur in any part of the lesion although it is most common in the capsule. Teeth and bone are rare, providing a link with teratomas. They form discrete masses which tend to compress rather than envelop adjacent vessels and nervous tissue. Dense adhesions to these local structures, from a foreign body, giant cell type meningeal reaction to leaked contents, are common. Rarely they may be multiple or associated with midline fusion defects such as cleft lip and spina bifida. They have been described with the Arnold–Chiari malformation. Occasional malignancy may arise [1].

Clinical features

Intracranial dermoids present with local and generalized symptoms of mass effect as with the epidermoid lesions, although the history tends to be more progressive. Pituitary dysfunction and visual symptoms are frequent with para- and suprasellar lesions. Meningitis is a more frequent event and may arise from infection tracking down a dermal sinus, or, aseptically following rupture. The latter reaction may be so severe as to induce seizures, vasospasm, infarction and even sudden death. Epilepsy is less frequent, as the temporal lobe is not so often involved and facial palsy and hemifacial spasm have not been reported [1,2].

Imaging

Defects and calcification are more commonly seen on skull X-ray than with epidermoids. Rounded and well delineated on CT scan (Fig. 37.2) they are uniformly hypodense (−20 to −40 HU). Capsular calcification is commonly seen. Rarely they are hyperdense and more rarely still does

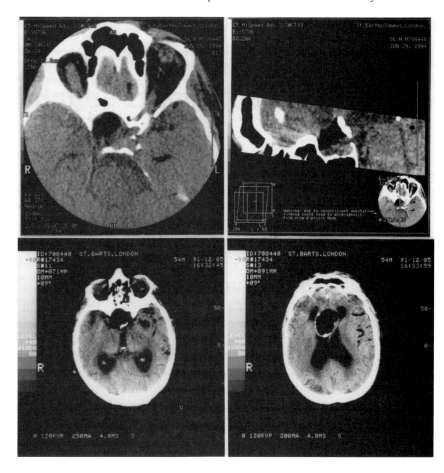

Fig. 37.2 CT scan of a suprasellar dermoid tumour. The four plates show a lesion arising above the sellar with extension into the fossa and up through the third ventricle to cause obstructive hydrocephalus. Calcification is seen in the wall and was visible on plain X-ray. Contents had leaked and can be seen around the temporal lobe and Sylvian fissure on the left. The patient was a 52-year-old male who presented with gradual cognitive failure, hypopituitarism and episodes of acute confusion. The lesion was successfully treated with stereotactic transventricular excision and hormone replacement.

anything other than peripheral enhancement arise with contrast. Hyperintense on T_1 they are either hypointense or inhomogeneously hyperintense on T_2 sequences with MRI. Following rupture, high-signal fat droplets may be seen throughout the subarachnoid spaces. They are avascular on angiography. The differential is that for epidermoids [4].

Treatment

Again treatment is surgical with a balance being drawn between the desire for complete removal and the knowledge that recurrence is slow in event of a remnant. Formal craniofacial procedures are occasionally required for the larger subfrontal lesions.

Prognosis

The prognosis is good although late recurrence is a feature.

Embryological origins and features

Whilst epidermoid and dermoid lesions may usually be clearly defined, on occasions the above features are less distinct. Close similarities may exist with craniopharyngiomas, simple epithelial cysts and Rathke's cleft cysts [1,2,4].

Harrison and colleagues [5] have recently proposed that these lesions be thought of as merely five common patterns in a continuum of cystic ectodermal derivatives. They provide compelling evidence of a common and ectodermal, embryological origin. They point to considerable overlap of both the histological and clinical features. Long follow-up studies refute the previously held views that Rathke's cleft cysts are not subject to recurrence and the rates for craniopharyngiomas far from being universally high have ranged to less than 10% for some series following radical excision. It is very likely this work will modify future classification and treatment design.

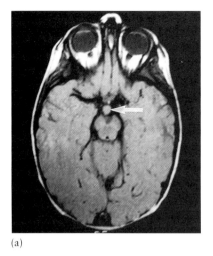 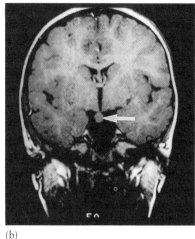 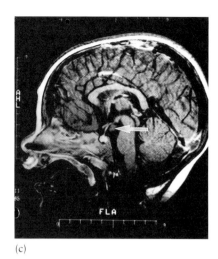

(a)   (b)   (c)

Fig. 38.1 (a) Axial, (b) coronal and (c) sagittal T_1-weighted (short TR) images of a pedunculated hypothalamic hamartoma (arrows).

harder to delineate [2]. HH do not enlarge over time and serial scans are not needed after diagnosis. In a young child with precocious puberty, a pedunculated mass below the hypothalamus is probably pathognomonic of an HH; sessile masses in such children are also more likely to be HH than gliomas.

Therapeutic options

There are no neurological consequences from untreated precocious puberty. Before the availability of effective medical treatment, patients with HH completed precocious puberty, lived sexually mature through childhood and became short-statured adults. The goal of both medical and surgical treatment is to halt the precocious puberty so that secondary sexual characteristics resolve and normal growth rate returns. If a child is diagnosed with precocious puberty and is within 1–2 years of normal pubertal age, it may be appropriate to withhold treatment if their projected height is similar to parental height [3].

Because puberty requires the pulsatile release of GnRH, it can be suppressed medically by the continuous administration of GnRH or GnRHa (analogue). GnRHa suppresses gonadotrophin and sex steroid levels, secondary sexual characteristics stabilize or reverse, and the rate of bone growth decelerates [1,4]. GnRHa is expensive (at least US$3600/year), it must be administered until normal pubertal age and it may not reverse the muscularity, increased appetite and adolescent personality in some patients. Short-acting GnRHa must be injected daily but a long-acting analogue is available and can be administered monthly. GnRHa has been used clinically for 14 years with no evident sequelae or undesirable side-effects.

Prior to 1980, surgical morbidity and mortality were unacceptably high, and the likelihood of cure was unacceptably low. In a review of 33 cases treated surgically after 1958, sub-total resections were done in 27 cases, and precocious puberty was alleviated in only one child [3]. Such sub-total resections are not effective treatment. In the past 15 years, however, effective microsurgical resections have been reported. Pedunculated and small, sessile HH, generally less than 15 mm in diameter, can be resected via a subtemporal approach, and if the hamartoma is resected, puberty ceases [5]. Several recent reports indicate no mortality and low morbidity. Advantages of resection include not being dependent on GnRHa for years, lower cost and virtually complete resolution of symptoms; the disadvantages include the need for a major operation and its neurological risks, particularly the risk of diplopia. The risk of diplopia may be reduced if electromyograms of muscles innervated by the oculomotor nerve are monitored intra-operatively. If MRI demonstrates a large HH where total resection seems unlikely without inordinate risks, the patient should not be treated surgically. Some authors have questioned the effects of HH resections in young children on their subsequent puberty. We have resected HH in five children and precocius puberty has ceased [5]. These children have been followed-up for 1.5–11.5 years (mean 6 years) with no recurrence of symptoms; one child has had normal pubertal development at a normal pubertal age.

Gelastic seizures have been treated by HH resections, by focal cortical resections and by anterior corpus callosum resections, but the results have been inconsistent.

References

1. Mahachoklertwattana P, Kaplan SL, Grumbach MM. The luteinizing hormone-releasing hormone-secreting hypothalamic hamartoma is a congenital malformation: natural history. *J. Clin. Endocrinol. Metab.* 1993;77:118–24.
2. Lona Soto A, Takahashi M, Yamashita Y *et al.* MRI findings of hypothalamic hamartoma: report of five cases and review of the literature. *Comput. Med. Imaging Graph.* 1991;15:415–21.
3. Starceski PJ, Lee PA, Albright AL, Migeon CJ. Hypothalamic hamartomas and sexual precocity. Evaluation of treatment options. *Am. J. Dis. Child.* 1990;144:225–8.
4. Pescovitz OH, Comite F, Hench K *et al.* The NIH experience with precocious puberty: diagnostic subgroups and response to short-term luteinizing hormone releasing hormone analogue therapy. *J. Pediatr.* 1986;108:47–54.
5. Albright AL, Lee PA. Neurosurgical treatment of hypothalamic hamartomas causing precocious puberty. *J. Neurosurg.* 1993;78:77–82.

Cranial Ependymoma

MICHAEL BRADA AND STEPHEN F. SHEPHERD

Introduction

Typically a tumour of children and adolescents, intracranial ependymoma accounts for 9% of primary brain tumours in the first decade of life, 4% in the second and third decades, and only 1% beyond the age of 30 years. This contrasts with ependymoma of the spinal cord, which commonly presents in middle life and comprises 13% of primary tumours at this site. Intracranial ependymomas can arise in relation to any part of the ventricular system but occur twice as frequently in infratentorial than supratentorial regions. They may arise from the roof, floor or lateral recesses of the fourth ventricle. Supratentorial ependymomas originate from ependymal cells lining the third and lateral ventricles and are more likely to be anaplastic. Ependymomas may be found elsewhere within the cerebral hemispheres, probably arising from ependymal cell rests.

Pathology

Ependymomas are solid, cystic or papillary masses, apparently demarcated from the adjacent neural tissue. They are comprised of cells with regular, 'carrot-shaped' nuclei containing abundant granular chromatin. Blepharoblasts, the basal bodies of cilia, which stain with phosphotungstic acid-haematoxylin (PTAH), are pathognomonic of ependymoma. Cells are frequently arranged into rosettes or clusters. Ependymal rosettes consist of tumour cells aligned around a small central lumen; if they surround a blood vessel, they are described as pseudorosettes. About half of ependymomas contain neuroglial intermediate filament, glial fibrillary acidic protein (GFAP). Ependymomas frequently contain astrocytes, prominent areas of oligodendrocytes or distinct regions of each glial cell type.

Two grades of differentiation are recognized, a benign/differentiated and a malignant or anaplastic ependy-moma. The presence of increased cellularity and mitotic figures, pleomorphism, multiple nuclei, giant cells and necrosis in a monophasic ependymoma or any component of a mixed tumour classifies it as anaplastic. Increased cell density and increased number of mitoses have been associated with worse prognosis in supratentorial ependymomas [1], but it has not been confirmed in all studies [2]. This reflects interobserver variation in the classification of tumours by grade and limits the usefulness of histopathological grading in predicting prognosis.

Proliferation characteristics determined by labelling index (LI) and growth fraction may have additional prognostic value [3–5]. Patients with tumours with LIs > 1% determined by bromodeoxyuridine (BrDU) labelling have a higher relapse rate within 2 years of treatment than those with LIs < 1% [3]. BrDU LI also inversely correlates with disease-free interval.

Primitive neuroectodermal tumours (PNETs) containing ependymal cells are a separate entity [6] and not considered within the group of ependymomas even though originally classified as ependymoblastoma. They are composed of poorly differentiated neuroepithelial cells as well as ependymal rosettes or canals.

Subependymoma is a benign form of ependymoma usually found incidentally at autopsy, although occasionally found as symptomatic tumour. Subependymomas occur in the fourth ventricle, septum pellucidum, or cervical cord. Histologically they consist of fibrillary subependymal astrocytes in fine fibrillary background.

Abnormalities of chromosome 6 represent a non-random cytogenetic alteration in childhood central nervous system tumours [7]. The majority of ependymomas also exhibit other cytogenetic abnormalities [7–9], and the most frequent is monosomy 22 [8–10]. Chromosome 22 is considered the site of a putative ependymoma-suppressor gene which differs from the 22q tumour-suppressor gene involved in the evolution of some astrocytomas [11].

Childhood ependymoma and choroid plexus papilloma contain and express a segment of T-antigen gene related to the SV40 virus [12] which suggests a viral aetiology for some of these tumours.

Diagnosis

Symptoms of children or adults presenting with ependymoma vary with the location of the tumour. They include features of raised intracranial pressure and focal neurological deficit as in other space-occupying intracranial lesions. Fourth ventricle location leads to frequent presentation with hydrocephalus.

On imaging, ependymomas are usually semi-solid, semi-cystic, hyperdense, enhancing tumours, which in the posterior fossa location fill the fourth ventricle and are indistinguishable from PNET/medulloblastoma. In supratentorial location the proximity and attachment to the ventricular surfaces suggests the diagnosis. When not associated with ventricles the mass is not discernible from other gliomas.

The propensity for leptomeningeal spread is often overestimated. It occurs it up to 6% of patients at diagnosis [13]. Although relatively uncommon, spinal imaging with spinal magnetic resonance imaging (MRI) is considered necessary. Cerebrospinal fluid (CSF) cytology is usually performed following surgery and is also considered an important staging investigation. However, it is unreliable either as a marker of the presence of disseminated disease at diagnosis, or as a predictor of future CSF spread.

Treatment

Because of the relative rarity of intracranial ependymoma, the management is mostly based on consensus rather than information obtained from prospective studies.

Although surgery is not often considered a curative treatment and extensive resection is associated with high morbidity, most retrospective studies suggest that the best survival results are obtained following attempted complete excision [14–16]. Such procedures are described as 'gross total excision' and vary from the surgeon's description of the extent of resection to postoperative scanning evidence of the amount of residual disease. The extent of resection is considered important particularly in patients with 'low-grade' tumours [14]. However, when faced with a tumour that is technically not resectable it is not possible to assess the role of a radical attempt at tumour clearance compared to just symptomatic tumour debulking.

In the presence of hydrocephalus shunting is not contraindicated as there is no evidence of potential tumour dissemination through the shunt. If restoration of normal drainage is expected following tumour removal, shunting and its long-term problems may be avoided.

Despite the lack of formal comparison of surgery with and without radiotherapy the use of postoperative irradiation in patients with ependymoma is generally accepted as standard treatment. This is based on retrospective studies which demonstrate good long-term tumour control following partial tumour excision and radiotherapy [13,14].

Historically recommendations on the extent of radiotherapy have been based on the apparent pattern of spread. The proximity of ependymoma to ventricular surfaces has been equated with a tendency to seed through the CSF and this has been borne out in occasional cases. Analogy with medulloblastoma, which has a particularly high risk of dissemination, has led to a policy of craniospinal axis irradiation.

The overall risk of developing cranial or spinal metastases is 7% [17]. Distant spinal or cranial disease appears mostly in patients who also relapse at the primary site but the incidence also relates to high tumour grade and infratentorial tumour location. The addition of craniospinal axis irradiation to local radiotherapy has not been shown to decrease the risk of CSF seeding [17].

Radiotherapy should therefore aim to achieve primary tumour control and currently there is no evidence that adding wide-field craniospinal irradiation either reduces the small risk of CSF seeding or that such policy would improve survival [17]. The long-term morbidity of craniospinal irradiation in children, the lack of demonstrable benefit of wide-field irradiation and the association of distant seeding with failure of primary tumour has lead to the now widely accepted policy of localized radiotherapy alone.

There is little information about the efficacy of chemotherapy in ependymoma. From chemotherapy studies reporting less than ten patients with recurrent ependymoma the response rate to nitrosourea-containing chemotherapy is of the order of 20–30% [13]. This is not dissimilar to other glial tumours. However, the use of adjuvant 1-(2-chloroethyl)-3-cyclohexyl-1-nitrosourea (CCNU) and vincristine in patients with high-grade ependymoma in a randomized International Society of Paediatric Oncology (SIOP I) study was not associated with improved survival [18]. With platinum or carboplatin the response rate in children with recurrent ependymoma has been reported to be up to 40% [13]. In line with the policy of avoiding radiotherapy in children under 3 years of age, 25 young children with ependymoma were treated with cyclophosphamide and vincristine, alternating with cisplatin and etoposide. The response rate was 48% and

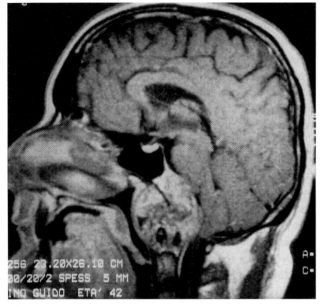

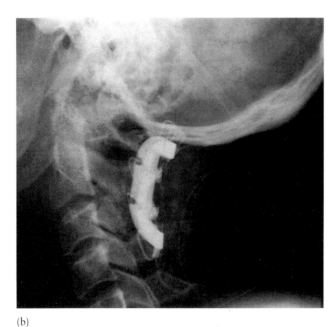

(a)

(b)

Fig. 40.2 (a) MRI demonstrating a large clivus chordoma.
(b) Postoperative radiograph. The titanium fixation system is fully compatible with MRI.

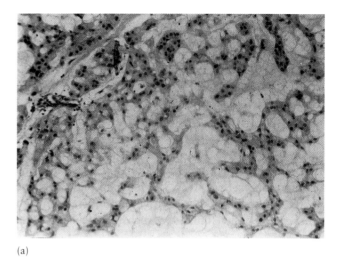

(a)

(b)

(c)

Fig. 40.3 Photomicrographs of a chordoma under high power.
(a) Haematoxylin and eosin stain. (b) The tumour cells are strongly positive on immunostaining for cytokeratin, and (c) for epithelial marker antigen. Arrows indicate representative staining cells.

histories. One group has the relatively indolent form with expected survival of at least a decade; a second group has an aggressive form with early recurrence and a high mortality.

Although they demonstrate usually benign histological features, the prognosis with clivus chordoma is poor. The reported mean survival of 11 untreated Swedish

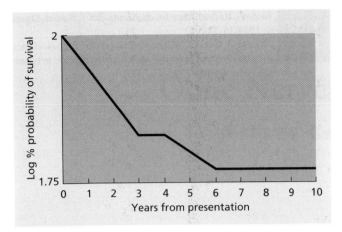

Fig. 40.4 Semilog plot of survival probability at intervals from diagnosis of intracranial chordoma. In this study the survival curve is not uniform, but has two segments of different gradient. This suggests that the population examined is composed of two subgroups with different mortality: one group with a median survival of less than 4 years, and a second group with an indolent disease process and much longer median survival. (Redrawn with permission from [2].)

patients in 1981 was less than 1 year. With treatment, long-term survival has changed little over the past 50 years, with reported mean survivals of between 19 and 56 months [3].

Radiation therapy

Radiation as an adjunct to surgery was suggested by Dahlin and MacCarty in 1952, although it is less clearly demonstrated that radiotherapy alone extends survival. Fuller and Bloom [4] showed some benefit in reducing disease progression but not survival, with tumour doses greater than 55 Gy compared to doses of less than 50 Gy. The effectiveness of conventional radiotherapy is limited by the inability to deliver an adequate therapeutic dose adjacent to critical structures, which include the brainstem, spinal cord, optic and other cranial nerves, temporal lobes, cerebellum and the major intracranial arteries [5]. Compared with skull base chordoma, sacral lesions have relatively longer rates of local control and this may relate to the higher tolerated radiation doses and efficacy of radical surgery.

In order to improve rates of local control in intracranial tumours, higher tumour doses have been achieved using the superior localizing properties of charged particles. Five-year survival rates of 55% with total radiation doses of 70 Gy have been reported. Localization may also be achieved with multiple-arc stereotactic radiotherapy.

Surgery

Radical surgery has an established role in the management of sacrococcygeal chordoma where tumour control rates of 54% have been achieved. At the skull base *en bloc* surgery is prohibited by the proximity of nervous and vascular elements. However, recent advances in surgical technique have led to the development of approaches through which the goal of radical surgery is becoming achievable. In tumours of the clivus, anterior extradural approaches are favoured involving transsphenoidal, transmaxillary and transoral procedures. If the tumour extends to the craniocervical junction, skeletal stability may be in jeopardy. Reconstruction techniques should employ titanium implants in order to allow for postoperative MRI (see Fig. 40.2b). The impact of radical surgery on patient survival is to be evaluated over the next decade.

Current management strategies

In the absence of definite evidence that immediate radiotherapy is beneficial, we suggest that the initial treatment of intracranial chordoma be limited to the most complete excision that is feasible for the individual patient. If disease recurs within five years, it could be supposed that the tumour is of an aggressive subtype. The patient would then be treated with further excision as appropriate, and radiotherapy, either with protons or using multiple-arc stereotactic techniques.

Conclusion

Without intervention, intracranial chordomas are rapidly fatal. However, conventional treatment has not significantly altered survival over the past 50 years. Due to the rarity of chordoma and the requirement for long-term follow-up the published series are retrospective, historical analyses. Comparisons between series are difficult to interpret because of the inclusion of unrelated skull base tumours, such as chondrosarcoma, in the survival data. With the advent of new therapeutic options including radical surgery and stereotactic and charged-particle radiotherapy, a prospective trial of treatment would yield valuable information on the management of these challenging tumours.

References

1. Oot R, Melville G, New P. The role of MR and CT in evaluating clival chordomas and chondrosarcomas. *Am. J. Radiol.* 1988;**151**:567–75.

Non-germinomatous germ-cell tumours

The standard therapy in NGGCTs remains craniospinal irradiation using the doses described above. The incidence of failure at all sites is higher in this group of patients. While the highest risk of failure appears to be at the primary site, this information is based predominantly on patients treated with local fields where there is the possibility of marginal failure. There is still a significant risk of distant cranial and spinal failure justifying craniospinal axis (CSA) irradiation in all patients. It is also important to consider that previously reported series may include pineal tumours without histological verification. This will therefore represent a heterogeneous patient group with different histological diagnoses. The results of treatment of NGGCT are at present poor and warrant examination of a combined modality approach using primary chemotherapy in addition to CSA irradiation (see below).

Chemotherapy

It is perhaps initially surprising that, in view of the success of combination chemotherapy in the management of gonadal GCTs, that chemotherapy has only been infrequently studied in intracranial GCT. This can be explained in part by the relative lack of central nervous system (CNS) penetration of the most active chemotherapy agents (e.g. cisplatinum, bleomycin) and the risks of potentiating late sequelae when sequenced closely with irradiation (e.g. cisplatinum and ototoxicity, methotrexate and cerebral necrosis). In addition the majority of chemotherapy studies have been used in the treatment of patients with relapsed disease. Used in this situation, successful chemotherapeutic salvage is unusual with the majority of patients experiencing partial response of up to 6–8 months' duration. The only exception to this observation is a higher rate of successful salvage of the few patients who relapse with systemic metastases alone seeding through a ventriculoperitoneal shunt.

More recent studies have reported the use of primary chemotherapy prior to definitive irradiation. This can exploit the disruption of the blood–brain barrier caused by the primary tumour prior to irradiation. Studies have used a number of drug regimens including single-agent high-dose cyclophosphamide and combination regimens including cisplatinum, carboplatin, high-dose methotrexate, vincristine, etoposide and bleomycin [15,16]. It is more controversial as to whether such primary chemotherapy penetrates fully to the leptomeninges and effectively treats the neuraxis.

The optimal drug regimen is, at present, not defined but should produce high response rates without deleterious interaction with definitive irradiation. Sebag-Montefiore and colleagues [13] reported the use of two courses of combination chemotherapy using vincristine, etoposide

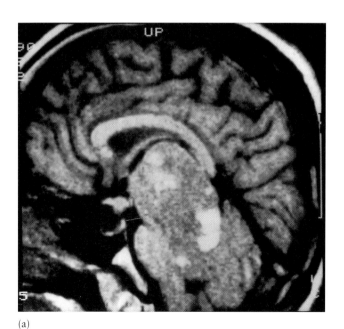
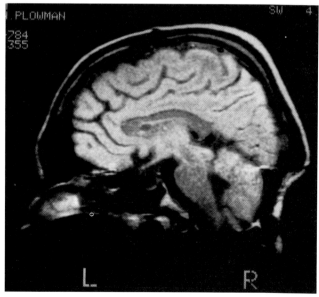

(a)   (b)

Fig. 43.2 Sagittal MRI scan showing: (a) large pineal germ-cell tumour prior to chemotherapy; and (b) complete response following two courses of chemotherapy.

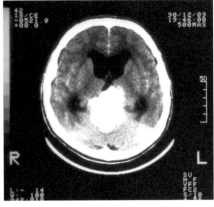 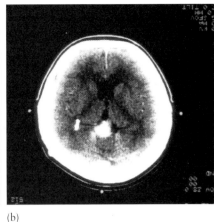

Fig. 43.3 Transaxial CT scan showing: (a) large pineal germ-cell tumour with contrast enhancement prior to chemotherapy; and (b) partial response following two courses of chemotherapy.

(a)   (b)

and carboplatin (used as being relatively safe drugs to administer prior to neuraxis radiotherapy) followed by response assessment prior to craniospinal irradiation. Complete response was seen in three out of four patients with germinoma (Fig. 43.2) and partial response in one out of two patients with NGGCT (Fig. 43.3). In the patients with germinoma who have achieved complete response on CT scan after two cycles of chemotherapy, the radiotherapy total dose is reduced (and a differential daily dose technique is employed (see below) [17].

In a phase II study of ten evaluable patients with germinoma, Allen and colleagues [14] used carboplatin 150 mg/m^2 given weekly for 4 weeks followed by a 2-week break. All patients responded, with complete response in seven patients (after two courses of chemotherapy in five patients and after four courses in two patients) and partial response was seen in three patients. Of seven patients eligible to receive a dose reduction (3060 cGy to the primary site, plus or minus 2160 cGy to the remaining craniospinal axis), this option was elected in five patients. One patient with localized germinoma who had complete response and reduced dose irradiation relapsed 5 months after local radiation with subarachnoid and peritoneal metastases with elevated tumour markers and died 23 months after diagnosis. The remaining ten patients are alive and disease-free after a median follow-up of 25 months.

Combination chemotherapy has been advocated as the main therapeutic modality for NGGCT. Smith and colleagues [18] reported their experience of combination chemotherapy in five patients using etoposide, cisplatinum, vincristine, methotrexate and bleomycin (EpPlt/OMB). Of the four patients with NGGCT, there were two complete responses, one partial response and one patient died of an intracranial catastrophe due to tumour enlargement which histologically demonstrated mature teratoma. The adverse close sequencing of radiation and high-dose methotrexate was seen in one patient (of two who received irradiation), with the development of a grand mal fit associated with periventricular changes on MRI compatible with leucoencephalopathy as a result of methotrexate following irradiation.

The optimal order of therapeutic modalities is unclear, but when chemotherapy is closely sequenced with irradiation it appears safer, and more logical, to deliver primary chemotherapy first (using the least 'interactive' drugs with irradiation) followed by neuraxis irradiation. Neuraxis irradiation should still be regarded as an essential component of therapy. The role of surgical debulking after primary chemotherapy is not yet established, although a trimodality approach (chemotherapy, surgery and radiotherapy) is being evaluated in phase II studies (see below).

Results of treatment

The reported survival rates for patients with pineal germinoma vary according to histological subtype and the proportion of patients with a histological or tumour marker verification. In the review of 208 cases by Fuller and colleagues [8], the 5-year survival for non-biopsied patients was 81%, for verified germinoma 76% and for verified NGGCT 36%. Hoffman and colleagues [2] reported the experience from Toronto Hospital for Sick Children spanning 37 years. Fifty-one patients with intracranial GCT were operated on, including 32 pineal tumours (five total resection, ten partial resection, 16 biopsy, one no surgery), of whom eight patients died in the postoperative period (all operated on prior to 1972). Forty-two patients received postoperative radiotherapy. The 5-year survival rate for patients with germinoma was 73.2%, and 33.3% for patients with NGGCT. In the Royal Marsden series, Dearnley and colleagues [19] reported a 69% 10-year overall survival rate and 86.5% cause-specific survival control. The surgical objective is total excision of the mural nodule; the cyst wall can be left undisturbed, thereby increasing the safety of the procedure without increasing the risk of recurrence. Preoperative embolization has been successfully used in selected cases of cerebellar haemangioblastomas and may also prove useful for those situated in or around the sella, providing that feeding vessels can be selectively catheterized and safely embolized.

The diagnosis of haemangioblastoma may be entertained only after intra-operative visualization of the tumour. Unexpected and dramatic bleeding is one of the more common encounters with sellar haemangioblastomas. If an intra-operative diagnosis of haemangioblastoma is suspected during the course of a trans-sphenoidal procedure, then complete excision of the mural nodule may still be feasible, provided the tumour is wholly situated below the sellar diaphragm. Should the tumour extend above the diaphragma, then it is wise to secure haemostasis, terminate the trans-sphenoidal procedure, and attempt a transcranial approach at a second sitting. In all cases a comprehensive diagnostic work-up to exclude VHL disease should be performed, including a detailed fundoscopic examination, careful scrutiny of neuroimaging studies to rule out multiple craniospinal lesions, a CT scan of the abdomen to exclude VHL-related tumours in the renal, adrenal and pancreatic areas, and a detailed pedigree analysis.

Prognosis

The prognosis for completely excised haemangioblastoma is generally favourable, with most patients enjoying long-term cure. Once totally removed these tumours seldom recur. Of the few tumours that do, repeat resection is often the most appropriate and effective therapeutic option. It is important to realize that recurrences may develop after long intervals of disease-free survival. Although the role of radiation therapy for partially removed tumours is unsettled, retrospective reports have suggested that doses of at least 5000 cGy do improve local control in patients with residual disease [8].

Haemangiopericytoma

General aspects and pathology

The haemangiopericytoma is an uncommon tumour of vascular origin, one presumed to arise from the pericyte, an enigmatic structural component of capillaries. Arising at virtually any site in the body, haemangiopericytomas most commonly involve the lower extremities and retroperitoneum. Although as many as 25% of haeman-

giopericytomas arise in the head and neck to involve such structures as the orbit, tongue, nose, nasopharynx, and paranasal sinuses [9], only a small fraction arise within the cranial cavity. Such intracranial examples are therefore rare and account for less than 1% of all intracranial tumours [10]. Of these, some may secondarily involve the sellar region from adjacent skull base sites; exceptionally few will arise primarily in the sella or suprasellar space. Like all haemangiopericytomas, those occurring in the sellar region are fully malignant neoplasms, ones notorious for both relentless local recurrence and a clear tendency for metastatic dissemination [11].

Histologically, haemangiopericytomas are highly cellular tumours, containing a monotonous population of round to oval cells chaotically disposed in tightly packed sheets [2,12]. Mitotic figures are encountered in small to moderate numbers, although their absolute frequency has not been found to be prognostically informative. Not surprisingly, vascular channels abound in this tumour, appearing as thin-walled and highly ramified vascular spaces whose cross-sectional profile has been described as 'staghorn' in appearance. The tumour's most distinctive feature is an extensive tracery of pericellular reticulin fibres which are seen to envelop individual tumour cells.

Clinical features

Haemangiopericytomas involving the sellar region do so primarily, or as the result of secondary extension from an adjacent skull base location; the latter appears more common. The literature concerning primary intra- or suprasellar haemangiopericytomas is scant, being restricted to five isolated case reports [11,13–16], and two additional cases identified among a large series of intracranial haemangiopericytomas [10]. Headache and visual disturbance are consistent symptoms, although individual patients have presented with signs of cavernous sinus involvement. Hypopituitarism, referable to compression of the pituitary is not a prominent presenting feature of sellar region haemangiopericytomas; if present, it is usually late in occurrence. Exceedingly unusual is an acromegalic presentation which, in a single instance, has been reported with a suprasellar haemangiopericytoma [15]. This case involved a middleaged woman who presented with acromegaly, amenorrhoea, visual loss, and simultaneous suprasellar and pulmonary haemangiopericytomas. Removal of the former not only normalized growth hormone (GH) levels, but immunohistochemical analysis of the tumour revealed cells immunoreactive for GH. This peculiar case aside, haemangiopericytomas are not considered hormonally active lesions, for their ultrastructure is devoid of the secretory organelles ordinarily present in hormone-secreting cells.

Radiologically, most haemangiopericytomas appear as diffusely enlarging, globular and well-circumscribed masses. Although CT and MRI provide a detailed anatomical diagnosis, these are non-specific investigations, ones incapable of distinguishing haemangiopericytomas from meningiomas. Erosion or destruction of bone may be observed; however hyperostosis is not a feature of haemangiopericytomas and its presence essentially excludes the diagnosis.

Management

All haemangiopericytomas, including those in the vicinity of the sella, are best managed by surgical resection followed by radiation therapy and meticulous long-term follow-up. Given their extreme vascularity, together with their frequent fibrous consistency, a transcranial procedure is generally safer, more effective, and overall, a far more strategic approach for sellar haemangiopericytomas than is a trans-sphenoidal one. The surgical objective is gross 'total' removal of all visible tumour, including the removal of an adequate dural perimeter at the site of attachment. In several series of intracranial haemangiopericytomas at all sites, including sellar and suprasellar ones, the rate of apparent complete resection ranged from 50 to 67% [12,17]. Whereas refinements in microsurgical techniques and instrumentation have reduced operative mortality to near zero in recent series, intraoperative haemorrhage continues to be an ongoing complication, one which seriously hampers attempts at gross total excision.

One of the most frustrating biological features of haemangiopericytomas relates to their relentless propensity for postoperative recurrence, despite 'complete' removal. Reconstituting themselves from seemingly insignificant and microscopic amounts of residual tissue, local symptomatic recurrence is an eventuality faced by the majority of haemangiopericytoma patients. In the largest series to date, 5-, 10- and 15-year actuarial recurrence rates were calculated as being 65, 76 and 85%, respectively; the average time to first recurrence was 51 months [10]. For incompletely resected tumours, symptomatic regrowth is virtually guaranteed. Given the aggressive biological profile, radiation therapy is indicated to forestall recurrence in all instances, regardless of the completeness of resection. Recurrences are best managed by repeat resection, preferably while still small and minimally symptomatic.

Prognosis

Given the limited number of sellar region haemangio-

pericytomas reported in the literature, it is difficult to draw long-term prognosis conclusions for haemangiopericytomas specifically at this site. Although the long-term prognosis for intracranial haemangiopericytomas is far more favourable than that of other malignant brain tumours, survival is adversely affected. Of the 44 patients in the Mayo Clinic series, 23 died directly as the result of their tumour [10]. The median time from initial operation to death was approximately 60 months. By actuarial analysis, the probability of tumour-related death was 33, 60 and 77% at 5, 10 and 15 years, respectively. Of the factors correlating with a favourable prognosis, radiation therapy after the initial resection proved the most powerful.

A second factor adversely affecting the prognosis of patients with haemangiopericytomas is metastatic dissemination. In fact, the regularity with which haemangiopericytomas give rise to extraneural metastases exceeds that of any other primary intracranial tumour. In order of frequency, the most common sites of extraneural dissemination are bone, lungs and liver [12]. Dissemination within the subarachnoid space occurs much less often, and has been reported with a sellar haemangiopericytoma [11]. It is important to acknowledge that metastatic deposits typically occur years after the diagnosis of the initial tumour, during which time many patients experience quality and symptom-free life. Meticulous clinical and radiological surveillance for metastatic disease is an essential aspect of the lifelong care required by these patients.

Cavernous haemangiomas

General aspects and pathology

Cavernous haemangiomas, while neither truly neoplastic in nature nor frequent in number, are probably the most common vascular 'tumour-like' lesion occurring in and around the sella. Generally regarded as malformative, hamartomatous growths, cavernous haemangiomas can arise at virtually any site within the craniospinal space [18]. The overwhelming majority are intra-axial lesions located within the cerebrum. Additional characteristic, but less common, sites include the brainstem, cerebellum and spinal cord. Many cavernous hemangiomas are asymptomatic lesions either incidentally discovered at autopsy or on MRI for complaints that are often unrelated to the lesion *per se*. Those that do genuinely produce symptoms do so in the form of seizures, focal neurological deficits, headache, or acute haemorrhage [19,20]. Relevant to this discussion, are the small numbers of cavernous haemangiomas that involve the sellar and parasellar regions. Taking origin about the optic nerve/chiasm, cavernous sinus, anterior third ventricle, adjacent

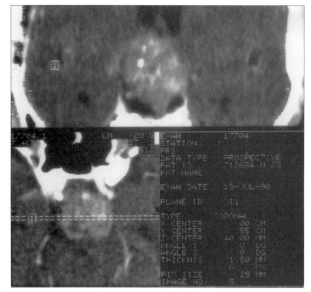

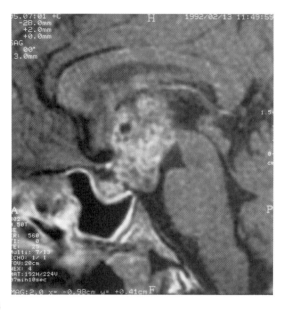

(a)

(b)

Fig. 44.2 (a) Coronal, and (b) sagittal computed tomography image of a patient with cavernous haemangioma and hypopituitarism.

diencephalon, or, rarely, the pituitary gland itself, parasellar cavernous haemangiomas can be the source of a number of localizing symptoms, including visual loss, pituitary and hypothalamic dysfunction, and cranial nerve palsies.

Cavernous haemangiomas are composed exclusively of thin-walled vessels. Grossly, they are unencapsulated, but well-circumscribed lesions whose fine nodular surface, purplish colour and overall appearance has been aptly likened to that of a mulberry [18]. Their size is variable, ranging from minute growths of barely macroscopic

proportions to lesions several centimetres in diameter. The texture of cavernous haemangiomas is also variable, ranging from soft, firm to gritty-hard, depending on the relative content of blood, thrombus, hyalinized tissue, cholesterol crystals or calcium deposits within the vascular spaces. As a rule, the surrounding brain is gliotic, yellow-stained, and replete with haemosiderin-laden macrophages—all telltale signs of prior, albeit occult, haemorrhage. On microscopic examination, one sees a honeycomb arrangement of thin-walled sinusoidal spaces that can be discerned as neither arterial nor venous in nature. Lacking both a smooth muscle component and an elastic layer, these thin-walled vessels consist only of a single endothelial layer, supported by varying amounts of extraluminal connective tissue. A key pathological feature of cavernous haemangiomas is the absence of any neural or glial tissue intervening in the vascular spaces, except perhaps at its very peripheral margins where the lesion interfaces with surrounding brain. In contrast to true arteriovenous malformations, these lesions are not serviced by any abnormal feeding arteries or draining veins. Despite their non-neoplastic nature, cavernous haemangiomas do exhibit an occasional capacity for expansile growth. Presumably the result of progressive thrombosis, organ-ization, hyalization, and/or repeat haemorrhage, simple mechanical expansion rather than true cellular prolifera-tion *per se*, likely account for periodic reports describing growth of cavernous haemangiomas.

Most examples are solitary and sporadic lesions occurring without known family history. A familial form of the disease, particularly among those of Mexican-American origin, has also been recognized [21,22].

Clinical features

The most common site of parasellar origin appears to be from within the cavernous sinus [23]. Predictably most patients with cavernous sinus haemangiomas present with various components of a cavernous sinus syndrome. Diplopia, ptosis and alterations in sensation of the face are expected presenting features. Less commonly medial extension of the lesion into the sella may cause compression of the pituitary gland with resultant hypopituitarism (Fig. 44.2). Occasionally, some may extend in an anterior direction to involve the superior orbital fissure and retro-orbital region, causing exoph-thalmos. Finally cavernous haemangiomas in this region may also extend in a superior direction to compress the chiasm and optic tracts to produce visual field defects. In most instances, these symptoms are slowly progressive, although some cases have been reported of acute haemorrhage within the lesion producing an abrupt onset of symptoms. Two recent, though retrospective studies, have indicated that the likelihood of spontaneous haemorrhage from cavernous haemangiomas of all sites is in the order of 0.25–0.7% per year [19,20]. Whereas cavernous haemangiomas occur with similar frequency between the sexes, those occurring in females appear more prone to undergo haemorrhage. Of the cavernous haemangiomas associated with clinically significant haemorrhage in the series of Robinson and colleagues [20], 86% occurred in women. In addition, cavernous haemangiomas appear especially prone to bleed during pregnancy.

A less frequent category of sellar region cavernous haemangiomas are those arising in the suprachiasmatic recess and anterior third ventricle. Such lesions have been known to produce chiasmal compression, hypothalamic dysfunction, hyperprolactinaemia, diabetes insipidus and hypopituitarism. Rarely, the lesions may be situated within the optic nerve or chiasm. They may be the source of progressive impairment of visual fields and/or acuity and sometimes produce a dramatic clinical presentation after undergoing acute haemorrhage. Aptly termed 'chiasmal apoplexy', the occurrence of haemorrhage into the chiasm or optic nerve is accompanied by acute visual loss, sudden headache, nausea and vomiting [24–27]. It is often difficult to distinguish this entity from the more common occurrence of subarachnoid haemorrhage, pituitary apoplexy, or haemorrhagic infarction of a non-pituitary sellar tumour.

Only very rarely have cavernous haemangiomas been described as arising from the pituitary fossa. In one instance, a giant pituitary cavernous haemangioma was reported as an incidental autopsy finding in an elderly patient who succumbed to metastatic breast cancer [28]. Despite filling the sella, compressing the pituitary gland and exhibiting marked suprasellar extension, the mass was seemingly asymptomatic. In another case, a 42-year-old man presented acutely with sudden headache, a visual field deficit and a seizure [29]. Imaging studies confirmed an enlarged and demineralized sella, and a transcranial procedure identified a haemorrhagic mass arising from the sella and compressing the optic nerve. After decompression for presumed pituitary apoplexy, the patient returned 8 years later with hypopituitarism, moderate hyperprolactinaemia and visual failure. An enhancing intra- and suprasellar mass was identified on CT scanning. A repeat decompression was performed and histological conformation of cavernous haemangioma was obtained.

Radiologically, cavernous haemangiomas at all sites have a fairly characteristic profile. Angiography may demonstrate a faint 'blush', although it is often absent and neither feeding arteries nor draining veins will be present. CT scanning, although occasionally suggestive, is seldom diagnostic. The typical pattern is that of a well-demarcated hyperdense area, which may exhibit calcification of varying degrees. The most sensitive test for cavernous haemangiomas, and often the only study necessary for securing their diagnosis, is MRI. On both T_1- and T_2-sequences, the MRI diagnostic criteria include a well-circumscribed lesion having a mottled central core of mixed signal intensity and a prominent surrounding rim of low signal intensity, indicative of haemosiderin deposition. Enhancement with gadolinium is minimal or absent. Of lesions located in the middle fossa and cavernous sinus, which secondarily involve the sella, bony erosion, enlargement or remodelling of the sella have all been reported [23,30].

Management

The management of cavernous haemangioma involving the sellar region is surgical resection. Unlike cavernous haemangiomas situated in the cerebrum, many of which are minimally symptomatic or incidentally discovered and often not in immediate need of treatment, most lesions involving the sella will be symptomatic at presentation, necessitating some form of surgical intervention. All cavernous haemangiomas in the region are best managed by a transcranial route. When safe to do so, the surgical objective should be total excision, for it is the only means to assure relief from future haemorrhage or regrowth.

Other 'vascular' lesions of the sellar region

The preceding discussion focused only on lesions of the sellar region that derive specifically from vascular elements. There are, however, a number of additional perisellar tumours, which cannot be considered truly vascular in origin, but are nonetheless known for their marked vascularity. In a few instances, the vascularity of these lesions manifests as spontaneous intratumoural haemorrhage, in others, it is recognized by intense contrast enhancement on imaging studies, and in most, it manifests as troublesome intra-operative bleeding.

Although not regarded as particularly vascular lesions, pituitary adenomas are well known for their occasional tendency to undergo apoplectic haemorrhagic infarction. Meningiomas of the sellar region, though seldom a source of spontaneous haemorrhage, are well known for their vascularity and tendency for intra-operative bleeding. The same also applied to granular cell tumours or 'choristomas' of the pituitary stalk. Several malignant sellar region tumours are also known for their vascularity.

Perhaps the most common of these are metastases to the sella, notably carcinomas arising from the breast, lung and prostate. Marked vascularity is also a feature of several tumours of the skull base and bony sella, such as giant cell tumour of the bone, juvenile angiofibroma, and the tumour-like condition, fibrous dysplasia. A final vascular lesion, one always deserving of some consideration in the differential diagnosis of a sellar region mass, is a cerebral aneurysm. The majority of aneurysms involving the sellar region derive from the intracavernous segment of the carotid artery, and less often, from the supraclinoid carotid and the anterior communicating artery complex. Their clinical picture may be indistinguishable from a non-functioning pituitary adenoma or other sellar mass. In addition to mimicking pituitary adenomas, aneurysms have also been known to coexist with pituitary adenomas. As reviewed by Weir [31], the incidence of coexisting pituitary adenomas and incidental cerebral aneurysms approaches 7.4%. GH-producing tumours, in particular, have been repeatedly reported to coexist with incidental aneurysms at a frequency beyond what would be expected by chance alone. The basis of this association is uncertain; because generalized arterial ectasia is a recognized feature of acromegaly, it has been speculated that the local effects of GH and/or insulin-like growth factor 1 may somehow predispose or contribute to aneurysm formation.

References

1. Huson SM, Harper PS, Hourihan MD *et al*. Cerebellar hemangioblastoma and von Hippel–Lindau disease. *Brain* 1986;**109**:1297–310.
2. Burger PC, Scheithauer BW, Vogel FS. *Surgical Pathology of the Nervous System and its Coverings*, 3rd edn. New York: Churchill Livingstone, 1991.
3. Rho Y-M. von Hippel–Lindau's disease. *Can. Med. Assoc. J.* 1969;**101**:135–42.
4. Dan NG, Smith DE. Pituitary hemangioblastoma in a patient with von Hippel–Lindau disease. *J. Neurosurg.* 1975;**42**:232–5.
5. O'Reilly GV, Rumbaugh CL, Bowens M, Kido DK, Naheedy MH. Supratentorial hemangioblastoma: the diagnostic roles of computed tomography and angiography. *Clin. Radiol.* 1981;**32**:389–92.
6. Grisoli F, Gambarelli D, Raybaud C, Guibout M, Leclercq T. Suprasellar hemangioblastoma. *Surg. Neurol.* 1984;**22**:257–62.
7. Neumann HPH, Eggert HR, Weigel K *et al*. Hemangioblastomas of the central nervous system. *J. Neurosurg.* 1989;**70**:24–30.
8. Smalley SR, Schomberg PJ, Earle JD *et al*. Radiotherapeutic considerations in the treatment of hemangioblastomas of the central nervous system. *Int. J. Radiat. Oncol. Biol. Phys.* 1990;**18**:1165–71.
9. Austin MB, Mills SE. Neoplasms and neoplasm-like lesions involving the skull base. *Ear Nose Throat J.* 1986;**65**:57–73.
10. Guthrie BL, Ebersold MJ, Scheithauer BW, Shaw EG. Meningeal hemangiopericytoma: histopathological features, treatment, and long-term follow-up of 44 cases. *Neurosurgery* 1989;**25**:514–22.
11. Kumar PP, Good RR, Skultety FM, Masih AS, McComb RD. Spinal metastases from pituitary hemangiopericytic meningioma. *Am. J. Clin. Oncol.* 1987;**10**:422–8.
12. Guthrie BL. Meningeal hemangiopericytomas: angioblastic meningiomas of Cushing and Eisenhardt. In Al-Mefty O (ed.). *Meningiomas*. New York: Raven Press, 1991:181–6.
13. Orf G. Angioretikulom der sella turcica. *Acta Neurochir. (Wien)* 1970;**23**:63–78.
14. Mangiardi JR, Flamm ES, Cravioto H, Fisher B. Hemangiopericytoma of the pituitary fossa: case report. *Neurosurgery* 1983;**13**:58–62.
15. Yokota M, Tani E, Yukio M *et al*. Acromegaly associated with suprasellar and pulmonary hemangiopericytomas. *J. Neurosurg.* 1985;**62**:767–71.
16. Nikonov AA, Matsko DE. Pituitary hemangiopericytoma. *Arch. Patol.* 1985;**47**:79–83.
17. Jaaskelainen J, Servo A, Haltia M, Wahlstrom T, Valtonen S. Intracranial hemangiopericytoma: radiology, surgery, radiotherapy, and outcome in 21 patients. *Surg. Neurol.* 1985;**23**:227–36.
18. Russell DS, Rubinstein LJ. Tumors and tumor-like lesions of maldevelopmental origin. In Russell DS, Rubinstein LJ. *Pathology of Tumours of the Nervous System*, 5th edn. Baltimore: Williams and Wilkins, 1989:664–765.
19. Del Curling O, Kelly DL, Elster AD, Craven TE. An analysis of the natural history of cavernous angiomas. *J. Neurosurg.* 1991;**75**:702–8.
20. Robinson JR, Awad IA, Little JR. Natural history of cavernous angioma. *J. Neurosurg.* 1991;**75**:709–14.
21. Rigamonti D, Hadley MN, Drayer BP *et al*. Cerebral cavernous malformations. Incidence and familial occurrence. *N. Engl. J. Med.* 1988; **319**: 343–7.
22. Gunel M, Awad IA, Finberg K *et al*. A founder mutation as a cause of cerebral cavernous malformation in Hispanic Americans. *N. Engl. J. Med.* 1996; **334**: 946–51.
23. Linskey ME, Sekhar LN. Cavernous sinus hemangiomas: a series, a review, and a hypothesis. *Neurosurgery* 1992;**30**:101–7.
24. Maitland CG, Abiko S, Hoyt WF, Wilson CB, Okamura T. Chiasmal apoplexy: report of four cases. *J. Neurosurg.* 1982;**56**:118–22.
25. Mohr G, Hardy J, Gauvin P. Chiasmal apoplexy due to ruptured cavernous hemangiomas of the optic chiasm. *Surg. Neurol.* 1985;**24**:636–40.
26. Corboy JR, Galetta SL. Familial cavernous angiomas manifesting with an acute chiasmal syndrome. *Am. J. Ophthalmol.* 1989;**108**:245–50.
27. Ferreira NP, Ferreira MP. Optic nerve apoplexy caused by a cavernous angioma: case report. *Neurosurgery* 1992;**30**:262–4.
28. Sansone ME, Liwnicz BH, Mandybur TI. Giant pituitary cavernous hemangioma. *J. Neurosurg.* 1980;**53**: 124–6.
29. Buonaguidi R, Canapicci R, Mimassi N, Ferdeghini M. Intrasellar cavernous hemangioma. *Neurosurgery* 1984;**14**:732–4.
30. Kawai K, Fukui M, Tanaka A, Kuramoto S, Kitamura K. Extracerebral cavernous hemangiomas of the middle fossa. *Surg. Neurol.* 1978;**8**:19–25.
31. Weir B. Pituitary tumours and aneurysm: case report and review of the literature. *Neurosurgery* 1992;**30**:585–91.

45

Langerhans' Cell Histiocytosis

MICHAEL G. CHEN

Introduction

Endocrinopathies resulting from Langerhans' cell histiocytosis (LCH) are among the striking features of this disease complex, previously called histiocytosis X. In spite of advances in recognizing pathological similarities between Letterer–Siwe disease, Hand–Schüller–Christian disease and eosinophilic granuloma and in identifying the Langerhans' cell as the pathognomonic finding in lesions of LCH, much remains to be learned about the aetiology, pathogenesis and effective therapy of this clinically heterogeneous collection of diseases. In keeping with the theme of this monograph, this chapter will focus on the endocrinological manifestations of LCH; natural history and epidemiology, diagnosis and staging, and therapy.

Epidemiology and natural history

The precise incidence of LCH is not known, but estimates in children have been reported in the range of 1–10 cases/ 2 000 000 children per year. Several large series report that more than 50% of LCH occurs in children between the ages of 1 and 15 years; the disease can be present at birth and can occur in patients over 60 years of age [1]. Endocrine dysfunctions are seen principally in the chronic, disseminated form of LCH, characterized by multifocal eosinophilic granulomas in bone, skin, lung and brain (including the meninges), but uncommonly in the unifocal eosinophilic granuloma form of LCH or in the rapidly progressive form of LCH seen in very young children. The most frequent endocrine abnormalities are diabetes insipidus (DI) and growth retardation, estimated to develop in one-third to one-half of patients with LCH [2].

Depending on the series, the prevalence of DI in LCH varies between 5 and 50%. In an 8-year study by the Pediatric Oncology Group [3], an intermediate group of patients corresponding to the chronic, disseminated form of LCH (neither good risk nor poor risk LCH) was studied. This subgroup was characterized either by progression of old lesions or development of new lesions after diagnosis without development of organ dysfunction, and comprised 53 patients. Eight presented with DI and 15 later developed soft tissue progression manifest as DI (total occurrence of 43%). This is to be compared to an 8% incidence in the good risk group (no disease progression) and 14% incidence in the poor risk group (fatal outcome). In adult patients the clinical symptoms of DI may precede the bone and soft tissue lesions of LCH by many months and make diagnosis exceedingly difficult.

Diagnosis and staging

Clinical studies necessary for the accurate diagnosis and staging of this relatively rare disorder are summarized by Lavin and Osband [4], and include screening for DI by the water deprivation test of Miller as detailed in Braunstein and Kohler [2]. In our series of 47 patients with DI, the diagnosis of DI in 12 patients (26%) predated the diagnosis of LCH. In ten patients (21%), the diagnoses were concurrent, and in 25 patients (53%) the diagnosis of DI occurred after the diagnosis of LCH [5].

In children with LCH, Braunstein and Kohler have studied growth retardation resulting in the short stature [2]. Growth hormone deficiency and DI in LCH patients are considered to be secondary to hypothalamic infiltration by the Langerhans' cells and/or histiocytosis involvement of meninges adjacent to the pituitary. Other rarer endocrinopathies such as hypogonadism, hyperprolactinaemia, and panhypopituitarism have also been reported [2]. In our series of 47 patients with DI, eight had growth hormone deficiency and six had panhypopituitarism [5]. Berry and Becton have reviewed rare extrahypothalamic central nervous system (CNS) manifestations of the disease presenting as cerebral and cerebellar dysfunction

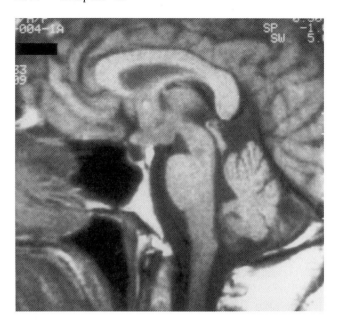

Fig. 45.1 MRI sagittal scan showing Langerhans' cell histiocytosis involvement of the hypothalamus and mammillary bodies in a patient who had diabetes insipidus and a severe hypothalamic syndrome involving fluid balance abnormalities and memory loss.

[1]. Computed tomography (CT) and magnetic resonance imaging (MRI) are useful in detecting the more common hypothalamic as well as less common hemispheric sites of disease involvement (Fig. 45.1).

Principles of therapy

In the absence of organ dysfunction or systemic involvement, LCH can exhibit a relatively indolent course and may go into spontaneous remission. Solitary bone lesions can be treated surgically by a variety of techniques depending on the bone involved. Simple injection of the bone lesions with methylprednisolone can be effective. Postoperative radiotherapy in low dose, such as 600–1000 cGy in 200 cGy daily fractions, has been employed successfully for persistent or relapsing bone lesions or for bone lesions difficult to access surgically because of site or in the interest of cosmesis.

In patients with multifocal LCH or organ dysfunction, particularly with hypothalamic/pituitary involvement and DI, the role of radiotherapy is more controversial. Greenberger and coworkers [6] and we [5] have reported outcomes in 21 and 28 LCH patients with DI, respectively, irradiated to low dose (approximately 800–1600 cGy total dose in 150–200 cGy daily fractions) to restricted fields covering the sella turcica, suprasellar region and hypothalamus. They reported that eight (38%) patients showed a decreased requirement for pitressin (four completely discontinued the drug); we found a 36% overall response rate (22% complete and 14% partial responses) using a similar analysis. Both studies emphasize the importance of rapid institution of therapy within 7–10 days of diagnosis.

Other investigators [2,7] do not agree that radiotherapy has any efficacy in arresting or reversing the DI of LCH, possibly because radiotherapy in their series was administered too late following diagnosis of DI. Large doses of glucocorticoids can transiently improve DI as well as the bone and visceral lesions of LCH. However, except in occasional patients, chemotherapeutic drugs have not been found to alter the course of DI [2,7]. Unfortunately, endocrinopathies due to LCH are not often therapeutically reversible; prompt recognition of endocrine deficiencies and appropriate hormonal replacement therapy remain the mainstays of treatment [2].

Complications of therapy in children, particularly late effects such as growth and developmental failure, neurological deficits and secondary malignancies, remain significant concerns and demand continued search for more effective, less toxic forms of therapy. We agree that radiotherapy in conventional doses to cranial bone lesions or for DI could theoretically cause damage to the hypothalamic/pituitary axis or induce second malignancies such as thyroid cancer, but that these risks are small compared to the morbidity of the disease process itself.

References

1. Berry BH, Becton DL. Natural history of histiocytosis-X. *Hematol. Oncol. Clin. North Am.* 1987;**1**:23–34.
2. Braunstein GD, Kohler PO. Endocrine manifestations of histiocytosis. *Am. J. Pediatr. Hematol. Oncol.* 1981;**3**:67–75.
3. Berry DH, Gresik MV, Humphrey GB *et al.* Natural history of histiocytosis X: a Pediatric Oncology Group study. *Med. Pediatr. Oncol.* 1986;**14**:1–5.
4. Lavin PT, Osband ME. Evaluating the role of therapy in histiocytosis-X; clinical studies, staging and scoring. *Hematol. Oncol. Clin. North Am.* 1987;**1**:35–47.
5. Minehan KJ, Chen MG, Zimmerman D *et al.* Radiation therapy for diabetes insipidus caused by Langerhans cell histiocytosis. *Int. J. Radiat. Oncol. Biol. Phys.* 1992;**23**:519–24.
6. Greenberger JS, Cassady JR, Jaffe N, Vawter G, Crocker AC. Radiation therapy in patients with histiocytosis: management of diabetes insipidus and bone lesions. *Int. J. Radiat. Oncol. Biol. Phys.* 1979;**5**:1749–55.
7. Dunger DB, Broadbent V, Yeoman E *et al.* The frequency and natural history of diabetes insipidus in children with Langerhans-cell histiocytosis. *N. Engl. J. Med.* 1989;**321**:1157–62.

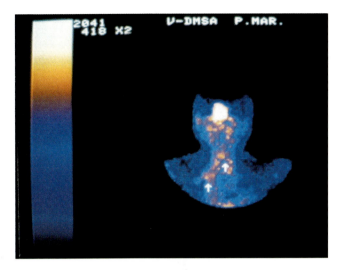

Plate 14.1 Medullary carcinoma of the thyroid, tumour recurrence: ^{99m}Tc-pentavalent dimercaptosuccinic acid scan showing increased uptake at the sites of disease (small white arrows).

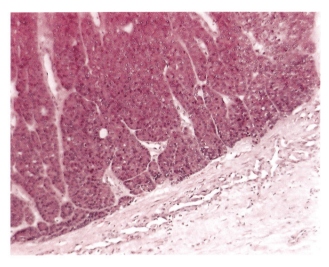

Plate 17.1 Follicular adenoma of the thyroid. The borders of this cellular nodule are well defined and there is no evidence of capsular or vascular invasion.

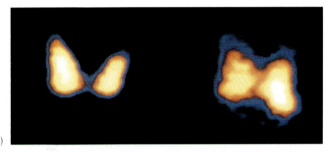

(a)

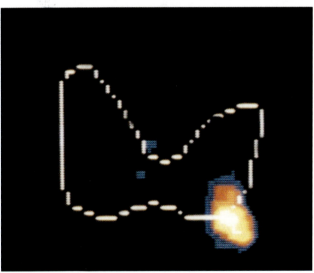

(b)

Plate 14.2 Parathyroid adenoma in the left inferior parathyroid gland: ^{99m}Tc-methoxyisobutylisonitrile (^{99m}Tc-MIBI)/technetium-99m pertechnetate (^{99m}TcO$_4$) double-tracer technique. (a) ^{99m}TcO$_4$ image on the left, and ^{99m}Tc-MIBI image on the right. (b) Subtraction image showing high uptake in the parathyroid adenoma. The white line marks the position of the thyroid lobes.

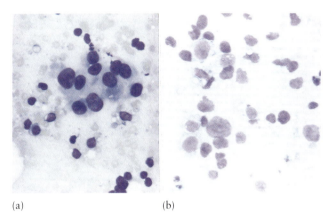

(a)   (b)

Plate 19.1 Thyroid fine needle aspiration cytology (FNAC). (a) A cluster of follicular epithelial cells with enlarged nuclei which vary in size. These appearances, together with the absence of colloid and the association with lymphocytes, which are seen in the background, are typical of Hashimoto's thyroiditis. (b) Enlarged, paler-staining pleomorphic cells with malignant nuclear features that include macronucleoli. The loss of cell cohesion and the disrupted cytoplasm are indications of malignant lymphoma. (Courtesy of Dr Elizabeth Hudson.)

[*facing page 272*]

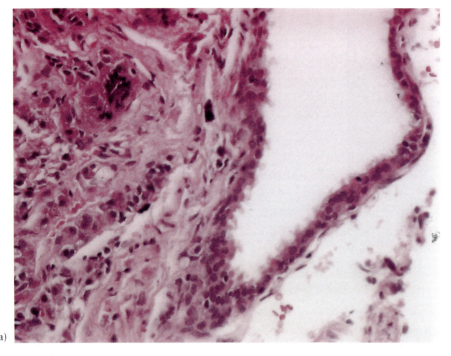

(a)

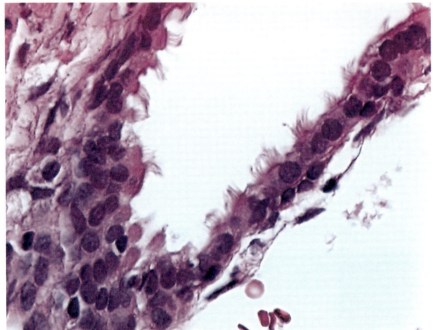

(b)

Plate 25.1 (a) A Rathke's pouch cyst of the pituitary. Anterior pituitary cells are present alongside a cystic space lined by cuboidal cells (b), many of which have long cilia.

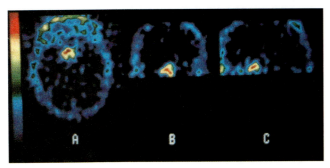
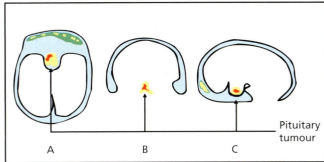

Plate 31.1 Brain SPET images after three-step immunoscintigraphy with antichromogranin A monoclonal antibody (MoAb A11) in a patient with a non-functioning pituitary adenoma. There is a high uptake at the tumour site 2 hours after [^{99}Tc] PnAO-biotin administration. Images: (A) transaxial; (B) coronal; (C) sagittal. (Courtesy of Dr A.G. Siccardi, University of Milan; from Colombo *et al.* 1993, with permission.)

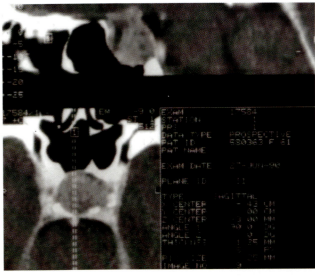

(a)

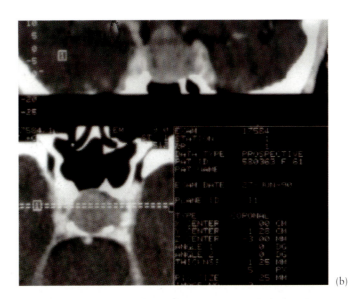

(b)

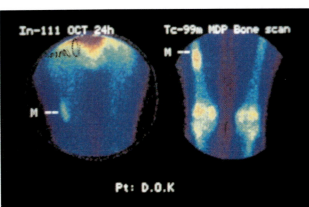

(c)

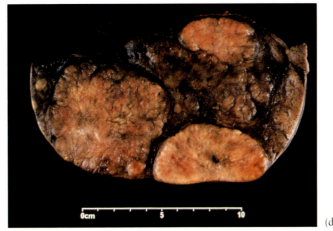

(d)

Plate 34.1 Sagittal (a), coronal (b) CT scan of a pituitary tumour showing a recurrence after initial surgery associated with marked hyperprolactinaemia. The bone scan shows appearances consistent with metastases; subsequent histology and immunostaining showed these to be both in (c) the femur and (d) the liver. Serum prolactin was 4200 mu/l at presentation and rose to 40×10^6 mu/l at death.

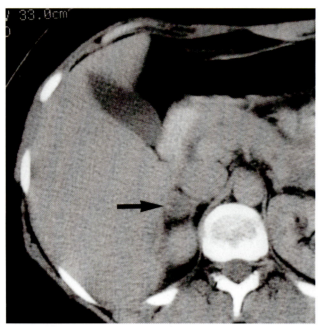

(a)

Plate 47.1 Incidentally discovered, non-functioning adrenal adenoma. (a) CT scan showing a small right adrenal mass of low soft tissue density (arrow). (b) ^{75}Se 6β-selenomethyl-19-norcholesterol scintigraphy showing high uptake in the mass.

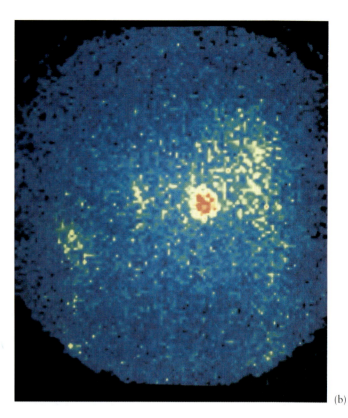

(b)

Plate 51.1 Primary pigmented nodular adrenocortical disease in a patient with Cushing's syndrome.

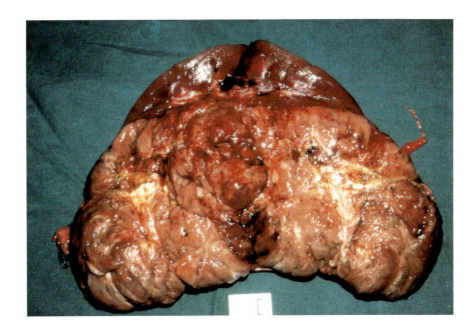

Plate 52.1 A left suprarenal tumour associated with high levels of testosterone and other steroids after surgical removal. The tumour has been bisected to reveal the cut surface. Note that it is very large, heterogeneous and vascular.

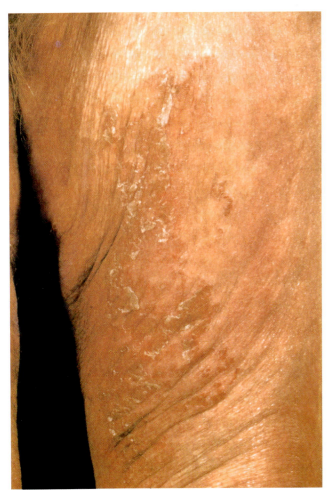

Plate 62.1 Necrolytic migratory erythema: encrusting of an area of erythema below the left groin.

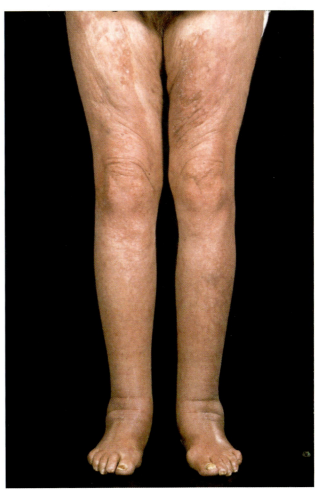

Plate 62.2 Necrolytic migratory erythema: lesions at different stages of evolution—new areas of erythema migrating from the groins, permanent hyperpigmentation of the distal extremities.

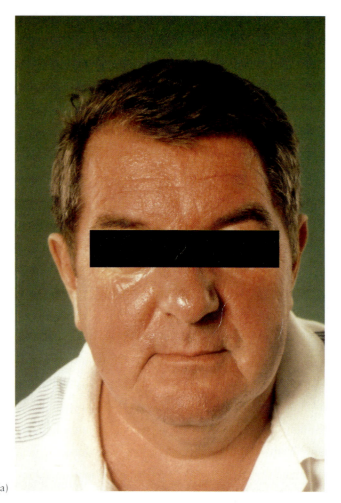

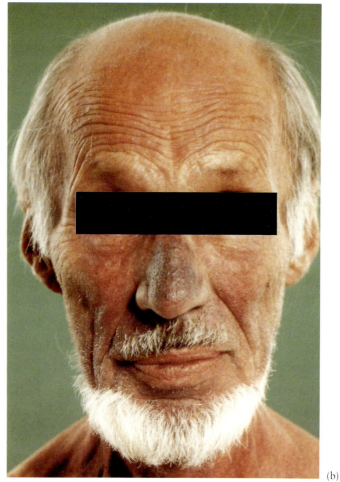

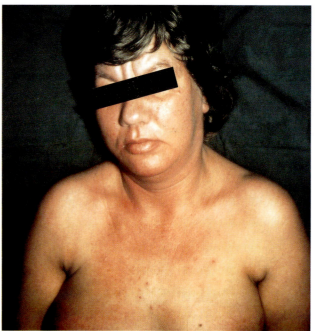

Plate 67.1 (a) A patient with a classic carcinoid flush related to a midgut carcinoid. (b) A patient with a long-standing carcinoid syndrome with heavily dilated veins on the nose. (c) A patient with a bronchial carcinoid and the carcinoid syndrome with concomitant release of serotonin and histamine. Notice the swelling of the face and lacrimation.

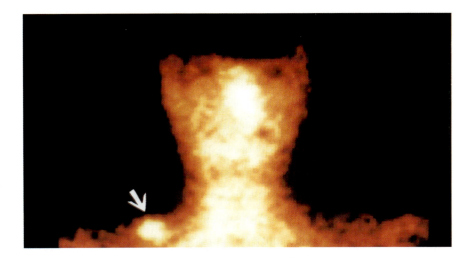

Plate 67.2 Indium-111 diethylenetriamine penta-acetic acid octreotide scintigraphy of a patient with a carcinoid tumour and metastasis in the left supraclavical fossa. The metastasis was only 0.5 cm at removal.

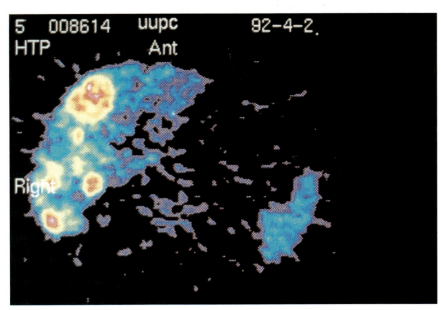

Plate 67.3 Positron emission tomography of a patient with a midgut carcinoid and liver metastases. Note the increased uptake of 5-hydroxytryptophan in several liver metastases, many of them not seen on computed tomography scans.

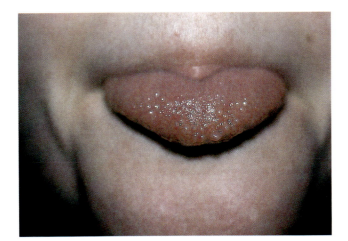

Plate 71.1 Oral ganglioneuromas of the tongue in a patient with multiple endocrine neoplasia type 2b.

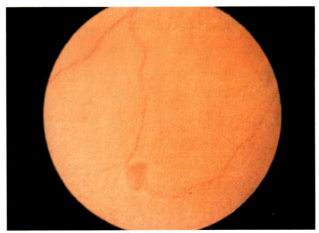

Plate 72.1 Haemangioblastoma situated at the periphery of the retina. Vessels can be seen entering and leaving the lesion.

46

Neurosarcoid

DONALD MITCHELL

Introduction

Sarcoidosis of the nervous system is associated with neuropathy and widespread involvement of the brain, spinal cord and meninges.

The salient features of the neuropathies are transient, often fluctuating lower motor neurone palsy. The facial nerve is the most frequent cranial nerve manifestation and may be bilateral. It may be associated with uveitis or parotid gland enlargement. In most cases the palsy recovers, although other manifestations of sarcoidosis may persist. Meningeal involvement can occur in the olfactory and other cranial nerves, most often the second, seventh and eight. The hypothalamus and pituitary gland may also be affected by meningeal disease.

Papilloedema may result from raised intracranial pressure due to granulomatous infiltration of basal meninges; unilateral papilloedema may result from infiltration within the optic foramen. Both divisions of the eighth cranial nerve are often involved usually by extensive, widespread and persistent granulomatous changes at the base of the brain. Involvement of the glossopharyngeal or vagus nerves may result in dysphagia or paresis of one or both vocal cords. Peripheral as well as cranial nerves may be affected; the peripheral neuropathy may present as a mononeuritis or as a more widespread sensory neuropathy.

The meninges, brain and, less frequently, the spinal cord may also be involved. The meninges principally over the base of the brain but often extending into the sulci over the brain and cerebellum become thickened by cellular infiltration with nodules arising from confluent granulomas. Local infiltrations by granulomas within the brain substance which may arise in any part of the brain, especially the hypothalamus and brain stem, may give rise to focal symptoms. These tumour-like masses may occasionally arise without evidence of meningeal involvement. The adventitia, the media and, more rarely, the intima of the blood vessels are involved by granulomatous infiltration to a greater or lesser extent and are often associated with granulomatous changes in other organs, although failure to find the latter does not negate a diagnosis of sarcoidosis if the histological changes in the brain are characteristic and are distributed in a recognized pattern. Occasionally, the vascular changes may simulate giant cell granulomatous angiitis or may be categorized only as granulomatous angiitis of the central nervous system and may be unrelated to sarcoidosis.

Granulomatous infiltration may impede the flow of cerebrospinal fluid (CSF) from the subarachnoid space at the base of the brain, at the outflow from the fourth ventricle or in the region of the aquaduct, giving rise to increased intracranial pressure.

Hypothalamic syndromes may give rise to diabetes insipidus, obesity, disturbances of sleep pattern and temperature regulation. Deficient anterior pituitary function may also occur; thus, features due to deficiencies in anterior pituitary hormones and in hypothalamic releasing hormones and disturbances of neuroregulatory function may arise.

Focal or generalized convulsions may be associated with neurological signs initially suggestive of cerebral tumour and pyramidal tract signs may be present. With extensive involvement of the nervous system, hemiparesis may occur; similarly, deterioration of intellectual function may be observed. A relatively few patients, in whom findings attributable to involvement of the spinal cord or its meninges, have also been reported. Accordingly, sarcoidosis of the nervous system may produce clinical pictures closely mimicking a wide variety of other disorders. Salient among these are multiple sclerosis, malignant lymphoma or other cerebral tumour and tuberculoma. More rarely, the presenting picture may mimic amyotrophic sclerosis, progressive multifocal leucoencephalopathy or myasthenia gravis [1].

Diagnosis

Clinical examination will provide reference to the presence of any lymphadenopathy, skin, ocular, conjunctival or nasal lesion and to any accessible tissue suitable for biopsy. It should be noted that visual evoked responses may be prolonged, as in multiple sclerosis.

Tuberculin testing may be helpful provided that account is taken of the patient's country of origin, age, ethnic group and of any previous evidence of bacille Calmette–Guérin (BCG) vaccination, tuberculosis or close contact with tuberculosis. Absent or weak tuberculin sensitivity is commonly found but the presence of even quite strong tuberculin sensitivity does not necessarily preclude a diagnosis of sarcoidosis. A chest radiograph is essential and occasionally an ultrasound of the abdomen and/or pelvis will assist in the detection of splenic enlargement or of enlarged para-aortic or pelvic lymph nodes.

Provided that clinical grounds justify the delay of four weeks incurred between its insertion and biopsy of the test site, a Kveim test may provide histological support, although rates of Kveim reactivity fall off with increasing duration of disease. Similarly, the serum and/or CSF angiotensin 1-converting enzyme (ACE) may be significantly elevated. Such findings provide a helpful marker of disease activity, although significantly raised levels may occasionally be found in other inflammatory and malignant disorders including tuberculosis and predominantly epithelioid cell lymphomas.

The CSF pressure, protein content and cell count are usually altered in accordance with the nature and site of the abnormality. In general, involvement of the basal cerebral meninges, with or without intracerebral deposits, will give rise to a more pronounced cellular pleocytosis (mainly lymphocytes) and raised protein content than those in which the lesion is restricted to one or more deposits in the brain substance. When the spinal cord or meninges are involved, the protein content may be significantly more elevated with or without cellular abnormality or pleocytosis. As in multiple sclerosis oligoclonal bands may be present in central nervous system (CNS) sarcoid. In any of these presentations the CSF glucose may be low and occasionally there is no CSF abnormality.

Gallium citrate (^{67}Ga) is taken up at sites of active sarcoidosis (and also by other inflammatory and malignant diseases); where scanning is appropriate it may reveal a characteristic pattern of uptake in lacrimal, parotid and/or submandibular glands, mediastinum and/or lungs. Additional extrathoracic sites of uptake may also be noted. Such positive findings assist in diagnosis and give additional information with regard to disease activity.

Magnetic resonance imaging (MRI) and computed tomography (CT) have complementary roles in the

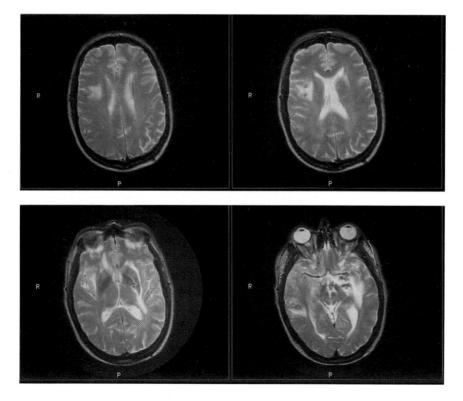

Fig. 46.1 Extensive areas of high signal mainly in the periventricular regions. Appearances entirely compatible with neurosarcoidosis.

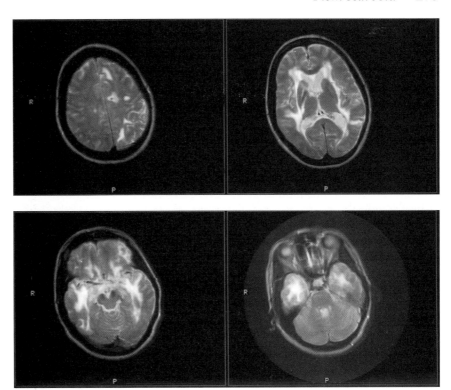

Fig. 46.2 Neurosarcoidosis. There are extensive areas of increased signal involving the left internal capsule, the posterior part of the right frontal lobe, and the left temporal lobe.

investigation of neurosarcoidosis. MRI is the best means of detecting parenchymal lesions and lesions in the posterior fossa, whereas contrast-enhanced CT is more useful in detecting diffuse meningeal involvement. MRI is useful in following response to treatment, with advantages over CT of no cumulative radiation dosage [2]. The most frequent MRI findings are periventricular abnormalities but these are non-specific and their differential diagnosis includes multiple sclerosis and other inflammatory and non-inflammatory cerebral vascular disease (Figs 46.1, 46.2). The accessibility of such lesions and the risks that may be associated with brain biopsy will be considered where appropriate in consultation with a neuroradiologist and neurosurgeon.

Treatment

High doses of oral prednisolone of the order of 60–80 mg daily are usually required for the initial treatment of severe neurological sarcoidosis. Subsequently, doses of the order of 40 mg daily for several months are often needed to maintain optimal suppression, with the consequent risk of serious side-effects. The life-threatening implications of fits in neurosarcoid are such that anticonvulsant therapy is often mandatory [3]. Unfortunately, anticonvulsant drugs are inducers of hepatic microsomal enzymes, which reduce the efficacy of steroids when given orally.

Intravenous 'pulses' of methylprednisolone do not incur this penalty and also mitigate the Cushingoid side-effects usually associated with prolonged, high-dose, oral prednisolone therapy [4]. Clearly, the frequency and dose of 'pulsed' i.v. methylprednisolone in combination with oral prednisolone therapy must be that which is considered optimal for individual patients when so severely afflicted as to warrant this approach, and must avoid the induction of steroid mania.

Typically, 1 g methylprednisolone admixed in 250 ml saline is given by slow intravenous drip over about 45 minutes (to avoid a metallic taste which otherwise may occur) on the same day of each week for eight consecutive weeks. Oral prednisolone is given in association with this in a dose of 20 mg daily during the first week, thereafter tailing slowly, and if clinically appropriate, to a dosage of 20 mg/0 mg on alternate days towards the end of this initial phase of combined treatment. Clearly, there are a few desperately ill patients in whom it is justifiable to give an initial period of 'pulsed' i.v. methylprednisolone, for example, 1 g daily for four or more days before recourse to weekly combined i.v./oral therapy. Subsequently, treatment with oral prednisolone alone or in combination with i.v. methylprednisolone given in smaller doses of 500 or 250 mg, at more widely spaced intervals, usually biweekly, must depend upon one's assessment as to the regimen of treatment that constitutes the smallest overall dosage of prednisolone given in the most sparing manner that proves adequate to maintain optimal suppression of the neurosarcoidosis.

It is probable that treatment with oral prednisolone will need to be continued, with tailing of dosage as judged mainly by clinical progress, MRI and/or CT scan, together with other parameters as appropriate to the individual patient for a period of 1–2 years, or more. The need for measurement of bone density should be carefully assessed; likewise regular careful surveillance is essential to alert one to the likelihood of any resurgence of the neurosarcoidosis during the tailing of the dosage of prednisolone or in the months following the termination of treatment. Only very rarely, in the presence of a high degree of tuberculin sensitivity or of other features suggestive of clinically occult mycobacterial infection, is antituberculous cover necessary. In this eventuality isoniazid should be used in a dosage of 150–300 mg daily during the initial months of treatment with corticosteroids. This avoids impairment of the therapeutic efficacy of oral prednisolone, which would otherwise be incurred by rifampicin or pyrazinamide.

Other so-called 'second-line' drugs may be used in combination with corticosteroids for their efficacy in suppressing sarcoidosis and thereby as 'steroid-sparing' agents. Principal among these drugs are hydroxychloroquine, methotrexate, azathioprine and cyclosporin. Of these, the use of hydroxychloroquine in low dose, 200 mg daily, and methotrexate in a single dose of the order of 10 mg once weekly and azathioprine, initially in a dose of 100 mg, increasing to 150 mg daily, are well established. Hydroxychloroquine in a dose of not more than 200 mg daily can be given without prior recourse to detailed ophthalmological examination, but is not usually continued for longer than 9 months to 1 year except in exceptional circumstances. The use of methotrexate or azathioprine necessitates regular routine blood counts to safeguard against the potential of these drugs to depress the bone marrow. Customarily it is used in conjunction with prednisolone and/or other suppressive agents over a period of 4–6 months, but can be continued for longer given adequate safeguards. Similarly, cyclosporin (with due regard to pretreatment and subsequent blood urea and creatinine levels) may be used in combination with corticosteroids or other immunosuppressant drugs. The initial dose is of the order of 9 mg/ kg daily adjusted thereafter to maintain blood trough levels of between 150 and 200 ng/l; it has been used with beneficial effect, but in the absence of a formal trial it is difficult to evaluate the results of treatment with this drug in these poor prognostic groups [5,6]. Recently, there

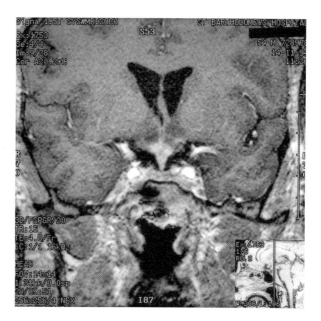

Fig. 46.3 MRI coronal T_1-weighted image after gadolinium i.v. showing hypothalamic involvement with sarcoidosis. The patient also had hilar lymph node involvement with a severe hypothalamic syndrome of panhypopituitarism, somnolence and memory deficit.

have been reports of possible beneficial effects from radiotherapy. It is possible that a trial of fractionated low-dose external beam radiotherapy to the whole brain or spinal cord may be justified where conventional measures have failed [7, 8].

Hypothalamic sarcoidosis (Fig. 46.3) can present a very difficult challenge. The endocrine effects of anterior panhypopituitarism and diabetes insipidus are compounded by often severe problems of water balance because of absent thirst, somnolence and poor memory. Frequently the mass is extremely resistant to treatment with steroids, other drugs or radiotherapy. Alternatively, the mass may respond to large doses of glucocorticoids and these have severe side-effects.

References

1. Scadding JG, Mitchell DN. *Sarcoidosis*, 2nd edn. London: Chapman and Hall, 1985.
2. Miller DH, Kendall BE, Barter G *et al*. Magnetic resonance imaging in central nervous system sarcoidosis. *Neurology* 1988;38:378–83.
3. Delaney P. Neurologic manifestations of sarcoidosis: review of the literature, with a report of 23 cases. *Ann. Intern. Med.* 1977;87:336–45.
4. Allen RKA, Mevory J. Intravenous pulse methylprednisolone in the successful treatment of severe sarcoid polyneuropathy with pulmonary involvement. *Aust. NZ J. Med.* 1988;15:45–6.

5. Cunnah D, Chew S, Wass J. Cyclosporin for central nervous system sarcoidosis. *Am. J. Med.* 1988;**85**:580–1.

6. Mitchell DN, Mitchell DM (eds). Sarcoidosis. In *Recent Advances in Respiratory Medicine: Sarcoidosis*. London: Churchill Livingstone, 1991:185–202.

7. Bejar JM, Kirby GR, Ziegler DK *et al*. Treatment of central nervous system sarcoidosis with radiotherapy. *Ann. Neurol.* 1985;**15**:258–60.

8. Martin N, Debroucher T, Mompoint D *et al*. Sarcoidosis of the pineal region; CT and MR studies. *J. Comput. Assist. Tomogr.* 1989;**13**:110–12.

4

ADRENAL AND GONADAL TUMOURS

approximately two standard deviations greater than the mean. Adrenal limbs greater than 5 mm can therefore be considered enlarged [14].

Adrenal disorders will be discussed in the context of clinical syndromes and problems.

Cushing's syndrome

ACTH-dependent Cushing's syndrome

In ACTH-dependent Cushing's syndrome the adrenal glands become hyperplastic, the largest glands tending to occur when there is an ectopic source of ACTH. Two types of adrenal hyperplasia are seen pathologically: smooth (diffuse) and nodular [15,16]. Smooth hyperplasia is more common, and may be obvious or not detectable on CT: a normal CT cannot therefore exclude the diagnosis. Nodular hyperplasia is much less common, and the nodularity can be micro- or macronodular. In the latter there is enlargement of the glands on CT, with one or more nodules. If one of the nodules is dominant, it may reach up to 4 cm, and may be mistaken for an adrenal adenoma, conflicting with the biochemical evidence of ACTH-dependent disease [8,15,17,18].

Having established a biochemical diagnosis of ACTH-dependent Cushing's syndrome, with or without radiological evidence of adrenal hyperplasia, the clinician must liaise with the radiologist in order to locate the ACTH source.

Pituitary adenoma

The reader is referred to Chapter 24 for information on pituitary imaging where MRI is the lead modality.

Ectopic ACTH source

The investigation of patients with 'occult' ectopic ACTH production represents a major challenge, since the clinical, biochemical and radiological features are often indistinguishable from pituitary-dependent Cushing's syndrome [19,20]. The radiological investigation requires great attention to detail since the tumours responsible are often small. Systemic venous sampling is frequently needed to provide functional information, especially when a small or equivocal lesion is detected on imaging. This technique requires specialized biochemistry services.

The most common site of the source of 'occult' ACTH production is in the chest, accounting for 79% of cases in one series [20]. The most common cause is a small bronchial carcinoid [21]. Other sources include thymic carcinoid, medullary carcinoma of the thyroid, pancreatic

islet cell tumour and phaeochromocytoma [21,22]. If the chest X-ray is normal, CT of the chest should be performed, as it is the most sensitive method for detecting small lung nodules. The thymus and remaining mediastinum can be examined at the same time. Bronchial carcinoid tumours responsible for ACTH tend to be small, ranging in size between 3 mm and 1.5 cm. Thus, they are often difficult to distinguish on imaging from other pulmonary nodules such as granulomata or hamartomas. Carcinoid tumours tend to be vascular, so occasionally enhancement after contrast can help distinguish them from granulomata and hamartomas. Nevertheless, care should always be exercised not to dismiss the smallest focal lung opacities. Although CT is highly sensitive it is relatively non-specific, so, when doubt exists, some recommend repeat CT every 6 months when tests are negative [21].

If the occult source is not found within the chest, careful ultrasound and CT examination of the pancreas should be performed, looking for the primary tumour, and of the liver, for metastases [20].

Systemic venous sampling is frequently performed in difficult cases. Even if it does not demonstrate the location of the ACTH source, the information is often useful. In patients shown to have a small intrapulmonary lesion on chest X-ray or CT, a negative systemic venous sampling, which does not sample the pulmonary circulation, focuses the attention on the intrapulmonary lesion as the potential source [20]. It should be noted, however, that elevated ACTH levels in the thymic vein may be due to hormone production by a bronchial carcinoid, mediastinal metastases, thymic carcinoid or diffuse thymic hyperplasia [23].

ACTH-independent Cushing's syndrome

ACTH-independent Cushing's syndrome is due to autonomous adrenal production of cortisol. In order of frequency, this may be due to adrenocortical adenoma, adrenal carcinoma and primary pigmented nodular adrenocortical disease.

Adrenocortical adenoma

An adrenal adenoma accounts for approximately 20% of all cases of Cushing's syndrome. They are best detected on CT but are also visualized on MRI, scintigraphy and sometimes ultrasound. On CT an adenoma appears as a well defined, rounded nodule, frequently greater than 2 cm in size at diagnosis [3,5,24], and of either low or soft tissue density. The contralateral adrenal gland tends to appear normal, but on occasion may look atrophic due to the low circulating ACTH levels [8].

MRI readily demonstrates adrenal adenomas, which tend to have homogeneous low signal intensity on T_1-weighted images. Adenomas may have signal similar to, or lower than, liver on T_2-weighted sequences [25–28] but some hyperfunctioning adenomas have higher T_2 signal intensity [4,29]. After intravenous gadolinium, over 90% of adenomas demonstrate a thin, hyperintense rim [30].

The detection of an adrenal mass in a patient with Cushing's syndrome does not necessarily indicate adenoma as the cause: such a mass carries a differential diagnosis including an incidental non-functioning adenoma, dominant nodule in macronodular hyperplasia, metastasis from an unrelated malignancy, phaeochromocytoma producing ACTH and a metastasis from a malignant ACTH-producing carcinoma [8,17]. Having detected a mass, it is essential to assess the rest of the gland and the contralateral gland. If there is a suspicion of hyperplasia, the diagnosis may be ACTH-dependent macronodular hyperplasia.

Occasionally, scintigraphy with ^{75}Se 6β-selenomethyl-19-norcholesterol is used to lateralize the abnormal adrenal gland in Cushing's syndrome when other imaging is equivocal. This tracer is taken into the adrenal gland and esterified to form part of the cholesterol ester substrate from which adrenal steroid hormones are synthesized [31]. This technique is particularly useful for the localization of postadrenalectomy remnants, and is helpful in distinguishing bilateral hyperplasia from adenomata in those cases where biochemical and imaging data are indeterminate [32].

Adrenal carcinoma

Adrenal carcinoma tends to present with a larger adrenal mass than does adenoma, usually more than 6 cm in diameter [8], and often larger than 9 cm at presentation [33]. On CT, such tumours often demonstrate central necrosis, irregular margins, thick rim enhancement and invasion into local structures including liver (Fig. 47.1) [34,35]. Calcification is seen in about 25% of cases [33,34]. Adrenal carcinoma is of lower signal intensity than liver on T_1-weighted MRI, and higher signal intensity on T_2 [6]. The tumours spread to regional lymph nodes, liver, lung and bone. Direct growth along the adrenal vein into the inferior vena cava (IVC) and right atrium is well documented [36]. All of these features are demonstrable on ultrasound, CT or MRI. Ultrasound [37] or MRI best determine the upper extent of thrombus, but neither will distinguish between tumour and blood in the thrombus [37]. CT is currently the most sensitive method for detection of pulmonary metastases [6]. The longitudinal

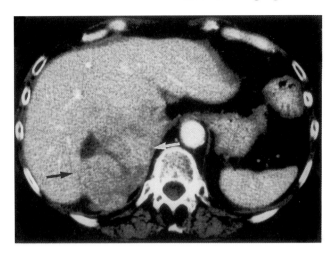

Fig. 47.1 Adrenal carcinoma. Contrast-enhanced CT showing 10 cm mass (arrows) arising in the right adrenal, with irregular enhancement pattern. The tumour is infiltrating the inferior vena cava.

representation on ultrasound or MRI is best suited to demonstrating the interface between the mass and the liver on the right side, and the spleen on the left.

Primary pigmented nodular adrenocortical disease (PPNAD)

PPNAD is a rare cause of Cushing's syndrome, with little in the literature regarding the imaging. The adrenal glands contain multiple, unencapsulated cortical nodules, which function autonomously, the intervening cortex being atrophied due to the low ACTH levels [38]. The condition occurs in younger patients and may be associated with Carney's complex (cardiac myxomas, skin pigmentation, giant calcifying Sertoli cell tumours of the testis, myxomas of the breast and subcutaneous tissues, and growth hormone-producing tumours) where PPNAD occurs in 45% of cases [39]. In these young patients, severe osteoporosis can be a striking feature, and should alert to the diagnosis of PPNAD. Earlier studies showed no abnormal features of the adrenals on CT, but with improvement in scanners and 5 mm collimation, Doppman and colleagues [38] were able to show small nodules in five out of six patients. Atrophy of the intervening adrenal tissue gives a characteristic 'string of beads' appearance. The nodules tend to have lower signal intensity than surrounding adrenal tissue on T_1- and T_2-weighted MRI. However, imaging may not detect the nodules, and in the absence of gradients on petrosal venous sampling, a presumptive diagnosis of PPNAD may be confirmed by bilateral adrenal uptake on scintigraphy [38].

Conn's syndrome (primary aldosteronism)

In common with other adrenocortical adenomas, Conn's adenomas tend to be well defined and of low or soft tissue density on CT (Fig. 47.2a). Conn's adenomas are more likely to have low density (less than 0 Hounsfield units) than other adenomas, the reason for this being unclear [40]. Due to their endocrine function, they tend to present whilst still small. The mean size is around 1.6–1.8 cm [24,41]. About 15–20% of adenomas are less than 1 cm

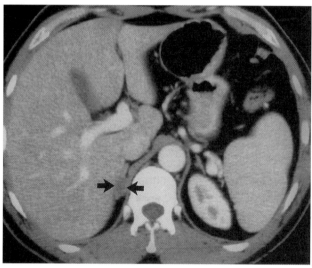

(a)

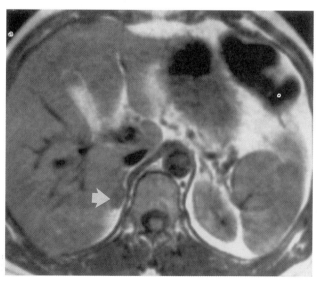

(b)

Fig. 47.2 Conn's adenoma. (a) Contrast-enhanced CT showing a 1.5 cm nodule in the limb of the right adrenal (arrows). (b) T$_1$-weighted MRI in the same patient showing low signal intensity (arrow).

in diameter (micronodules), which can be overlooked, but should not be missed with 5 mm collimation scanning [8]. The sensitivity of CT for the detection of adenomas is reported to be between 70 and 90% [5,42–4]. In our institution we have found a sensitivity of 100% but with an accuracy of 81% and positive predictive value of 83% [45]. Doppman and colleagues [43] report a similar positive predictive value. When there are several non-functioning adenomas in the presence of a functioning adenoma, a misdiagnosis of adrenal hyperplasia can be made [8]. As in Cushing's syndrome, a dominant nodule in hyperplasia can also be mistaken for an adenoma. In cases of hyperplasia, the glands appear normal on CT in 60% [5].

Adrenal venous sampling for aldosterone levels is very accurate in the preoperative diagnosis of Conn's syndrome. However, the cummulative failure rate for catheterization of the right adrenal vein is 26% [46]. A sensitivity of between 70 and 100% is achievable if the operator can catheterize both adrenal veins [43,45,46], with a positive predictive value of 90% [45].

^{75}Se 6β-selenomethyl-19-norcholesterol imaging may be performed to lateralize a Conn's adenoma when other investigations produce equivocal or conflicting results [32]. Scintigraphy after dexamethasone suppression was introduced by Conn and colleagues [47] in an attempt to accentuate the abnormal tracer uptake. In a study using the functionally equivalent ^{131}I-6β-iodomethylnorcholesterol (NP59), imaging after dexamethasone suppression improved the sensitivity and specificity from 68 and 63% to 87 and 89%, respectively [48]. However, using dexamethasone has the disadvantage of not differentiating between bilateral hyperplasia and normality [32].

MRI has not routinely been used to study aldosterone-producing adenomas, and there is little in the literature regarding their appearance. To date there are no specific characteristics to distinguish them from other adenomas on MRI (see Fig. 47.2b) [8].

Virilization

Virilization may be due to congenital adrenocortical hyperplasia (CAH), adrenal adenoma, adrenocortical carcinoma and extra-adrenal pathologies (polycystic ovary syndrome and gonadal tumours).

CAH is characterized by an inborn enzyme deficiency causing a partial block in adrenocortical steroid synthesis. The resultant chronic increase in ACTH levels stimulates the adrenal cortex leading to marked hyperplasia of the zona fasciculata-reticularis. The glands are grossly enlarged at diagnosis, enabling them to be imaged by ultrasound,

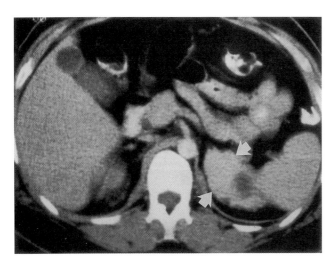

Fig. 47.3 Congenital adrenocortical hyperplasia. The left adrenal gland is grossly enlarged (arrows). On a different CT image, the right adrenal was similarly enlarged.

CT or MRI (Fig. 47.3) [49]. They often enhance inhomogeneously after intravenous contrast injection and can be mass-like, indistinguishable from carcinoma. Rarely, long-term ACTH stimulation in CAH may lead to transformation of the adrenal hyperplasia into an adenoma or sometimes a carcinoma. This is a complication that occurs in patients who have had untreated CAH for many years, and therefore is a distinct clinical group to those with primary virilizing adrenal tumours [49–51].

A primary virilizing adenoma or carcinoma is usually greater than 2 cm in diameter. The imaging characteristics are as already described for other adrenal adenomas and carcinomas (Fig. 47.4) [5,8]. The important distinction to make on imaging is between CAH and primary adrenal tumour. This is usually easily achieved by ultrasound and/or MRI. In these young patients, it is preferable to avoid CT if possible, on account of the ionizing radiation. Scintigraphy is not routinely indicated in the assessment of these patients but demonstration of unilateral or bilateral tracer uptake may provide useful information in some cases.

Imaging in a patient with virilization must also extend to exclude a primary tumour in the ovaries or testes. Again, ultrasound and MRI are the modalities of choice.

Phaeochromocytoma and paraganglionomas

Phaeochromocytoma is a tumour of paraganglion cells. Ninety-eight percent of phaeochromocytomas arise in the abdomen, and 90% of these are in the adrenal medulla, but they may arise anywhere in the autonomic nervous system [52]. Of the extra-adrenal phaeochromocytomas, most arise within the paravertebral sympathetic ganglia, in the organ of Zuckerkandl or, rarely, in the urinary bladder [8]. Ninety percent are sporadic, the remainder being inherited as an isolated disorder or as part of a multiple endocrine neoplasia syndrome (MEN type 2a or 2b), neurofibromatosis (Fig. 47.5) or von Hippel–Lindau syndrome. Phaeochromocytomas are multiple in 10% of sporadic cases and approximately 30% of cases when associated with a systemic disease [8,53]. Approximately 10% of phaeochromocytomas are malignant; the malignancy rate rising to 40% in extra-adrenal tumours [54]. The distinction between benign and malignant is very difficult, even histologically, malignancy often being diagnosed as a result of the tumour behaviour. Adrenal paraganglionomas are far more likely to be hormonally active than sympathetic or parasympathetic chain paraganglionomas [55].

Sporadic cases of phaeochromocytoma usually present with hormonal effects, but approximately 50% of cases associated with MEN are found as a result of a search [8].

Scintigraphy

MIBG is an aralkylguanidine which resembles noradrenaline and concentrates in sympatho-adrenal tissue. MIBG is therefore used for imaging tumours of neural crest origin, particularly phaeochromocytomas and paraganglionomas (Figs 47.6, 47.7). Since the whole body is imaged, ^{123}I-MIBG (or ^{131}I-MIBG) scintigraphy is extremely useful in the detection of extra-adrenal tumours. Metastatic lesions may be detected, most commonly in the skeleton, but also in the liver, lymph nodes, peritoneum and lung [56]. The functional nature of the information helps identify recurrent tumour within postoperative scar tissue [49]. MIBG may be labelled with ^{123}I or ^{131}I, but the former has many advantages, including reduced patient dose and better imaging characteristics. ^{123}I-MIBG provides better demonstration of small or metastatic lesions [57]. [123]I is therefore the primary scintigraphic diagnostic tool, and is performed as an essential prelude to ^{131}I-MIBG therapy. Standard bone scintigraphy is, however, still the most sensitive method for the detection of bone metastases [58].

Many studies report the use of ^{131}I-MIBG as opposed to ^{123}I-MIBG. The quoted sensitivity of ^{131}I-MIBG scintigraphy in detecting functioning phaeochromocytomas is around 90%, and the specificity 92–99% [16,56,59–63]. ^{111}In-pentetreotide may also be used. For the detection of paraganglionomas with ^{131}I-MIBG and ^{111}In-pentetreotide, the sensitivities are 89% and 97%

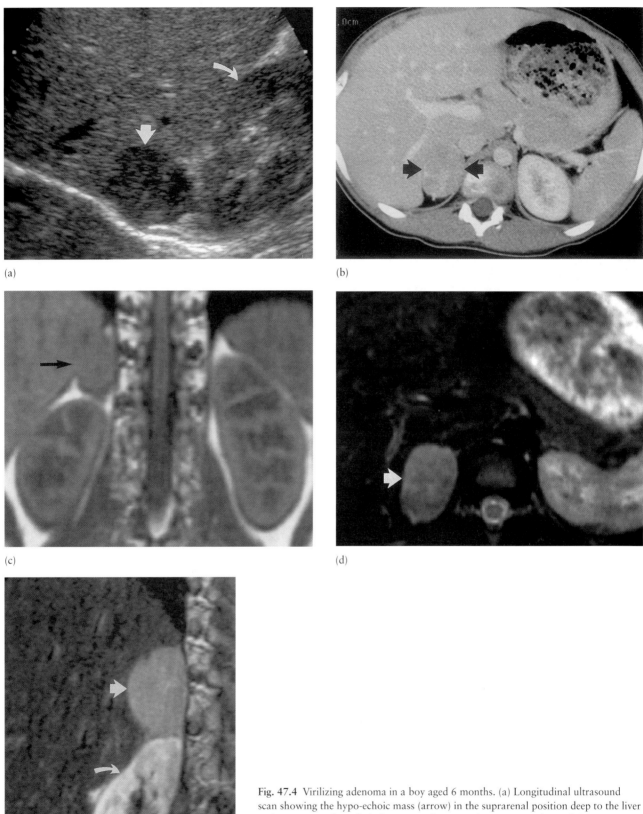

Fig. 47.4 Virilizing adenoma in a boy aged 6 months. (a) Longitudinal ultrasound scan showing the hypo-echoic mass (arrow) in the suprarenal position deep to the liver and superior to the right kidney (curved arrow). (b) Contrast-enhanced CT demonstrating the right adrenal mass (arrows) with slightly inhomogeneous enhancement pattern. (c) T_1-weighted MRI in coronal plane. The adenoma (arrow) has similar signal intensity to adjacent liver. (d) T_2-weighted MRI in axial plane. The adenoma has high signal on T_2-weighted images (arrow). (e) T_2-weighted MRI in sagittal plane. This technique effectively demonstrates the high signal adenoma (arrow) to be separate from the kidney (curved arrow).

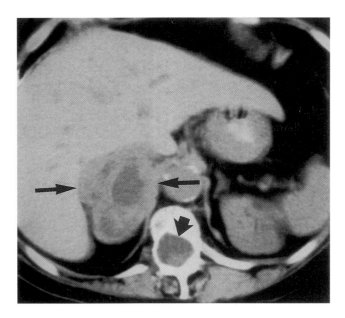

Fig. 47.5 Right adrenal phaeochromocytoma and dural ectasia in a patient with neurofibromatosis type I. Contrast-enhanced CT shows the large inhomogeneous phaeochromocytoma (long arrows). Dural ectasia is causing widening of the spinal canal (short arrow).

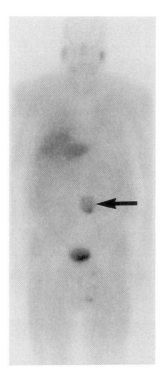

Fig. 47.7 Paraganglionoma. ^{123}I-MIBG scan showing abnormal accumulation of tracer in the left paraspinal region (arrow).

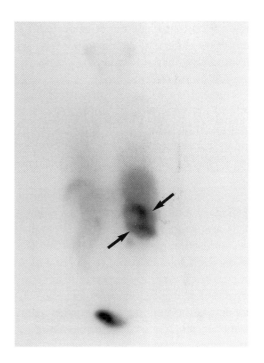

Fig. 47.6 Phaeochromocytoma. ^{123}I-MIBG whole body scan, posterior view, showing a right-sided phaeochromocytoma (arrows).

respectively [63]. With ^{111}In-pentetreotide imaging, high uptake in the kidneys masks small adrenal sites of disease [64]. False-positives can produce diagnostic problems, so correlation of scintigraphic findings with CT and MRI is important [49]. Scintigraphy is a sensitive method in this context, so where clinical and biochemical evidence for a neural crest tumour is equivocal, a negative ^{123}I-MIBG excludes the need for further imaging investigations. Where the evidence for such a tumour is strong and the ^{123}I-MIBG scan is negative, further imaging should be performed. Where scintigraphy demonstrates metastatic disease, CT and MRI is unlikely to alter the clinical management. The disadvantages of MIBG scintigraphy are the lack of anatomical detail and the high cost of the radiopharmaceutical.

Computed tomography (CT)

Phaeochromocytomas tend to be large at the time of diagnosis with an average size of 5 cm, rarely smaller than 3 cm [5]. When found as a result of screening of patients at risk, they may be smaller [16]. On pre-contrast-enhanced CT they are usually of soft tissue attenuation, similar to liver, sometimes with central low attenuation due to necrosis or cystic change (see Fig. 47.5) [65]. Calcification occurs but is not common. After intravenous contrast medium they enhance markedly (Fig. 47.8a), as do paraganglionomas (Fig. 47.9a). Since there is an unpredictable noradrenaline response to contrast injection in patients with phaeochromocytoma, with attendant risk of hypertensive crisis, α-blockade prophylaxis is given

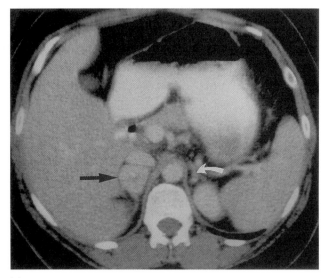

(a)

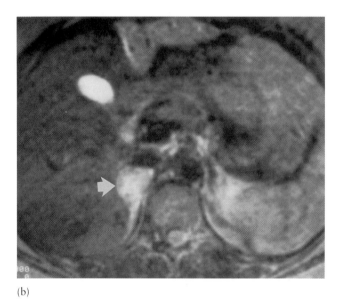

(b)

Fig. 47.8 Phaeochromocytoma. (a) Contrast-enhanced CT showing the right adrenal mass (black arrow), which enhances almost to the same degree as the major vessels. A normal adrenal gland is seen on the left (white arrow). (b) Axial T_2-weighted MRI showing the mass to have very high signal (arrow).

before scanning [66]. This reaction was recorded with older ionic contrast media, however, and has not been definitely shown to occur with newer non-ionic media.

CT is very accurate in the detection of adrenal phaeochromocytomas, with reported sensitivities up to 90–100% [65,67]. The sensitivity is equivalent to that of MRI and scintigraphy. However, in the detection of extra-adrenal phaeochromocytomas and recurrent tumours, CT is not as sensitive as MRI or scintigraphy [55,68,69]. Quint and colleagues [68] reported CT to

have a sensitivity of 57%, and MRI 86% in the detection of recurrent tumour.

Magnetic resonance imaging

On T_1-weighted images phaeochromocytomas show signal similar in intensity to liver, or slightly lower, and fairly consistently very high signal on T_2-weighted images (Figs 47.8b, 47.10b, 47.11d, 47.12c) [4,16,25,26,68,70]. This pattern, although not always present [28], helps distinguish a phaeochromocytoma from a benign adenoma. Phaeochromocytomas also demonstrate enhancement after intravenous gadolinium-diethylenetriamine penta-acetic acid (DTPA). MRI appears to be equivalent to CT in diagnosing adrenal phaeochromocytomas, but more accurate in detecting extra-adrenal and recurrent phaeochromocytomas. When the biochemistry is equivocal, MRI may be more specific than CT at distinguishing between cortical adenoma and phaeochromocytoma [25,26,28,71].

Neuroblastoma and ganglioneuroblastoma

Eighty-five percent of these tumours occur in children less than 5 years of age. Neuroblastomas may arise anywhere along the sympathetic chain, but between 50 and 80% arise within the adrenal medulla. Neuroblastomas are usually large at presentation, and may be disseminated to liver, bone, bone marrow, lymph nodes and other organs. Ultrasound is frequently the first investigation for a child with an abdominal mass, and neuroblastomas are readily demonstrated by this method. The multiplanar nature of ultrasound may help to show the mass to be separate from the kidney, even though the tumour may invade the kidney, making distinction from Wilms' tumour difficult. CT and, more recently, MRI are the main imaging modalities used in staging and documenting the extent of the tumour. Ultrasound is mainly reserved for the follow-up of patients during therapy for neuroblastoma [8].

CT features of neuroblastoma are of a large mass, often extending across the midline to engulf the aorta and its major branches (Fig. 47.13). Neuroblastoma is said to displace the aorta anteriorly more frequently than Wilm's tumour. Another feature to help distinguish neuroblastoma from a Wilm's tumour is that of calcification, which is more common in neuroblastoma and may show a characteristic rim distribution [72]. Inhomogeneous enhancement after intravenous contrast is usual. CT is invaluable in the planning and execution of a biopsy [73].

MRI has become a modality of choice for staging of the disease, with good contrast between the very high-signal tumour and the surrounding tissues on T_2-weighted

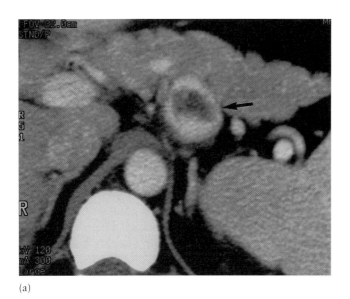

(a)

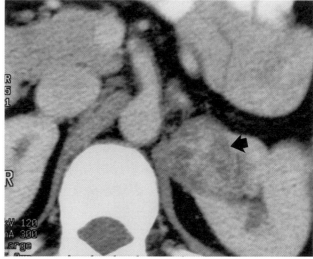

(b)

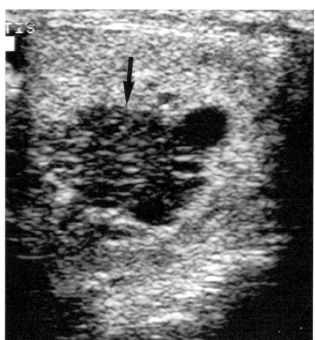

Fig. 47.9 Paraganglionoma, renal cell carcinoma and epididymal adenomas in a patient with von Hippel–Lindau disease.
(a) Contrast-enhanced CT showing the markedly enhancing paraganglioma (arrow) just deep to the pancreas, related to the coeliac vessels. (b) A further image from the same CT investigation as in (a), showing a renal cell carcinoma in the medial aspect of the left kidney (arrow). (c) Scrotal ultrasound in the same patient showing an epididymal adenoma (arrow).

(c)

images, and multiplanar imaging capability [49,74]. These factors help to identify those patients with stage 1 and 2 disease [72]. Extension into the spinal canal of a paraspinal tumour characteristically produces a dumb-bell configuration which is well demonstrated on MRI without the need for myelography.

Neuroblastomas and ganglioneuroblastomas may be imaged using ^{123}I-MIBG or ^{131}I-MIBG scintigraphy, playing a complementary role to MRI and CT. Scintigraphy has the advantage of being able to detect metastases and, due to this, may be more accurate than MRI or CT in some cases [69]. The reported cumulative sensitivity of ^{131}I-MIBG for the detection of neuroblastoma in 779 patients is 92%, with a specificity of nearly 100% [63]. ^{99m}Tc-methyl diphosphonate is still the most sensitive method for detecting skeletal metastases [72]. Where the tumour and its metastases are ^{123}I-MIBG avid, ^{131}I-MIBG therapy is an option. ^{111}In-pentetreotide imaging has also been used for neuroblastoma, but the sensitivity (77%) is not as high as with ^{131}I-MIBG [63].

The information gained from CT and/or MRI, skeletal scintigraphy, bone marrow aspirate and clinical data will

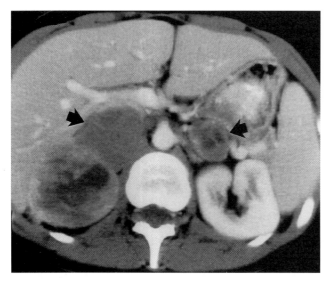

(a)

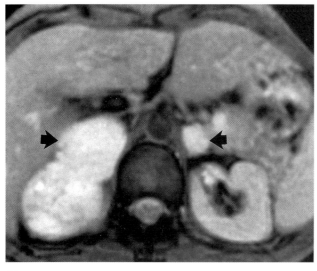

(b)

Fig. 47.10 Bilateral phaeochromocytomas in a patient with multiple endocrine neoplasia type 2a (MEN-2a). (a) Contrast-enhanced CT showing bilateral adrenal masses (arrows). The mass on the right is invading the kidney. (b) T$_2$-weighted MRI showing the masses to be of very high signal intensity, characteristic of phaeochromocytomas (arrows).

accurately stage at least 95% of patients with thoraco-abdominal neuroblastomas [74].

Incidentally discovered adrenal masses

At autopsy, the adrenal glands have been found to contain grossly visible adenomas in 2–9% of patients, and microscopic nodules in up to 50% [75]. Nodules measuring 1–3 cm are found incidentally in a significant number of abdominal CT examinations, making an incidentally discovered or unsuspected adrenal mass a diagnostic problem [75,76]. The differential diagnosis for the mass in the absence of any biochemical information is long, the most important being hyperfunctioning or non-hyperfunctioning adenoma, adenocarcinoma, metastasis, phaeochromocytoma, lymphoma, adrenal haemorrhage, abscess and myelolipoma. The nature of any biochemical abnormality dictates further management [8]. Clearly, a non-functioning mass poses the most difficulty.

After assessment of function, the size of the mass is the next most important consideration. A mass that is larger than 5 cm has a significant chance of being a carcinoma which may be cured by resection. For this reason, most masses this size will be removed. A mass that is 3 cm in diameter or less is usually benign if there is no known malignancy, especially if the CT features of an adenoma are present. Most masses less than 3 cm in size are followed-up by CT or MRI to monitor change. If the imaging features are markedly atypical for an adenoma, the mass may be biopsied [8]. Masses measuring between 3 and 5 cm form an indeterminate group where management varies from institution to institution. In our hospital, they are followed-up by CT or MRI after 6 months unless there are features atypical of an adenoma, in which case the mass is biopsied or removed. Biopsy is best carried out under CT guidance.

On CT, a non-hyperfunctioning adenoma typically shows as a well-defined, rounded homogeneous mass, with relatively low soft tissue density (0–30 Hounsfield units; Fig. 47.14a). Calcification can occur but is uncommon. Central haemorrhage or necrosis is rare [29]. After intravenous contrast enhancement, adenomas sometimes show punctate enhancement with a thin or absent rim (Fig. 47.14a). Metastases and carcinomas tend to enhance with a thick and irregular rim. Some authors claim a high positive predictive value based on these CT appearances [35].

MRI signal characteristics may provide further evidence for the benign nature of a mass, but no absolute criteria exist. Non-hyperfunctioning adenomas tend to have relatively low signal on T$_2$-weighted images, similar to, or lower than liver (Fig. 47.15c). Metastases and carcinomas have a higher signal on T$_2$, and phaeochromocytomas a very high signal [25,26,28]. As with CT contrast enhancement, adenomas tend to show thin rim enhancement after gadolinium, and metastases thick irregular rim enhancement [30]. These criteria are statistically valid, but signal characteristic overlap between the pathologies is such that an absolute diagnosis cannot be made on MRI in any one case [4,12,27]. Guidelines derived at 0.5 T signal strength are not necessarily applicable at 1.5 T [28].

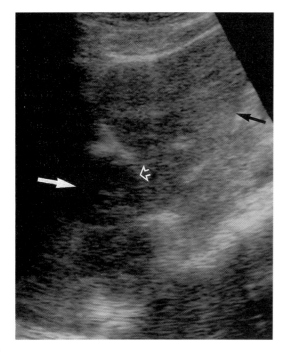

(a)

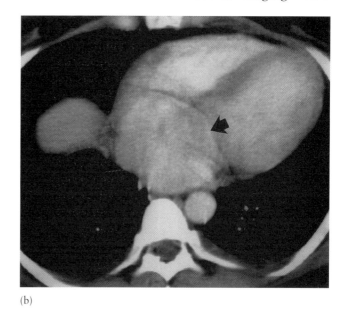

(b)

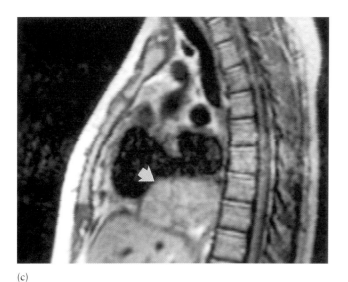

(c)

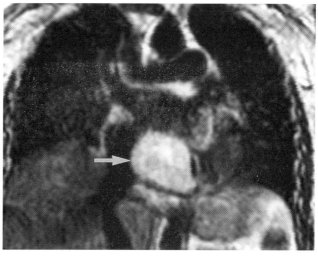

(d)

Fig. 47.11 Intracardiac phaeochromocytoma. (a) Longitudinal ultrasound scan showing a mass (white arrow) above the diaphragm (open arrow) and the left lobe of the liver (black arrow). (b) Contrast-enhanced CT. The mass (arrow), which occupies much of the left atrium, enhances to a similar degree to the blood in the other chambers, thus masking its presence on CT. (c) Sagittal T_1-weighted MRI. The tumour (arrow) has similar signal intensity to the subadjacent liver. (d) T_2-weighted coronal MRI through the chest demonstrating very high signal intensity in the tumour (arrow).

The more recent MRI technique of chemical shift imaging is showing improved but not absolute differentiation between adrenal masses [12]. MR spectroscopy has been used to demonstrate the lipid content of adrenal masses, a lipid content of 10% or more indicating a mass to be benign, but this technique is not in clinical use [77]. Adrenal haemorrhage has a very variable signal on T_2-weighted images, probably related to the marked changes in T_2 relaxation time that are known to occur during the evolution of haematoma [28].

^{75}Se 6β-selenomethyl-19-norcholesterol scintigraphy may demonstrate increased uptake in a non-functioning adenoma (see Plate 47.1, between pp. 272 and 273). If the uptake is greater in the abnormal gland than in the

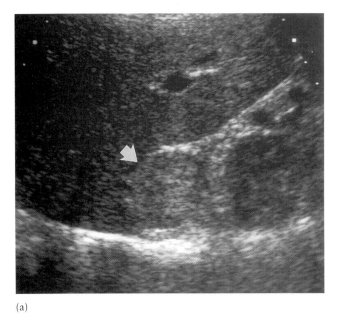

(a)

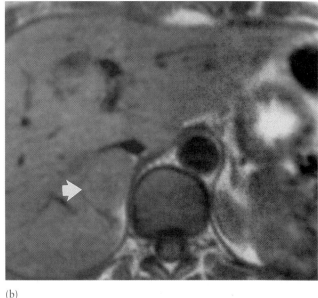

(b)

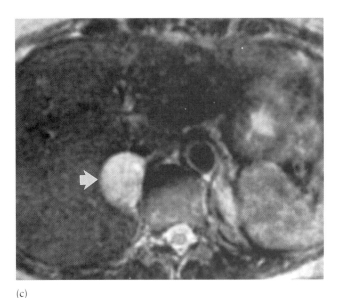

(c)

Fig. 47.12 Phaeochromocytoma. (a) Longitudinal ultrasound showing rounded mass in the adrenal area (arrow). (b) T_1-weighted MRI showing the mass (arrow) to be of similar signal intensity to liver. (c) T_2-weighted MRI at the same level showing the mass (arrow) to have high signal.

contralateral gland, this is further assurance that the mass is benign [78]. Absence of uptake is not specific, however, since neither a cyst, a haematoma, nor an inflammatory mass will take up tracer [29].

Adrenal metastases

Even when there is a known primary elsewhere, it has been shown that a unilateral adrenal mass is still more likely to be a small adenoma than a metastasis. In a CT series of 330 patients with small-cell carcinoma of the lung, adenomas were twice as frequent as metastases [79]. When the patient does not have a present or past

malignancy, a unilateral adrenal mass seldom, if ever, represents a metastasis [5,35]. Some authors have drawn attention to an increased incidence of adenomas in patients with renal cell carcinoma [80]. Metastases may be of any size and configuration, and are often unilateral rather than bilateral. When an adrenal mass is greater than 3 cm in diameter, it is more likely to represent metastasis than adenoma in an oncology patient [79]. On MRI, metastases tend to have a higher signal than adenomas on T_2-weighted images, and to show thick and irregular rim enhancement after contrast on both MRI and CT [25,30,35,81]. The discovery of an indeterminate adrenal mass in a patient with a known malignancy

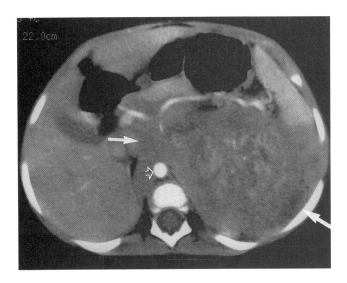

Fig. 47.13 Neuroblastoma. Contrast-enhanced CT showing a large mass in the left of the abdomen with inhomogeneous enhancement (white arrows). The mass has spread across the midline to engulf the aorta (open arrow) and coeliac axis vessels.

may lead to an adrenal biopsy, which is best performed under CT guidance. This is probably the most common indication for an adrenal biopsy [82].

Adrenal hyperplasia occurs in the presence of malignancy of many types, detectable on CT (Fig. 47.16) [83,84]. The degree of hyperplasia has been shown not to be linked to the stage of tumour, and is not thought to be due to the presence of metastases. The mechanism for this phenomenon is not well understood, but may be due to the production of factors by the tumour [84].

Primary adrenal lymphoma is very rare [8]. Involvement of the adrenal glands in widespread non-Hodgkin's lymphoma, however, is relatively common, being detected radiographically in approximately 4% of cases. On CT this appears as masses of soft tissue attenuation (Fig. 47.17), showing slight enhancement after administration of intravenous contrast.

Adrenal myelolipoma

Adrenal myelolipoma is a rare, benign neoplasm composed of adipose and haematopoietic tissue. The imaging features are usually characteristic, allowing the radiologist to make a confident diagnosis. They are frequently discovered incidentally during imaging for another indication, but they characteristically present with pain due to haemorrhage or necrosis within the tumour [85,86]. If of sufficient size (approximately 4 cm), ultrasound will show a highly echogenic mass (Fig. 47.18a). Myelolipomas are best assessed by CT scanning, where fat density (Fig.

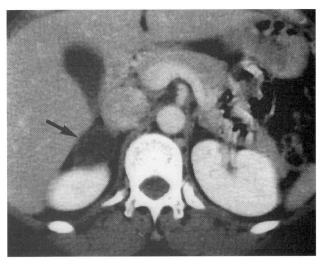

(a)

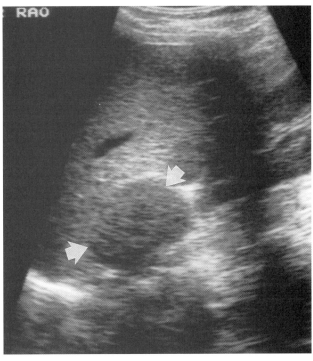

(b)

Fig. 47.14 Non-functioning adrenal adenoma. (a) Contrast-enhanced CT scan demonstrating a right adrenal mass of low attenuation (arrow). A very thin rim of enhancement can just be seen. (b) Longitudinal ultrasound scan showing the mass to be solid (arrows).

47.18b) and haemorrhage, if this has occurred, can be demonstrated. Other fat-containing tumours in the retroperitoneum, such as lipoma, liposarcoma and renal angiomyelolipoma may mimic the appearances [86]. Engulfment of normal periadrenal adipose tissue by a

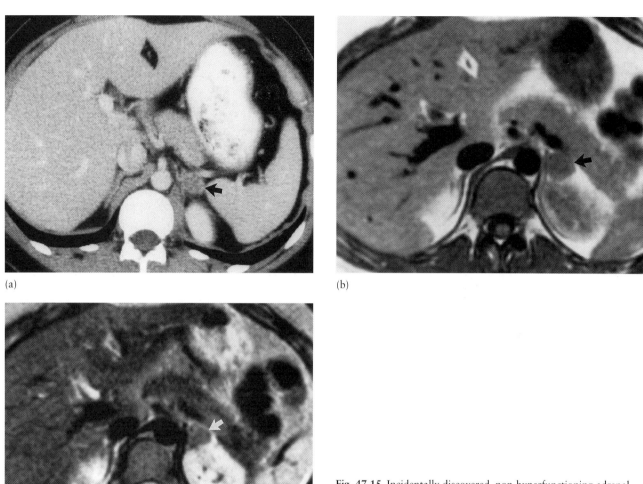

(a)

(b)

(c)

Fig. 47.15 Incidentally discovered, non-hyperfunctioning adrenal adenoma. (a) Contrast-enhanced CT showing 1.8 cm left adrenal mass (arrow). (b) T_1-weighted MRI showing the mass to be of intermediate signal (arrow). (c) T_2-weighted fast spin echo MRI: the mass is of low signal (arrow).

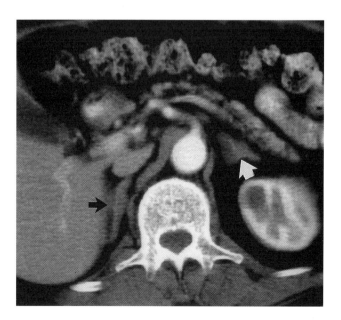

Fig. 47.16 Bilateral adrenal hyperplasia in malignancy. Contrast-enhanced CT in a patient with chondrosarcoma. There is diffuse enlargement of both adrenals (arrows).

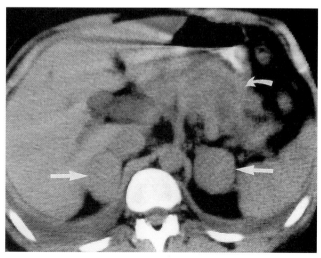

Fig. 47.17 Lymphoma involving the adrenal glands. CT scan showing masses in both adrenal glands (arrows). A large lymph node mass is also seen around the coeliac axis (curved arrow).

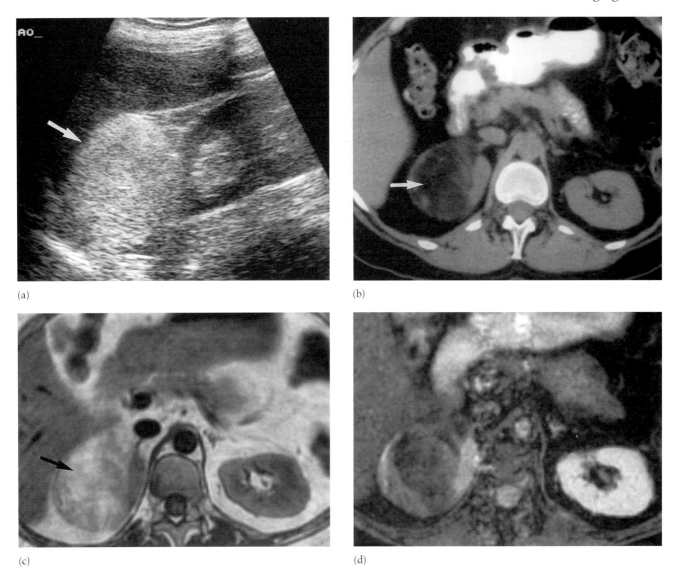

(a)

(b)

(c)

(d)

Fig. 47.18 Adrenal myelolipoma. (a) Longitudinal ultrasound scan showing a large hyperechoic adrenal mass (arrow). (b) CT scan in the same patient demonstrating fat density within the mass (arrow). (c) T_1-weighted MRI showing the high signal of fat within the lesion (arrow). (d) T_2-weighted MRI with fat suppression showing the loss of signal within the fat.

malignant adrenal mass may also mimic a fat-containing tumour [5]. If the fat component of the myelolipoma is small, the attenuation value may only be moderately low (0–30 Hounsfield units), and it may not be possible to distinguish from other adrenal masses [87].

Adrenal cyst

Cysts of the adrenal glands are uncommon, and are usually found incidentally. There are several types of cyst, the most frequent being endothelial cysts (45%) [8]. These may be lymphatic or angiomatous, the former probably arising as a result of a blocked lymph duct. Remaining cysts are epithelial, parasitic (echinococcus), and pseudocysts (39% of all cysts), which are presumed to result from haemorrhage [29].

Ultrasonography will demonstrate the cystic nature of an adrenal mass. Unlike benign renal cysts, adrenal cysts commonly have a thick wall, and pseudocysts may have internal septa [29]. CT will readily demonstrate the mass, but since an adenoma can have low density with Hounsfield numbers identical to a cyst, CT cannot reliably distinguish between cyst and adenoma. Ultrasound or MRI must be employed to differentiate. Malignancy in a cystic mass is difficult to exclude, and follow-up or cyst fluid aspiration cytology may be required.

References

1. Dunnick NR, Schaner EG, Doppman JL *et al*. Computed tomography in adrenal tumors. *Am. J. Roentgenol.* 1979;**132**:43–6.

2. Eghrari M, McLoughlin MJ, Rosen IE *et al*. The role of computed tomography in assessment of tumoral pathology of the adrenal glands. *J. Comput. Ass. Tomogr.* 1980;**4**(1):71–7.

3. Adams JE, Johnson RJ, Rickards D, Isherwood I. Computed tomography in adrenal disease. *Clin. Radiol.* 1983;**34**:39–49.

4. Falke THM, te Strake L, Shaff MI *et al*. MR imaging of the adrenals: correlation with computed tomography. *J. Comput. Assist. Tomogr.* 1986;**10**:242–53.

5. Moulton Jonathan S, Moulton Jeffrey S. CT of the adrenal glands. *Semin. Roentgenol.* 1988;**28**:288–303.

6. Dunnick NR. Adrenal carcinoma. *Radiol. Clin. North Am.* 1994;**32**(1):99–108.

7. White EM, Edelman RR, Stark DD *et al*. Surface coil MR imaging of abdominal viscera. Part II. The adrenal glands. *Radiology* 1985;**157**;431–6.

8. Reznek RH, Armstrong P. Imaging in endocrinology: the adrenal gland. *Clin. Endocrinol.* 1994;**40**:561–76.

9. Saini S, Stark DD, Rzedzian RR *et al*. Forty-millisecond MR imaging of the abdomen at 2.0 T. *Radiology* 1989;**173**:111–16.

10. Stehling MJ, Howseman AM, Ordidge RJ *et al*. Whole-body echo-planar MR imaging at 0.5 T. *Radiology* 1989;**170**:257–63.

11. Mirowitz SA, Lee JKT, Brown JL *et al*. Rapid acquisition spin-echo (RASE) MR imaging: a new technique for reduction of artifacts and acquisition time. *Radiology*, 1990;**175**:131–5.

12. Reinig JW, Stutley JE, Leonhardt CM *et al*. Differentiation of adrenal masses with MR imaging: comparison of techniques. *Radiology* 1994;**192**:41–6.

13. Hawkins LA, Britton KE, Shapiro B. Selenium 75 selenomethyl cholesterol: a new agent for quantitative scintigraphy of the adrenals: physical aspects. *Br. J. Radiol.* 1980;**53**:883–9.

14. Vincent JM, Morrison ID, Armstrong P, Reznek RH. The size of normal adrenal glands on computed tomography. *Clin. Radiol.* 1994;**49**:453–5. (Erratum *Clin. Radiol.* 1994;**50**:202.)

15. Smals AGH, Pieters GFFM, van Haelst UJG, Kloppenborg PWC. Macronodular adrenocortical hyperplasia in long-standing Cushing's disease. *J. Clin. Endocrinol. Metab.* 1984;**58**:25–31.

16. Francis IR, Gross MD, Shapiro B, Korobkin M, Quint LE. Integrated imaging of adrenal disease. *Radiology* 1992;**184**:1–13.

17. Aron DC, Findling JW, Fitzgerald PA *et al*. Pituitary ACTH dependency of nodular adrenal hyperplasia in Cushing's syndrome. *Am. J. Med.* 1981;**71**:302–6.

18. Doppman JL, Miller DL, Dwyer AJ *et al*. Macronodular adrenal hyperplasia in Cushing Disease. *Radiology* 1988;**166**:347–52.

19. Findling JW, Tyrrell JB. Occult ectopic secretion of corticotrophin. *Arch. Intern. Med.* 1986;**146**:929–33.

20. Vincent JM, Trainer PJ, Reznek RH *et al*. The radiological investigation of occult ectopic ACTH-dependent Cushing's syndrome. *Clin. Radiol.* 1993;**48**:11–17.

21. Doppman JL, Nieman L, Miller DL *et al*. Ectopic adrenocorticotrophic hormone syndrome: localization studies in 28 patients. *Radiology* 1989;**172**:115–24.

22. Imura H, Matsukura S, Yamamoto H *et al*. Studies on ectopic ACTH-producing tumors II. Clinical and biochemical features of 30 cases. *Cancer* 1975;**35**:1430–7.

23. Doppman JL, Pass HI, Nieman LK *et al*. Corticotrophin-secreting carcinoid tumors of the thymus: diagnostic unreliability of thymic venous sampling. *Radiology* 1992;**184**:71–4.

24. Dunnick NR, Doppman JL, Gill JR *et al*. Localization of functional adrenal tumors by computed tomography and venous sampling. *Radiology* 1982;**142**:429–33.

25. Glazer GM, Woolsey EJ, Borrello J *et al*. Adrenal tissue characterization using MR imaging. *Radiology* 1986;**158**:73–9.

26. Reinig JW, Doppman JL, Dwyer AJ, Frank J. MRI of indeterminate adrenal masses. *Am. J. Roentgenol.* 1986;**147**:493–6.

27. Chang A, Glazer HS, Lee JKT, Ling D, Heiken JP. Adrenal gland: MR imaging. *Radiology* 1987;**163**:123–8.

28. Kier R, McCarthy S. MR characterization of adrenal masses: field strength and pulse sequence considerations. *Radiology* 1989;**171**:671–4.

29. Dunnick NR. Adrenal imaging: current status. *Am. J. Roentgenol.* 1990;**154**:927–36.

30. Ichikawa T, Ohmoto K, Uchiyama G *et al*. Adrenal adenomas: characteristic hyperintense rim sign on fat-saturated spin-echo MR images. *Radiology* 1994;**193**:247–50.

31. Sandler MP, Delbeke D. Radionuclides in endocrine imaging. *Radiol. Clin. North Am.* 1993;**31**(4):909–21.

32. Shapiro B, Britton KE, Hawkins LA, Edwards CRW. Clinical experience with ⁷⁵Se selenomethylcholesterol adrenal imaging. *Clin. Endocrinol.* 1981;**15**:19–27.

33. Dunnick NR, Heaston D, Halvorsen R, Moore AV, Korobkin M. CT appearance of adrenal cortical carcinoma. *J. Comput. Assist. Tomogr.* 1982;**6**(5):978–82.

34. Fishman EK, Deutch BM, Hartman DS *et al*. Primary adrenocortical carcinoma: CT evaluation with clinical correlation. *Am. J. Roentgenol.* 1987;**148**:531–5.

35. Berland LL, Koslin DB, Kenney PJ, Stanley RJ, Lee JY. Differentiation between small benign and malignant adrenal masses with dynamic incremented CT. *Am. J. Roentgenol.* 1988;**151**:95–101.

36. Dunnick NR, Doppman JL, Geelhoed GW. Intravenous extension of endocrine tumors. *Am. J. Roentgenol.* 1980;**135**:471–6.

37. Didier D, Racle A, Etievent JP, Weill F. Tumor thrombus of the inferior vena cava secondary to malignant abdominal neoplasms: US and CT evaluation. *Radiology* 1987;**162**:83–9.

38. Doppman JL, Travis WD, Nieman L *et al*. Cushing syndrome due to primary pigmented nodular adrenocortical disease: findings at CT and MRI imaging. *Radiology* 1989;**172**:415–20.

39. Carney JA, Hruska LS, Beauchamp GD, Gordon H. Dominant inheritance of the complex of myxomas, spotty pigmentation, and endocrine overactivity. *Mayo Clin. Proc.* 1986;**61**:165–72.

40. Miyake H, Maeda H, Tashiro M *et al*. CT of adrenal tumours: frequency and clinical significance of low-attenuation lesions. *Am. J. Roentgenol.* 1989;**152**:1005–7.

41. Geisinger MA, Zelch MG, Bravo EL *et al*. Primary hyperaldosteronism: comparison of CT, adrenal venography, and venous sampling. *Am. J. Roentgenol.* 1983;**141**:299–302.

42. Ikeda DM, Francis IR, Glazer GM *et al*. The detection of adrenal tumors and hyperplasia in patients with primary aldosteronism: comparison of scintigraphy, CT, and MR imaging. *Am. J. Roentgenol.* 1989;**153**:301–6.

43. Doppman JL, Gill JR, Miller DL *et al*. Distinction between hyperaldosteronism due to bilateral hyperplasia and unilateral aldosteronoma: reliability of CT. *Radiology* 1992;**184**:677–82.

44. Dunnick NR, Leight GS, Roubidoux MA *et al*. CT in the diagnosis

of primary aldosteronism: sensitivity in 29 patients. *Am. J. Roentgenol.* 1993;**160**:321–4.

45. Goldin J, Sheaves R, Reznek RH *et al.* The role of computed tomography and venous sampling in the investigation of hyper-aldosteronism (Conn's syndrome). *Clin. Radiol.* 1993;**48**:357.

46. Young WF, Hogan MJ, Klee GG, Grant CS, van Heerden JA. Primary aldosteronism: diagnosis and treatment. *Mayo Clin. Proc.* 1990;**65**:96–110.

47. Conn JW, Cohen EL, Herwig KR. The dexamethasone-modified adrenal scintiscan in hyporeninemic aldosteronism (tumor versus hyperplasia). A comparison with adrenal venography and adrenal venous aldosterone. *J. Lab. Clin. Med.* 1976;**88**:841–56.

48. Gross MD, Shapiro B, Grekin RJ *et al.* Scintigraphic localiz-ation of adrenal lesions in primary aldosteronism. *Am. J. Med.* 1984;**77**:839–44.

49. Gross MD, Falke THM, Shapiro B, Sandler MP. Adrenal glands. In Sandler MP, Patton JA, Gross MD, Shapiro B, Falke THM (eds). *Endocrine Imaging*. Norwalk, Connecticut: Appleton and Lange, 1992:271–349.

50. Pang S, Becker D, Cotelingam J, Foley TP, Drash AL. Adrenocortical tumor in a patient with congenital adrenal hyperplasia due to 21-hydroxylase deficiency. *Pediatrics* 1981;**68**(2):242–6.

51. Falke THM, van Seters AP, Schaberg A, Moolenaar AJ. Computed tomography in untreated adults with virilising congenital cortical hyperplasia. *Clin. Radiol.* 1986;**37**:155–60.

52. Radin DR, Ralls PW, Boswell WD *et al.* Phaeochromocytoma: detection by unenhanced CT. *Am. J. Roentgenol.* 1986;**146**:741–4.

53. Horton WA, Wong V, Eldridge R. Von Hippel–Lindau disease. *Arch. Intern. Med.* 1976;**136**:769–77.

54. Van Heerden JA, Sheps SG, Hamberger B *et al.* Phaeochromo-cytoma: current status and changing trends. *Surgery* 1982;**91**:367–73.

55. Dunn GD, Brown MJ, Sapsford RN *et al.* Functioning middle mediastinal paraganglionoma (Phaeochromocytoma) associated with intercarotid paraganglionomas. *Lancet* 1986;**1**:1061–4.

56. Shapiro B, Sisson JC, Lloyd R *et al.* Malignant phaeochro-mocytoma: clinical biochemical and scintigraphic characterization. *Clin. Endocrinol.* 1984;**20**:189–203.

57. Lynn MD, Shapiro B, Sisson JC *et al.* Portrayal of phaeo-chromocytoma and normal human adrenal medulla by *m*-[123I]iodobenzylguanidine: concise communication. *J. Nucl. Med.* 1984;**25**:436–40.

58. Lynn MD, Braunstein EM, Wahl RL *et al.* Bone metastases in phaeochromocytoma: comparative studies of efficacy of imaging. *Radiology* 1986;**160**:701–6.

59. Ackery DM, Tippett PA, Condon BR, Sutton HE, Wyeth P. New approach to the localisation of phaeochromocytoma: imaging with iodine-131-meta-iodobenzylguanidine. *Br. Med. J.* 1984;**288**:1587–91.

60. Chatal JF, Charbonnel B. Comparison of iodobenzylguanidine imaging with computed tomography in locating phaeochromo-cytoma. *J. Clin. Endocrinol. Metab.* 1985;**61**:769–72.

61. Shapiro B, Copp JE, Sisson JC *et al.* Iodine-131 metaiodo-benzylguanidine for the locating of suspected phaeochromocytoma: experience in 400 cases. *J. Nucl. Med.* 1985;**26**:575–85.

62. Gross MD, Shapiro B. Scintigraphic studies in adrenal hypertension. *Semin. Nucl. Med.* 1989;**19**:122–43.

63. Hoefnagel CA. Metaiodobenzylguanidine and somatostatin in oncology: role in the management of neural crest tumours. *Eur. J. Nucl. Med.* 1994;**21**:561–81.

64. Krenning EP, Kwekkeboom DJ, Bakker WH *et al.* Somatostatin receptor scintigraphy with [111In-DTPA-D-Phe]- and [123I-Tyr]-octreotide: the Rotterdam experience with more than 1000 patients. *Eur. J. Nucl. Med.* 1993;**20**:716–31.

65. Welch TJ, Sheedy PF, van Heerden JA *et al.* Phaeochromo-cytoma: value of computed tomography. *Radiology* 1983;**148**:501–3.

66. Raisanen J, Shapiro B, Glazer GM, Desai S, Sisson JC. Plasma catecholamines in phaeochromocytoma: effect of urographic con-trast media. *Am. J. Roentgenol.* 1984;**143**:43–6.

67. Francis IR, Glazer GM, Shapiro B, Sisson JC, Gross BH. Com-plementary roles of CT and 131I-MIBG scintigraphy in diagnosing phaeochromocytoma. *Am. J. Roentgenol.* 1983;**141**:719–25.

68. Quint LE, Glazer GM, Francis IR, Shapiro B, Chenevert TL. Phaeochromocytoma and paraganglionoma: comparison of MR imaging with CT and I-131 MIBG scintigraphy. *Radiology* 1987;**165**:89–93.

69. Bomanji J, Conry BG, Britton KE, Reznek RH. Imaging neural crest tumours with 123I-metaiodobenzylguanidine and X-ray computed tomography: a comparative study. *Clin. Radiol.* 1988;**39**:502–6.

70. Fink IJ, Reinig JW, Dwyer AJ *et al.* MR imaging of phaeo-chromocytomas. *J. Comput. Assist. Tomogr.* 1985;**9**:454–8.

71. Lee MJ, Hahn PF, Papanicolaou N *et al.* Benign and malignant adrenal masses: CT distinction with attenuation coefficients, size, and observer analysis. *Radiology* 1991;**179**:415–18.

72. Ng YY, Kingston JE. The role of radiology in the staging of neuroblastoma. *Clin. Radiol.* 1993;**47**:226–35.

73. Kuhns LR. Computed tomography of the retroperitoneum in children. *Radiol. Clin. North Am.* 1981;**19**:495–501.

74. Merten DF, Gold SH. Radiologic staging of thoracoabdominal tumors in childhood. *Radiol. Clin. North Am.* 1994;**32**(1):133–49.

75. Glazer HS, Weyman PJ, Sagel SS, Levitt RG, McClennan BL. Nonfunctioning adrenal masses: incidental discovery on computed tomography. *Am. J. Roentgenol.* 1982;**139**:81–5.

76. Mitnick JS, Bosniak MA, Megibow AJ, Naidich DP. Non-functioning adrenal adenomas discovered incidentally on computed tomography. *Radiology* 1983;**148**:495–9.

77. Leroy-Willig A, Bittoun J, Luton JP *et al. In vivo* MR spectroscopic imaging of the adrenal glands: distinction between adenomas and carcinomas larger than 15 mm based on lipid content. *Am. J. Roentgenol.* 1989;**153**:771–3.

78. Gross MD, Wilton GP, Shapiro B *et al.* Functional scintigraphic evaluation of the silent adrenal mass. *J. Nucl. Med.* 1987;**28**:1401–7.

79. Oliver TW, Bernardino ME, Miller JI *et al.* Isolated adrenal masses in nonsmall-cell bronchogenic carcinoma. *Radiology* 1984;**153**:217–18.

80. Ambos MA, Bosniak MA, Lefleur RS, Mitty HA. Adrenal adenoma associated with renal cell carcinoma. *Am. J. Roentgenol.* 1981;**136**:81–4.

81. Reinig JW, Doppman JL, Dwyer AJ, Johnson AR, Knop RH. Distinction between adrenal adenomas and metastases using MR imaging. *J. Comput. Assist. Tomogr.* 1985;**9**:898–901.

82. Welch TJ, Sheedy PF, Stephens DH, Johnson CM, Swensen SJ. Percutaneous adrenal biopsy: review of a 10-year experience. *Radiology* 1994;**193**:341–4.

83. Parker TG, Sommers SC. Adrenal cortical hyperplasia accom-panying cancer. *Arch. Surg.* 1956;**72**:495–9.

84. Vincent JM, Morrison ID, Armstrong P, Reznek RH. Com-

puted tomography of diffuse, non-metastatic enlargement of the adrenal glands in patients with malignant disease. *Clin. Radiol.* 1994;**49**:456–60.

85. Fink DW, Wurtzebach LR. Symptomatic myelolipoma of the adrenal. Report of a case with computed tomographic evaluation. *Radiology* 1980;**134**:451–2.

86. Pagana TJ, Karasick SJ, Karasick D, Stahlgren LH. Myelolipoma of the adrenal gland. *Am. J. Surg.* 1981;**141**:282–5.

87. Musante F, Derchi LE, Zappasodi F *et al.* Myelolipoma of the adrenal gland: sonographic and CT features. *Am. J. Roentgenol.* 1988;**151**:961–4.

Phaeochromocytoma

PIERRE-MARC G. BOULOUX AND MAZIN FAKEEH

Introduction

Catecholamine-secreting tumours originating in the adrenal medulla are called phaeochromocytoma; those arising in extra-adrenal tissues, notably ganglia and chromaffin remnants, are termed paragangliomas. The tumours are rare, and account for < 0.1% of causes of hypertension. Catecholamine-secreting tumours occur with equal frequency in both sexes and at any age from childhood to the seventies, though most often in the third and fourth decade. The dominant secretory products of the tumours are the catecholamines (noradrenaline, adrenaline, dopamine, L-dihydroxyphenylalanine (L-dopa)) and a variety of biologically active neuropeptides. Their constant or episodic secretion is responsible for the protean and often alarming manifestations of the disease. Most phaeochromocytomas are found at post mortem, and symptoms may antedate the diagnosis by many years [1].

Aetiology

Tumours are sporadic in 90% of cases, and inherited in 10%. Between 10 and 12% of tumours are malignant. Inherited tumours may be bilateral and may originate from hyperplastic adrenal medullary tissue. A number of syndromes, notably the multiple endocrine neoplasia (MEN) type 2a and 2b and the neurocristopathic disorders, are associated with these tumours. The latter include the von Hippel–Lindau and Sturge–Weber syndromes, and neurofibromatosis type 1 (NF-1). The latter is a genetically dominantly inherited disorder affecting approximately one in 3500 individuals, the molecular biology of which has been recently elucidated. The NF-1 gene encodes a member of the GTPase activating peptide (GAP) family of ras regulatory proteins. The GAP-related domain of the NF-1 encoded protein (neurofibromin) can stimulate the GTPase activity of p21 ras in vitro, suggesting that neurofibromin normally acts as a ras-dependent signal transduction pathway. NF-1 is likely to be a tumour-suppressor gene. Phaeochromocytoma in MEN-2a is associated with hyperparathyroidism and medullary carcinoma of the thyroid. When associated with a marfanoid habitus, intestinal ganglioneuromatosis, thickened corneal nerves and mucosal neuromas the term MEN-2b is used. These are both autosomal dominant conditions.

The molecular basis of phaeochromocytoma has recently been elucidated with the demonstration of ret proto-oncogene mutations within tumours. ret is 80 kb long and encodes a putative tyrosine kinase receptor. Its endogenous ligand may be the recently characterized glial cell line-derived neurotrophic factor (GDNF). Its extracellular calcium-binding domain is similar to that of cadherins, with a cysteine-rich region proximal to the transmembrane domain. Patients with MEN-2a have germline mutations in these cysteines which probably represent the first example of a dominant effect initiating an oncogenic mechanism in man. Adrenomedullary hyperplasia appears to be an invariable precursor of phaeochromocytomas in MEN-2a and b. Whereas the gene for ret is on chromosome 10, it is evident that mutations in critical loci on chromosome 17 (NF-1) and 3 (von Hippel–Lindau, see Chapter 72) may also lead to tumourous transformation of the adrenal medulla.

Presentation

Sustained hypertension resistant to conventional treatment (particularly beta-blockade), hypertensive crises with malignant hypertension, hypertensive encephalopathy, and paroxysmal episodes or spells suggestive of seizure disorder, anxiety attacks or hyperventilation should lead to suspicion of the presence of a catecholamine-secreting tumour. In childhood, tumours are often bilateral, and may be associated with mottling of the skin, renal artery stenosis, and curiously polyuria and polydipsia. The hallmark of these tumours is however the 'crisis'.

Phaeochromocytoma crisis

The phaeochromocytoma crisis is the physiological consequence of abrupt catecholamine (or other biologically active neuropeptide) release from the tumour, and the subsequent stimulation of adrenoceptors throughout the body. Headache (80%), throbbing or constant when present may be frontal or occipital. Diaphoresis, palpitations, a feeling of apprehension, with discomfort in the chest or abdomen, and blanching/flushing, especially in the face, may also occur (Table 48.1). Blood pressure may rise alarmingly, either with reflex bradycardia (noradrenaline secretion) or tachycardia (adrenaline secretion). Such crises may last from a few minutes to several hours. Factors that may trigger them include movements that may disturb the abdominal viscera, lifting, straining and bending. More often however, crises occur without any obvious precipitant. The precise mechanism of catecholamine release is unknown, but is most likely due to niduses of infarction within the tumour.

Hypertension may therefore be truly paroxysmal (25–40% cases) or constant. It is usually severe and occasionally malignant with retinopathy, left ventricular hypertrophy, proteinuria and secondary aldosteronism. Since the centrally acting α_2- agonist clonidine depresses blood pressure in patients with phaeochromocytoma, it seems likely that neurogenic mechanisms may also be operating in maintaining the elevated blood pressure.

In addition to the secretion of the catecholamines noradrenaline, adrenaline and dopamine, phaeochromocytomas can also secrete L-dopa, and many neuropeptides, many of which are biologically active, and may contribute to the protean manifestations of these tumours. These include enkephalins, vasoactive intestinal polypeptide (VIP), calcitonin gene-related peptide (CGRP), endothelin, renin, adrenocorticotrophic hormone (ACTH), and neuropeptide Y (Table 48.2). Chromogranin A, a component

of the secretory vesicle, is usually co-secreted with catecholamines, and its prolonged half-life, in contrast to the catecholamines themselves ($t_{1/2}$ 90 seconds), has led to its use in the diagnosis of phaeochromocytomas.

Other distinctive features of phaeochromocytoma include orthostatic hypotension (reduced circulating volume together with down-regulation of alpha receptors), shock, chest pain with angina pectoris, heart failure (occasional dilated cardiomyopathy), neurogenic pulmonary oedema, sweating, heat intolerance, weight loss, carbohydrate intolerance, hypercalcaemia, increased haematocrit and constipation (occasionally mimicking pseudo-obstruction).

Drug-induced crises are also encountered (Table 48.3). Drugs that may precipitate a crisis include propranolol, naloxone, opiates, histamine, corticotrophin, saralasin, glucagon, metoclopramide, droperidol and pancuronium and radiographic contrast media.

Table 48.1 Clinical features of phaeochromocytoma

Feature	Occurrence (%)
Hypertension (paroxysmal or constant)	95
Headache	80
Palpitations/tachycardia	64
Excessive perspiration	64
Anxiety, perspiration	28
Tremor	28
Pallor	25
Chest or abdominal pains	18
Nausea, vomiting	15
Malaise	10
Weight loss	<5
Postural hypotension	<5
Hypertensive retinopathy (grade IV)	<25

Table 48.2 Non-catecholamine phaeochromocytoma secretory products

Corticotrophin
Melanocyte-stimulating hormone
Endorphins
Enkephalins
Somatostatin
Vasoactive intestinal peptide (VIP)
Insulin
Calcitonin
Cholecystokinin
Parathormone-related protein
Neurone specific enolase
Vasopressin
Human growth hormone-releasing hormone (hGHRH)
Substance P
Motilin
Galanin
Neuropeptide Y

Table 48.3 Drugs capable of inducing a phaeochromocytoma crisis

Propranolol
Naloxone
Metoclopramide
Glucagon
Tyramine
Histamine
Guanethidine
Saralasin
Cytotoxic drugs
Tricyclic antidepressants
Phenothiazines
Corticotrophin

Pathological features

Lesions are most often solitary, usually less than 10 cm, and the cut surface usually shows areas of haemorrhage and necrosis. Microscopically the tumour is composed of large pleomorphic chromaffin cells. About 10% of tumours are malignant, as evidenced by local invasion or metastases. Familial tumours are usually multinodular (reflecting their multicentric origin). Aneuploidy of tumours reflect potential malignant behaviour. Extra-adrenal lesions (paragangliomas) occur in and about the sympathetic ganglia in locations that parallel the anatomical distribution of extra-adrenal chromaffin tissue. Most are intra-abdominal, but they may occur in the posterior mediastinum, within the heart or pericardium, and in the cervical region. They have a greater tendency to display malignant behaviour. With the exception of tumours arising from the organs of Zuckerkandl (situated on the side of the abdominal aorta), which may secrete both noradrenaline and adrenaline, most paragangliomas secrete noradrenaline only. Within the tumours, feedback inhibition of tyrosine hydroxylase enzyme by noradrenaline may be defective; subsequent high synthetic rate of catecholamines with faulty storage within the chromaffin granules results in their markedly increased turnover rate.

Small tumours are generally intra-adrenal and predominantly adrenaline secreting. Symptoms of hypermetabolism and glucose intolerance may predominate with these tumours. The larger tumours tend to be predominantly noradrenaline secreting, a consequence of direct vascular supply and the absence of high local concentrations of cortisol, required for the induction of phenylethanolamine-*N*-methyl transferase (PNMT) (and thus methylation of noradrenaline into adrenaline).

Tumour size correlates inversely with the ratio of free catecholamines to catecholamine metabolites in urine. Thus small tumours have a relatively low metabolic conversion of catecholamines to their metabolites,with, as a consequence, a relatively higher amount of urinary free catecholamines. Conversely large tumours have a high metabolite/free catecholamine ratio.

Diagnostic tests

Urinary measurements

The diagnosis depends first and foremost on clinical suspicion, and subsequently on the demonstration of inappropriately high levels of either circulating or urinary free catecholamines or their metabolites in a hypertensive or symptomatic patient [2]. A large number of conditions

Table 48.4 Differential diagnosis of phaeochromocytoma

Hyperadrenergic essential
hypertension (pseudophaeochromocytoma)
Anxiety attacks
Hyperventilation
Thyrotoxicosis
Monoamine oxidase (MAO) inhibitors
Clonidine withdrawal
Alcohol withdrawal
Subarachnoid haemorrhage
Excess caffeine intake
Acute intermittent porphyria
Tabetic crises
Lead poisoning

can mimic phaeochromocytoma, and these must be borne in mind (Table 48.4). Until recently, diagnosis rested on the demonstration of elevated urinary monodeaminated and catecholamine 'o' methyl transferase (COMT) methylated metabolites vanillyl mandelic acid (VMA) and/or metanephrines (normetadrenaline and metadrenaline) determined in acidified urine by colorimetric assays. The sensitivity of metanephrine measurement is around 80–84%, and that of VMA nearer 65%. Because of the poor sensitivity and specificity of urinary catecholamine metabolites, the measurement of urinary free catecholamines is now favoured, usually measured in acidified urine by high-performance liquid chromatography with electrochemical detection (HPLC-ECD). In a symptomatic patient, sensitivity approaches 100%. The high levels of urinary free catecholamines usually mean that assay sensitivity is not a problem. Although 24-hour samples are conventionally analysed, shorter collection times (e.g. nocturnal collection, 1-hour samples, or spot urine samples) may also enable diagnosis. Measurement of increased urinary dopamine and homovanillic acid may indicate the presence of a malignant lesion.

The usual upper limit of normal for VMA is 35 μmol/day (7 mg/day), and for metanephrines 5 μmol/day (1 mg/day).

The usual normal range for a 24-hour urinary-free noradrenaline is < 675 nmol/day, adrenaline < 275 nmol/day. Urinary dopamine is dependent on salt intake and is of little diagnostic value.

Plasma catecholamine measurement

Plasma catecholamine estimations have been used less commonly because of technical difficulties in their measurement.

Levels should be measured under carefully controlled conditions, with the subject supine having been cannulated 30 minutes before sampling. Blood is drawn into a lithium heparin tube, immediately cold spun, and the plasma stored at –70°C until assay. With HPLC-ECD, the catecholamines are adsorbed onto acidified alumina under alkaline conditions after sample spiking with a known amount of the internal standard dihydroxybenzylamine (DHBA). Back extraction of the catecholamines is usually with 0.5 mol phosphoric acid. An aliquot of the acid extract is then loaded onto a 3μ ODS (octa-deca silane) reversed phase column, and chromatographed. The catecholamines are measured by electrochemical detection, and the plasma concentration computed after correction for recovery of DHBA. Noradrenaline measurement does not pose a problem with sensitivity, but the detection limits with both colorimetric and amperometric detection is around 80 pmol for adrenaline, the coefficient of variation at this range being in the order of 15%. Small phaeochromocytomas may secrete adrenaline only, but levels generally exceed 0.8 nmol/l, when assay sensitivity is not limiting. Normal supine noradrenaline is 0.3–2.8 nmol/l and adrenaline 0.17–0.52 nmol/l.

Plasma catecholamines are invariably well outside the normal range when sampled during a phaeochromocytoma crisis. This is the one situation when sensitivity and specificity are greatest. Further, the presence of normal plasma catecholamines in a hypertensive patient effectively rules out a catecholamine-secreting tumour as the cause of hypertension.

Suppressive tests

Since anxiety may elevate particularly circulating adrenaline into a grey zone, patients with adrenaline levels of 0.8–2.0 nmol/l often pose a diagnostic problem. A suppressive test with pentolinium (2.5 mg i.v. at time 0, and plasma catecholamines at 0 and 10 minutes) may distinguish between autonomous (i.e. tumorous = non-suppression) and physiological (stress-mediated) elevation (suppression into the low normal range) of catecholamines. The centrally active α_2-adrenergic agonist clonidine (200 μg orally at time 0, and plasma catecholamines sampled at time 0, 120 and 180 min) has also been used in these instances, non-suppression being suggestive of a tumour [3]. The clonidine suppression test may increase the sensitivity and specificity of plasma catecholamine measurement. It has been reported to have a 97% sensitivity with only a 1.5% false-positive rate in patients with essential hypertension. It may also be used as part of an overnight urinary catecholamine test, when non-suppression of urinary catecholamines is indicative of phaeochromocytoma.

Provocative tests

Provocative tests are rarely employed now and were designed to make the diagnosis in patients with paroxysmal symptoms who were normotensive at the time of investigation. Histamine (50 μg) and tyramine (1 mg) given intravenously will trigger an exaggerated pressor response associated with a sharp rise in plasma catecholamines in patients with phaeochromocytoma compared with controls. Glucagon (1 mg i.v.), which acts directly on tumour tissue (which in contrast to the normal adrenal medulla bears its receptor), has the greatest sensitivity and specificity. Its role can now only be justified in situations where symptomatology is genuinely paroxysmal, and there is strong clinical suspicion of a lesion being present, as, for example, in a MEN syndrome. The test should only be performed under these circumstances following alpha- and beta-blockade, using plasma catecholamines as the response parameter.

Adrenolytic tests

A sharp fall in blood pressure following i.v. injection of the mixed α_1- and α_2-antagonist phentolamine may suggest the diagnosis. The usual initial test dose is 0.5 mg. In the absence of a dramatic fall in blood pressure, the remaining 4.5 mg is given as an i.v. bolus. The test is considered positive if the fall in systolic blood pressure exceeds 35 mmHg and the diastolic 25 mmHg, beginning within 3 minutes of the i.v. bolus.

Chromogranin A measurement

Of the many neuropeptides that are co-stored and co-secreted with catecholamines, chromogranin A and B and neuropeptide Y have been used in diagnosis [4]. Chromogranin A (CgA) is the major soluble protein in the core of chromaffin vesicles, and may play a role in neurosecretory protein trafficking. Because of its longer plasma half-life, CgA has been used in the diagnosis of phaeochromocytoma, with a reported sensitivity of 83% and specificity of 96%. Plasma CgA is a predictor of tumour size and overall catecholamine production. It has also been used (83% specificity and 100% sensitivity) in the detection of familial lesions in the von Hippel–Lindau syndrome. Chromogranin A measurements are unreliable when severe renal impairment is present.

Platelet catecholamines

Platelet catecholamine concentrations may be used to distinguish phaeochromocytoma from non-phaeochromocytoma because platelet catecholamine content may be less susceptible to rapid changes than plasma catecholamine levels. This test is not however in widespread use.

Fine needle aspiration

Although reported as a sensitive and specific test, fine-needle aspiration is potentially hazardous.

Imaging of tumours

Biochemical evidence of a phaeochromocytoma should be followed by imaging for tumour localization [5]. Computed tomography (CT) scanning and magnetic resonance imaging (MRI) have largely superseded the older techniques of intravenous urography and arteriography (Fig. 48.1). CT scanning (93% sensitivity) lacks tissue specificity, being unable to distinguish between phaeochromocytoma, adrenal adenomas and myelolipomas. CT/MRI imaging of the adrenals should initially be performed however (see Chapter 47). Most adrenal tumours will fall well within the limit of resolution of both methods (0.5–1.0 cm), MRI classically yielding a bright, hyperintense signal on the T_2 setting with almost 100% sensitivity. MRI shows higher specificity because of better tissue characterization, further enhanced by the use of gadolinium. The newer technique of chemical shift fast low-angle shot MRI may allow discrimination between adrenocortical adenomas, metastatic tumours and phaeochromocytoma. Intravenous contrast should not be given to the naive patient without prior full alpha-blockade with phenoxybenzamine (20 mg tds orally) and beta-blockade (40 mg tds propranolol), given in that order. As an added precaution, i.v. phenoxybenzamine 0.5 mg/kg given in 100 ml 5% dextrose over 4 hours should be infused i.v. for 2–3 consecutive days prior to any invasive procedure. 90% of catecholamine-secreting tumours are adrenal and will be visualized by the above methods. The remainder, so called paragangliomas, can occur anywhere within the sympathetic chain. They may be branchiomeric (intercarotid, jugulotympanic, orbital, laryngeal, aortico-pulmonary, coronary, pulmonary), intravagal, aortico-sympathetic (neck, thoracic, abdominal) or visceral autonomic (atria of heart, urinary bladder, liver hilum, mesenteric vessels). When the adrenal CT/MRI scan is normal, and there is strong biochemical evidence of a catecholamine-secreting lesion, MRI scanning of the rest of the body should be performed. The technique is particularly useful in demonstrating intracardiac phaeochromocytomas.

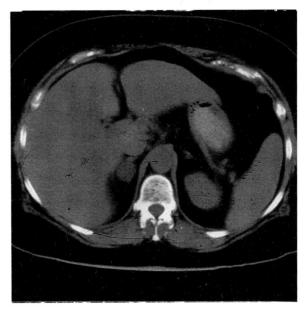

(a)

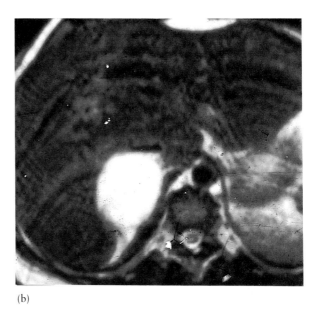

(b)

Fig. 48.1 (a) CT of a right adrenal phaeochromocytoma found incidentally. (b) MRI T_2-weighted image of a right adrenal phaeochromocytoma.

^{123}I-MIBG scanning and venous sampling

Where there is unequivocal biochemical evidence of a catecholamine-secreting tumour, but a negative CT/MRI scan, two additional approaches are helpful. Metaiodobenzylguanidine (^{123}I-MIBG) scanning, using the guanethidine-like chromaffin-seeking compound may visualize the lesion in up to 75% of tumours, enabling scanning of the whole body. When used for preoperative localization ^{123}I-MIBG has a sensitivity of 85–90% and

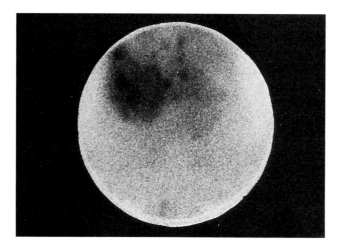

Fig. 48.2 ^{123}I-MIBG scan of upper abdomen in a patient harbouring metastatic phaeochromocytoma lesions in the liver.

a specificity of more than 95%. ^{123}I-MIBG produces better images than ^{131}I-MIBG because of its physical properties, enabling performance of single-photon emission tomography. MIBG scanning is particularly useful for detection of metastatic disease (Fig. 48.2). Tricyclic antidepressants and labetalol may interfere with MIBG scanning giving false-negative results. Only tumours with abundant neuro-secretory granules take up MIBG. When a tumour cannot be adequately visualized by the above modalities, positron emission tomography performed after administration of either hydroxyephedrine (a radionuclide that concentrates in adrenergic nerve terminals) or 2-[^{18}F]-fluoro-2-deoxy-D-glucose (the accumulation of which is an index of tumour activity) may aid in correct localization of tumours.

Alternatively, venous sampling may be performed. The latter will provide absolute confirmation that a suspicious mass is truly the source of catecholamine secretion, but should not be performed without the prior absence of alpha- and beta-blockade.

Venous sampling is also useful to confirm or refute the diagnosis of bilateral adrenal phaeochromocytomas when a lesion is seen on each side on imaging. Usually the plasma adrenaline : noradrenaline ratio in the adrenal venous effluent is between 4 and 10 under 'basal' conditions. The reversal of this ratio is therefore strongly suggestive of adrenomedullary pathology.

Treatment of phaeochromocytoma

The treatment of phaeochromocytoma is primarily by surgical extirpation, undertaken only after adequate alpha- and beta-blockade (see above). Successful tumour excision is associated with normalization of blood

pressure in 75% of patients, and disappearance of the crises [6]. Some 10% of tumours are malignant at the time of presentation, as evidenced by metastatic lesions within lymph nodes, lungs or bones, and liver. Metastases may be visualized by ^{123}I-MIBG scanning, and will usually be confirmed by elevated free urinary catecholamine post-primary excision, but non-secretory metastases have been described.

Surgical therapy

Blood pressure should be normalized for at least 2 weeks prior to surgery, and all patients should have central venous pressure monitoring and intra-arterial blood pressure monitoring during anaesthesia and surgery. Meperidine and the short-acting barbiturates are suitable for pre-anaesthetic preparation. Just before induction, 5 mg i.v. phentolamine is given to prevent a pressor crisis. Thiopentone and succinyl choline are recommended for induction, and nitrous oxide and meperidine or fentanyl as anaesthetic agents. The abdomen is opened via a vertical or horizontal incision, enabling the surgeon to explore the entire abdomen. The venous drainage of any mass should be clamped before any manipulation is undertaken. Sodium nitroprusside, lignocaine, plasma expanders, intravenous phentolamine and propranolol should be available in the event of sudden changes in blood pressure or cardiac rhythm. As successful tumour extirpation is usually followed by hypotension, it is as well to transfuse patients pre-operatively if the haematocrit has fallen significantly with adrenoceptor blockade.

Medical therapy of malignant tumours

In contrast to the 5-year survival rate of 96% for patients with benign lesions, malignant phaeochromocytoma carries a 44% survival rate. In the latter case, combined alpha- and beta-blockade may prove inadequate, and the tyrosine hydroxylase inhibitor α-methylparatyrosine in doses of 1–2 g/day may control symptoms. Symptoms of Parkinsonism have been described in some cases with this drug. The advent of ^{131}I-MIBG therapy for malignant tumours holds promise. In our experience, therapy doses of 5550 MBq (150 mCi) given at intervals (to a maximum dose of 33750 MBq (900 mCi) has led to regression of metastatic deposits and the slow normalization of plasma catecholamine levels. Cytotoxic therapy has also been used in disseminated lesions; although transient, often dramatic, results have been obtained with cyclophosphamide, vincristine and dacarbazine, longer term results are generally disappointing [7].

Long-term phaeochromocytoma follow-up

Because the incidence of malignancy in phaeochromocytoma may be underestimated, it is wise to perform annual urinary free catecholamines in all patients for at least 5 years after surgical excision. The reappearance of elevated urinary free catecholamines should then prompt re-investigation, with a further MIBG scan.

References

1. Stein PP, Black HR. A simplified approach to phaeochromocytoma. A review of the literature and report of one institution's experience. *Medicine (Baltimore)* 1991;70:46–66.
2. Sheps GS, Jiang N-D, Klee GG. Diagnostic evaluation of phaeochromocytoma. *Endocrinol. Metab. Clin. North Am.* 1988;17:397–415.
3. Sjoberg RJ, Simcic KJ, Kidd GS. The clonidine suppression test for phaeochromocytoma. A review of its utility and pitfalls. *Arch. Intern. Med.*1992;152:1193–7.
4. Hsiao RJ, Parmer RJ, Takiyuddin MA, O'Connor DT. Chromogranin A storage and secretion: sensitivity and specificity for the diagnosis of phaeochromocytoma. *Medicine (Baltimore)* 1991;70:33–45.
5. Francis IR, Gross MD, Shapiro B, Korobkin M, Quint LE. Integrated imaging of adrenal disease. *Radiology* 1992;184:1–13.
6. Dequattro V, Myers M, Campese VM. Phaeochromocytoma: diagnosis and therapy. In DeGroot L. (ed.) *Endocrinology.* Philadelphia: W.B. Saunders, 1989:1780–97.
7. Averbuch SD, Steakley CS, Young RC *et al.* Malignant phaeochromocytomas: effective treatment with a combination of cyclophosphamide, vincristine and dacarbazine. *Ann. Intern. Med.* 1988;109:267–71.

Neuroblastoma

BRUNO DE BERNARDI, CLAUDIA MILANACCIO
AND MAURO OCCHI

Introduction

The term neuroblastoma refers to a group of malignant tumours of early childhood originating from cells of the primitive autonomic nervous system. Over 80% of patients with neuroblastoma secrete abnormal amounts of sympathetic amines, mainly adrenaline and noradrenaline, indicating that the tumour preferentially affects the sympathetic component of the autonomic nervous system.

The overall incidence in children up to 15 years of age is between 8 and 10 per million per year. It accounts for approximately 10% of all paediatric malignancies, ranking third in frequency after acute leukaemias and tumours of the central nervous system. It is, however, the most frequent tumour of the first 5 years of life with a median age at diagnosis close to 2 years. In addition more than a half of the tumours diagnosed in the neonatal period are neuroblastomas [1].

Remarkable progress has been made in the last two decades in the understanding of the oncogenesis and biological characteristics of this tumour [2]. Unfortunately this progress has so far only led to marginal improvements in therapy.

From a clinical viewpoint, neuroblastoma has a number of peculiarities, making it one of the most intriguing of human cancers; for example, its prognosis is much better in infants compared to older children irrespective of disease extension and more than half the children present with widespread disease. Also, and especially in the youngest of patients, the disease may regress spontaneously despite dissemination. Unfortunately, unlike other childhood tumours, the cure rate has not been significantly improved by modern multimodal approaches.

The combination of a high metastatic rate at presentation and a poor prognosis make neuroblastoma a commonly frustrating experience for paediatric oncologists. This has provided the stimulus for both basic and clinical research focused on treatment of this tumour. Thus, recent progress has been made by the adoption by a number of international centres of common criteria for diagnosis and treatment. This international agreement has been facilitated by the Forbeck Foundation leading to the formulation of the International Neuroblastoma Staging System (INSS) [3].

There are still a number of important unanswered questions and clinicians are actively pursuing further objectives in neuroblastoma treatment. In particular it is hoped that biochemical or radiological screening may lead to earlier diagnosis, and also that reliable risk factors can be identified. More effective and specific therapies are required and methods to detect minimal residual disease are being evaluated.

Clinical presentation

Two-thirds of neuroblastomas present with an abdominal mass, which may be either centrally or laterally located. The tumour arises from the diversity of sympathetic tissue within the abdomen such as the adrenal medulla and paravertebral ganglia (Figs 49.1 and 49.2). Symptoms depend on the organs compressed by the tumour. When palpable, the tumour is appreciated as a hard, fixed, irregular, non-tender mass.

In 20% of cases the tumour arises in the lateral posterior mediastinum. This may be asymptomatic and discovered on a routine chest X-ray or respiratory symptoms may result. The neck and pelvis are primary tumour sites in no more than 2–5% of patients. In the former case the tumour usually mimics enlarged lymph nodes and histological confirmation of a neuroblastoma is revealed unexpectedly. Tumours arising from the pelvis may present with bowel and/or bladder dysfunction.

More than half the patients have disseminated disease at the time of diagnosis, with the skeleton and bone marrow being most often infiltrated by the tumour. Disease spread is often associated with non-specific symptoms such as pallor, anorexia and subtle changes in personality. This period may precede the detection of a tumour mass by several weeks or months or even remain the only evidence of the disease. This explains why in some cases there is a significant delay between the initial presentation and confirmation of the diagnosis. This is especially so when the primary tumour mass remains small and occurs in such sites as the upper retroperitoneum which is difficult to detect by clinical examination.

The connection existing between the sympathetic nervous system and the spinal cord is thought to influence the propensity of neuroblastomas to infiltrate the intervertebral foramina (Fig. 49.3). While this is detected in magnetic resonance imaging (MRI) in approximately one-third of patients, only 7–10% have symptomatic spinal cord compression. Early detection of this phenomenon is essential because the tumour may rapidly compromise the cord and thus cause irreversible paraplegia. Unfortunately, the symptoms of spinal cord compression are difficult to detect in small children and particular attention should be paid to examining for limb hypotonia.

In 1–2% of cases, neuroblastoma presents with myoclonic encephalopathy (Fig. 49.4). The typical clinical

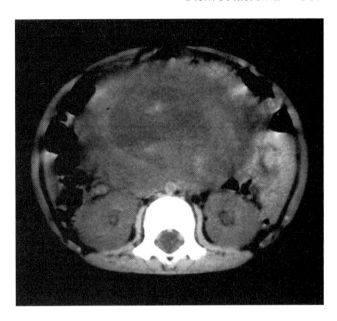

Fig. 49.2 CT scan, axial view, showing a large inhomogeneous retroperitoneal mass encasing the aorta, coeliac axis and mesenteric vessels.

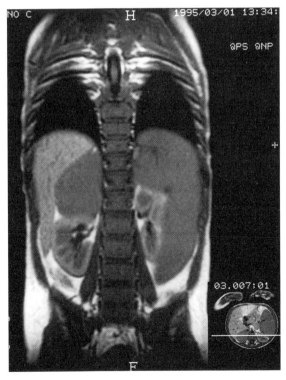

Fig. 49.1 MRI, T₁-weighted image showing a right-sided homogeneous suprarenal neuroblastoma. There is an enormous splenomegaly secondary to portal vein thrombosis.

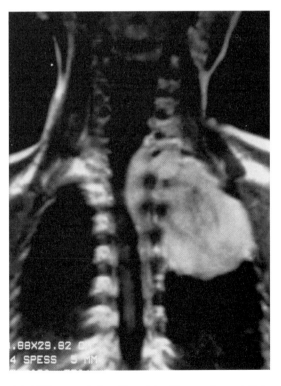

Fig. 49.3 MRI, coronal view; T₁-weighted image after gadolinium administration. A large mass occupies the apical region of the left hemithorax and entering the spinal canal between the levels of the D1 and D5 foramina. The patient was neurologically asymptomatic.

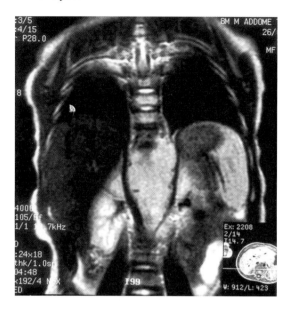

Fig. 49.4 MRI, coronal view, T_1-weighted image showing a fusiform thoraco-abdominal neuroblastoma in a 1-year-old infant with myoclonic encephalopathy.

signs include ataxia, myoclonic movements and erratic nystagmus ('dancing eyes' and 'dancing feet' syndrome). These symptoms may even precede the detection of a tumour mass and are thought to be due to autoimmune mechanisms involving the cerebellum and reticular system.

An even rarer presentation of neuroblastoma is with watery diarrhoea due to production by the tumour of vasoactive intestinal polypeptide (VIP). These symptoms usually regress after surgical resection of the tumour or after the administration of chemotherapy.

Diagnosis and diagnostic work-up

A noteworthy development in the study of this tumour has been the recent adoption by the major cooperative groups of common criteria to diagnose the disease, and to evaluate its extension and response to therapy. This international agreement has been facilitated by the Forbeck Foundation and the formulation of the (INSS) [3]. According to this system, the diagnosis of neuroblastoma requires histological confirmation. This is preferentially performed on tumour tissue derived by surgical intervention. However, especially in severely compromised patients, a Tru-cut or fine-needle aspiration cytology may provide adequate amounts of tissue. Although undifferentiated tumours may be confused with other entities of the small blue-cell tumour family (rhabdomyosarcoma, lymphoma, Ewing's sarcoma, peripheral neuroepithelioma, etc.), the pathologist may

be helped by a number of ancillary techniques, such as immunohistochemistry, electron microscopy and molecular biological studies. In the few cases in which histology cannot be obtained, the diagnosis may be based on the combination of unequivocal bone marrow infiltration (classical 'pseudorosettes' in the aspirates and/or tumour cell aggregates should be identified) and abnormal catecholamine metabolite excretion (Table 49.1). Neuroblastoma tissue can synthesize and catabolize catecholamines, resulting in increased urinary excretion of homovanillic acid (HVA), the main metabolite of dopamine, and vanillyl mandelic acid (VMA), the main metabolite of epinephrine and norepinephrine. The measurement of urinary VMA and HVA, and more recently, dopamine, detects at least 90% of patients with neuroblastoma.

A careful work-up at diagnosis aiming to define the precise disease extension is mandatory to plan proper therapy. The INSS provides clear guidelines for this (Table 49.2). Study of primary tumour requires MRI or computed tomography (CT) scan to evaluate the relationship with the vasculature and any intraspinal extension. Special attention is to be paid to the search for bone marrow infiltration and skeletal involvement. Proper marrow evaluation should include morphological, histological and immunocytological studies of marrow aspirates and trephine biopsies from both posterior iliac crests. Bone involvement will be best documented with ^{131}I and/or ^{125}I metaiodobenzylguanidine (MIBG) scintigraphy. A [99m]technetium scan, however, may detect bone lesions missed by MIBG and is mandatory in the few patients with negative MIBG scan.

The serum assay of some biochemical tumour markers, such as lactate dehydrogenase (LDH), ferritin, neurone-specific enolase, chromogranin A and GD2 ganglioside, is helpful in that these data correlate with tumour aggressiveness and response to therapy.

On the basis of quality of initial surgery and of results of diagnostic work-up, the patient is assigned a stage number from 1 to 4 according to INSS criteria (Table 49.3). Stages 1–2 define a localized tumour, stage 3 a

Table 49.1 Diagnosis of neuroblastoma

Established if:
unequivocal pathological diagnosis is made from tumour tissue by light microscopy (with or without immunohistology, electron microscopy, increased urine or serum catecholamines or metabolites)

or if:
bone marrow aspirate or trephine biopsy contains unequivocal tumour cells (e.g. syncytia or immunocytologically positive clumps of cells) and increased urine or serum catecholamines or metabolites

Table 49.2 Assessment of extent of disease

Tumour site	Recommended tests
Primary tumour	CT and/or MRI scan, MIBG scan
Metastatic sites	
Bone marrow	Bilateral posterior iliac crest marrow aspirates and trephine (core) bone marrow biopsies required to exclude marrow involvement. A single positive site documents marrow involvement. Core biopsies must contain at least 1 cm of marrow (excluding cartilage) to be considered adequate
Bone	MIBG scan; ^{99m}Tc scan required if MIBG scan negative, and plain radiographs of positive lesions are recommended
Lymph nodes	Clinical examination (palpable nodes), confirmed histologically. CT scan for non-palpable nodes (3D measurements)
Abdomen/liver	CT and/or MRI scan
Chest	Anteroposterior and lateral chest radiographs. CT/MRI necessary if chest radiograph positive, or if abdominal mass/nodes extend into chest

CT, computed tomography; MIBG, metaiodobenzylguanidine; MRI, magnetic resonance imaging.

Table 49.3 International Neuroblastoma Staging System (INSS)

Stage	Definition
1	Localized tumour with complete gross excision, with or without microscopic residual disease; representative ipsilateral lymph nodes negative for tumour microscopically (nodes attached to and removed with the primary tumour may be positive)
2A	Localized tumour with incomplete gross excision; representative ipsilateral non-adherent lymph nodes negative for tumour microscopically
2B	Localized tumour with or without complete gross excision, with ipsilateral non-adherent lymph nodes positive for tumour. Enlarged contralateral lymph nodes must be negative microscopically
3	Unresectable unilateral tumour infiltrating across the midline, with or without regional lymph node involvement; or localized unilateral tumour with contralateral regional lymph node involvement; or midline tumour with bilateral extension by infiltration (unresectable) or by lymph node involvement
4	Any primary tumour with dissemination to distant lymph nodes, bone, bone marrow, liver, skin and/or other organs (except as defined for stage 4s)
4s	Localized primary tumour (as defined for stages 1, 2A or 2B), with dissemination limited to skin, liver, and/or bone marrow (limited to infants < 1 year of age)

Table 49.4 Stage distribution of 195 children with neuroblastoma according to the International Neuroblastoma Staging System (INSS) (from the Italian Neuroblastoma Registry)

INSS stage	Patients	
	Number	%
1	29	15
2A	9	5
2B	18	9
3	39	20
4	87	45
4s	13	6
Total	195	100

tumour that infiltrates across the midline and/or invades the contralateral nodes, stage 4 the disease that has spread to distant sites, and stage 4s a special entity that affects infants and tends to regress spontaneously despite dissemination to liver, skin and bone marrow (in any combination). The proportion of patients for each INSS stage in the recent Italian experience is depicted in Table 49.4 (unpublished data).

Therapy

The management of children with neuroblastoma remains one of the most important challenges in paediatric oncology. It currently depends on age and disease extension. However, biological characteristics will probably have a growing role in defining subgroups of patients requiring specific treatments.

Surgery is most effective in low stages, while chemotherapy followed by resection of primary tumour is the most common strategy for advanced stages. Radiation therapy appears useless in stages 1–2 and of undefined value in advanced stages. Stage 4s does not require therapy unless life-threatening progression occurs.

Localized operable disease (INSS stage 1 and 2)

Localized operable disease involves about 20% of neuroblastomas, and includes patients with macroscopically resected tumour (stage 1) and tumour incompletely resected without or with infiltration of regional lymph nodes (stages 2A and 2B, respectively), but no midline infiltration. The outcome for these patients is favourable, with 5-year survival above 80% with little or no postoperative chemotherapy. However, between 15 and 20% do relapse and thus require aggressive therapy to be saved [4]. The characteristics associated with higher risk of relapse are poorly known. In addition, it is not

Confirming the diagnosis

Almost all patients with primary hyperaldosteronism have subnormal supine and erect PRA over a 4-hour upright period, and corresponding high plasma aldosterone concentrations (PAC) (Fig. 50.1). Ideally these should be measured two weeks off antihypertensive therapy, which itself modulates the renin–angiotensin–aldosterone system. Because of severe hypertension, however, this may not always be possible; prazosin interferes least with the renin–angiotensin–aldosterone axis and may be given. The physician should consult closely with an endocrinologist and the local laboratory for appropriate reference values, but in the authors institution a plasma aldosterone of > 550 pmol/l (radioimmunoassay) in the face of a concomitant supine/erect PRA of < 0.5 or < 1.5 ng angiotensin I/ml per hour respectively is probably diagnostic. Several workers argue that sensitivity is increased further if either 24-hour urinary aldosterone is measured or if the plasma PAC/PRA ratio is calculated. Again these will depend on the local assays and expertise available. If aldosterone levels are normal, then these should be repeated having restored serum potassium above 3.0 mmol/l, as hypokalaemia can suppress aldosterone secretion [3].

Failure of plasma aldosterone to suppress after an oral sodium load (2–3 g/day for 4 days) or following a saline

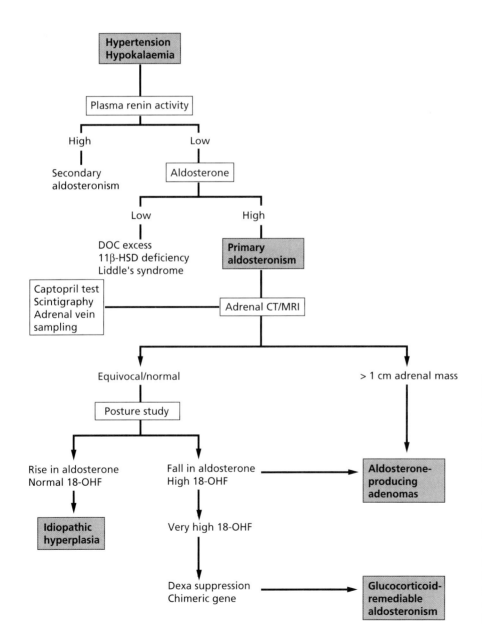

Fig. 50.1 Suggested flow chart for the investigation of a patient with hypertension and hypokalaemia. A sensible modification of this scheme is to measure plasma renin activity, aldosterone, cortisol and 18-hydroxycortisol (18-OHF) initially across the posture study (08.00h supine, 12.00h erect) on two separate occasions. Having confirmed the diagnosis of primary aldosteronism biochemically, adrenal computed tomography (CT) or magnetic resonance imaging (MRI) should be carried out. The captopril test, adrenal scintigraphy and adrenal vein sampling can be used as adjunct tests. DOC, deoxycorticosterone; HSD, hydroxysteroid dehydrogenase.

infusion (0.9% saline for 2 hours) have been used to confirm autonomy of secretion, but are not necessary in the majority of cases.

Distinction between the subtypes and localization

Because the treatment of APA, IHA and GRA vary, it is essential to distinguish them correctly. In general the clinical picture of patients with APA differs from that of patients with IHA because of more severe hypertension, more profound hypokalaemia, and higher plasma and urinary aldosterone levels but this in itself is insufficient to distinguish between the subgroups. Hormone studies, pharmacological tests, imaging techniques and sometimes catheter studies are used in the diagnostic differentiation of APA from IHA and GRA [3,5] (see Fig. 50.1).

Posture studies

Posture studies carried out over a 4-hour period are most helpful in distinguishing between APA and IHA and, when performed correctly, have an overall accuracy of 80–85% [7]. It takes advantage of the fact that in APA aldosterone secretion is sensitive to changes in ACTH, while in IHA aldosterone secretion is sensitive to changes in angiotensin II levels. Baseline plasma renin, aldosterone and cortisol are drawn at 08.00h. The patient is then ambulant for 4 hours after which the measurements are repeated. In patients with IHA, the postambulatory aldosterone level is higher than the baseline value (approximately 33%) due to stimulation from angiotensin II which increases with ambulation. In contrast, in patients with APA, the 4-hour postambulatory aldosterone level is the same or slightly lower than the baseline measurement due to the circadian decrease in ACTH levels. This diurnal decrease in ACTH levels is confirmed by a decrease in cortisol levels over the test period, but if the cortisol value at 12.00 h is higher than at 08.00 h then the test is not valid.

18-hydroxycortisol and -corticosterone

18-hydroxycortisol (18-OHF) is formed in the human adrenal cortex through 18-hydroxylation of circulating cortisol. 18-hydroxycorticosterone (18-OHB) is considered either the immediate precursor of aldosterone or a separate end-product formed after 18-hydroxylation of corticosterone. Both circulating and urinary 18-OHF and 18-OHB are found to be highest in GRA >> APA > IHA [8,9]. Indeed the best biochemical marker for GRA is an elevated plasma or urinary 18-OHF value, although most studies, but not all, do indicate some crossover in 18-OHF levels in patients with APA and IHA. The

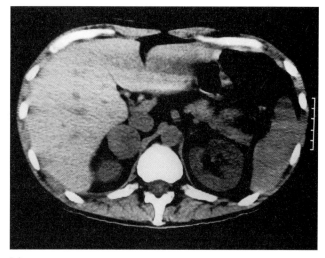

(a)

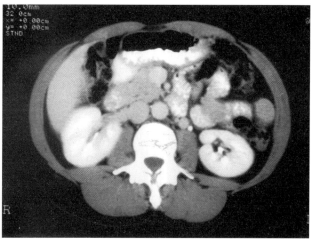

(b)

Fig. 50.2 Adrenal CT scans of two patients with primary aldosteronism showing: (a) a large 3 × 3 cm right adrenal adenoma, and (b) bilateral adrenal hyperplasia.

predictability of 18-OHF is similar to that of 18-OHB, but since the amount of 18-OHF excreted in the urine is far greater than 18-OHB, the former is perhaps a more suitable marker.

Captopril test

The captopril test is performed in the sitting position. Plasma aldosterone is measured basally and 60 minutes following the administration of the angiotensin-converting enzyme inhibitor, captopril. The inhibition of angiotensin II production results in a fall in plasma aldosterone in patients with IHA, but levels are unchanged in APA [3].

Radiological investigations

Radiological investigations are required to localize an adenoma preoperatively, and may be needed in difficult cases to differentiate APA from IHA. This can be accomplished by computed tomography (CT) scan of the adrenal gland, scintigraphy with radiolabelled iodocholesterol and adrenal vein sampling. However, because of the high incidence of non-functioning adrenal 'incidentalomas', it is essential that some form of biochemical confirmation of primary aldosteronism has been made prior to embarking on radiological studies.

Adrenal CT scanning

CT is a non-invasive procedure and is the initial step in localization with a sensitivity of > 85% for adenomas larger than 1 cm (Fig. 50.2). Magnetic resonance imaging (MRI) may be more sensitive for smaller adenomas. Patients who have adenomas > 3 cm in diameter should be suspected of having an aldosterone-producing carcinoma. Patients with IHA have either normal-appearing glands or changes consistent with bilateral nodular hyperplasia. As stated above, 2–8% of the population have small benign non-functioning adenomas, and the finding of a mass on CT/MRI is not necessarily synonymous with APA [10].

Adrenal scintigraphy with radiolabelled iodocholesterol

Adrenal imaging with iodocholesterol (^{131}I-6-β-iodomethyl-19-norcholesterol, NP-59) provides a non-invasive means of differentiating patients with APA from those with IHA and identifies the site of the adenoma when present. NP-59 accumulates rapidly in the adrenals, and scintigraphy is carried out 5 days after administration. Sensitivity and specificity is increased if the patient is given dexamethasone 1.0–1.5 mg/day for 6 days starting 24 hours prior to the administration of the isotope. Patients with APA concentrate radioactivity at the site of the tumour, whereas patients with IHA usually show diffuse uptake. Aldosterone-producing carcinomas show little or no radioactivity. The overall diagnostic accuracy of NP-59 scanning is approximately 72% [10].

Adrenal vein sampling

Bilateral adrenal venous sampling is still the most accurate test for localizing APAs. However, it is invasive, technically demanding and requires skill and experience. There is an appreciable incidence of complications, including venous thrombosis and extravasation of dye

leading to adrenal insufficiency. It is therefore only performed when hormonal studies, CT imaging and/or iodocholesterol scanning yield conflicting results. The normal adrenal venous aldosterone concentration is 200–600 ng/dl. In an APA the ratio of ipsilateral to contralateral aldosterone is usually greater than 10 : 1. The accuracy of catheter placement can be evaluated by obtaining simultaneous basal or ACTH-stimulated adrenal venous cortisol levels.

Treatment

Surgery

When a functional unilateral adrenal adenoma is confirmed, the treatment of choice is a unilateral adrenalectomy. Cure rates (defined as normotension and normokalaemia postoperatively) vary, but a review of 694 cases indicated a cure rate of 69%. In the case of a cure, potassium levels are normalized rapidly after surgery, blood pressure returns to normal within a few days in 50% of cases, but takes considerably longer (months) in others. In the future, laparoscopic adrenalectomy may replace open adrenalectomy for smaller tumours. Patients should be adequately prepared preoperatively (ideally for 6 weeks) with spironolactone or amiloride (see below) and the blood pressure response to these agents preoperatively has been used as a predictor of response to adrenalectomy. If the patient is not adequately blocked, there is the anaesthetic risk of hypokalaemia and hypertension, but perhaps more importantly of a mineralocorticoid deficiency state postoperatively. If preoperative medical therapy has been inadequate and the renin–angiotensin drive to aldosterone secretion from the 'normal' contralateral adrenal remains suppressed, there is a real risk of hyperkalaemia postoperatively. This may be exacerbated by spironolactone which has a long half-life and may still be effective for several days after discontinuation of the drug. Rarely these adenomas may secrete aldosterone and cortisol and for the same reasons glucocorticoid deficiency has also been reported postoperatively. Thus the pre- and postoperative management of these patients should involve careful liaison between the surgeon and endocrinologist.

Surgery is effective in less than 20% of cases of IHA and should therefore be avoided.

Medical therapy

Medical therapy is indicated in all patients pre-operatively and long-term for patients who are unsuitable surgical candidates or who have IHA or GRA. One of the first-line agents is the mineralocorticoid receptor antagonist, spironolactone. Doses are given initially as 100 mg/day, increasing as required to a maximum of 400 mg/day. This is usually extremely effective in correcting hypokalaemia, although as stated above it may take some time for blood pressure to fall to normal. Spironolactone, particularly in high doses inhibits testosterone biosynthesis and peripheral androgen action resulting in gynaecomastia (often painful), reduced libido and erectile impotence in males and menstrual irregularity in females. Other side-effects include nausea and abdominal pain. Amiloride can be used as a first-line agent or in patients intolerant of spironolactone. Doses starting at 10 mg/day often need to be increased to 30–40 mg/day. Side-effects are rare but include headache, fatigue and nausea. In the rare patient who is intolerant of spironolactone and amiloride, triamterene can be used in doses of 100–300 mg/day.

Patients with GRA should be treated with dexamethasone designed to suppress endogenous ACTH levels. Some patients with GRA are very sensitive to dexamethasone requiring only 0.5 mg/day, which is best given as a single dose at night. Higher doses may be required but careful monitoring of plasma potassium, aldosterone and blood pressure should be undertaken to prevent overtreatment.

Antihypertensive therapy is frequently required in addition to the above medications. Because intracellular calcium is an important second messenger in the synthesis and action of aldosterone, calcium antagonists such as nifedipine and verapamil have been used with good success. Aldosterone secretion in patients with IHA is extremely sensitive to circulating angiotensin II and perhaps the most effective antihypertensive in such patients are the angiotensin-converting enzyme (ACE) inhibitors.

Aetiology

Aldosterone-producing adenomas

The cause of APAs remains unknown. A familial basis for the condition has been described by some authors. Several putative factors have been excluded. McCune–Albright syndrome may result in adrenal adenomas (usually causing Cushing's syndrome), but no $G_s\alpha$ G-protein abnormalities (which is mutated in McCune–Albright syndrome) have been documented in sporadic adrenal tumours. More recent studies have concentrated on oncogenes in the development of adrenal adenomas. *p53* is a tumour-suppressor gene that regulates cell growth and differentiation, probably by regulating cellular GTP concentrations. Mutations in *p53* result in the over-

expression of G-protein-regulated genes, and whilst *p53* mutations have been documented in one study in 11/13 APA, it is not yet clear whether such mutations are a primary or secondary phenomenon [11].

Glucocorticoid-remediable aldosteronism

Our understanding of the aetiology of GRA has increased significantly in the recent months with the description of the full molecular characterization of GRA [12,13]. Perhaps more importantly, for the first time a single gene mutation has been linked with the development of hypertension and is probably far more common than was first thought. The synthesis of aldosterone in the adrenal zona glomerulosa requires the action of two distinct but related P_{450} enzymes, 11β-hydroxylase and aldosterone synthase. The genes encoding these enzymes have been cloned (*CYP 11β1* and *CYP 11β2* respectively), are 95% homologous and lie in close proximity to each other on chromosome 8q22. In the normal zona fasciculata, aldo synthase is absent and therefore aldosterone is not synthesized. Both corticosterone and cortisol are synthesized under the control of ACTH which regulates 11β-hydroxylase. In the zona glomerulosa, 17α-hydroxylase activity is absent and cortisol cannot be made. Corticosterone (B), however, can be metabolized further to 18-OHB and aldosterone by aldo synthase which is regulated primarily by angiotensin II. GRA is now known to occur because of a gene rearrangement event. Unequal crossover at meiosis between the related *CYP 11β1* and -2 genes results in a chimeric gene comprising 5′ sequences of 11β-hydroxylase and 3′ sequences of aldo synthase. Providing this break point occurs 5′ to exon 4 of the *CYP 11β2* gene then the chimeric gene will still possess 18-hydroxylase activity. This chimeric gene, which is aberrantly expressed in the zona fasciculata, has the ability therefore to synthesize aldosterone from corticosterone, but is now regulated by ACTH and not by angiotensin II. Furthermore this also accounts for the large secretion of 18-hydroxylated cortisol and corticosterone metabolites in GRA (Fig. 50.3).

GRA may be more prevalent than first realized. Several large kindreds have been reported since the molecular genetics have been elucidated. Furthermore, in a recent screen of young patients (< 25 years) with hypertension and patients with a family history of hypertension < 50 years of age, elevated 18-OHF excretion together with the chimeric gene was found in approximately 5% of individuals (R. Dluhy, personal communication). Many of these patients had normokalaemia for reasons which are not clear, but which makes the diagnosis difficult unless a strong index of suspicion is maintained. If these

(a)

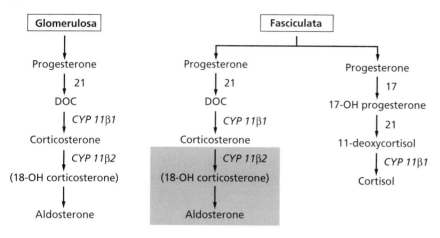

(b)

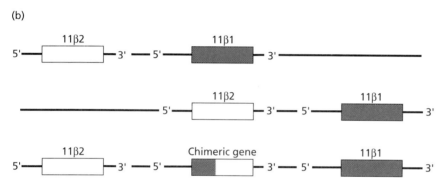

Fig. 50.3 An outline of the pathogenesis of glucocorticoid-remediable aldosteronism (GRA). In the normal adrenal, only the zona glomerulosa synthesizes aldosterone because it expresses aldo synthase (a product of the *CYP 11β2* gene). Both the zona glomerulosa and fasciculata express 11β-hydroxylase (a product of the *CYP 11β1* gene) but cortisol can be synthesized in the zona fasciculata because it expresses 17α-hydroxylase. GRA results from a chimeric gene which occurs because of an unequal crossover between the *CYP 11β1* and *CYP 11β2* genes at meiosis (b). This chimeric gene results in the expression of an enzyme in the zona fasciculata (boxed area in a) which can synthesize aldosterone from corticosterone but which is regulated by ACTH and not angiotensin II. DOC, deoxycorticosterone; OH, -hydroxy.

studies are confirmed then perhaps all young hypertensives should be screened for GRA irrespective of potassium levels.

References

1. Conn JW. Primary aldosteronism, a new clinical syndrome. *J. Lab. Clin. Med.* 1955;**45**:6–17.
2. Young WJ, Hogan MJ, Klee GG, Grant CS, vanHeerden JA. Primary aldosteronism: diagnosis and treatment. *Mayo Clin. Proc.* 1990;**65**:96–110.
3. Opocher G, Rocco S, Carpene G, Mantero F. Differential diagnosis in primary aldosteronism. *J. Steroid Biochem. Molec. Biol.* 1993;**45**:49–55.
4. Sutherland DJA, Ruse JL, Laidlaw JC. Hypertension, increased aldosterone secretion and low plasma renin activity relieved by dexamethasone. *Can. Med. Assoc. J.* 1966;**95**:1109–19.
5. Streeten DHP, Tomyez N, Anderson GH Jr. Reliability of screening methods for the diagnosis of primary aldosteronism. *Am. J. Med.* 1979;**67**:403–13.
6. Biglieri EG. Spectrum of mineralocorticoid hypertension. *Hypertension* 1991;**17**:251–61.
7. Fontes RG, Kater CE, Biglieri EG, Irony I. Reassessment of the predictive value of the postural stimulation test in primary aldosteronism. *Am. J. Hypertension* 1991;**4**:786–91.
8. Ulick S, Chu MD. Hypersecretion of a new corticosteroid, 18-hydroxycortisol in two types of adrenocortical hypertension. *Clin. Exp. Hypertension* 1982;**4**:1771–7.
9. Kem DC, Tang K, Hanson CS *et al*. The prediction of anatomical morphology of primary aldosteronism using serum 18-hydroxycorticosterone levels. *J. Clin. Endocrinol. Metab.* 1985;**60**:67–73.
10. Ikeda DM, Francis IR, Glazer GM *et al*. The detection of adrenal tumours and hyperplasia in patients with primary aldosteronism; comparison of scintigraphy, CT and MR imaging. *Am. J. Radiol.* 1989;**153**:301–6.
11. Lin SL, Lee YJ, Tsai JH. Mutations of the p53 gene in human functional adrenal neoplasms. *J. Clin. Endocrinol. Metab.* 1994;**78**:483–91.
12. Lifton RP, Dluhy RG, Powers M *et al*. A chimaeric 11β-hydroxylase/aldosterone synthase gene causes glucocorticoid-remediable aldosteronism and human hypertension. *Nature* 1992;**355**:262–5.
13. Pascoe L, Curnow KM, Slutsker L *et al*. Glucocorticoid-suppressible hyperaldosteronism results from hybrid genes created by unequal crossovers between CYP11β1 and CYP11β2. *Proc. Natl. Acad. Sci. USA* 1992;**89**:8327–31.

Adrenal Causes of Cushing's Syndrome

ROY HARPER AND A. BREW ATKINSON

Introduction

Cushing's syndrome is a constellation of clinical and biochemical abnormalities resulting from chronic excess of cortisol of any aetiology. There are two major classifications of the syndrome: adrenocorticotrophic hormone (ACTH)-dependent and ACTH-independent Cushing's syndrome. The presentation, investigation and treatment of ACTH-dependent Cushing's syndrome is discussed elsewhere. This chapter will consider the adrenal causes of Cushing's syndrome.

ACTH-independent Cushing's syndrome

There are a number of ACTH-independent causes of the syndrome (Table 51.1). Adrenal adenomas and carcinomas account for about 10–20% of all cases of Cushing's syndrome, with equal frequencies of adenoma and carcinoma in adults. These tumours are less common in men than in women. The majority of tumours arise spontaneously and are not associated with chronic ACTH stimulation. With small tumours the clinical picture is usually that of glucocorticoid excess, although purely virilizing or mixed adrenocortical adenomas may occur. Large tumours are more likely to be malignant and often show clinical evidence of both glucocorticoid excess and excess androgen production. Occasionally, adrenal carcinomas may also secrete aldosterone, deoxycorticosterone or oestrogens.

Presentation

The symptoms and signs of Cushing's syndrome are well known to clinicians. It is difficult to rival the excellent description of the disease provided by Harvey Cushing himself [1]. Cushing described a patient with cessation of menses, increasing obesity, headache, nausea, vomiting and palpitations, purpuric outbreaks, a definite growth of hair on the face with thinning of the hair on the scalp, muscular weakness and backache. On physical examination the patient was undersized, kyphotic and of most extraordinary appearance. Her round face was dusky and cyanosed with an abnormal growth of hair, particularly noticeable on the sides of the forehead, upper lip and chin. Her abdomen had the appearance of a full-term pregnancy. The breasts were hypertrophied and pendulous, and there were pads of fat over the supraclavicular and posterior cervical regions. The cyanotic appearance of the skin was particularly apparent over the body and lower extremities which were spotted by subcutaneous ecchymoses. Numerous purple striae were present over the stretched skin and a fine hirsuties was present over the back, hips and around the umbilicus. The skin, which everywhere was rough and dry, showed considerable pigmentation. The peculiar tense and painful adiposity affecting face, neck and trunk was in marked contrast to her comparatively spare extremities.

As well as the classic features described above, other abnormalities have been reported in Cushing's syndrome. Hypertension, diabetes mellitus and osteoporosis are prevalent. An increased incidence of opportunistic infections such as cryptococcosis, aspergillosis, nocardiosis and *Pneumocystis carinii* pneumonia have been reported, with the signs and symptoms of infection often masked by the hypercortisolism. The prevalence of the various signs and symptoms has been well reviewed [2,3]. It is not often possible to differentiate between the various causes of Cushing's syndrome on the basis of symptoms and signs alone but certain features may suggest a specific aetiology. Adrenal adenomas usually present with a clinical picture of mild hypercortisolism of a gradual onset. Androgenic manifestations such as hirsutism are usually absent. With adrenal carcinomas, clinical features of glucocorticoid and androgen hypersecretion have a much more rapid onset and are rapidly progressive. Hypercortisolism is usually marked. Hypokalaemia is common.

Table 51.1 ACTH-independent causes of Cushing's syndrome

Iatrogenic: treatment with glucocorticoids
Adrenocortical adenoma
Adrenocortical carcinoma
Adrenocortical macronodular hyperplasia (partially
    ACTH-dependent)
Pigmented nodular adrenocortical disease

Abdominal pain, abdominal masses and evidence of hepatic or pulmonary metastases are common at diagnosis.

Diagnosis of Cushing's syndrome

The diagnosis of Cushing's syndrome is the first essential step in investigation prior to proceeding to differential diagnosis (see Chapter 30).

Differential diagnosis

Having established the diagnosis of Cushing's syndrome, one proceeds to differential diagnosis [4,5]. Proper treatment of Cushing's syndrome depends crucially on establishing the precise aetiology. The mainstays of the differential diagnostic tests have been the high-dose dexamethasone suppression test, the metyrapone test, and measurement of plasma ACTH, potassium and dehydroepiandrosterone sulphate (DHEA-S). More recently, computerized tomography (CT) and magnetic resonance imaging (MRI) of the adrenal glands, bilateral inferior petrosal sampling for ACTH levels, and the plasma cortisol response to exogenous corticotrophic hormone (CRH) have been added.

Whereas it is often difficult to establish precisely the site of abnormality in ACTH-dependent Cushing's syndrome, there is usually no great difficulty in establishing the differential diagnosis of ACTH-independent Cushing's syndrome. Primary adrenal lesions can be readily identified using the combination of CT scans of the adrenals and the demonstration of undetectable or very low plasma ACTH levels. In addition, there is generally no suppression of cortisol with high-dose dexamethasone, no rise in plasma 11-deoxycortisol or urinary steroids following metyrapone, and no response of cortisol to CRH. Both adrenal adenomas and carcinomas causing Cushing's syndrome are readily apparent on CT scan [6].

CT scanning produces excellent delineation of the adrenal gland morphology because of the characteristically abundant perinephric and adrenal fat in Cushing's syndrome. Adrenal cortical adenomas producing Cushing's syndrome are usually larger than 2 cm and are of low tissue density on CT. The contralateral gland usually appears normal but can appear atrophic secondary to the feedback reduction in ACTH levels. The differential diagnosis for an adrenal mass in a patient with Cushing's syndrome includes a phaeochromocytoma producing ACTH, a metastasis from an ectopic ACTH carcinoma, an incidental mass such as a non-functioning adenoma or a metastasis from a known or unknown primary tumour. Adrenal scintigraphy with cholesterol-based radiopharmaceuticals such as ^{75}Se-selenocholesterol or NP-59 can also be used to image unilateral functional adenomas with absence of radiopharmaceutical in the contralateral gland. However, this is not usually necessary.

Adrenal carcinomas generally exceed 6 cm on CT scanning. They are often heterogeneous with areas of necrosis and calcification. Some carcinomas may be smaller and resemble adenomas. Carcinomas invade adjacent organs such as the liver (Fig. 51.1). Such invasion can be assessed using ultrasonography, CT and MRI scanning. Direct invasion into the inferior vena cava, involvement of regional lymph nodes and metastases to the liver, lung and bone can all occur. Adrenal cortical carcinomas show no uptake of cholesterol-based radiopharmaceuticals unless they are well differentiated, which is rare.

MRI will readily identify functioning adrenal adenomas and carcinomas but does not appear to adequately differentiate adenoma from carcinoma on the basis of relative signal intensities. MRI sequences that reflect adrenal lipid content may be more useful for distinguishing benign from malignant adenomas. Advances in fine needle aspiration technology may also allow improvements in diagnostic accuracy.

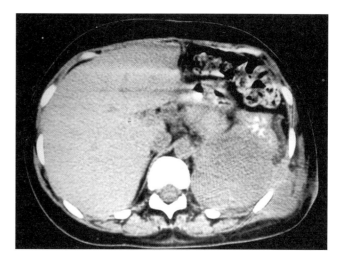

Fig. 51.1 This shows a large left-sided adrenal carcinoma with invasion of surrounding tissues.

In adrenocortical macronodular hyperplasia, a rare cause of Cushing's syndrome, patients typically have bilateral large adrenal nodules of varying size but often up to several centimetres in diameter. These nodules often coexist with a hyperplastic adrenal cortex. ACTH levels tend to be low or undetectable and cortical levels fail to show 50% suppression during a high-dose dexamethasone suppression test. Similar biochemical features are found in primary pigmented nodular adrenocortical disease (see Plate 51.1, between pp. 272 and 273), another rare cause of Cushing's syndrome, in which the adrenal glands show multiple, small, deeply pigmented adrenal nodules. This condition may be familial and can be associated with mesenchymal tumours (myxomas), pigmented skin lesions, spotty facial pigmentation, testicular and pituitary tumours (Carney's complex) [7]. It is important to be aware of these rare conditions, as nodular hyperplasia of the adrenals with a solitary or dominant nodule may be misdiagnosed as a hyperfunctioning adrenal adenoma.

Pathophysiology and molecular biology of adrenal causes of Cushing's syndrome

The precise pathophysiology of these conditions is poorly understood. The development of autonomous nodules within a hyperplastic adrenal gland, with subsequent regression of an initial pituitary adenoma may explain the phenomenon of adrenocortical macronodular hyperplasia. ACTH-receptor antibodies may be important in adrenocortical hyperfunction in pigmented nodular adrenocortical disease [7]. Inappropriate sensitivity of the adrenal glands to normal postprandial increases in gastric inhibitory polypeptide produces adrenal hyperplasia and a novel form of Cushing's syndrome that is food-dependent [8].

The molecular and genetic basis of adrenal adenoma and carcinoma, however, remains poorly understood. Adrenal carcinomas appear to be monoclonal in origin [9] although their pathogenesis may involve multiple genetic changes. Mutations of the tumour-suppressor gene *p53* have been reported in two studies and this tumour is a feature of the Li Fraumeni syndrome in which there is inheritance of germline mutations in *p53*, which results in the development of a variety of carcinomas in affected individuals [10]. Mutations of *p53* and the *ras* oncogene have also been sought unsuccessfully in adrenocortical adenomas.

Activating mutations of the ACTH receptor have also recently been excluded as a common factor in the pathogenesis of adrenal tumours [11], although there is some evidence that cAMP-dependent mitogenic pathways may be important, in that activating mutations in the cyclase inhibitory G$_i$α subunit have been detected in both adenomas and occasional carcinoma. However, our knowledge of the molecular biology of these tumours remains incomplete and much work remains to be done to show any proof of similarity to other cancers that may allow more rational selection of chemotherapeutic regimens in the future.

Treatment of adrenal causes of Cushing's syndrome

Adrenal adenomas can be successfully treated by unilateral adrenalectomy. The prognosis is excellent. Postoperatively, all patients have adrenal insufficiency because of suppression of ACTH secretion and hence of the contralateral adrenal gland. Adequate glucocorticoid replacement therapy is therefore mandatory but mineralocorticoid therapy is not usually required. Glucocorticoid therapy must be continued until complete recovery of the hypothalamic–pituitary–adrenal axis has occurred. This can take up to or even longer than 24 months.

Treatment of adrenocortical carcinoma is much less satisfactory and the mortality rate is high. Many patients have widespread metastases at the time of diagnosis. Extensive surgery, if possible, is the first step in therapy, serving to reduce the tumour mass and the degree of hypercortisolism. Curative surgery should result in absent steroid secretion since the pituitary output of ACTH is suppressed. Persisting non-suppressible plasma cortisol following surgery indicates residual metastatic tumour.

After operation, mitotane is usually employed [12]. It is given in doses of between 6 and 12 g daily, but severe side-effects (nausea, vomiting, diarrhoea) limit its use in high doses in many patients. Because mitotane affects the metabolism of cortisol, plasma cortisol or urinary free cortisol should be monitored in these patients and, if necessary, dexamethasone given as replacement steroid therapy.

Metyrapone and aminoglutethimide can also be given in attempts to control steroid hypersecretion, and ketoconazole should also be considered. 5-Fluorouracil has also been used as combination therapy. Suramin, a polysulphonated naphthylurea, has recently been used in the treatment of adrenal carcinoma. This drug preferentially accumulates in adrenal cells and may have therapeutic efficacy as a single agent. Further evaluation of this interesting compound will be of interest. More recently, three of 18 patients whose tumours were refractory to other chemotherapeutic agents, had partial tumour responses to oral gossypol, a spermatotoxin that inhibits the growth of human adrenocortical tumours in nude mice [13].

Despite aggressive management the outlook is poor. The 5-year survival rate was reported in one older series as 31% but in other studies mean survival time after therapy was only 10.3 months. In a recent study of 105 patients with adrenocortical carcinoma the average duration of symptoms before diagnosis was 8.7 months [14]. At the time of diagnosis 68% had endocrine symptoms and 30% had distant metastases. The median disease-free interval after surgery was 12.1 months and the median survival time 14.5 months, with a 5-year survival of 22%. Age over 40 and the presence of metastases at diagnosis indicated a poor prognosis. Although mitotane was generally effective in controlling hormonal hypersecretion, it did not have a significant effect on survival.

Conclusion

Cushing's syndrome is an unusual and unpleasant condition, which carries a high mortality if undetected or untreated. Following careful assessment and confirmation of hypercortisolism by biochemical means, it is imperative to accurately define the underlying cause. ACTH-independent Cushing's syndrome accounts for up to 20% of cases and can usually be readily distinguished from ACTH-dependent causes. Radiological and other imaging techniques help further define the underlying aetiology, which is most often an adrenal adenoma or carcinoma. Surgical treatment of adrenal adenomas is highly successful. In stark contrast, adrenal carcinomas bring a very poor prognosis but combined surgical and chemotherapeutic treatment may help improve survival. Better agents are urgently required.

References

1. Cushing H. The basophil adenomas of the pituitary body and their clinical manifestations (pituitary basophilism). *Bull. Johns Hopkins Hosp.* 1932;**50**:137–95.
2. Crapo L. Cushing's syndrome: a review of diagnostic tests. *Metabolism* 1979;**28**:955–7.
3. Besser GM, Edwards CRW. Cushing's syndrome. *Clin. Endocrinol. Metab.* 1972;**1**:451–90.
4. Trainer PJ, Grossman A. The diagnosis and differential diagnosis of Cushing's syndrome. *Clin. Endocrinol.* 1991;**34**:317–30.
5. Atkinson AB. Cushing's syndrome. In Robertson JIS (ed.). *Handbook of Hypertension, Vol 15. Clinical Hypertension.* Oxford: Elsevier Science Publishers, 1992:390–419.
6. Chan FL, Wang C. Imaging for adrenal tumours. *Clin. Endocrinol. Metab.* 1989;**3**:153–89.
7. Young WF, Carney JA, Musa BU *et al.* Familial Cushing's syndrome due to primary pigmented nodular adrenocortical disease. Reinvestigation 50 years later. *N. Engl. J. Med.* 1989;**321**:1659–64.
8. Reznik Y, Allali-Zerah V, Chayvialle JA *et al.* Food-dependent Cushing's syndrome mediated by aberrant adrenal sensitivity to gastric inhibitory polypeptide. *N. Engl. J. Med.* 1992;**327**:981–6.
9. Gicquel C, Leblond-Francillard M, Bertagna X *et al.* Clonal analysis of human adrenocortical carcinomas and secreting adenomas. *Clin. Endocrinol.* 1994;**40**:465–77.
10. Reincke M, Karl M, Travis WH *et al. p53* mutations in human adrenocortical neoplasms: immunohistochemical and molecular studies. *J. Clin. Endocrinol. Metab.* 1994;**78**:790–4.
11. Light K, Jenkins PJ, Weber A *et al.* Are activating mutations of the adrenocorticotropin receptor involved in adrenal cortical neoplasia? *Life Sci.* 1995;**56**:1523–7.
12. Miller JW, Crapo L. The medical treatment of Cushing's syndrome. *Endocr. Rev.* 1993;**14**:443–58.
13. Flack MR, Pyle RG, Mullen NM *et al.* Oral gossypol in the treatment of metastatic adrenal cancer. *J. Clin. Endocrinol. Metab.* 1993;**76**:1019–24.
14. Luton JP, Cerdas S, Billaud L *et al.* Clinical features of adrenocortical carcinoma, prognostic factors and the effect of mitotane treatment. *N. Engl. J. Med.* 1990;**322**:1195–2001.

Androgen-secreting Tumours

DIANA HAMILTON-FAIRLEY AND STEPHEN FRANKS

Introduction

Androgen-secreting tumours (ASTs) are very rare. The origin of the tumour is either the ovary or the adrenal gland. The tumours may be benign or malignant but in the majority of cases they are benign. They are more commonly found in younger women; 75% of ovarian ASTs occur in women under the age of 30 [1] and over 50% of adrenal ASTs arise in women under the age of 50 [2].

Ovarian ASTs are more common than adrenal ones and represent 0.4% of all ovarian tumours or 1.8% of solid, benign ovarian tumours. The nomenclature of the tumours that arise in the ovary has varied widely over the years, reflecting theories as to their origin within the ovary as well as describing their similarity to androgen-producing cells of the adrenal gland and testis.

The classification of the majority of the ovarian ASTs (Table 52.1) can be divided into two types: the sex cord stromal cell tumours and adrenal-like tumours.

The sex cord stromal cell tumours, which show a testicular direction of differentiation, are now called Sertoli–Leydig cell tumours (SLCTs). They were previously referred to as arrhenoblastomas, androblastomas or gynandroblastomas. Although these terms implied masculinization, some of the tumours are non-functioning and some produce oestrogen. The adrenal-like tumours of the ovary had an even greater number of names, some indicative of the high lipoid content of the cells that is typical of the adrenal fasciculata, for example virilizing lipoid cell tumour, adrenal-rest tumour, luteoma, adrenal cortical carcinoma of the ovary, androblastoma diffusum and hypernephroma. The classification of the adrenal ASTs is more simple since it refers solely to the benign or malignant nature of the tumour and which is therefore called either an adrenal adenoma or adenocarcinoma. The malignant potential of both adrenal and ovarian tumours depends on their degree of differentiation. Generally, the larger the tumour, the more likely it is to be malignant.

The aim of this chapter is to deal with the clinical aspects of these tumours and we will discuss their presentation, diagnosis, treatment and prognosis.

Presentation

Women with these tumours commonly present with varying degrees of virilization (Table 52.2), although Young and Scully [1] reported a prevalence of definite androgenic manifestations of only 34% in patients with SCLTs. The time interval from the onset of symptoms to referral to a specialist varies enormously, in one series the range was 6 months to 9 years. They may occasionally present as a consequence of local symptoms of the tumour itself.

Women with a large adrenal mass may present with loin or back pain, while ovarian tumours may rupture or become torted causing pain and/or peritonism. Ovarian tumours rarely present with pressure symptoms secondary to tumour size.

Hirsutism is the most common presenting symptom with increased hair growth on the face, predominantly on the upper lip and chin, a male pattern estucheon on the abdomen, hair around the nipples and on the back. Menstrual disturbance, secondary amenorrhoea or oligomenorrhoea, are also common and women may present with primary or secondary infertility. A smaller proportion of women will present with other signs of virilization including acne, male-pattern baldness, deepening of the voice, clitoromegaly, change in body habitus including breast atrophy.

The history is important in reaching the diagnosis since the patient has usually noticed a fairly sudden onset of symptoms having previously not had any signs of virilization or menstrual irregularity. This is in contrast to

Table 52.1 Classification of androgen-secreting tumours

	Old terms	New terms
Ovary		
Sex cord stromal tumours	Arrhenoblastomas Androblastomas Gynandroblastomas	Sertoli–Leydig cell tumours (SLCTs)
Adrenal-like tumours	Virilizing lipoid cell tumour Adrenal rest tumour Luteoma Androblastoma diffusum Hypernephroma Adrenal–cortical carcinoma of the ovary	Adrenal-like tumours of the ovary
Adrenal		
Benign		Adenoma
Malignant		Adenocarcinoma

Table 52.2 Presenting symptoms

Virilization
Hirsutism
Acne
Male-pattern baldness
Voice change
Clitoromegaly
Breast atrophy

Menstrual disturbance
Oligomenorrhoea
Secondary amenorrhoea
Polymenorrhoea

Other (less frequent)
Pain
Oedema
Cushingoid signs/symptoms (50% of adrenal tumours)
Deep venous thrombosis
Fatigue
Abdominal swelling

conditions such as polycystic ovary syndrome (PCOS) where hirsutism and menstrual disturbance are often present from puberty or shortly thereafter.

On examination, a record should be made of signs of virilization using the Ferriman–Gallwey score to classify hirsutism. This method provides an objective measure of hirsutism which can be used for follow-up, since greater than 90% of the patients will lose all signs of virilization (except voice change) once the tumour has been removed. Signs of adrenal cortical overactivity should also be looked for since in the largest series of adrenal-like tumours of the ovary (58 cases) [3] 50% were Cushingoid in appearance, with a moon-face, striae,

atrophy of the skin, ecchymoses, buffalo hump and central obesity.

Examination of the abdomen and pelvis may be unremarkable since the tumours are usually small, with 40% measuring less than 5 cm but a few may reach a much greater size; the largest ovarian Sertoli–Leydig cell tumour reported from a series of 200 cases measured 51 cm (average 13.5 cm) in diameter [1].

Diagnosis

The aim of diagnostic tests in women who present with virilization is to differentiate those women with an underlying benign biochemical abnormality, such as women with PCOS or congenital adrenal hyperplasia (CAH), from those with a tumour that requires surgical removal. In those women with a tumour, the site of production of the androgens is all important and so tests must look for both an adrenal or an ovarian cause. The tests include hormone profiles and imaging of adrenals or ovaries by ultrasound, venography, computed tomography (CT) or magnetic resonance imaging (MRI). When imaging yields uncertain results, selective catheterization and sampling of adrenal or ovarian veins may be required for localization.

Hormone profiles

In women with a virilizing tumour, testosterone is usually raised. The levels are usually significantly higher in those tumours that are malignant, whilst benign tumours produce androgen concentrations that may also be very high but can be indistinguishable from non-neoplastic causes of virilization such as PCOS and

CAH. The levels of the other androgens can vary enormously and may not assist in identifying the source of the androgens. Figure 52.1 shows the biosynthesis of androgens both in the ovary and adrenal. The overproduction of androgens by these tumours does not follow any particular pattern, with each tumour appearing to use different steroidal pathways and, more importantly, to show variable responses to dynamic hormonal manipulation [4]. Non-steroidal hormones may also be produced by these tumours; for example, there has been a case report of prorenin secretion by an ovarian tumour.

In both ovarian and adrenal ASTs overproduction of testosterone is usually the key diagnostic test (Fig. 52.2). The concentration of testosterone is usually more than twice the upper limit of the normal range (0.5–2.6 nmol/l), unlike that in women with PCOS who usually have levels of < 5 nmol/l. A serum testosterone level in the male range (> 10 nmol/l) should be regarded as indicative of a tumour until proved otherwise. The other androgens, including androstenedione (A4), dehydroepiandrosterone (DHEA) and its sulphate (DHEA-S), and 17α-hydroxyprogesterone (17-OHP), have all been reported to be raised in both ovarian and adrenal tumours, although a raised DHEA or DHEA-S is more likely to be from an adrenal rather than an ovarian tumour. In women with CAH the concentrations of the androgen precursors, particularly 17-OHP, tend to be proportionately higher than the testosterone concentrations and will rise still further during a stimulation

test with adrenocorticotrophic hormone (ACTH). Some of the tumours also produce cortisol and 11-deoxycortisol. This is more commonly found in adrenal tumours but has been reported in ovarian adrenal-like tumours [5]. These tests alone therefore will not separate an adrenal from an ovarian tumour nor will they assist in excluding a diagnosis of PCOS or CAH. The addition of measuring luteinizing hormone (LH) and follicle-stimulating hormone (FSH) shows no consistent pattern in either ovarian or adrenal ASTs and is therefore not of any further diagnostic assistance. In women with a short history of hirsutism and/or a serum testosterone of > 5 nmol/l, a 24-hour urine free cortisol measurement should be performed to screen for hypercortisolism of pituitary or adrenal origin. If Cushing's syndrome is suspected, a low-dose dexamethasone suppression test should be performed.

Further investigation involves examination of the pituitary–adrenal axis to determine whether the tumour is responsive to pituitary control or whether it is functioning autonomously. Dexamethasone 2 mg at night for 5 days should be given to suppress the pituitary–adrenal axis. While the cortisol pathway is suppressed after only two doses of dexamethasone, the androgen pathway usually requires 5 days to show a response. In general, ovarian Sertoli–Leydig tumours will not show any suppression of androgen production in response to dexamethasone, whilst the benign adrenal and ovarian adrenal-like tumours often do. This is not universal and tumours of the ovary and, less commonly, the adrenal

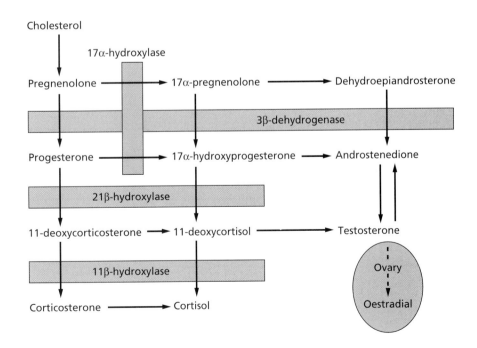

Fig. 52.1 Androgen biosynthesis in the adrenal gland and ovary.

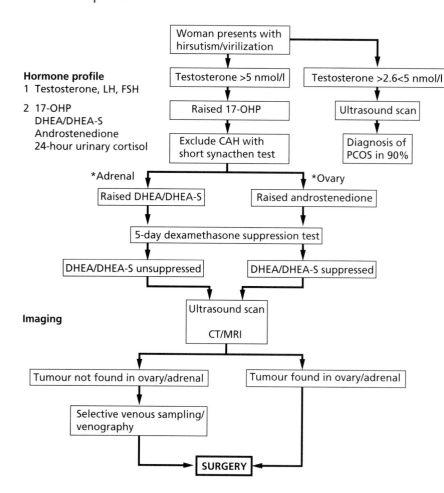

Hormone profile
1 Testosterone, LH, FSH

2 17-OHP
  DHEA/DHEA-S
  Androstenedione
  24-hour urinary cortisol

Imaging

Fig. 52.2 Investigation of androgen-secreting tumours. *The demarcation between the ovary and adrenal is not absolute and a normal result does not exclude a tumour at the other site. CAH, congenital adrenal hyperplasia; CT, computed tomography; DHEA-S, dehydroepiandrosterone sulphate; FSH, follicle-stimulating hormone; LH, luteinizing hormone; MRI, magnetic resonance imaging; 17-OHP, 17-hydroxyprogesterone; PCOS, polycystic ovary syndrome.

have been shown to have LH and human chorionic gonadotrophin (hCG) receptors so that they will respond to hCG but will not alter their androgen production by manipulation of ACTH. It should also be noted that the response to dexamethasone will not reliably distinguish adrenal tumours from adrenal-like tumours of the ovary.

Diagnostic imaging

Imaging techniques that have been used include ultrasound, of both the ovary and the adrenal, venography, CT and MRI of the abdomen and pelvis. All these techniques are able to detect a tumour of > 2 cm in diameter with a greater than 95% accuracy but no routine scanning method has a high degree of accuracy for tumours smaller than 1 cm. In general, MRI or CT are the methods of first choice for detection of suspected adrenal tumours and high-resolution ultrasound is the most appropriate first-line investigation of ovarian tumours.

Transvaginal ultrasound has been found to be useful in the detection of ovarian tumours greater than 1 cm

in diameter [6]. The usefulness of ultrasound for the detection of small tumours is limited by the fact that a polycystic morphology does not necessarily mean that PCOS is the diagnosis. Polycystic ovaries may be detected in subjects with other causes of hyperandrogenism including CAH and ASTs. Since tumours are rare and polycystic ovaries are so common, the latter diagnosis is usually correct but in women with testosterone concentrations in excess of 5 nmol/l further tests to exclude a tumour should be pursued. The smaller ovarian tumours tend to be well differentiated and therefore of low malignant potential.

In cases where it remains uncertain whether the adrenal or ovary is the source of excess androgen production or if the tumour has not been clearly lateralized by imaging techniques, it may be necessary to perform selective, transfemoral venous sampling from ovarian and adrenal vessels [6].

Treatment and prognosis

Medical treatment has little place in the treatment

of these tumours. Chemotherapy or radiotherapy are rarely effective in treatment of malignant ASTs. The only curative therapy is surgical removal, usually in the form of an adrenalectomy, ovarian cystectomy or oophorectomy. Histology will reveal whether or not the tumour is benign or malignant. The degree of differentiation determines the prognosis. All of the well differentiated ovarian SLCT tumours in Young and Scully's series [1] presented as stage Ia compared with 52% of the poorly differentiated tumours. In those tumours with heterologous elements or classified as retiform 80% presented as stage Ia. The incidence of stage II and III disease was 2.5% of all SLCTs and these were confined entirely to the poorly differentiated, heterologous and retiform groups.

As far as adrenal tumours are concerned, prognosis is based on the differentiation of the disease, age of the patient and extent of the disease. In a series of 156 adrenal carcinomas it was found that people under the age of 30 and/or those with ASTs had a better prognosis. The largest group presented with stage II disease and, following surgery, had a 53% actuarial 5-year-survival rate. These data refer to all adrenal tumours and not solely to ASTs [7].

Following surgical removal, hirsutism will regress but deepening of the voice, male-pattern baldness and clitoromegaly may show only minimal improvement. Recurrence of hirsutism and other signs of virilization usually indicate tumour recurrence, which is most likely in the first year following surgery of a malignant/poorly differentiated tumour.

The prognosis for the patient following surgery is determined entirely by the malignant potential of the tumour. In 12 women with adrenal carcinoma only two presented without metastases and these were the only two still alive 30 and 55 months postoperatively. The remainder died, seven within 1 year of presentation, two at 3 years and one after 7.5 years [2]. Those women with adrenal adenomas have an extremely good prognosis following surgery, although they may require adrenal replacement therapy.

The survival of women with ovarian SLCTs depends on the stage at presentation, whether the cyst had ruptured prior to surgery, which was associated with malignancy, and the size of the tumour, since the larger ones were more likely to be malignant. The number of mitoses per 10 high power fields (hpf) was also significant with a much poorer survival rate if more than 15 mitoses per 10 hpf was present [1]. Twenty-three women with well differentiated tumours were alive and well an average of 6 years (6 months – 23 years) after surgery. In 111 women whose tumours showed moderate differentiation 80

were followed-up for between 1 and 23 years. Sixty-nine of the women were alive and disease-free an average of 6 years postoperatively. Twenty-seven women were found to have poorly differentiated tumours. Five women were reported alive and disease-free of 22 women followed up for 1–15 years (average 7 years), three were alive with tumour (2–27 years) following surgery and fourteen had died between 9 months and 17 years postoperatively.

Postoperative adjuvant therapy, whether combination chemotherapy, radiotherapy or both for malignant ovarian or adrenal tumours does not seem to alter the prognosis. In Young and Scully's series [1] several different regimens were tried but survival was not improved.

Case report

The case of Mrs H.Y. illustrates the principles of investigation and management of ASTs.

Case history

She presented to the gynaecological endocrine clinic at the age of 32 with a history of secondary infertility. She had been amenorrhoeic for 10 months and had noticed the onset of acne and mild hirsutism 6 months prior to presentation. Initial investigations suggested a diagnosis of PCOS; she had polycystic ovaries on ultrasound, the serum LH concentration was at the upper limit of normal (11 iu/l) with a normal level of FSH (4.5 iu/l). However her initial serum testosterone concentration was greatly elevated at 11 nmol/l (normal range 0.5–3.0 nmol/l). This was repeated and found again to be in the male range at 15 nmol/l.

Further investigations were then undertaken; the androstenedione level was grossly elevated (770 nmol/l, normal < 9.0), serum 17-OHP was also increased (23 nmol/l, normal < 12) but, crucially, the high levels of both serum DHEA-S (108 nmol/l, normal < 9) and urinary free cortisol (1110 nmol/24, normal < 300) pointed to an adrenal cause of hyperandrogenaemia (although, as indicated above, an adrenal-like tumour of the ovary cannot be excluded).

A CT scan of the adrenals was performed and this showed a very large tumour in the left renal region, displacing the left kidney (Fig. 52.3). She then underwent surgery at which the tumour, some 10 cm in diameter, was found to be adherent to the left kidney (see Plate 52.1, between pp. 272 and 273). Consequently, both the tumour and the kidney were removed. Histological examination confirmed the presence of a steroidogenically active tumour. Although it was well encapsulated, there

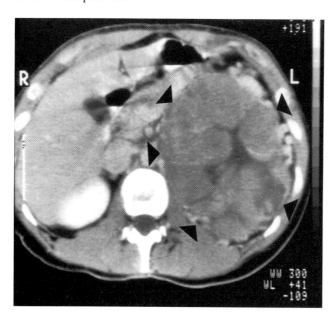

Fig. 52.3 CT scan of the abdomen showing a very large left suprarenal tumour (arrows).

were many mitotic figures and evidence of microvascular invasion, features highly suggestive of a carcinoma.

Following surgery, she enjoyed clinical and biochemical remission. The serum androgens were normalized, there was resolution of her acne and hirsutism and return of ovulatory menses. Indeed she was able to conceive after spontaneous ovulation. Sadly, but not unexpectedly, her symptoms returned 2 years later and an ultrasound scan of her liver revealed the presence of tumour metastases. Partial hepatectomy produced a further but temporary remission and despite attempted chemotherapy, she died a few months later, some 4 years after the initial presentation. Fortunately, the distressing symptoms of hyperandrogenism had been controlled by the administration of the anti-androgen cyproterone acetate.

Comment

The important diagnostic point of this case was the short history of hirsutism and acne, even though these symptoms were initially mild and much less important to the patient than her anovulatory infertility. Indeed, the original clinical diagnosis was PCOS but, as discussed earlier in this chapter, the ultrasound appearance of polycystic ovaries is not specific to PCOS and may occur in other hyperandrogenic states including CAH and ovarian or adrenal tumours.

The most significant of the initial tests was the greatly elevated serum testosterone. As discussed in a previous section, a testosterone level in the male range (> 10 nmol/l) strongly suggests the presence of an AST. Subsequent tests showed enormously raised concentrations of androstenedione (the major secretory product of the tumour) and, importantly for localization, greatly elevated levels of DHEA-S in serum and cortisol in the 24-h urine collection. These findings, without the need for dynamic tests, suggested an underlying adrenal tumour which was all too readily visible on CT scanning. Tumours of this size are almost always malignant and so it was no surprise to find evidence of this on histology, even though there was no clinical evidence of metastases at the time of surgery. Nevertheless, the only chance of cure is surgery and for some time she derived considerable benefit from adrenalectomy. Unfortunately, these tumours are rarely radio- or chemosensitive, as proved to be the case here, but the quality of her remaining life was improved by management of hyperandrogenic symptoms with anti-androgen therapy.

Conclusion

ASTs are very rare. They usually present with signs of virilization. They may arise in the adrenal gland or the ovary. The hormone profile and response to dexamethasone does not always reflect accurately the site of the tumour and unless readily found by imaging techniques, selective venous sampling should be performed prior to surgery. Surgical excision is the treatment of choice but in both adrenal and ovarian tumours the prognosis in malignant tumours is invariably poor in spite of radiotherapy and chemotherapy.

References

1. Young RH, Scully RE. Ovarian Sertoli–Leydig cell tumours. *Am. J. Surg. Pathol.* 1985;**9**:543–69.
2. Derksen J, Nagesser SK, Meinders AE, Haak HR, Van de Welde CJH. Identification of virilising adrenal tumours in hirsute women. *N. Engl. J. Med.* 1994;**331**:968–73.
3. Pedowitz P, Pomerance W. Adrenal-like tumours of the ovary. Review of the literature and report of 2 new cases. *Obstet. Gynecol.* 1962;**19**:183–94.
4. Gabrilove JL, Seman AT, Sabet R, Mitty HA, Nicolis GL. Virilizing adrenal adenoma with studies on the steroid content of the adrenal venous effluent and a review of the literature. *Endocr. Rev.* 1981;**2**:462–70.
5. Freeman DA. Steroid hormone producing tumours in man. *Endocr. Rev.* 1986;**7**:204–20.
6. Lobo RA. Ovarian hyperandrogenism and androgen producing tumours. *Endocrinol. Metab. Clin. North Am.* 1991;**20**:773–805.
7. Icard P, Chapuis Y, Andreassian B, Bernard A, Proye C. Adrenocortical carcinoma in surgically treated patients: a retrospective study on 156 cases by the French Association of Endocrine Surgery. *Surgery* 1992;**112**:972–9.

53

Imaging of Functioning Gonadal Disorders

IAIN D. MORRISON, RODNEY H. REZNEK AND
JAMSHED B. BOMANJI

Functioning testicular tumours

The majority of testicular masses are neoplasms, and most extratesticular scrotal masses are inflammatory or benign. Investigations that reliably distinguish between intra- and extratesticular masses are, therefore, of particular value in the evaluation of scrotal abnormalities. Ultrasound is the first investigation of choice, being readily available, inexpensive and with no harmful effects. 7.5 MHz or 10 MHz probes provide excellent spatial resolution down to 0.5 mm, and around 90% of scrotal abnormalities can be categorized into intra- or extratesticular subgroups in this way [1]. Subsidiary extratesticular findings such as skin thickness, epididymal enlargement and hydrocele do not help categorize an intratesticular mass [2].

The various types of malignant testicular mass and functioning non-germ-cell tumours cannot be distinguished from each other on ultrasonographic grounds. In general, testicular neoplasms are hypo-echoic compared with normal testis. Seminomas are classically of uniform hypo-echoic texture, teratomas tend to show greater disorganization of the tissues, cystic spaces, focal highly reflective areas, and areas of calcification. Highly reflective focal areas are also seen frequently in embryonal carcinomas [3]. Sensitivity and specificity of ultrasound for the detection of testicular tumours is in the region of 95%.

Magnetic resonance imaging (MRI) provides clear delineation of scrotal contents with no radiation dose, but is not widely performed owing to the effectiveness of ultrasound. A surface coil is suspended 1–2 cm above the scrotal skin. The testicular tissue is of uniformly high signal intensity on T_2-weighted images, and the tunica albuginea forms a low signal capsule around the testis [4]. Intratesticular masses are of lower signal than surrounding normal testis. Although the contrast resolution of MRI is excellent, the spatial resolution of ultrasound is far better. MRI is as good as ultrasound at distinguishing

between intra- and extratesticular abnormalities. In one study the two modalities were compared in the diagnosis and staging of testicular tumours in 23 patients. MRI correctly sited the abnormalities in all patients, and demonstrated intratesticular lesions in four patients where ultrasound had given a false-negative result. The missed abnormalities consisted of two cases of leukaemic involvement, one of lymphoma and one Leydig cell tumour. In two of the cases, ultrasound had shown the affected testis to be enlarged, but of similar echogenicity to the contralateral testis. Neither modality reliably differentiated benign from malignant disorders, and both were disappointing in terms of staging accuracy [5]. At present, ultrasound is the imaging modality of choice, and MRI should be used when the abnormality is thought to be diffuse and infiltrative.

Computed tomography (CT) is the modality of choice for the assessment of nodal and distal spread of malignant testicular tumours, but has no role in the initial diagnosis or characterization of a testicular abnormality.

Functioning ovarian pathologies

Polycystic ovary syndrome

The radiological diagnosis of polycystic ovary syndrome (PCOS) is made using ultrasound, either transabdominally, or, more accurately, transvaginally. The classic description is of bilaterally enlarged ovaries of two to five times normal volume, with multiple cysts in a subcortical position, each measuring less than 1 cm. However, up to 30% of women with the clinical syndrome have normal ovaries on ultrasound [6].

MRI is also very effective in the demonstration of polycystic ovaries. On T_2-weighted images the peripherally situated cysts show as well defined spheres of high signal in enlarged ovaries (Fig. 53.1). The cysts are of low signal intensity on T_1-weighted images, consistent

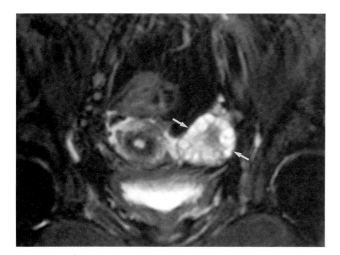

Fig. 53.1 Polycystic ovary syndrome. Coronal plane T_2-weighted MRI scan showing the left ovary (arrows) adjacent to the uterus with numerous peripherally sited cysts which are of high signal intensity.

with their fluid contents. The uterus may also be seen to be of reduced size with the reduced signal of hypoplasia on T_2-weighted images [7]. CT is not useful in the assessment of PCOS since the cysts are shown less clearly, and the investigation carries a significant radiation dose.

Stromal hyperthecosis of the ovary is a hyperplastic disorder, which produces similar clinical and radiological features to PCOS. The diagnosis, which can only be made histologically, is important since the treatment of the two disorders is different. Bilateral oophorectomy may be necessary to halt the progressive virilization seen in stromal hyperthecosis [7].

Functioning ovarian tumours

Ovarian tumours that cause virilization include Sertoli–Leydig cell tumours (SLCTs), the rare lipoid cell tumours and Brenner tumours [7]. Granulosa-theca cell tumours are the most common oestrogen-producing tumours, but may also release testosterone. Ultrasound, CT and MRI demonstrate solid unilateral ovarian masses, but there are no specific features to help distinguish one type of tumour from another.

MRI has the advantage over CT of improved differentiation between uterine and adnexal masses, and no ionizing radiation is involved. MRI does not have an established role in the management of ovarian neoplasms

that are of indeterminate cause on ultrasound, but some workers claim MRI to be more accurate than ultrasound in distinguishing benign from malignant ovarian neoplasms [8]. The accuracy in diagnosing ovarian carcinoma is similar for CT and MRI [9]. CT is better than ultrasound at assessing malignant tumours for involvement of the pelvic side-wall, mesentery, and lymph nodes in the pelvis and retroperitoneum, but an alarming degree of peritoneal or recurrent disease can be missed by CT. An indium-111-labelled monoclonal antibody has been used successfully to image ovarian carcinoma [10], and may be particularly useful for detecting disease recurrence. Radioisotope studies are not shown to be of any benefit in the assessment of functioning ovarian disorders.

Benign tumours cannot be reliably distinguished from malignant tumours on imaging grounds, either by ultrasound, CT or MRI. When an ovarian mass is discovered, management consists of early surgery, so imaging is of limited value except as a staging procedure.

References

1. Entwisle KG, Ayers AB. Imaging of the scrotum and testes. *Imaging* 1992;**4**:107–16.
2. Feld R, Middleton WD. Recent advances in sonography of the testis and scrotum. *Radiol. Clin. North Am.* 1992;**30**(5):1033–51.
3. Fowler R, Imaging the testis and scrotal structures. *Clin. Radiol.* 1990;**41**:81–5.
4. Nagle CE, Freitas JE. Scrotal imaging. In Sandler MP, Patton JA, Gross MD, Shapiro B, Falke THM (eds). *Endocrine Imaging.* Norwalk, Connecticut: Appleton and Lange, 1992:377–403.
5. Thurnher S, Hricak H, Carroll PR, Pobiel RS, Filly RA. Imaging the testis: comparison between MR imaging and US. *Radiology* 1988;**167**:631–6.
6. Yeh HC, Futterweit W, Thornton JC. Polycystic ovarian disease: US features in 104 patients. *Radiology* 1987;**163**:111.
7. Occhipinti KA, Frankel SD, Hricak H. The ovary. Computed tomography and magnetic resonance imaging. *Radiol. Clin. North Am.* 1993;**31**(5):1115–32.
8. Outwater EK, Dunton CJ. Imaging of the ovary and adnexa: clinical issues and applications of MR imaging. *Radiology* 1995;**194**:1–18.
9. Buist MR, Golding RP, Berger CW *et al.* Comparative evaluation of diagnostic methods in ovarian carcinoma with emphasis on CT and MRI. *Gynaecol. Oncol.* 1994;**52**:191–8.
10. Massuger LFAG, Kenemans P, Claessens RAMJ *et al.* Immuno-scintigraphy of ovarian cancer with indium-111-labelled OV-TL 3 F(ab')$_2$ monoclonal antibody. *J. Nucl. Med.* 1990;**31**:1802–10.

54

Ovarian Tumours

ROBIN A.F. CRAWFORD AND JOHN H. SHEPHERD

Introduction

Ovarian cancer is the fifth most common cancer in women, with nearly 6000 new cases occurring each year in the UK. Mortality rates from ovarian cancer have increased since the beginning of the century for the group aged over 40 years. This may, in part, be related to more accurate diagnosis, but as survival rates have not improved significantly it is clear that there is also an increase in incidence. The UK has the highest incidence rate in Europe (155 cases per million) with a mortality rate of 150 per million. Although women with early stage disease have a 5-year survival rate of up to 90%, overall less than one-third of patients live for 5 years and the survival curve continues to fall even after this time. Ovarian cancer accounts for 6% of all cancer deaths. The deaths attributable to ovarian cancer are greater in number than for all other gynaecological malignancies combined.

Ovarian cancer is more common in the industrialized countries. Unceasing ovulation is associated with an increased risk of ovarian cancer. Nulliparous women, including those with involuntary infertility and possibly those undertaking ovarian stimulation, are also at increased risk of ovarian malignancy. Conversely, the combined oral contraceptive, which suppresses ovulation, reduces the risk of developing the disease by 10% after 1 year and 50% after 5 years. Similarly, there is a reduced incidence in multiparous women, and for those women who have had tubal ligation or even hysterectomy with ovarian conservation. Familial ovarian cancer accounts for less than 5% of all ovarian cancer cases but the lifetime risk of ovarian cancer for the woman with one first-degree relative who has died of the disease triples to 5% and increases to 7% with two affected relatives.

Pathology

The pathology of primary ovarian cancer includes tumours originating from the serosal surface of the ovary, the germ cell, the sex cords and the ovarian stroma. Although epithelial cancers are the most common type, accounting for more than 60% of all ovarian tumours, the age range of the various subtypes of ovarian tumours is different. The germ-cell type accounts for 60% of tumours in women younger than 20 years of age and only 5% of ovarian cancers in the postmenopausal group. Conversely, the epithelial group accounts for 82% of the tumours in the postmenopausal age group, with only 14% of epithelial cancers occurring before 40 years. From this age distribution, it is clear that in a young woman (aged less than 40 years) with adnexal pathology, the full range of tumour markers, including α fetoprotein (AFP) and human chorionic gonadotrophin (hCG), should be recorded to determine whether a curable germ-cell tumour is present.

Serous carcinoma accounts for 40–50% of epithelial tumours, endometrioid tumours account for 15–30%, mucinous type for 5–15% and the clear cell variant for up to 10%. Approximately 60% of serous tumours are bilateral compared to 30% endometrioid and 20% mucinous. The germ-cell tumours may show all forms of differentiation from the dysgerminoma with almost no differentiation, through non-gestational choriocarcinoma with trophoblastic differentiation secreting hCG, yolk sac tumours with extra-embryonic differentiation and secreting AFP, to teratomas that have differentiated along embryonic lines. Sex cord stromal malignancies are relatively rare. Sex cord tumours include granulosa cell tumours, which secrete oestrogen and the useful marker dimeric inhibin, as well as Sertoli–Leydig cell tumours, which may secrete testosterone. Brenner tumours are uncommon, solid, fibro-epithelial tumours with nests of transitional cells. In the malignant variant, they are a transitional cell carcinoma of the ovary.

Metastases from ovarian tumours spread by direct extension, exfoliation of clonogenic cells into the peritoneal

331

fluid and lymphatic invasion. Metastatic invasion of the ovary by other cancers is surprisingly common; the Krukenberg tumour is associated with a mucinous cancer usually originating from the stomach but can also arise from the breast, colon or gall bladder.

A further subset of ovarian cancer pathology is called borderline or 'low-malignant potential'. Nearly 15% of epithelial and 20% of mucinous tumours will be of borderline histology. The borderline tumour appears malignant but obvious invasion of the stroma is lacking. This type of tumour is characterized by an excellent prognosis if confined to the pelvis and a relative resistance to chemotherapy.

Tumour markers

Tumour markers are widely used in the diagnosis and management of women with ovarian cancer. CA-125 is an antigenic determinant of a high molecular weight glycoprotein expressed by epithelial ovarian tumours and by other tissues of Müllerian origin, which is recognized by the monoclonal antibody OC-125. A serum CA-125 greater than 35 u/ml is considered elevated and it is raised in 80% of women preoperatively who have epithelial ovarian cancer. It is also raised in a number of benign conditions such as endometriosis, peritoneal inflammation (e.g. pelvic inflammatory disease), pregnancy and liver disease. It is not so useful for mucinous tumours and only 50% of women with stage I ovarian cancer have elevated levels. The use of other ovarian markers such as OVX-1 and markers more specific for other tumours (CA-19.9, CA-15.3 and carcinoembryonic antigen (CEA)) may increase the value of tumour marker estimation preoperatively. The secretion of various markers such as AFP, hCG and inhibin by the relatively rare teratomas and sex cord tumours is helpful, both for diagnosis and for monitoring treatment. There is value in using CA-125 in follow-up for epithelial tumours. If the patient has an early-stage tumour and she is treated with surgery alone, the rise in CA-125 gives an important lead-time of up to 3 months prior to clinical detection of disease. This allows adjuvant chemotherapy to be used when the disease volume is small.

In advanced disease, the CA-125 gives a measure of the response to chemotherapy as well as a marker for recurrence. Although there is a lead-time prior to clinically obvious disease in these women with advanced disease who have had a complete response to chemotherapy, second-line regimens are not offered until the woman is symptomatic because the treatment of recurrence is only palliative. Tumour markers in non-epithelial cancers are very useful. AFP, hCG and lactate dehydrogenase are indicated in germ-cell tumours and allow very accurate assessment of tumour activity. In view of the young age of these women and that fertility-sparing surgery is often used, these tumour markers are valuable for assessing physiological cysts which frequently appear on the remaining ovary.

Screening

The two screening procedures available for ovarian cancer are serum tumour marker estimations and pelvic ultrasound. The sensitivity and specificity of a bimanual pelvic examination, even when performed by a specialist, are too low for this to form part of a useful screening test. The use of a panel of complementary tumour markers in the initial screening test, with transvaginal sonography with colour Doppler to assess a positive initial screen, may refine screening. However, the natural history of ovarian cancer in its early stages is not clear. There is no evidence to show that early detection reduces mortality. In the high-risk group with a family history of cancer, a genetic marker (the breast–ovarian cancer families frequently have a BRCA-1 mutation on 17q or a BRCA-2 mutation on 13q), that is useful for screening, is a possibility. Unfortunately, the removal of the ovaries does not entirely prevent an ovarian cancer-like condition called carcinoma peritoneii. Also known as primary peritoneal carcinomatosis, it is treated in similar fashion to ovarian cancer.

Presentation

Early-stage disease is usually asymptomatic. There is even a small but significant incidence (up to 3.7%) of ovarian cancer in women with adnexal masses thought to be benign on ultrasound and laparoscopy. Seventy percent of women present with widespread abdominal disease (stage III) (Table 54.1). They present with vague symptoms such as abdominal pain and swelling, dyspepsia, bloating, constipation, vaginal bleeding and bowel obstruction. Physical signs include ascites, a pelvic and/or an abdominal mass and pleural effusions.

Prognostic features

Prognostic features in ovarian cancer can help to determine the management. Accepted factors include FIGO stage (the patients with more advanced stage do worse), performance status (the poorer the status the worse the outcome), age (the older the woman the worse the outcome, especially over 70 years), tumour differentiation (if poorly differentiated the outcome is worse), the

Table 54.1 The FIGO staging definitions for carcinoma of the ovary [1] and the 5-year survival rate [2]. The 5-year survival rate for all stages is 35–42%

Stage	Description	% surviving 5 years
I	Limited to the ovaries	70–100
a	Limited to one ovary with no ascites or tumour on the external surface	
b	Limited to both ovaries	
c	Either of above with positive cytology from ascites or peritoneal washings, or tumour on the surface of the capsule or cyst ruptured	
II	Pelvic extension	55–63
a	Extension to the uterus and/or tubes	
b	Extension to other pelvic tissues	
c	Either of the above with positive cytology from ascites or peritoneal washings, or tumour on the surface of the capsule or cyst ruptured	
III	Tumour outside the pelvis	10–27
a	Microscopic involvement of extrapelvic peritoneum	
b	Deposits of tumour ≤ 2 cm in abdomen	
c	Deposits of tumour ≥ 2 cm in abdomen and/or positive lymphadenopathy	
IV	Distant metastases including parenchymal liver involvement or cytologically positive pleural effusion	3–5

presence of ascites and residual tumour present following surgery (the best outcome is in those women with only microscopic amounts of residual disease remaining). Other features that appear to be significant are the tumour ploidy (aneuploid tumours have a worse prognosis), histological cell type (clear cell and mucinous types have a worse prognosis) and the clinician performing the initial surgery (gynaecological oncologist in the USA and possibly in the UK having better survival results than a general obstetrician/gynaecologist, who, in turn, has better results than a general surgeon) and the place of follow-up (women treated and followed-up in a combined clinic with a specialized gynaecologist and a medical oncologist do better than in a general clinic).

Treatment

Surgery plays a major role in the management of ovarian cancer [3]. At operation the diagnosis is confirmed (histology of the tumour removed), the disease can be appropriately staged (see Table 54.1) and therapy started. At this staging operation, the extent of the disease is

documented. Peritoneal cytology or ascites is sent for examination and multiple biopsies of the peritoneum are performed, including from the diaphragm. A lymphadenectomy may be useful in apparently early-stage disease as micrometastases would down-stage the woman to stage IIIc. Usually a bilateral oophorectomy, total abdominal hysterectomy, including the Fallopian tubes and cervix, and an infracolic omentectomy are performed at the primary surgery. Other tumour masses are removed if possible. The importance of accurate staging is that the stage will determine the prognosis and the subsequent therapy.

Surgery in the treatment of women with early-stage disease can be curative. This surgery includes removing the affected ovary, sampling the contralateral ovary and completing a full staging procedure. In the woman who has completed her family, it is sensible to remove the contralateral ovary and perform a hysterectomy. Although the prognostic significance of intra-operative tumour rupture appears not to be as important as previously believed, it is appropriate to excise the malignant cyst without spillage. This is of significance if the mass is being removed laparoscopically. Since the early 1970s, gynaecologists have been trying to reduce or completely remove the tumour bulk in advanced disease and this is called cytoreduction. Primary surgery is that performed at the initial staging. Interval surgery refers to an operation in those women who have had unresectable or unresected disease at primary surgery who then have a course of chemotherapy (three to four cycles) and then a planned attempt at aggressive surgery. Secondary surgery includes all the other aspects, such as the second-look procedure (an operation performed when the patient has had primary surgery, adjuvant chemotherapy and then achieved a clinical complete response), secondary cytoreductive and palliative surgery. The impact of primary cytoreduction on survival appeared to be significant based on retrospective data. However, the published work does not conclusively support the hypothesis that survival is improved by reducing tumour bulk with aggressive surgery (possible in 10–15% of all women with stage III disease), and that there is a definite survival advantage. Reducing the size of tumour to less than 1–2 cm in size also appears to help survival and this is possible in a further 30–40% of cases. The remaining women with stage III disease fall into the group who are suboptimally debulked. In the quest to remove the tumour plaques leading to this optimal cytoreduction, surgeons have tried peritoneal stripping, bowel resection and the removal of other organs affected by the cancer. This does not appear to be beneficial and it is thought that aspects of the tumour biology allow the surgeon to remove all the cancer in one woman and not in the next. However, other benefits of this surgery include the relief of symptoms and improvement in the quality of life. The value of the cytoreduction is the subject of several prospective studies in the UK and the results of these are awaited. It appears that there may be some role for interval debulking surgery after initial chemotherapy following minimal surgery. The second-look procedure is currently not used in the UK as there is no survival advantage. In woman with a complete pathological response, there is a false-negative rate with recurrence in up to 35% of patients.

The gynaecologist must be aware of the chemosensitivity of the germ-cell tumours and be prepared to perform conservative surgery in a young woman with an undiagnosed ovarian cancer. Preoperative tumour markers and referral to a specialist centre are mandatory for these women, in whom cure can now be expected.

Chemotherapy for germ-cell tumours has been very successful. Using the tumour markers to monitor response, aggressive combination chemotherapy such as bleomycin, etoposide and cisplatin (BEP) has cured 70% or more of these women, with their fertility being preserved. The dysgerminoma is very radiosensitive but is now also treated with chemotherapy so that fertility is preserved.

In epithelial ovarian cancers, the results of chemotherapy have not been so dramatic. It is clear that the treatment needs to include a platinum compound, as this is the single most active agent against epithelial ovarian cancer. With poor activity and concerns over the effects on the bone marrow and the long-term risk of leukaemia in the few survivors, there is now little place for chlorambucil or treosulfan. An oral platinum agent is on trial, which may be applicable for the very elderly or frail. However, carboplatin is extremely well tolerated when given using the Calvert formula based on the glomerular filtration rate (GFR). Although it was thought that carboplatin and cisplatin were directly interchangeable, this may not be the case in long-term survival [4]. It also appears that there is a survival advantage using combination chemotherapy over single-agent treatment. This combination adds in cyclophosphamide and Adriamycin to cisplatin. The dose intensity and total dose are being reviewed at present. Initially, it was felt that high-dose intensity was beneficial but the mature data shows the survival curves are now converging.

Platinum resistance does occur and this is where new drugs have been introduced such as the taxanes, gemcitabine and the topoisomerase-1 inhibitors. The taxanes include paclitaxel and docetaxel. Paclitaxel (derived from the bark of the Pacific yew tree) has shown significant crossreactivity in these patients who progress through standard treatment. The success of this drug is such that it is now being offered as first-line treatment in the USA in combination with cisplatin to women with advanced disease. One drawback of paclitaxel is the high cost of the drug. Docetaxel (a semisynthetic derivative from the needles of the European yew tree) has shown response rates of 25% in the face of platinum resistance. There appears to be a suggestion that consolidation treatment in conjunction with peripheral stem cell rescue similar to regimens in breast cancer may be useful in good prognosis cases. This would lead to a stratified treatment protocol with aggressive chemotherapy with an intent to cure in the good prognosis group and palliative chemotherapy with minimal side-effects in the poor prognosis group. Radiotherapy and intraperitoneal therapy have little role to play in the management of either early stage or advanced disease in the UK at present.

Conclusion

Ovarian cancer, a major killer of women in the UK, still represents a challenge in the 1990s. Advances are being made both to prevent the disease via screening and to treat the disease with better surgical and chemotherapeutic regimen which may improve survival and quality of life.

References

1. Crawford RAF, Shepherd JH. FIGO staging of gynaecological malignancies. *Contemp. Rev. Obstet. Gynaecol.* 1994;6:137–41.
2. Venesmaa P. Epithelial ovarian cancer: impact of surgery and chemotherapy on survival during 1977–1990. *Obstet. Gynecol.* 1994;84:8–11.
3. Cannistra SA. Medical progress: cancer of the ovary. *N. Engl. J. Med.* 1994;329:1550–9.
4. Neijt JP. Advances in chemotherapy of gynecologic cancer. *Curr. Opin. Oncol.* 1994;6:531–8.

55

Testicular Germ-cell Tumours

R. TIMOTHY D. OLIVER

Introduction

There is little dispute that the stem cells, which are the source of more than 90% of testicular cancer in young adults, the spermatogonia, are hormone dependent. Equally the occurrence of ectopic endocrinopathy from inappropriate hormone production by this group of tumours now collectively known as germ-cell cancers (GCCs) was discovered long before those from other tumour sites. This was because the Aschheim Zondek test for ovulation in frogs enabled the demonstration of what subsequently became known as human chorionic gonadotrophin (hCG) in males with testis cancer and gynaecomastia [1].

Despite this, apart from the demonstration of carcinoma-*in-situ*, changes in a small minority of biopsies from men with infertility [2] and more than 90% of GCCs [3], in recent years there has been very little input from endocrinologists into either the pathogenesis of testis cancer or its treatment. With an overall cure rate today in excess of 95% [4], one might question whether there was any need. However, late follow-up of cured patients demonstrates that 20% develop second non-testicular cancers within 20 years of radiation [5] when their average age would be only 55, while after excessive dosage of etoposide in excess of 1% develop leukaemias [6]. After cisplatin, hypertension, vascular and hearing problems are well documented late effects [7,8]. This is leading to considerable pressure to do trials risking less treatment in the more curable good risk patients, which is not without risk, as the 10% worse survival in trials of carboplatin [9] and similar worse results in trials to justify stopping use of bleomycin [10], illustrate.

It is the aim of this chapter to focus on the relevance of modern endocrinology to pathogenesis and treatment of testicular GCC and attempt to identify areas for the future where there may be a case for involvement of endocrinologists in development of new strategies for this disease.

Geographical epidemiology

Testis germ-cell tumours are the most frequent malignancy in males in Caucasian populations between the age of 20 and 34, when the lifetime risk is one in 500. In Asian, and particularly African, populations they are very rare, with the exception of the New Zealand Maori [11]. Germ-cell tumours are exceptionally rare prior to puberty, although there is a small peak in the first year of life, presumably reflecting the influence of intrauterine hormone milieus. It is this observation which may explain why the clinical behaviour of these tumours is more like a delayed paediatric tumour than an early-onset adult tumour in terms of response to chemotherapy and radiotherapy.

The peak age incidence in adults (20–45 years) precisely coincides with the period of maximum sexual activity in the male and recently, coincident with evidence of earlier onset of puberty and evidence of earlier onset of regular sexual activity, the incidence has begun to peak earlier, providing compelling evidence to suggest that the tumour, at least initially, must have some dependence on hormone factors.

Atrophy-induced gonadotrophin drive as the final common pathway of testis tumour development

As Table 55.1 demonstrates there has been a worldwide decline in sperm count [12] coincident with the rising incidence of GCC [13]. This is leading to increasing acceptance that gonadal atrophy with loss of feedback inhibition of the hypothalamus and increased gonadotrophin drive, thus allowing less time for repair of DNA

Table 55.1 Danish testis cancer incidence and overview of literature reports on sperm counts during the last 50 years (after [12])

Years	Incidence ($\times 10^5$)*	Number of studies†	Median of reported mean sperm count ($\times 10^6$/ml)	Proportion with sperm count $> 100 \times 10^6$/ml (%)
<1960	4.7	10 (1612)	107	46
1960–81	6.3	20 (2651)	84	25
1982–90	8.6	31 (10 679)	72	17

* From [13].
† n = Total number of cases in study.

damage, may be the final common pathway in tumour development [14,15]. Support for this comes from the demonstration that more than 70% of patients have evidence of reduced spermatogenesis from their contralateral 'normal' testis (Table 55.2).

That chemical-induced atrophy could be a factor comes from the discovery that military dogs returning from Vietnam after exposure to Agent Orange had an increased incidence of seminoma [13] and in addition to reduced sperm counts [17], one study of returning members of the armed forces also found an increased risk of GCC [18]. Attention has also focused on other agricultural organochlorine chemicals as possible contributing factors. They are well known to cause damage to the germinal epithelium [17] and also chronic immune suppression [19], which, in the setting of massive accidental overdose such as occurred in Bophal and in Minnesota, can be associated with the development of a human immuno-deficiency virus (HIV)-negative type of acquired immune deficiency syndrome (AIDS). The observation from Israel that substantial reduction (greater than 90%) in the levels of this group of chemicals in milk between 1976 and 1986 was associated with a 28% reduction in breast cancer in women under the age of 45 and 19% in women between 45 and 64 [20], may provide an explanation as to why one study has observed a significant association between consumption of milk and risk of GCC [21], while a report from Denmark has claimed that organic food farmers have higher than average sperm counts [22].

That agricultural organochlorine compounds are not the only gonadal atrophogens involved comes from the recently published results from a case control epidemiological risk factor study involving 794 patients and controls [23,24]. The observation of a significant association with testicular trauma, always held in suspicion because of recall bias, and orchitis, venereal disease and infertility points to the fact that there may be multiple interacting atrophogens involved. The observation from the same studies that early puberty and a sedentary lifestyle increase risk, while late onset of puberty and more than average exercise (known from studies in women to reduce gonadotrophin production and reduce breast cancer risk) is protective (Table 55.3), provided added evidence that gonadotrophin drive is important in development of these tumours.

There have been two reports suggesting that serum follicle-stimulating hormone (FSH) levels may be of prognostic significance in the clinical behaviour of GCC. The first from Norway [25] demonstrated that patients with an elevated FSH had a higher than average risk

Table 55.2 Semen analysis in normal males and patients with germ-cell tumours [16]

	Number of cases	Sperm count Median count ($\times 10^6$/ml)	$< 20 \times 10^6$/ml (%)	20–40 $\times 10^6$/ml (%)	$> 40 \times 10^6$/ml (%)
Normal male:					
Fertile	104	84.0	11.5	11.5	77
Infertile	53	10.0	68.0	8.0	28
Testis tumour:					
stage I on surveillance	16	7.5	75.0	0.0	25
Metastatic prechemotherapy	24	10.0	71.0	8.0	21
Metastatic postchemotherapy	27	7.0	70.0	7.0	22

Table 55.3 UK Testicular Cancer Study Group risk factors in testis tumour and control population (after [23, 24])

Risk factor	Number in group	Percentage	χ^2 for trend
Voice broke ≤ 13 years			
Testis tumour	552	47	6.7
Neighbourhood control	550	40	
Started shaving ≤ 16 years			
Testis tumour	749	49	7.2
Neighbourhood control	757	43	
First nocturnal emission at ≤ 14 years			
Testis tumour	652	57	4.6
Neighbourhood control	628	51	
Sexual activity at age 20 > 2–3/week			
Testis tumour	689	72	4.9
Neighbourhood control	692	67	
Exercise at time of diagnosis < 4 h/week			
Testis cancer	794	73	3.4
Neighbourhood control	793	69	
Sitting at time of diagnosis > 10 h/day			
Testis cancer	793	29	7.9
Neighbourhood control	794	23	

for the development of tumours in the contralateral testis, and Hornac and colleagues, in a report from Slovakia, demonstrated that patients with raised FSH on surveillance have a higher risk of relapse [26]. This suggests that the early stages of GCC, which as the next section indicates could include seminoma, may be hormone dependent.

The only factor that does not fit with this hypothesis is the observation that germ-cell tumour incidence decreases after its peak at 30–35 years when FSH levels are rising in association with declining sperm count. A possible explanation could be that the vulnerable stem cells or the Sertoli cells become menopausal and are switched off or exhausted at this stage or there is an organ resistance to FSH. Recent evidence that inhibin has a wide pleotrophic tumour-suppressive effect provides one avenue in need of further investigation to explain this paradox.

There are two therapeutic options that might emerge from these observations on the prognostic significance of elevated FSH on development of metastases and tumours in the contralateral testis. The first is that such patients at diagnosis might benefit from automatic use of testosterone replacement, even in patients not suffering

loss of libido, to suppress the hypothalamus and reduce gonadotrophin drive. The second therapeutic option that could be explored arising out of these observations is the possibility of using short-term total androgen blockade to treat carcinoma-*in-situ*. Old experimental animal data [27], now supported from some recent clinical observations [28,29] emerging from study of the effects of hormone treatment on the immune system (i.e. its ability to induce lymphocytosis and thymic regeneration), suggests that endocrine therapy might have an immunoadjuvant effect, which could enable short-term endocrine therapy completely to reject premalignant cells. It has been speculated that this may explain why some patients with prostate cancer can have durable remissions after stopping hor-mone therapy [30].

Modern views on GCC pathology

It is increasingly accepted that most tissue cell growth is regulated in an endocrine manner by positive growth factors stimulating growth and negative inhibitors of growth (so-called suppressor genes) inhibiting replication and enhancing cellular differentiation. Understanding this endocrinology is increasingly important in cancer as mutation in the set of genes called cellular oncogenes (so called because mutated forms of these genes were found in oncogenic viruses), leads to increased growth of cancers as do deletions of DNA material controlling suppressor genes [31].

It is now more than 15 years since the early cytogenetic data of Atkin first led to the suggestion that nonseminomas with a modal DNA content of 2.8 N may, at least in part, arise by clonal evolution from seminoma with a modal DNA content of 3.6 N in association with chromosomal loss [16]. The subsequent discovery of premalignant carcinoma-*in-situ* lesions in testis biopsies from men with infertility, and the association of this pathological feature with all types of GCC (Table 55.4) has been particularly important for understanding the cytogenetics. This was because these cells had higher chromosome numbers than both seminoma and nonseminoma and a minority of tumours containing both seminoma and non-seminoma elements had a gradient in DNA content between carcinoma-*in-situ*, seminoma and non-seminoma components [33]. This led to the conclusion that in the majority of patients the chromosomal loss occurred before development of the solid tumour element.

It is clear from reviewing the data presented in Table 55.5 that for all parameters examined patients with combined seminoma/non-seminoma display characteristics that are intermediate between those of pure seminoma

Table 55.4 Risk factors for carcinoma-*in-situ* (CIS) (after [32])

Subpopulation	Prevalence of CIS
General Danish male population	< 0.8%
Cryptorchidism	2.0–3.0%
Infertility	0.4–1.1%
Unilateral GCC*	5.0–6.0%
Unilateral GCC†	94.0%
Extragonadal GCC	35.0%
Androgen insensitivity	25.0% (4/12)
Gonadal dysgenesis	High (4/4)

* Contralateral testis.
† Ipsilateral testis.
GCC, germ-cell cancer.

and pure non-seminoma. It is this gradient, taken with the morphological similarity between seminoma cells and the spermatogonia, that justifies applying the principles used in grading other solid cancers to seminoma and considering it as grade 1 or well-differentiated GCC (G1 GCC) with respect to its cell of origin [34]. On this basis, combined tumours with both cell types would be considered as grade 2 or intermediate differentiated GCC (G2 GCC) and pure non-seminoma (so-called malignant teratoma in the British Testicular Tumour Panel classification) without any cells resembling the differentiated stem cell would be considered as undifferentiated or grade 3 GCC (G3 GCC).

Although this scheme explains very clearly the relationship between seminoma and the embryonal carcinoma elements it does not explain the occurrence of extra-embryonic tissue such as trophoblast and yolk sac or fetal tissues such as cartilage, glandular or neural elements. The increasing frequency with which immunocytochemistry is identifying these elements in other solid tumours such as bladder cancer [35] and classifying them as metaplastic components provides a possible solution for improving the precision of classification in combination with a grading classification. The report from Murty and colleagues that GCC with somatic elements have a higher level of loss of heterozygosity than other GCC [36] provides a justification for considering the clonal grading evolution and fetal/somatic tissue differentiation as two separate dimensions of GCC development.

Contribution of immune response to prognostication of metastatic seminoma

Although considerable scepticism persists about the practical relevance of the concept of immune surveillance in cancer, the 60% durable complete remission of patients with superficial bladder cancer treated by intravesical bacille Calmette–Guérin (BCG) and its durability correlating with degree of interleukin-2 induction, the high response rate of wart-virus-induced tumours to α-interferon and the occurrence of up to 5% durable (more than 5 years) complete remission of terminal renal cell

Table 55.5 Combined tumours as an intermediate prognosis subgroup of testicular germ-cell tumours [34]

Group	Seminoma (*n* = 248) (%)	Combined seminoma/ non-seminoma (*n* = 116) (%)	Non-seminoma (*n* = 241) (%)
Proportion presenting in stage I	79	51	41
Relapse stage I after adjuvant chemotherapy	1	6	0
Relapse stage I after surveillance only	23	31	38
Primary cure of all metastatic patients	91	93	86
Proportion of metastatic cases with high markers	0	16	21
Cure rate low markers	91	94	92
Cure rate high markers	–	89	65

The median age for stage I patients with: seminoma is 36 years; non-seminoma, 29 years; combined seminoma/non-seminoma 31 years. The median age for metastatic patients with: seminoma is 42 years; non-seminoma, 29 years; combined seminoma/non-seminoma 37 years.

cancer and melanoma patients after interleukin-2 regimens, are the most convincing evidence that even today there are limited areas of gain from immunotherapy (for review see [37]). The evidence that the survival of cancer patients might be improved if it were possible to reduce the immunosuppression occurring after prolonged anaesthesia for surgical procedures, blood transfusion, pregnancy or in heavy smokers provide additional reasons for clinical awareness of the relevance of immune suppression (for review see [37]), over and above its effect in HIV-positive and transplant patients [38]. New evidence that the durable cure rate after chemotherapy of the curable cancers such as Hodgkin's disease [39] and high-grade non-Hodgkin's lymphoma [40] but also including GCC [41] in immune-deprived patients, is substantially lower than in patients with a normal immune response, even after exclusion of those patients dying from infectious complications, provides added evidence for the importance of antitumour immune response.

As discussed earlier (see p. 338), seminoma is the germ-cell tumour of which the morphology most closely resembles the original starting stem cell, the spermatogonium, and can therefore be functionally considered as well differentiated. This tumour's excessive levels of lymphocyte infiltrate [42] and high frequency of spontaneous regression [16] has long been well established. The idea discussed earlier that GCC develop in a clonal way [16] in association with chromosomal loss from near tetraploid carcinoma-*in-situ* via seminoma (DNA content 3.6 N) and combined tumours (mixed content populations) to embryonal carcinoma (DNA content 2.8 N), fits closely to the accepted clonal evolution with increasing escape from immune surveillance from grade 1 to grade 3 tumours in other adult cancers and explains why seminoma like other grade 1 tumours such as superficial bladder cancer demonstrates more evidence for the importance of antitumour immune response.

Clinical use of oncofetal markers

Although known about for a long time since the advent of the Aschheim Zondek test [1], the real era of tumour markers began with the advent of radioimmunoassays and today use of such assays is an integral part of patient management. Marker decline rate at the appropriate half-life (36 hours for human chorionic gonadotrophin (β-hCG) and 6 days for α-fetoprotein) after orchidectomy in patients without obvious metastases is a routine way to establish the absence of metastasis and in some centres also for response of metastases to chemotherapy [43], although this is more disputed because many patients with metastases develop posttreatment surges due to tumour

lysis [44]. The third main area is in detection of relapse, although it cannot be relied on totally as one-third of relapses are marker-negative and are picked up by scans [45].

Although α-fetoprotein and β-hCG are the most frequently used tumour markers for clinical monitoring of patients, other markers have been used to a lesser extent. The most valuable is lactic dehydrogenase (LDH), particularly the isoform LDH-1 [46], which in clinical practice is most easily defined by the assay for hydroxy-butyric dehydrogenase (HBD) performed at a temperature of 37°C. This, as well as predicting patients with a high risk of metastases resistant to chemotherapy, is also paradoxically positive in seminoma patients, who by definition are hCG and α-fetoprotein negative. Placental alkaline phosphatase is another marker that is specific for seminoma [47], although false-positives in smokers have limited the reliability of the assay.

Currently, as far as prognostication is concerned, tumour marker levels are proving more important than actual anatomical volume of metastases in defining a prognostic index to identify patients with high, intermediate and low chance of cure by modern chemotherapy [48].

Clinical behaviour and response to treatment

The last 80 years has seen the overall cure rate of testicular GCC rise from 15 to 95%. Although a major part of this has occurred in the last 10 years since the introduction of cisplatin-based chemotherapy (Fig. 55.1), there has been a continuous improvement since the end of the 19th century. Table 55.6 summarizes the results by stage and histology subgroup and Table 55.7 lists the current standard and experimental approaches.

Metastatic disease

During the last 15 years of curative chemotherapy for GCC as summarized in Table 55.8, there have been four principal schools of chemotherapy development (for review see [49]), although large-scale clinical trials have now established a consensus that the combination of bleomycin, etoposide and cisplatin (BEP) developed by the substitution of etoposide instead of vinblastine in Einhorn's original platinum, vinblastine and bleomycin (PVB) regimen [50,51], is the most effective and this is now the standard for all stages and histological subgroups. This is a 3–5 day treatment normally given as an in-patient for four courses. Although total alopecia is universal and cumulative lethargy and anaemia result in the patient being unable to work during the 3 months of

342   *Chapter 55*

Table 55.10 Relapse and area under curve (AUC) optimization of carboplatin dose for germ-cell cancer (after [55])

AUC	Number of cases	Relapse rate (%)
< 4.0	8	50
4–4.5	20	10
4.6–5.0	73	4
> 5.0	20	0

Early-stage tumours

Although many centres still routinely use radiation for stage I seminoma, the recent reports that 20% of these young patients may develop second tumours by 20 years [5] and the success of chemotherapy in metastatic seminoma, where bulky metastases could be cured with cisplatin alone [14], has led to trials using two, and, more recently, a single course of carboplatin as an adjuvant [56]. To date with 106 patients followed for 2 years or more, of whom more than 30 have been followed for 5 years, there has only been one relapse. This is at least as good, possibly better, than radiation (Fig. 55.2), which is associated with a 3–5% relapse rate, although it is too early to know if the incidence of late effects has been reduced.

Today, patients are being diagnosed earlier with smaller tumours [57]. The demonstration in patients who had such extensive disease that they were unfit for orchidectomy, that chemotherapy can cure primary tumours as well as metastases has led to increasing interest in using chemotherapy as treatment for primary tumours [57]. This, as well as saving patients from having to undergo orchidectomy if they have a tumour in a solitary testis,

could also be of value to the 75% who have some degree of atrophy in their contralateral testis. Reports of successful parenting after treatment of tumours in solitary testis [58] is providing powerful justification for such studies.

Conclusion

The equisite chemosensitivity of GCC is demonstrated by the fact that even in the third-line setting there are drugs that can cure one in five patients, while in the earliest stage of the disease, that is stage I seminoma, a 25% risk of relapse has been eliminated by a single dose of carboplatin. Today overall more than 95% of patients presenting with a testicular GCC can expect to be cured by orchidectomy combined with BEP for patients with metastases. It is clear that the last 15 years have seen a revolution in treatment of this tumour, although with the demonstration that testis-conserving chemotherapy is possible and the development of less toxic drugs for use as an out-patient, there remain important clinical studies that will stimulate interest in this tumour for a long time to come.

The advances of the last decade in molecular biology have also transformed our understanding of the genetics of development of testicular GCC, with increasing support for the view that clonal evolution from carcinoma-*in-situ* through seminoma and combined seminoma/non-seminoma to pure non-seminoma is a realistic possibility to explain the myriad of cell types found in this group of tumours.

It is, however, in the epidemiology and specifically in understanding the role in tumour development of gonadotrophin and sex hormone driven proliferation of germ cells under circumstances of chemical, viral and

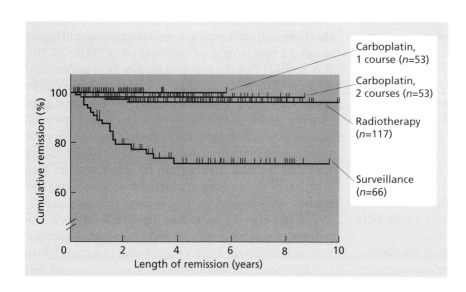

Fig. 55.2 Stage I seminoma relapse-free survival after radiotherapy, adjuvant carboplatin or surveillance.

traumatic atrophic damage that is of increasing interest to the endocrinologist. In addition at the therapeutic level the possibility of using short-term endocrine treatment for the premalignant changes is another area with potential for interesting collaboration between oncologists and endocrinologists in the next decade.

References

1. Ferguson RS. Quantitative behaviour of prolan A in teratoma testis. *Am. J. Cancer* 1933;**18**:269–95.
2. Skakkbaek NE. Possible carcinoma-*in-situ* of the testis. *Lancet* 1972;**2**:516–17.
3. Jacobsen GK, Henriksen OB, von der Maase H. Carcinoma *in-situ* of testicular tissue adjacent to malignant germ cell tumours. A study of 105 cases. *Cancer* 1981;**47**:2260–2.
4. Oliver RTD, Fowler CG. Testis. In Allen-Mersch TG (ed.). *Bailey and Love Companion Series: Surgical Oncology.* London: Chapman and Hall, 1995:267–89.
5. van Leeuwen FE, Stiggelbout AM, Vandenbeltdusebout AW *et al.* Second tumours after radiation treatment of testicular germ-cell tumors. *J. Clin. Oncol.* 1993;**11**:2286–7.
6. Boshoff CB, Begent RHJ, Oliver RTD *et al.* Secondary tumours following etoposide containing therapy for germ cell cancer. *Ann. Oncol.* 1994;**6**:35–40.
7. Hansen SW, Groth S, Dawgaard G, Rossing N, Rorth M. Long term effects on renal function and blood pressure of treatment with cisplatin, vinblastine and bleomycin in patients with germ cell cancer. *J. Clin. Oncol.* 1988;**6**:1728–31.
8. Gietema JA, Devries EGE, Sleijfer DT. Increased incidence of cardiovascular risk factors in cured testicular cancer patients. *J. Clin. Oncol.* 1992;**10**:1652.
9. Horwich A, Sleijfer D. Carboplatin-based chemotherapy in good prognosis metastatic non seminoma of the testis (NSGCT): an interim report of an MRC/EORTC randomised trial. *Eur. J. Cancer Proc. ECCO 7* 1993;**29A**:1350 (abstr).
10. Loehrer PJ, Elson P, Johnson DH *et al.* A randomised trial of cisplatin plus etoposide with or without bleomycin in favorable prognosis disseminated germ cell tumours. *Proc. ASCO* 1991;**10**:169, (abstr. 540).
11. Wilkinson TJ, Colls BM, Schluter PJ. Increased incidence of germ cell testicular cancer in New Zealand Maoris. *Br. J. Cancer* 1992;**65**:769–71.
12. Carlsen E, Giwercman A, Keiding N, Skakkebaek NE. Evidence for decreasing quality of semen during the past 50 years. *Br. Med. J.* 1992;**305**:609–12.
13. Møller H. Clues to the aetiology of testicular germ cell tumours from descriptive epidemiology. *Eur. Urol.* 1993;**23**:8–15.
14. Oliver RTD, Love S, Ong J. Alternatives to radiotherapy in management of seminoma. *Br. J. Urol.* 1990;**65**:61–7.
15. Oliver RTD. Atrophy, hormones, genes and viruses in aetiological germ cell tumours. *Cancer Surv.* 1990;**9**:263–8.
16. Oliver RTD. Clues from natural history and results of treatment supporting the monoclonal origin of germ cell tumours. *Cancer Surv.* 1990;**9**:332–68.
17. Destefano F, Annest JL, Kresnow M. Semen characteristics of Vietnam veterans. *Reprod. Toxicol.* 1989;**3**:165–73.
18. Tarone RE, Hayes HM, Hoover RN, Rosenthal JF. Service in Vietnam and risk of testicular cancer. *J. Nat. Cancer Inst.* 1990;**83**:1497–9.
19. Bekesi J, Roboz J, Solomon S *et al.* Altered immune function in Michigan residents exposed to polybrominated biphenyls. *Immunotoxicology* 1983;**1**:181–91.
20. Westin JB, Richter E. The Israeli breast cancer anomaly. *Ann. NY Acad. Sci.* 1990;**609**:269–79.
21. Davies T, Ruya E, Palmer R. Diet and testicular cancer. *Br. J. Cancer* 1996; (in press).
22. Abell A. Organic food and sperm counts in men. *Lancet* 1994;**343**:1498.
23. Chilvers CED, Forman D, Oliver RTD, Pike MC and the Testicular Cancer Study Group. Social, behavioural and medical factors in the aetiology of testicular cancer: results from the UK study. *Br. J. Cancer* 1994;**70**:513–20.
24. Forman D, Chilvers C, Oliver R, Pike M. The aetiology of testicular cancer: association with congenital abnormalities, age at puberty, infertility and exercise. *Br. Med. J.* 1994;**308**:1393–9.
25. Hoff Wanderas E, Fossa SD, Heilo A, Stenwig AE, Norman N. Serum follicle stimulating hormone — predictor of cancer in the remaining testis in patients with unilateral testicular cancer. *Br. J. Cancer* 1990;**66**:315–17.
26. Hornac M, Zvara V, Oridus D. La 'Surveillance' de temeurs non-seminomateuses de testicule. *Ann. Urol.* 1992;**26**:306–10.
27. Grossman CJ. Interactions between the gonadal-steroids and the immune system. *Science* 1985;**227**:257–61.
28. Oliver RTD, Joseph JV, Gallagher CJ. Castration-induced lymphocytosis in prostate cancer: possible evidence for gonad/thymus endocrine interaction in man. *Urol. Int.* 1995;**54**(4):226.
29. Sperandio P, Tomio P, Oliver RTD, Fiorentino MV, Pagano F. Gonadal atrophy as a cause of thymic hyyperplasia after chemotherapy. *Br. J. Cancer* 1996 (in press).
30. Oliver R, Gallagher C. Intermittent endocrine therapy and its potential for chemoprevention of prostate cancer. *Cancer Surv.* 1995;**23**:191.
31. Vogelstein B, Fearon ER, Hamilton SR *et al.* Genetic alterations during colorectal-tumor development. *N. Engl. J. Med.* 1988;**319**:527–32.
32. Giwercman A, von der Maase H, Skakkebaek NE. Epidemiological and clinical aspects of carcinoma *in situ* of the testis. *Eur. Urol.* 1993;**23**:104–14.
33. Oosterhuis JW, Gillis AJM, van Putten WJL, de Jong B, Looijenga LHJ. Interphase cytogenetics of carcinoma *in situ* of the testis. *Eur. Urol.* 1993;**23**:16–22.
34. Oliver RTD, Leahy M, Ong J. Combined seminoma/non-seminoma should be considered as intermediate grade germ cell cancer (GCC). *Eur. J. Cancer* 1995;**31A**:1392–4.
35. Oliver RTD, Nouri AME, Crosby D *et al.* Biological significance of beta hCG, HLA and other membrane antigen expression on bladder tumours and their relationship to tumour infiltrating lymphocytes (TIL). *J. Immunogenet.* 1989;**16**:381–90.
36. Murty VVVS, Bosi G, Houldsworth J *et al.* Allelic loss and somatic differentiation in human male germ cell tumors. *Oncogene* 1994;**9**:2245–51.
37. Oliver RTD, Nouri AME. T cell immune response to cancer in humans and its relevance for immunodiagnosis and therapy. *Cancer Surv.* 1991;**13**:173–204.
38. Penn I. Cancers complicating organ transplantation. *N. Engl. J. Med.* 1990;**323**:1967–8.
39. Levy R, Colonna P, Tournani J. Human immunodeficiency virus associated with Hodgkin's disease: report of 45 cases from the French Registry of HIV associated tumours. *Leuk. Lymphoma* 1995;**16**:451.
40. Gill P, Levine A, Krailo M. AIDS related malignant lymphoma:

results of prospective treatment trials. *J. Clin. Oncol.* 1987;5:1322–8.

41. Vaccher E, Bernardi D, Errante D *et al.* Treatments of testicular germ-cell tumours in patients with HIV infection: the GICAT experience. *Ann. Oncol.* 1994;5:3(abstr. 06).

42. Marshall AME, Dayan AD. Immunological reaction in man against certain tumours. *Lancet* 1964;2:1102–3.

43. Toner GG, Geller NL, Tom C *et al.* Serum tumour marker half life during chemotherapy. *Cancer Res.* 1990;50:5904–10.

44. Kohn JRD, Raghaven D. Tumour markers in malignant germ cell tumours. In Peckham M (ed.) *The Management of Testicular Tumours.* London: Edward Arnold, 1981:50–69.

45. Freedman LS, Parkinson MC, Jones WG *et al.* Histopathology in the prediction of relapse of patients with stage 1 testicular teratoma treated by orchidectomy alone. On behalf of MRC Testicular Tumour Subgroup (Urological Working Party). *Lancet* 1987;2:294–8.

46. Von Eyben FE, Blaabjerg O, Madsen EL *et al.* Serum lactate dehydrogenase isoenzyme-1 and tumour volume are indicators of response to treatment and predictors of prognosis in metastatic testicular germ cell tumours. *Eur. J. Cancer* 1992;29:664–8.

47. Tucker DF, Oliver RTD, Travers P, Bodmer WF. Serum marker potential of placental alkaline phosphatase-like activity in testicular germ cell tumours evaluated by H17E2 monoclonal antibody assay. *Br. J. Cancer* 1985;51:631–9.

48. Mead GM, Stenning SP, Cullen MH *et al.* The Second Medical Research Study of prognostic factors in nonseminomatous germ cell tumours. *Clin. Oncol.* 1992;10:85–94.

49. Oliver RTD, Gallagher CJ. Intermittent endocrine therapy and its potential for chemoprevention of prostate cancer. *Cancer Surv.* 1995;23:191–207.

50. Einhorn LH, Donohue JP. *Cis*-diaminodichloroplatinum, vinblastine, and bleomycin combination chemotherapy in disseminated testicular cancer. *Ann. Intern. Med.* 1977;87:293–8.

51. Peckham MJ, Barrett A, Liew KH *et al.* The treatment of metastatic germ-cell testicular tumours with bleomycin, etoposide and cisplatin (BEP). *Br. J. Cancer* 1983;47:613–19.

52. Motzer RJ, Bosl GJ. High-dose chemotherapy for resistant germ cell tumors: recent advances and future directions. *J. Natl. Cancer Inst.* 1992;84:1703–9.

53. Mead GM. International consensus on prognostic factor clarification of metastatic germ cell tumour. *Proc. Am. Soc. Clin. Oncol.* 1995;14:235(abstr. 615).

54. Jodrell DI, Egorin MJ, Canetta RM. Relationships between carboplatin exposure and tumour response and toxicity in patients with ovarian cancer. *J. Clin. Oncol.* 1992;10:520–8.

55. Childs WJ, Nicholls EJ, Horwich A. The optimisation of carboplatin dose in carboplatin, etoposide and bleomycin combination chemotherapy for good prognosis metastatic non-seminomatous germ cell tumours of the testis. *Ann. Oncol.* 1992;3:291–6.

56. Oliver RTD, Edmonds P, Ong JYH *et al.* Pilot studies of 2 and 1 course carboplatin as adjuvant for stage I seminoma: should it be tested in a randomised trial against radiotherapy? *Int. J. Rad. Oncol. Biol. Phys.* 1994;29:3–8.

57. Oliver R, Ong J, Blandy J, Altman D. Testis conservation studies in germ cell cancer justified by improved primary chemotherapy response and reduced delay 1978–1994. *Br. J. Urol.* 1996; (in press).

58. Sobeh M, Jenkins BJ, Paris AMI, Oliver RTD. Partial orchidectomy for secondary testis tumours. *Eur. J. Surg. Oncol.* 1994;20:585–6.

56

Neoplasia and Intersex States

MARIA E. STREET, DAVID LOWE AND MARTIN O. SAVAGE

Introduction

Disorders of sexual differentiation lead to states of clinical intersexuality which are characterized by abnormal internal or external genital structures. The basic defects are present during the process of fetal sexual differentiation and the child presents either at birth with ambiguous external genitalia or, more rarely, at puberty because of abnormal development. The classification of patients with intersex states is based on the karyotype and the morphology and differentiation of the fetal gonads. The most simple classification is shown in Table 56.1.

An important aspect of intersex disorders is the widely recognized association between certain of these conditions and gonadal neoplasia [1]. Their occurrence appears principally related to the presence of dysgenetic gonadal tissue and Y chromosomal material [2]. The most frequent neoplasms are of germ-cell origin [3]. This chapter reviews the intersex disorders that confer risk of neoplasm formation and the principal forms of neoplasia. We also discuss the prevention and management of these tumours.

Physiology of fetal sexual differentiation

It is important to have a basic knowledge of the sexual differentiation of the fetus because this provides the theoretical basis for the investigation and classification of the intersex conditions. Both female and male gonads originate from a gonadal primordium, the gonadal ridge, which is progressively colonized by primordial germ cells originating in the stalk of the allantois. In the male, primordial Sertoli cells develop at this stage and aggregate to form sex cords in which germ cells become enclosed. The testis as a structure can be recognized from the seventh week of gestation. The Sertoli cells then begin to secrete the anti-Müllerian hormone (AMH) which inhibits Müllerian structure development. Stro-

mal Leydig cells become active at 8 weeks and produce testosterone, which is responsible for the virilization of the Wolffian duct derivatives, that is the vasa deferentia, seminal vesicles and epididymides.

The principal genes encoding for the male sexual differentiation are carried on the Y chromosome. Currently the best candidate for the testis-determining factor (TDF) appears to be the *SRY* gene [4], which is close to the pseudoautosomal boundary of the Y chromosome. Hormones, principally AMH, and other genes on autosomal chromosomes are also probably involved in the process. In normal males Müllerian regression occurs between 8 and 12 weeks of gestation. The virilization of tissues such as the urogenital sinus and the external genitalia, which normally have 5-α-reductase activity, depends on dihydrotestosterone rather than testosterone alone.

Normal female sexual differentiation requires two normal X chromosomes. In the female gonadal blastema, oogonia and somatic cells are mixed until the second month of gestation. The production of oestrogen by the granulosa cells begins after 8 weeks of gestation, and the Fallopian tubes, uterus and upper part of the vagina originate from the Müllerian ducts. The vagina forms, after the degeneration of the Wolffian ducts, at the site of the Müllerian tubercle at the level of the urogenital sinus. Labia majora originate from the dorsal commissure and the urethral folds give rise to the labia minora. The primordial phallus develops into the clitoris. In both males and females genital development is completed by 20 weeks of fetal life.

Gonadal dysgenesis

In gonadal dysgenesis one or both of the gonads are 'streak gonads', consisting of gonadal-type fibrous tissue. Some classifications include gonads with areas of recognizable but poorly formed testicular or ovarian elements in this fibrous tissue, but these are better considered as

Table 56.1 Classification of patients with intersex states

Female pseudohermaphrodites
Virilization of genetic females with ovaries

Male pseudohermaphrodites
Incomplete virilization of genetic males
with testes

True hermaphrodites
Individuals with both ovarian and
testicular tissue

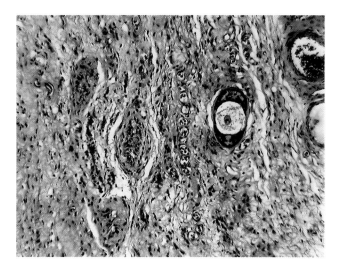

Fig. 56.1 An ovotestis, which is composed of sclerosed testicular tubules lined by Sertoli cells only (left of centre) and developing Graffian follicles containing oocytes (right of centre).

pseudohermaphrodite gonads (see below). Gonadal dysgenesis occurs as a result of an unknown defect in the cytogenetic control of gonadal differentiation. Some authors state that a 'streak gonad' must be devoid of germ cells, but as gonadoblastomas and dysgerminoma/seminoma have been reported in these organs, this cannot be considered essential [5]. The terms 'dysgenetic testis' and 'dysgenetic ovary' refer to gonads in which sufficient differentiation has occurred in a streak gonad to allow categorization of the gonad type; they are composed of dense gonadal-type fibrous tissue in which small numbers of immature testicular cords or primitive ovarian follicles are present (Fig. 56.1) [5].

Pure gonadal dysgenesis

These patients usually have a female phenotype without external genital ambiguity and the female internal genitalia are normal except for the gonads. There are bilateral streak gonads and the karyotype may be either 46XY or 46XX. Malignant germ-cell tumours have been described, especially in XY subjects, where 20–30% of the patients develop gonadoblastomas.

Gonadal dysgenesis of 46XY type may be inherited as an X-linked recessive or male-limited autosomal dominant condition. A subgroup has balanced translocations on the X chromosome. In XY pure gonadal dysgenesis as many as five different histological subtypes of germ-cell malignancies have been described, namely gonadoblastoma, germinoma, mature teratoma, malignant teratoma undifferentiated (embryonal carcinoma), and yolk sac tumour [6]. Familial germ-cell tumours are recognized in kinships with pure gonadal dysgenesis.

Mixed gonadal dysgenesis

The features of mixed gonadal dysgenesis are a unilateral testis and contralateral streak gonad. Persistent Müllerian structures are present due to decreased production of AMH, usually by the streak gonad. External genitalia are often ambiguous, but may range from normal female to normal male in appearance [7]. Phenotypic females may present with virilization.

The most common karyotype is 45XO/46XY mosaicism, a Y chromosome being present in all patients. Due to the XO cells, features of Turner's syndrome may be present. Germ-cell tumours are common in these patients and in one series seven of 15 patients had gonadal tumours. Gonadoblastoma, germinoma, malignant intratubular germ-cell neoplasia and gonadal stromal tumour have been described [7]. The most common tumour is gonadoblastoma.

Male pseudohermaphroditism

The only recognizable gonadal element in subjects with male pseudohermaphroditism is testicular tissue, which is almost always found bilaterally. The anatomical sexual differentiation can vary from normal female appearance to male genitalia with perineal hypospadias. The karyotype is 46XY. The main aetiological groups are described below.

Testosterone biosynthetic defects

Testosterone biosynthetic defects are characterized by inadequate testosterone secretion by the testes. The gonads are not prone to develop malignancies, although adrenal cortical cell rests in the gonads may mimic tumours.

5-α-reductase deficiency

Individuals with 5-α-reductase deficiency are unable to convert testosterone to dihydrotestosterone and are phenotypically female until puberty when virilization occurs. Gonadal tumours have not been described in these patients.

Testicular feminization syndrome

Testicular feminization syndrome, also known as androgen insensitivity syndrome, results from qualitative defects in androgen binding, usually related to mutations of the androgen-receptor gene. The phenotype is essentially female and testes are usually undescended. Leydig and Sertoli cells may be hyperplastic. At puberty breast development occurs, but pubic and axillary hair is often scanty and menstruation is absent owing to suppression of Müllerian structures.

Several gonadal neoplasms have been described in these patients (Table 56.2) [3]. Dysgerminoma/seminoma is very rare in childhood but has a high incidence in adults with this condition [8]. Intratubular germ-cell neoplasia (carcinoma-*in-situ*) has been described in prepubertal children with androgen insensitivity [9].

Dysgenetic male pseudohermaphroditism

Dysgenetic testes secrete so little testosterone and AMH that Müllerian structures persist, and result in ambiguous genitalia and cryptorchidism. Gonadoblastoma and invasive germ-cell tumours have been described, particularly in intra-abdominal or inguinal testes. These occur rarely during the prepubertal period but with increasing incidence after puberty.

True hermaphroditism

The diagnosis of ture hermaphroditism is based on the presence in a person of both ovarian and testicular tissues. These may coexist in one or both gonads (ovotestes) (see Figs 56.1 and 56.2) or be separate as a testis and

Table 56.2 Disorders of sexual differentiation predisposing to gonadal neoplasia

Gonadal dysgenesis
Mixed gonadal dysgenesis
Dysgenetic male pseudohermaphroditism
Pure gonadal dysgenesis
True hermaphroditism
Testicular feminization

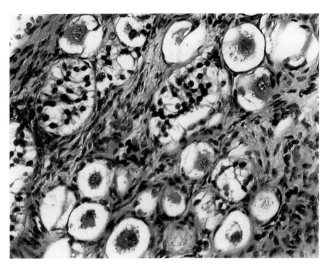

Fig. 56.2 An ovotestis in which the gonadal components are more intimately mixed than in Fig. 56.1. There are numerous very large oocytes in the stroma around testicular tubules containing Sertoli cells only (upper and left field).

a contralateral ovary. The presence of densely cellular, spindle-celled stroma is a common feature in both gonads. In the ovotestis the oocytes are usually in the cortical area surrounded by dense fibrous tissue and the testicular elements are in the central medullary area. The most common combination of gonads is an ovotestis with a contralateral ovary, followed by bilateral ovotestes.

Most true hermaphrodites are 46XX. About one-third are 46XX/46XY mosaics. The demonstration of a Y chromosome is associated with a two- to threefold increase in frequency of testis rather than ovotestis formation [7], together with an increased risk of gonadal neoplasia.

Gonadoblastoma, dysgerminoma/seminoma, teratoma, Brenner tumour, mucinous cystadenoma and gynandroblastoma have all been described in these patients. In a very large series of patients [10] dysgerminoma was the most frequent malignancy and was thought to arise from a pre-existing gonadoblastoma. Gonadoblastomas have also been reported in the testicular component of an ovotestis of a 46XX patient [5].

Individual neoplasias (Table 56.3)

Intratubular germ-cell neoplasia

All malignant tumours are thought to arise from intratubular germ-cell neoplasia or carcinoma-*in-situ*, which is characterized histologically by large atypical germ cells with vesicular nuclei, prominent nucleoli and

Table 56.3 Neoplasms occurring in patients with abnormal sexual differentiation

Gonadal dysgenesis true hermaphroditism	Testicular feminization
Germ-cell tumours	
Germ-cell neoplasia-*in-situ*	Germ-cell neoplasia-*in-situ*
Dysgerminoma/seminoma	Dysgerminoma/seminoma
MTU/embryonal carcinoma	Sertoli cell tumour
Gonadoblastoma	
Yolk sac tumour	
Sex cord tumour	
Juvenile granulosa cell tumour	

MTU, malignant teratoma undifferentiated.

accumulation of glycogen in the cytoplasm (Fig. 56.3). Positive staining with placental alkaline phosphatase has been demonstrated.

Recently 102 patients, prepubertal and pubertal, with various intersex states were reviewed in order to assess the frequency of this lesion [11]. Altogether the frequency was 6%. The overall incidence in androgen-insensitivity syndrome was 5–10%, the risk increasing with age to 33% at 50 years of age. The tumour was more frequently bilateral. Intratubular germ-cell neoplasia was occasionally found to be associated with other neoplasms. In the patients with gonadal dysgenesis the frequency of tumours ranged from 9 to 25%. In mixed gonadal dysgenesis the risk of developing a tumour is 10% at the age of 20 years, and 19% at 30 years of age. In true hermaphroditism 2.6% of cases had intratubular germ-cell neoplasia [11].

Gonadoblastoma

Gonadoblastoma is the most common malignancy in individuals with dysgenetic gonads. In about 50% of cases it is associated with seminoma [11]. Gonadoblastoma is believed to represent a pre-invasive change in the dysgenetic gonad and about one-fifth of the tumours are discovered because of microscopic examination of a streak gonad. The dimensions of a gonadoblastoma are very variable and may range from microscopic to several centimetres in size. This tumour has been described in very young children, but the most commonly affected ages are in the second and third decades. Phenotypic females with dysgenetic gonads and a Y chromosome are the most affected subjects.

A gonadoblastoma Y gene has been postulated to predispose to the tumour and is thought to lie on the long arm of the Y chromosome separate from the TDF [2].

Histologically, gonadoblastomas are composed of islands of two cell types, germ cells and sex-cord-derived cells which resemble Sertoli cells or granulosa cells. The sex-cord cells have approximately the same relation with the germ cells as in a normal follicle or testicular tubule; they either surround the germ cells or are randomly interspersed between them (Fig. 56.4). The

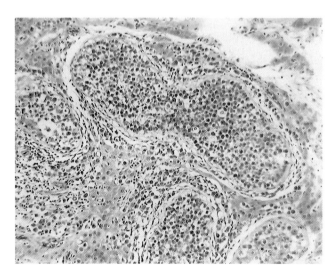

Fig. 56.3 Intratubular germ-cell neoplasia in a patient who had invasive germinoma in the same gonad. The tubules are packed with large, atypical germ cells, and there is a lymphocytic infiltrate in the immediately adjacent stroma.

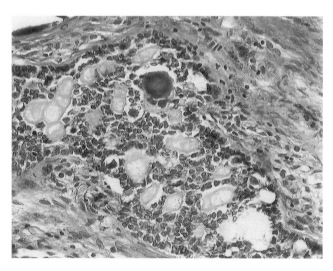

Fig. 56.4 An island of gonadoblastoma in a dysgenetic gonad that had Y chromosomal material. There are cords of Sertoli cells around cystic spaces and collections of collagen, and occasional germ cells are also present. Psammoma bodies (upper centre field) are commonly found in gonadoblastoma.

diagnosis of gonadoblastoma depends on finding these two cell types, but in over half the cases Leydig cells are present in the adjacent gonadal stroma, particularly in patients over 15 years old. Rounded collections of basement membrane-like material develop in the tumour islands and occasionally can entirely obliterate the tumour cells. Hyalinization and calcification are common in the basement membrane material. When an invasive malignancy such as dysgerminoma/seminoma develops, it has the same histological characteristics as its much more common counterpart arising in an apparently normal adult gonad. The prognosis for patients with pure gonadoblastoma is excellent provided that both gonads are excised.

Dysgerminoma/seminoma

Dysgerminoma/seminoma is an invasive malignant tumour composed of neoplastic germ cells (Fig. 56.5). When the tumour arises in a gonadoblastoma, the Sertoli and Leydig cells of the latter do not form part of the invasive neoplasm. The prognosis is good as metastases occur late and the tumours are radiosensitive. Patients most at risk are those with pure gonadal dysgenesis, mixed gonadal dysgenesis and dysgenetic male pseudohermaphroditism, especially when Y chromosomal material is present. Postpubertal patients with testicular feminization are also at risk, although the incidence of invasive malignancy is lower.

Choriocarcinoma, malignant teratoma undifferentiated (embryonal carcinoma) and yolk sac tumour

Choriocarcinoma, malignant teratoma undifferentiated (embryonal carcinoma) and yolk sac tumour are rare, aggressive germ-cell tumours which may also occur in patients with dysgenetic gonads and a Y chromosome. Differentiation of germ cells into trophoblast or structures resembling the yolk sac of the human embryo occurs in choriocarcinoma and yolk sac tumour (Fig. 56.6) respectively; when there is no differentiation into these patterns and no mature tissues are present, the tumour is classified as a malignant teratoma undifferentiated (MTU; called embryonal carcinoma in the American literature). Tumour markers such as β-human chorionic gonadotrophin (β-hCG), α-fetoprotein, human placental lactogen and placental alkaline phosphatase may be present in the patient's serum or demonstrable in histological sections. Testicular yolk sac tumour has also been reported in an intra-abdominal gonad in a patient with the persistent Müllerian duct syndrome.

Patients with abnormal sexual development who have developed gonadal neoplasia: personal series

The clinical details and gonadal histology of seven patients with abnormal sexual differentiation who had histological evidence of germ-cell neoplasia are shown in Table 56.4. In two patients (cases 1 and 2) the neoplasia occurred during the prepubertal period. In a third (case 3), clinical

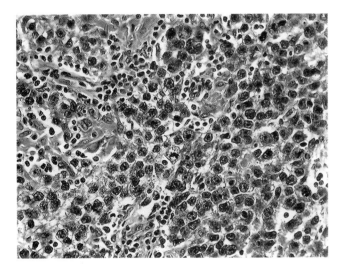

Fig. 56.5 Invasive germinoma in a dysgenetic gonad from a patient with an XY karyotype. The tumour cells are large with vesicular nuclei and clear cytoplasm. A mitotic figure is present (centre field). Between the tumour cells is an infiltrate of lymphocytes, a characteristic finding in germinoma.

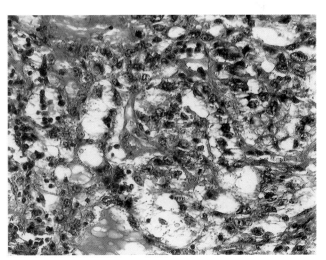

Fig. 56.6 Yolk sac tumour in a gonad with gonadoblastoma (not shown in field). The tumour cells are bizarre and arranged in sheets and there are poor attempts at gland formation.

Table 56.4 Clinical details and gonadal histology of patients with germ-cell neoplasia: personal experience

Patient	Age (years)	Karyotype	External genitalia	Gender	Diagnosis	Site of neoplastic gonad	Histology
1	7	XY	Ambiguous	F	DMP	Abdominal	Gonadoblastoma
2	11	XY	Ambiguous	M	DMP	Inguinal	Gonadoblastoma (bilateral), seminoma
3	12	XY	Ambiguous	F	DMP	Abdominal	Gonadoblastoma, seminoma, yolk sac tumour, choriocarcinoma
4	19	XY	Ambiguous	M	DMP	Inguinal	Carcinoma-*in-situ*, gonadoblastoma,
5	14	XY	Female	F	PGD	Abdominal	Dysgerminoma
6	16	XY	Female (clitoromegaly)	F	Ovarian dysgenesis	Abdominal	Gonadoblastoma, dysgerminoma
7	17	XX	Male	M	True hermaphroditism	Inguinal	Carcinoma-*in-situ*, gonadoblastoma (bilateral)

DMP, dysgenetic male pseudohermaphroditism; PGP, pure gonadal dysgenesis.

virilization occurred, presumably due to androgen secretion by the Leydig cells in the gonadoblastoma element of the mixed tumour. In each case the neoplastic gonad was either intra-abdominal or inguinal. In three patients (cases 3, 5 and 6) the tumour presented clinically as an abdominal mass; in the four other patients it was detected microscopically in the gonadectomy specimens.

Clinical presentation

Gonadal tumours can present clinically in children with abnormal sexual differentiation but they are usually found incidentally. Most reported cases of germ-cell neoplasia were microscopic and detected histologically in a gonad that had been removed or biopsied. This was particularly true of germ-cell neoplasia-*in-situ* and gonadoblastoma. When this is so, tumour would almost certainly not be detectable clinically or by palpation. Gonadoblastoma may also present as an abdominal mass, as may invasive malignant tumours.

The presence of abdominal pain and nausea may indicate torsion of a gonadal neoplasm. Rare presenting symptoms and signs may be pain, abdominal swelling or pelvic mass. Metastases may be present at the time of diagnosis in highly malignant germ-cell neoplasms such as choriocarcinoma or yolk sac tumour. Germ-cell tumours almost always occur in gonads that are undescended, intra-abdominal gonads being the most susceptible (see Table 56.4).

Age of gonadal tumour occurrence

The age range of gonadal tumours in patients with inter-

sex is wide. The incidence increases with increasing age, particularly after puberty. Manuel and colleagues [8] reviewed the age incidence of neoplasia in 320 patients with ambiguous genitalia and a Y chromosome. They found that gonadal tumours in patients with gonadal dysgenesis can occur before puberty but the incidence increases sharply at and after puberty in all forms of intersex with impaired gonadal differentiation. This is supported by the findings in our own series in which tumours occurred in five peripubertal patients between the ages of 12 and 19 years (see Table 56.4).

There are several reports in the literature of germ-cell neoplasia occurring in intersex states as a congenital tumour in infancy and in early childhood.

Prevention and management

The most important step in the prevention of gonadal tumours is to define the pathogenesis of the particular disorder correctly so that the risk of the patient developing malignancy can be assessed. In childhood there is a serious risk of neoplasia arising in dysgenetic gonads, in contrast to other forms of intersex in which the risk is appreciably less. In the testicular feminization syndrome, for example, germ-cell neoplasms are rare in the prepubertal child. If the diagnosis of an androgen-receptor defect or a testosterone biosynthesis defect cannot be made, further investigations are required, including ultrasound, computed tomography (CT) scan or laparotomy to define the internal urogenital organs and gonadal biopsy to look for evidence of gonadal dysgenesis.

Whether gonadectomy should be performed in early childhood in patients with abnormal sexual differentiation can be difficult to decide. It has been suggested that all dysgenetic testes should be removed and, certainly, when a gonadoblastoma is found on gonadal biopsy bilateral gonadectomy is essential. On the other hand, bilateral orchiectomy can cause serious psychological problems in peripubertal and postpubertal boys, and we do not have such an inflexible policy. Even when there is carcinoma-*in-situ* in peripubertal patients with testicular feminization, the risk of invasive malignancy appears to be extremely small [3].

Our practice is determined by:

1 the assigned gender of the patient;

2 the presence of dysgenetic gonads;

3 the position of the gonads.

If the child has been brought up as a girl, the gonads should be removed in infancy irrespective of their site. If the child has been reared as a boy, the testes should be removed during childhood if they are dysgenetic and not normally descended in the scrotum. Surgical manoeuvres to bring a gonad into the scrotum with the aim of preserving endocrine function are usually not worthwhile. Dysgenetic testes are unlikely to secrete normal adult concentrations of testosterone and cannot produce normal numbers of spermatozoa. These factors, together with the risk of malignancy, favour early gonadectomy. This is followed at an appropriate time by androgen-replacement therapy to induce puberty and maintain normal adult concentrations of serum testosterone, with prosthetic testicular implants in suitable cases.

If the testes are fully descended and of approximately normal size, the risk of malignancy is less. The advantages and drawbacks of retaining the gonads and the results of implantation of prosthetic testes are discussed with the patient if he is old enough to understand. If there is the possibility of psychological problems arising from castration, the gonads are left *in situ* and regular clinical examination is performed. The patient, if old enough, can be taught to examine his own gonads as a further check.

Finally, in familial pure gonadal dysgenesis the karyotype of all phenotypic female siblings of the propositus should be obtained. If an XY pattern is found, prophylactic gonadectomy should be performed in these patients because of the high risk of malignancy in this condition.

References

1. Verp MS, Simpson JL. Abnormal sexual differentiation and neoplasia. *Cancer Genet. Cytogenet.* 1987;**25**:191–218.
2. Page DC. Hypothesis: a Y-chromosomal gene causes gonadoblastoma in dysgenetic gonads. *Development* 1987;**101**(Suppl.):151–5.
3. Scully RE. Neoplasia associated with anomalous sexual development and abnormal sex chromosomes. *Pediatr. Adolesc. Endocrinol.* 1981;**8**:203–17.
4. Josso N. Sexual differentiation. In Grossman A (ed.). *Clinical Endocrinology*. Oxford: Blackwell Scientific Publications, 1992:737–44.
5. Savage MO, Lowe DG. Gonadal neoplasia and abnormal sexual differentiation. *Clin. Endocrinol.* 1990;**32**:519–33.
6. Bremer GL, Land JA, Tiebosch A, Van der Putten. Five different histological subtypes of germ cell malignancies in an XY female. *Gynaecol. Oncol.* 1993;**50**:247–8.
7. Robboy SJ, Miller T, Donahoe PK *et al.* Dysgenesis of testicular and streak gonads in the syndrome of mixed gonadal dysgenesis: perspective derived from a clinopathologic analysis of twenty-one cases. *Hum. Pathol.* 1982;**13**:700–16.
8. Manuel M, Katayama KP, Jones HW. The age of occurrence of gonadal tumours in intersex patients with a Y chromosome. *Am. J. Obstet. Gynecol.* 1976;**124**:293–300.
9. Müller J. Morphometry and histology of gonads from twelve children and adolescents with the androgen insensitivity (testicular feminization) syndrome. *J. Clin. Endocrinol. Metab.* 1984;**59**:785–9.
10. Van Niekerk WA. True hermaphroditism: an analytic review with a report of three new cases. *Am. J. Obstet. Gynecol.* 1976;**126**:890–904.
11. Ramani P, Yeung CK, Habeebu SSM. Testicular intratubular germ cell neoplasia in children and adolescents with intersex. *Am. J. Surg. Pathol.* 1993;**17**(11):1124–33.
12. Donahoe PK, Crawford JD, Hendren WH. Mixed gonadal dysgenesis, pathogenesis and management. *J. Pediatr. Surg.* 1979;**14**:287–300.

Gestational Trophoblastic Neoplasia

JOHN L. LEWIS JR

Introduction

Gestational trophoblastic neoplasia (GTN) is a disease category which includes a continuum of tumours that arise in the fetal chorion during various types of pregnancy [1]. Histologically they are categorized as one of two types of hydatidiform mole (partial or complete), gestational choriocarcinoma or placental site trophoblastic tumour (PSTT). The latter is the rarest form of GTN. They are of particular significance to the merging disciplines of oncology and endocrinology for two reasons.

1 The use of methotrexate in 1955 reproducibly to cure patients with metastatic GTN was the first demonstration of curative chemotherapy.

2 These tumours (except PSTT) always produce human chorionic gonadotrophin (hCG) in amounts proportional to the volume of viable tumour, thus making this hormone an ideal tumour marker.

In addition to these characteristics of curability with chemotherapy and consistent production of hCG, GTN was recognized as arising in tissue that is genetically different from the host. Since they are fetal in origin, they can carry paternal antigens derived from the male partner. To the extent that the paternal antigens differ from those of the maternal host, there is the potential for an immune response to somatic antigens in the tumour which were contributed by the male partner. When the curability of these tumours was first demonstrated, it was assumed by many that this success was based on synergism between the cytotoxic chemotherapy and immunological rejection based on a response to the paternal antigens. In fact, the immune response to the antigens in these tumours is usually tolerance rather than rejection, thus allowing persistence of this partially 'foreign' tissue, just as its normal counterpart, placenta, persists due to specific tolerance.

From the viewpoint of this publication, it is of interest that the initial use of methotrexate in patients with metastatic GTN by Hertz and his colleagues [2] took place in an endocrine department (Endocrinology Branch, National Cancer Institute (NCI), National Institutes of Health (NIH), Bethesda, Maryland). These investigators were studying hormone-producing neoplasms arising in various organs (pituitary, adrenal, ovary, testes and other sites), as well as tumours that responded to hormonal manipulation (usually breast or prostate cancer). When methotrexate was first used, the evidence for its effectiveness was initially obtained from measuring the decrease in urinary gonadotrophins. It would be difficult to find a closer relationship between oncology and endocrinology.

Histopathological diagnoses

As discussed above, there are four recognized histopathological diagnoses of gestational trophoblastic neoplasia: complete hydatidiform mole, partial hydatidiform mole, gestational choriocarcinoma and placental site trophoblastic tumour.

Complete and partial hydatidiform moles

Complete and partial hydatidiform moles present as abnormal pregnancies ending in a first or second trimester abortion. They differ in several respects: histopathological characteristics, cytogenetic constitution, obstetric presentation and likelihood of developing 'malignant' sequelae. The latter is defined as persistence of molar tissue after evacuation of the uterus, resulting in progressive growth, rising hCG levels, or the actual development of malignant choriocarcinoma from molar tissue. Table 57.1 summarizes the difference between these two forms of hydatidiform mole.

Table 57.1 Comparison of partial and complete hydatidiform moles (from [1] with permission)

Characteristics	Partial mole	Complete mole
Cytogenetic analysis	Triploidy; 69,XXX most common	Diploidy; 46,XX most common
	Paternal and maternal origin	Paternal origin
Pathology		
Hydropic villi	Focal, variable	Diffuse, often marked
Trophoblastic proliferation	Focal, slight	Diffuse, variable
Fetus, amnion, fetal erythrocytes	Present	Absent
Clinical		
'Mole' clinical, ultrasound diagnosis	Rare	Common
Uterus large for gestational dates	Rare	25–50%
Theca lutein cysts	Rare	25–35%
Malignant sequelae	< 10%	20%

Gestational choriocarcinoma

Gestational choriocarcinoma is a highly malignant tumour consisting of malignant cells derived from the two types of trophoblastic cells forming the fetal chorion: syncytial and cytotrophoblastic cells. Although similar cells can be found in the trophoblastic epithelium covering molar villi, when villi are present it is classified as a molar pregnancy, and when only malignant trophoblastic cells are seen without villi, it is choriocarcinoma. Why the presence of villi is associated with a more benign prognosis is not known. Gestational choriocarcinoma is always associated with haemorrhage and necrosis and readily invades host vessels. The histopathological pattern found in gestational choriocarcinoma is not unique to tumours of placental origin, for similar tissue can be found in testicular and ovarian germ-cell tumours.

Placental site trophoblastic tumours

Placental site trophoblastic tumour is also of placental origin but varies in several important ways. It has only one cell type, the so-called intermediate trophoblast. It can follow any type of pregnancy. It is slow to metastasize but is quite resistant to chemotherapy. Its production of hCG is variable and does not correlate with the amount of tumour. Some of these tumours produce little or no hCG. They are more likely to produce human placental lactogen. Their clinical course is unpredictable. Some are cured with only a curettage. If the tumour persists after curettage, hysterectomy should be considered. Fortunately, this is the rarest of all forms of GTN.

Antecedent pregnancies

Gestational trophoblastic neoplasms arise in various types of pregnancies, most of which are clinically recognized as abnormal. The most common are molar pregnancies, but these tumours can also arise in abortions, ectopic pregnancies and full-term, apparently normal pregnancies.

Most patients with GTN who require chemotherapy have had the tumour arise in a molar pregnancy. Approximately 10–20% of patients will need chemotherapy after evacuation of a molar pregnancy because of an hCG level that increases after an original decrease. However, as many as 5% of patients with a molar pregnancy will eventually develop histologically confirmable choriocarcinoma if not treated because of hCG elevation only. In the initial 5-year report of the first 63 patients with metastatic GTN treated at the NIH with methotrexate [3], it was possible to determine the relative incidence of types of pregnancy leading to the metastatic disease. Forty-six percent followed molar pregnancies, 30% followed a non-molar abortion and 24% followed delivery of an infant at term. Significantly, all patients who died of progressive, drug-resistant disease had choriocarcinoma at autopsy, regardless of type of antecedent pregnancy.

Clinical surveillance of patients who have had a molar pregnancy is the only practical method to decrease the development of metastatic GTN. Because molar pregnancies are clinically detectable and account for more than half of the patients with GTN who require chemotherapy, it is reasonable to follow hCG levels at 2-week intervals in all patients who have had a molar pregnancy until they become normal or remain elevated and require treatment.

A much greater problem is detecting gestational choriocarcinoma that follows an abortion or normal term delivery. The very low incidence of choriocarcinoma following these pregnancies makes following hCG levels impractical. They are usually detected when metastases become symptomatic. Sites of initial metastases in descending order are lung, vagina, brain, liver, gastrointestinal tract and kidney. Because the interval between the pregnancy event and the development of metastatic disease can be months to years and the tumours are so rare, many clinicians do not consider the possibility of trophoblastic tumour when evaluating a patient with what turns out to be metastatic GTN. One useful dictum: any woman of reproductive age who has an undiagnosed tumour or unexplained bleeding from any organ other than the uterus should undergo one sensitive hCG assay to determine whether she has the rare, but highly curable, gestational choriocarcinoma. It is a clinical tragedy when metastatic GTN is first diagnosed at autopsy.

Classification of gestational trophoblastic neoplasms

Classification or staging of patients with GTN has been controversial since chemotherapy was first used [4]. Almost all staging systems for cancers arising as solid tumours are based on the histology and location of the tumours. Tumour cell characteristics, such as differentiation and characteristics of local growth patterns, may also be included. However, this type of staging has not been very useful in GTN. There are several reasons for this. As noted before, choriocarcinoma can arise from molar tissue, aborted tissue, or an apparently normal placenta. In fact, there are reports of choriocarcinoma being present in metastatic sites when molar tissue or a normal placenta is still in the uterus. Also, there is little benefit in biopsying metastatic sites if a molar pregnancy has occurred and the appearance of metastases is associated with a rising hCG level.

The staging classification that first gained acceptance in the USA was the scheme developed at the NIH [5] which assigned patients with metastatic GTN into two categories ('good prognosis' and 'bad prognosis'), based on the site of metastases, levels of hCG excretion at the onset of treatment, and duration of time elapsed between the pregnancy event and diagnosis of GTN. Early treatment, low hCG levels and metastases limited to the lungs or pelvis were associated with a 'good prognosis,' or low risk of failing to be cured by single-agent chemotherapy. Patients with non-metastatic disease were not

included in the classification because none were treated with chemotherapy at the beginning of this clinical series and were not added later because they were essentially all curable. This classification down-played the importance of determining histology in metastasis sites but emphasized the hormonal activity and duration of disease as being important.

In 1976, Bagshawe [6] introduced a much more comprehensive classification scheme based on factors associated with multiple patient and tumour characteristics. The prognostic importance of the parameters in predicting response to chemotherapy was calculated by retrospective review of outcomes in the extensive clinical trials in GTN carried out at Charing Cross Hospital. This original scheme has been simplified and accepted by the World Health Organization (WHO) [7] as a 'scoring system based on prognostic factors' for patients with gestational trophoblastic disease. (The terms 'gestational trophoblastic disease', 'gestational trophoblastic neoplasia' and 'gestational trophoblastic tumours' are used by different authors basically to include the same conditions, although some do not include non-metastatic disease or molar patients who do not require chemotherapy.) The WHO classification is listed in Table 57.2.

Both of these classification schemes have a characteristic that separates them from all standard staging

Table 57.2 World Health Organization scoring system based on prognostic factors (from [4] with permission)

Prognostic factor	Score*			
	1	2	3	4
Age (years)	≤ 39	> 39		
Antecedent pregnancy	HM	Abortion	Term	
Interval (months)	4	4–6	7–12	12
hCG (i.u./l)	10^3	10^3–10^4	10^4–10^5	10^5
ABO groups (female × male)		O × A A × O	B AB	
Largest tumour		3–5 cm	5 cm	
Site of metastases		Spleen, liver	GI tract, liver	Brain
Number of metastases		1–4	4–8	8
Prior chemotherapy			Single drug	Two or more drugs

* Total score for a patient determines risk category. It is derived by adding individual scores in each prognostic category. Low risk, ≤ 4; medium risk, 5–7; high risk, ≥ 8.
GI, gastrointestinal; hCG, human chorionic gonadotrophin; HM, hydatidiform mole.

systems. Patients can be assigned to a new risk category if they are not cured by their prior therapy; for example, one parameter in the WHO scoring system is 'prior chemotherapy'. A score of 3 is assigned if the patient has received only one drug regimen and 4 if they have received two or more different regimens. In no other staging system are patients reassigned because of treatment failure.

Treatment and results

The selection of appropriate chemotherapy is the most important decision to be made in a patient with GTN [7]. Because there are several effective drugs that can be used individually and in various combinations, the goal is to use the least toxic therapy that does not jeopardize the likelihood of the patient being cured.

Low-risk patients (WHO score of ≤ 4)

Low-risk patients can be treated with relatively non-toxic chemotherapy and all should be cured. That most commonly used is methotrexate with folinic acid 'rescue', which significantly reduces toxicity. Dactinomycin may be selected for patients with abnormalities of liver or renal function. Combination chemotherapy may be required in the minority of patients whose disease is not cleared with initial treatment.

Medium-risk patients (WHO score 5–7)

Patients in the medium-risk category are best treated initially with combination chemotherapy. The combination used most often has been M.C. Li's 'triple therapy' [8], consisting of methotrexate, dactinomycin and an alkylating agent. Although originally used as therapy for testicular cancer, it is a mainstay in treatment of GTN patients. Folinic acid is added to the regimen to reduce toxicity, giving the so-called MAC III regimen. If these patients are treated initially and aggressively in a specialized centre, their cure rate should approach 100%.

High-risk patients (WHO score of ≥ 8)

The high-risk category still has a significant mortality rate. Deaths may occur early in treatment due to haemorrhage from extensive tumour growth in the brain, liver or intestinal tract. Late in treatment, drug resistance may develop and death is due to progressive tumour growth in the same organs as listed above, as well as the lung. Although the cure rates reported in these patients remained at about 50% with the MAC III regimen, Charing Cross investigators have reported an 80% cure

rate in these patients if their initial treatment is with the EMA-CO regimen [9]. This consists of a 2-day course of etoposide, methotrexate and dactinomycin, followed the next week by cyclophosphamide and Oncovin. The combination is remarkably well tolerated and can usually be continued for significant periods of time without interruption. Patients in this risk category require several courses of treatment, even after the hCG first reaches an apparently normal level.

The small group of patients who fail to be cured by EMA-CO represent the need and opportunity for identifying new, useful drugs for treating GTN [4]. Early reports have suggested that cisplatin, cytosine arabinoside and taxol may be useful. These patients have also utilized colony-stimulating factors, total parenteral nutrition and autologous bone marrow transplant.

Surgery has a role in the patients who develop resistant disease, for they will occasionally be cured by the surgical removal of a single focus of drug-resistant tumour, most often in the lung or brain. (Although not the subject of this presentation, surgery can be useful in other clinical settings: initial evaluation of a molar pregnancy, hysterectomy for resistant molar tissue not cured with single-agent chemotherapy, and procedures to treat haemorrhage or infections that develop during chemotherapy.)

The term 'cure' in patients with GTN is important, for the vast majority not only remain free of disease without further therapy, but they may resume relatively normal lives. Those with intact reproductive organs have a high success rate in subsequent pregnancies. With the exception of a slight increase in the incidence of first trimester miscarriage and in placenta accreta, the pregnancies differ little from those in normal women. No increase in fetal abnormalities has been reported. Equally importantly, there has been no increase in secondary malignancies in the women who received chemotherapy for GTN.

Human chorionic gonadotrophin

hCG is a glycoprotein hormone made by trophoblastic tissue in the placenta, all gestational trophoblastic neoplasms (except the rare placental site trophoblastic tumours), gonadal germ-cell tumours and various non-trophoblastic solid tumors (so-called 'ectopic production') such as stomach, breast, pancreas, lung and others. Its usefulness in patients with molar disease or gestational choriocarcinoma is based on the direct relationship between the amount of viable trophoblastic tissue and the level of hCG in the serum or excreted in urine. Thus, accurate measurement of hCG is necessary to establish the diagnosis of GTN, to monitor response to the

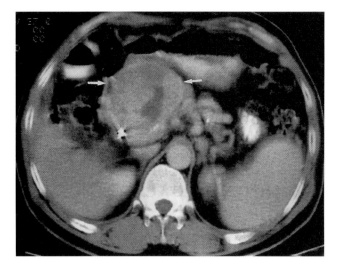

Fig. 58.1 Malignant non-functioning islet cell tumour. Contrast-enhanced CT scan showing an 8 cm mass in the head of the pancreas (arrows), which enhances irregularly.

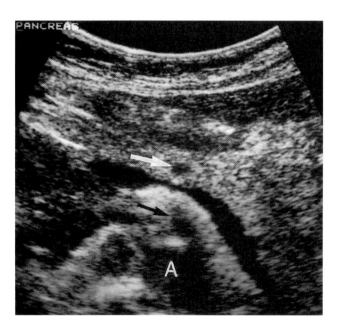

Fig. 58.2 Insulinoma. Transverse, transabdominal ultrasound scan showing a 7 mm insulinoma in the neck of the pancreas (white arrow). The mass is well defined and hypo-echoic. A, aorta; black arrow, superior mesenteric artery.

a potential blindspot for this technique [8]. However, endoscopic ultrasound requires very special expertise, specialized equipment, and is only available at a few institutions.

Intra-operative ultrasound

Before the development of modern radiological investigations, palpation of the pancreas at the time of surgery was the mainstay in the localization of islet cell tumours. Intra-operative ultrasound is an extension of this technique, using a high-frequency transducer applied directly to the pancreas. Tumours as small as 4 mm have been detected. In the detection of insulinomas this is a very effective technique, with a sensitivity of 90% [1]. Intra-operative palpation and ultrasound are complementary, the combination of the two techniques leading to the localization of 100% of solitary insulinomas with a mean size of 1.4 cm in a series of 44 patients [5]. In the case of multiple insulinomas, intra-operative ultrasound and continuous blood glucose monitoring to detect a rise after resection are required to localize all the tumours. With extrapancreatic gastrinomas, the sensitivity of intra-operative ultrasound falls, since tumours in the gastric or duodenal wall (an area where endoscopic ultrasound has an advantage) may not be visualized. Intra-operative ultrasound is also of use to the surgeon to help prevent damage to the biliary and pancreatic ducts. Intrapancreatic lymph nodes and ectopic pancreatic tissue in the duodenum are causes of false-positive results for both intra-operative ultrasound and palpation [9].

Computed tomography

CT is widely available, and, together with ultrasound, it forms the mainstay of general pancreatic imaging. The gland should be scanned both before and after intravenous contrast medium injection, ideally on a 'spiral' scanner in 5 mm or 3 mm intervals during a single breath-hold. Spiral scanning reduces respiratory artefact and allows for improved vascular enhancement when compared with conventional dynamic CT. Oral contrast medium is given to delineate the stomach, duodenal loop and jejunum.

Before contrast injection, an islet cell tumour may show as a disruption of the gland contour. Calcification is present in approximately 10% of islet cell tumours, and if present, tends to be discrete and nodular, and is associated with malignancy in 70% of cases. After contrast, islet cell tumours typically enhance more than surrounding pancreas, but they may not be visible on standard abdominal viewing windows, only becoming detectable on narrow windows (Figs 58.4 and 58.5, and see Fig. 58.7b). The radiologist must take care to manipulate the images on the operating console in

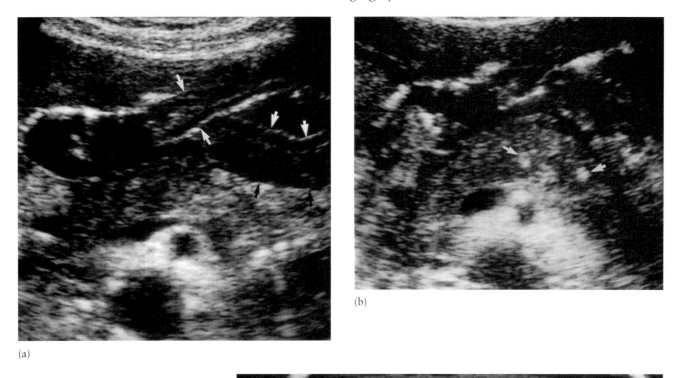

(a)

(b)

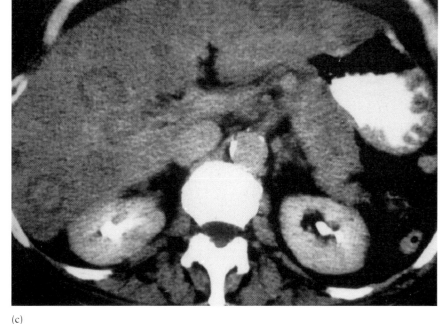

(c)

Fig. 58.3 Malignant gastrinoma. (a) Transabdominal ultrasound in the transverse plane. There is gross thickening of the gastric wall up to 2 cm (arrows). (b) Transverse ultrasound scan through the pancreas showing multiple small hyperechoic gastrinomas in the neck and body of the gland (arrows). (c) Contrast-enhanced CT scan in the same patient demonstrating multiple hepatic metastases. The pancreatic lesions were not shown on the CT scan.

order not to miss lesions. Hypodense lesions are rare. Tumours as small as 5 mm can be detected by contrast-enhanced CT. Non-functioning tumours tend to be large at diagnosis, and most are detected by CT. Large tumours are more likely to show necrosis and calcification.

Local lymph nodes and hepatic metastases may be demonstrated on CT. Hepatic metastases tend to be hypodense before and hyperdense after intravenous contrast medium due to increased vascularity. The blush may mask the presence of metastases relative to the

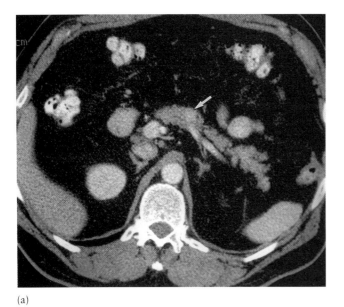

(a)

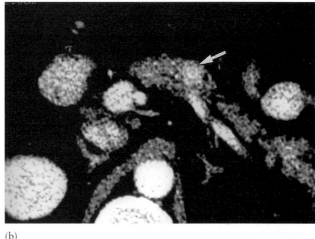

(b)

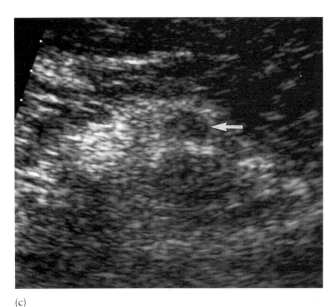

(c)

Fig. 58.4 Insulinoma. (a) Contrast-enhanced CT scan displayed on standard abdominal window settings. The insulinoma is only just seen in the body of the pancreas (arrow). (b) The same image as (a), but displayed on narrow window settings to emphasize the enhancement of the mass (arrow) compared with the pancreatic tissue. (c) The same mass demonstrated on ultrasound (arrow).

surrounding liver. Early enhancement-phase imaging or dual-phase imaging will help to avoid this pitfall. A solitary hepatic metastasis may be indistinguishable from a haemangioma.

The sensitivity of CT in the localization of islet cell tumours varies between studies, partly due to differences in patient selection and technique. Sensitivity figures quoted range from 42 to 78%. Galiber and colleagues [5] report CT sensitivity of 30% where single insulinomas are present, and only 8% for each insulinoma where multiple tumours are present. In general, sensitivities are below 50% for insulinomas, and above 50% for

gastrinomas. Significant advances in scanner technology have occurred since many of these studies were carried out. In our institution, using careful technique, we have found CT to be very sensitive for the localization of islet cell tumours, more so than somatostatin receptor scintigraphy [10].

CT scanning during intra-arterial injection of contrast medium through a coeliac axis or superior mesenteric artery catheter has been advocated, but the catheter produces CT streak artefacts which may obscure a tumour. This technique was used as a way of achieving improved pancreatic enhancement without using ex-

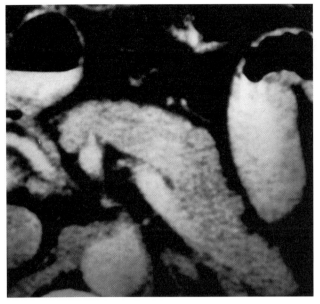

(a)

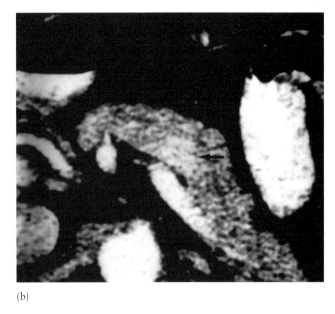

(b)

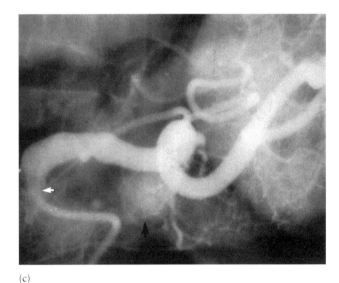

(c)

Fig. 58.5 Insulinoma. (a) Contrast-enhanced CT scan displayed on standard window settings. (b) The same image displayed on narrow windows, making the enhancing insulinoma more apparent (arrow). (c) Arteriogram in the same patient. The catheter tip is in the origin of the splenic artery (white arrow). The insulinoma shows as a characteristic blush (black arrow).

cessive doses of contrast medium when CT scanners were slow. Excellent enhancement is now achievable throughout the pancreas using dynamic spiral scanning after intravenous contrast, and so the technique is not widely used, and experience with it is limited.

Magnetic resonance imaging

Magnetic resonance imaging (MRI) of abdominal organs has improved with the development of rapid imaging sequences, respiratory gating, bowel contrast agents and breath-hold techniques. MRI is now an important

modality in the imaging of islet cell tumours. The appearance of the tumour will depend on the imaging sequence used. Most islet cell tumours are of low signal intensity on T_1-weighted images compared with normal pancreas, particularly on fat-suppressed images (Fig. 58.6a), although the tumour may be isointense. On T_2-weighted images, the tumours are usually hyperintense compared with normal pancreas (Fig. 58.6b), particularly gastrinomas [11]. As with contrast-enhanced CT, insulinomas enhance markedly with gadolinium reflecting their vascularity. Gastrinomas classically show ring enhancement with central low signal [11]. Islet cell

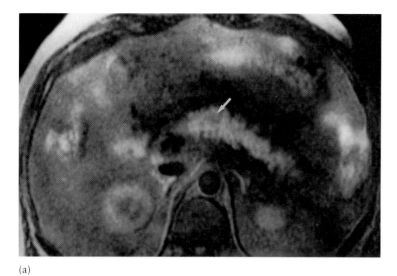

(a)

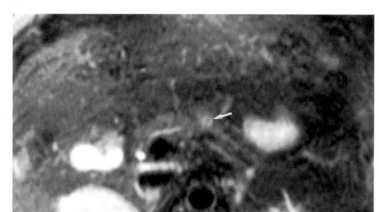

(b)

Fig. 58.6 Insulinoma. (a) T_1-weighted MRI with fat suppression showing a small mass (arrow) which is of lower signal intensity than the surrounding pancreas. (b) T_2-weighted fast spin echo image with fat suppression showing the mass (arrow) to be of higher signal intensity than surrounding pancreas.

tumours are of high signal intensity on short T_1 inversion recovery (STIR) imaging. Lymph node and hepatic metastasis tend to be of high signal on T_2-weighted images. These signal characteristics are also common to many other types of pancreatic pathology.

As MRI technology is still developing rapidly, data on the accuracy of MRI is sparse. However, to date, studies using conventional T_1- and T_2-weighted spin echo sequences have shown variable sensitivities for the localization of islet cell tumours. A more recent study has reported a sensitivity reaching 100% [12]. Semelka and colleagues found that small insulinomas were best demonstrated on dynamic contrast-enhanced fast low-angle shot (FLASH) images. However, results such as these are not universal. Sensitivities as low as 20% have been reported, but using relatively low field strength

magnets. Pisegna and colleagues [13] reported MRI sensitivity for detection of metastatic gastrinoma in the liver of 83%, but in the localization of primary gastrinoma in 32 patients, the sensitivity was only 25%. Even when combined with the results of CT and US, the sensitivity did not reach that of angiography (59%) [13].

Echoplanar imaging is a newer technique where images may be acquired during a single breath-hold, thus reducing respiratory motion artefact. Although reducing the signal-to-noise ratio, this technique also reduces movement artefact, and it is hoped that it will result in improved detection of islet cell tumours.

Radionucleotide imaging

Octreotide is a synthetic somatostatin analogue. A radio-

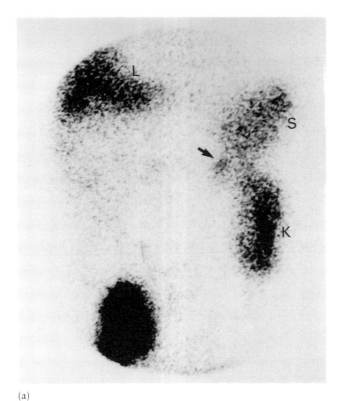

(a)

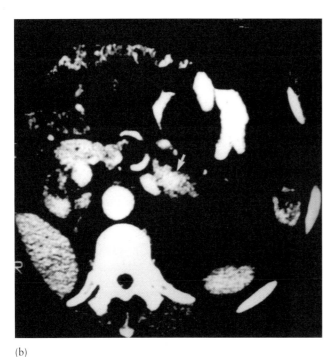

(b)

Fig. 58.7 Somatostatin receptor scintigraphy. (a) ^{111}In-pentetreotide scan showing an insulinoma (arrow) in the tail of the pancreas. Normal uptake is seen in the liver (L), spleen (S) and kidney (K). (b) Contrast-enhanced CT in the same patient showing the enhancing mass (arrow) which could only be detected on narrow window settings.

labelled derivative, ^{111}In-pentetreotide, binds to somatostatin receptors on primary and metastatic tumour cells which can then be imaged (Fig. 58.7a).

Tumours as small as 1 cm can be detected. In a study of 40 patients with neuroendocrine tumours, the tumour was visualized in 80% of patients [14]; in 40% of the patients, ^{111}In-pentetreotide imaging showed lesions not detected by ultrasonography, CT or MRI. Tumour masses shown by these latter imaging techniques were missed by ^{111}In-pentetreotide imaging in eight patients, some of them with large tumours. The conspicuity did not relate to tumour size, but to the density of somatostatin receptors. ^{111}In-pentetreotide imaging is particularly useful in detecting intra-abdominal and bone metastases. Other studies have shown that 68–86% of islet cell tumours can be detected, and a similar percentage of metastatic carcinoid tumours. In our institution, somatostatin receptor imaging is not as sensitive as CT, and so is not used as a first-line investigation. Somatostatin receptor imaging is especially useful, however, where an islet cell tumour is suspected but the CT is negative, where the CT scan is equivocal, or when the disease is disseminated [10]. The two investigations frequently complement each other.

In many instances, a positive scan predicts a favourable response to treatment with octreotide [15]. Unfortunately many insulinomas, and occasional gastrinomas, carcinoid tumours and vasoactive intestinal polypeptide (VIP)omas, do not express somatostatin receptors. Adenocarcinoma of the pancreas does not take up somatostatin analogues [15].

Arteriography

For many years pancreatic arteriography had been the method of choice for localizing insulinomas [16] and gastrinomas. Now, the technique is usually applied when initial investigations fail to demonstrate the suspected tumour, or are equivocal. Because such tumours are frequently small, meticulous attention to detail at arteriography is essential [17]. Selective injections are made into the coeliac axis and superior mesenteric artery, demonstrating the arterial anatomy of the pancreas. Branches supplying specific areas of the pancreas are then opacified, this being known as superselective or subselective arteriography. Many pancreatic lesions will be missed unless superselective studies are performed. Distension of the stomach with gas after smooth muscle relaxants reduces overlying bowel artefact.

The typical angiographic appearance of an islet cell tumour is a dense, circumscribed, homogeneous capillary blush appearing at 2–4 seconds and persisting for

12–16 seconds see (see Fig. 58.5c). Prominent draining veins have also been described, particularly with VIPomas [17].

In most studies where angiography is compared to ultrasound, CT, and MRI, angiography performs equal to or better than the other modalities individually.

The published rates for successful localization range from 29 to 90% for insulinomas, and 15 to 88% for gastrinomas [10,18]. Where multiple insulinomas are present and the detection of each is considered individually, the sensitivity falls to 29% [5]. In this latter study, arteriography still out-performed ultrasound and CT.

Venous sampling

Transhepatic portal venous sampling

Transhepatic portal venous sampling (TPVS) is an invasive method of islet cell tumour localization: the right portal vein is cannulated percutaneously, and a sheath approximately 2 mm in diameter is inserted into the hepatic track through which a catheter can be manipulated. Venous samples are drawn at 1 cm intervals along the splenic, superior mesenteric and portal veins for analysis. The site of each specimen is recorded on a map. A localized increase in hormone concentration indicates the site of tumour. Various criteria can be used to define the increase, but a hormone level two standard deviations above the portal vein mean level gives good results. Complications of the procedure are relatively frequent (9.2%) and it carries a mortality rate of 0.7%, so these risks should be taken into account when considering the investigation.

Several authors find TPVS more sensitive for tumour localization than angiography [4,18,19]. Some studies show a sensitivity for localization of gastrinomas of below 50% [20,21] but others give sensitivities of between 73 and 95% [18,19]. Vinick and colleagues found a poor correlation between the site of maximum hormone concentration and the location of the tumour. If only wishing to localize to one of three areas, pancreatic body and tail, gastrinoma triangle, or liver, then sensitivity of 94% can be achieved [21]. Rossi and colleagues reviewed the literature on TPVS in insulinomas, finding the sensitivity to be approximately 84% [17].

False-positive results are common in this technique. Where there are multifocal tumours or hepatic metastases, results can be difficult to interpret [17]. TPVS should not be performed shortly after diagnostic angiography since the latter may produce transient rises and falls in hormone levels.

Due to the invasive nature of the investigation, TPVS is not routinely performed, but is useful where other investigations are equivocal. It is particularly effective in localizing occult insulinomas [19].

Arterial stimulation venous sampling

This technique has been developed recently to improve detection of small islet cell tumours, which are frequently not localized preoperatively. The technique relies on selective intra-arterial injection of a secretagogue producing a detectable rise of hormone in the venous effluent when the branch supplying the tumour is injected. The secretagogue is calcium gluconate for localizing insulinomas, and secretin for gastrinomas [16,20].

There is very little data to derive figures for sensitivity and specificity, but Doppman and colleagues found a sensitivity for gastrinomas of 54% compared with 46% using TPVS [20]. Figures for insulinoma are not yet available, but Doppman and colleagues found abrupt rises in serum insulin levels after infusion of calcium gluconate into the supply artery in all of four cases, and no rise on infusion into an artery not supplying the tumour [16].

Conclusion

Most patients with suspected islet cell tumours will undergo ultrasound or CT as their first imaging investigation. These modalities will demonstrate the tumour and hepatic metastases in approximately 40% of gastrinomas, 80% of insulinomas and almost all other functioning and non-functioning tumours. Where these tests are equivocal or negative, MRI and/or arteriography may then be performed. Subsequent investigations depend on the local practice and the patient, but include TPVS and somatostatin receptor imaging. Endoscopic ultrasound is a very sensitive investigation which is gaining prominence. Finally, intra-operative palpation and ultrasound may locate the remaining tumours.

Carcinoid tumours

Diagnosis and therapy

The management of patients with malignant carcinoid syndrome depends on the presence of hepatic metastases. Imaging must therefore be directed to the sensitive detection of metastatic spread. Ultrasound is an effective modality in liver imaging, but poor views may be obtained in patients of a certain body habitus, and so CT scanning is the usual staging procedure. Metastatic carcinoid masses are usually multifocal showing enhancement after intravenous contrast medium, frequently with low attenuation centres due to necrosis, and may reach a great size. CT scanning has a reported sensitivity of 90% and greater for the detection of carcinoid liver metastases. MRI is at least as sensitive as CT; on T_1-weighted images, the lesions are usually iso-intense to surrounding liver, but of high signal on T_2-weighted images. Angiography is also a sensitive investigation, but is invasive, and is no longer indicated as a diagnostic procedure except when there is a plan to institute embolization therapy. Various substances have been used to embolize hepatic carcinoid metastases via selective arterial catheterization with good effect.

[111]In-pentetreotide has been used for imaging patients with carcinoid tumours, giving a sensitivity of 85%. Previously unsuspected extrahepatic sites of disease may be detected. Since pentetreotide scintigraphy demonstrates somatostatin receptor-positive tumours, the technique predicts which tumours would be suitable for octreotide therapy [15]. ^{123}I-labelled metaiodobenzylguanidine (MIBG) is also taken up by carcinoid tumours to varying degrees (Fig. 58.8), but is not as sensitive as pentetreotide imaging [15]. The main indication for diagnostic ^{123}I-MIBG is to evaluate these patients for possible palliative therapy with ^{131}I-MIBG.

Primary hepatic carcinoid is a rare tumour which tends to be hyperechoic on ultrasound. This tumour has similar findings on CT and MRI to metastatic carcinoid, but may have an apparent capsule which shows as low signal intensity on T_2-weighted MRI.

References

1. Gooding GAW. Adrenal, pancreatic, and scrotal ultrasound in endocrine disease. *Radiol. Clin. North Am.* 1993;**31**(5):1069–83.
2. Kent RB, van Heerden JA, Weiland LH. Nonfunctioning islet cell tumours. *Ann. Surg.* 1981;**193**:185–90.
3. King CMP, Reznek RH, Dacie JE, Wass JAH. Imaging islet cell tumours. *Clin. Radiol.* 1994;**49**:295–303.
4. Gunther RW, Klose KJ, Ruckert K *et al.* Localization of small islet-cell tumours. Preoperative and intraoperative ultrasound, computed tomography, arteriography, digital subtraction angiography, and pancreatic venous sampling. *Gastrointest. Radiol.* 1985;**10**:145–52.
5. Galiber AK, Reading CC, Charboneau JW *et al.* Localization of pancreatic insulinoma: comparison of pre- and intraoperative US with CT and angiography. *Radiology* 1988;**166**:405–8.
6. London JF, Shawker TH, Doppman JL *et al.* Zollinger-Ellison syndrome: prospective assessment of abdominal US in the localization of gastrinomas. *Radiology* 1991;**178**:763–7.
7. Rosch T, Lightdale CJ, Botet JF *et al.* Localization of pancreatic endocrine tumours by endoscopic ultrasonography. *N. Engl. J. Med.* 1992;**326**:1721–6.
8. Glover JR, Shorvon PJ, Lees WR. Endoscopic ultrasound for localisation of islet cell tumours. *Gut* 1992;**33**:108–10.
9. Norton JA, Cromack DT, Shawker TH *et al.* Intraoperative ultrasonographic localization of islet cell tumours. A prospective comparison to palpation. *Ann. Surg.* 1988;**207**:160–8.
10. King CMP, Reznek RH, Bomanji J *et al.* Imaging neuro-endocrine tumours with radiolabelled somatostatin analogues and X-ray computed tomography: a comparative study. *Clin. Radiol.* 1993;**48**:386–91.
11. Semelka RC, Ascher SM. MR imaging of the pancreas. *Radiology* 1993;**188**:593–602.
12. Semelka RC, Cumming MJ, Shoenut JP *et al.* Islet cell tumours: comparison of dynamic contrast-enhanced CT and MR imaging with dynamic gadolinium enhancement and fat suppression. *Radiology* 1993;**186**:799–802.
13. Pisegna JR, Doppman JL, Norton JA, Metz DC, Jensen RT. Prospective comparative study of ability of MR imaging and other imaging modalities to localize tumours in patients with Zollinger-Ellison syndrome. *Digest. Dis. Sci.* 1993;**38**:1318–28.
14. Scherubl H, Bader M, Fett U *et al.* Somatostatin-receptor imaging of neuroendocrine gastroenteropancreatic tumours. *Gastroenterology* 1993;**105**:1705–9.
15. Krenning EP, Kwekkeboom DJ, Bakker WH *et al.* Somatostatin receptor scintigraphy with [^{111}In-DTPA-D-Phe]- and [^{123}I-Tyr]-octreotide: the Rotterdam experience with more than 1000 patients. *Eur. J. Nucl. Med.* 1993;**20**:716–31.
16. Doppman JL, Miller DL, Chang R, Shawker TH, Gorden P, Norton JA. Insulinomas: localization with selective intraarterial injection of calcium. *Radiology* 1991;**178**:237–41.
17. Rossi P, Allison DJ, Bezzi M. Endocrine tumours of the pancreas. *Radiol. Clin. North Am.* 1989;**27**:129–61.

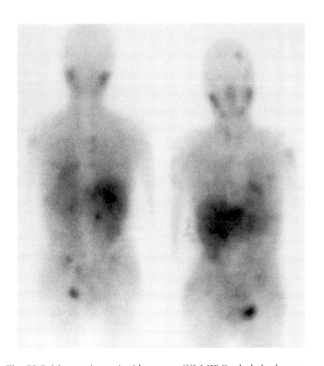

Fig. 58.8 Metastatic carcinoid tumour. ^{123}I-MIBG whole body scan, posterior and anterior views. Areas of increased tracer uptake are seen in the liver, skull, left chest, left humerus and left hemipelvis.

18. Roche A, Raisonnier A, Gillon-Savouret M-C. Pancreatic venous sampling and arteriography in localizing insulinomas and gastrinomas: procedure and results in 55 cases. *Radiology* 1982;**145**:621–7.

19. Fraker DL, Norton JA. Localization and resection of insulinomas and gastrinomas. *JAMA* 1988;**259**:3601–5.

20. Doppman JL, Miller DL, Chang R *et al.* Gastrinomas: localization by means of selective intraarterial injection of secretin. *Radiology* 1990;**174**:25–9.

21. Vinik AI, Moattari AR, Cho K, Thompson N. Transhepatic portal vein catheterization for localization of sporadic and MEN gastrinomas: a ten-year experience. *Surgery* 1990;**107**:246–55.

59

Classification of Neuroendocrine Tumours

ANNE E. BISHOP AND JULIA M. POLAK

Introduction

The concept of the endocrine system has expanded in recent years to encompass a spectrum of related cell types from classical endocrine cells, through paracrine, neuroendocrine, neurocrine and endothelial subsets to include the entire central and peripheral nervous systems. Components of this diffuse neuroendocrine system are found in almost every tissue investigated, but are particularly prominent in the gastrointestinal tract and pancreas, the thyroid (C cells), the adrenal medulla, the respiratory tract, the skin and the genitourinary system. Neuroendocrine tumours thus arise from all these tissues.

The diagnosis of neuroendocrine tumours can often depend on histological assessment. However, although some growth patterns are characteristic, conventional histology alone cannot be used to identify endocrine tumours as it gives no information on their products, and, in some cases (e.g. poorly differentiated carcinomas), cannot even differentiate between neuroendocrine and other neoplasms. Electron microscopy, histochemistry and, latterly, immunocytochemistry have provided the means for thorough classification of neuroendocrine tumours and now provide the basis for accurate diagnosis in routine histopathological practice. In addition, the information obtained from immunocytochemical detection of neuroendocrine tumour products is being augmented in numerous routine laboratories by *in situ* hybridization of nucleic acids.

This chapter describes the classification of the diffuse neuroendocrine system and its derivative tumours.

Specific neuroendocrine cell types

The general features of the various cell types of the normal diffuse neuroendocrine system are presented for brevity in Tables 59.1 and 59.2, which show the internationally accepted classification.

Neuroendocrine tumours of individual organs

Gastrointestinal tract

The main neuroendocrine tumours of the gastrointestinal tract are listed in Table 59.3, along with their major characteristics. In addition to those tumours listed, poorly differentiated neuroendocrine carcinomas, or small-cell carcinomas, can arise, mostly in the oesophagus, stomach and large bowel, from proto-endocrine cells. These tumours are not associated with any particular clinical syndrome.

Oesophagus

Neuroendocrine tumours are rare in the oesophagus and mainly comprise the neuroendocrine carcinomas described above. No consistent clinical syndrome is associated with neuroendocrine tumours of the oesophagus, although there have been rare reports of the production of inappropriate hormones (e.g. adrenocorticotrophic hormone (ACTH), serotonin).

Stomach

Neuroendocrine tumours of the stomach are more common and varied. The majority arise in the fundus/body and their functions have yet to be characterized fully. The incidence of gastric neuroendocrine tumours appears to be increasing, or detection and identification of this tumour type may have improved. In conditions of hypochlorhydria and resultant hypergastrinaemia, due to, for example, chronic atrophic gastritis or therapeutic blockade of gastric acid secretion, there can be hyperplasia, dysplasia and neoplasia of D_1/P, enterochromaffin (EC) and, most frequently, enterochromaffin-like (ECL) cells (Fig. 59.1). An internationally agreed classification

Table 59.1 Major neuroendocrine cells of the gastroenteropancreatic tract

| Cell | Pancreas | Stomach | | Small intestine | | Large intestine | Granules | Product |
		Oxyntic	Pyloric	Upper	Lower			
P	–	+	+	+	–	–	100–140 nm, round, e.d.	?
D₁	Rare	+	Rare	Rare	Rare	Rare	140–190 nm, round, e.d.	?
EC	–	+	+	+	+	+	Pleomorphic, e.d.	5-HT, motilin, substance P, neurokinins
D	+	+	+	+	+	+	260–370 nm, round, low e.d.	Somatostatin
B	+	–	–	–	–	–	200 nm, crystalline core	Insulin, C-peptide, amylin
A	+	–	–	–	–	–	300 nm, e.d. core, halo	Glucagon immunoreactants
PP	+	–	–	–	–	–	100–200 nm, round/oval, e.d. core and narrow halo	Pancreatic polypeptide
X	–	+	–	–	–	–	250 nm, round, e.d.	?
ECL	–	+	–	–	–	–	200 nm, vesicular or e.d.	Histamine
G	–	–	+	–	–	–	200–400 nm, vesicular to moderately e.d.	Gastrin (G17)
IG	–	–	–	+	–	–	200 nm, e.d.	Gastrin (G34)
I	–	–	–	+	–	–	250 nm, irregular, e.d.	CCK
S	–	–	–	+	–	–	250 nm, irregular, halo	Secretin
K	–	–	–	+	–	–	350 nm, round and irregular e.d.	GIP
Mo	–	–	–	+	–	–	?	Motilin
N	–	–	–	–	+	–	300 nm, round, moderately e.d.	Neurotensin
L	–	–	–	–	+	+	250 nm, round, moderately e.d.	Glucagon immunoreactants, PYY

CCK, cholecystokinin; e.d., electron dense; GIP, glucose-dependent insulinotropic peptide; 5-HT, 5-hydroxytryptamine or serotonin; PYY, peptide tyrosine tyrosine.

Table 59.2 Non-gastroenteropancreatic endocrine cells

Site	Cell type	Granules	Product(s)
Pituitary	Somatotroph	250–600 nm, round, e.d.	GH
	Lactotroph	150–2000 nm, round, irregular, e.d.	PRL
	Corticotroph	250–400 nm, irregular, varying e.d.	ACTH
	FSH gonadotroph	200–450 nm, round, e.d.	FSH
	LH gonadotroph	150–350 nm, round, e.d.	LH
	Thyrotroph	< 150 nm, round, e.d.	TSH
Thyroid	C	200–300 nm, round, e.d.	Calcitonin, CGRP, somatostatin, ACTH
Lung	P	100–140 nm, round, e.d.	?GRP
	D₁	140–190 nm, round, e.d.	?GRP
Adrenal	A	200 nm, e.d.	Adrenaline
	NA	200 nm, highly e.d.	Noradrenaline
Skin	Merkel cell	150–300 nm, round, e.d.	?
Prostate	EC+?	160–450 nm, round, pleomorphic	5-HT+?
Breast	?	?	?
Uterus	?	?	?
Thymus	?	?	?

ACTH, adrenocorticotrophic hormone; CGRP, calcitonin gene-related peptide; e.d., electron dense; FSH, follicle-stimulating hormone; GH, growth hormone; GRP, gastrin-releasing peptide; 5-HT, 5-hydroxytryptamine or serotonin; LH, luteinizing hormone; PRL, prolactin; TSH, thyroid-stimulating hormone.

of this sequence of gastric endocrine cell changes has been published by Solcia and colleagues [3]. Histologically, the tumours usually have a nested or trabecular architecture. ECL cells are particularly abundant in the oxyntic mucosa of the stomach and are susceptible to the trophic effects of gastrin. Thus, they constitute non-argentaffin carcinoids of the gastric/body fundus. No peptide has been identified in ECL cells. They are known to contain

Table 59.3 Characteristics of main neuroendocrine tumours of the gastrointestinal tract [1, 2]

Site	Main cell type	Product/s	Syndrome
Oesophagus	EC	Serotonin (rare)	Atypical carcinoid
	P	?ACTH	Cushing's
		Calcitonin (rare)	
Fundus	EC	Serotonin (rare)	Atypical carcinoid
	ECL	?Histamine	
	D_1/P	?	
	Inappropriate	ACTH	Cushing's
Antrum	G	Gastrin	ZE
	D	Somatostatin (rare)	MEN-2
	P/D_1	?	
	Inappropriate	ACTH	Cushing's
Small intestine	G/IG	Gastrin	ZE, MEN-1
	D	Somatostatin	MEN-2
	?Paraganglia	Somatostatin, PP	
	EC	Serotonin, tachykinins	Carcinoid
	P	?	
	Inappropriate	ACTH	Cushing's
Large intestine	L	Glucagon and related peptides, PYY	
	EC	Serotonin (rare)	
	D	Somatostatin (rare)	

ACTH, adrenocorticotrophic hormone; MEN, multiple endocrine neoplasia; PP, pancreatic polypeptide; PYY, peptide tyrosine tyrosine; ZE, Zollinger–Ellison.

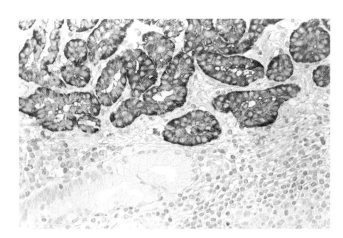

Fig. 59.1 Immunoreactivity for the general neuroendocrine marker chromogranin demonstrates the presence of an infiltrating neuroendocrine (enterochromaffin-like cell) tumour in the oxyntic mucosa of the stomach of a patient with chronic atrophic gastritis. (Haematoxylin counterstain, × 350.)

histamine in rodents and there have been isolated reports of the presence of histamine in normal human ECL cells and in the circulation of some patients with ECL cell carcinoids.

Although the gastric antrum is the major site for gastrin (G) cells in the normal gastrointestinal tract, very few (about 1%) gastrin-producing tumours have been described in the stomach, most occur in the pancreas (see later) or duodenum. When they do occur in the stomach, they are often associated with the Zollinger–Ellison or gastrinoma syndrome.

Small intestine

A large proportion of patients with a gastrin-producing tumour have the multiple endocrine neoplasia (MEN) 1 syndrome [4]. When hypergastrinaemia is detected in MEN-1 patients it is usually thought to be due to a pancreatic tumour. However, it appears that the duodenum may be the major site for these tumours (Fig. 59.2), an observation which may explain the failure to locate a gastrin-secreting pancreatic tumour in some cases. Not all G cell tumours of the duodenum give rise to the gastrinoma syndrome, as some clinically silent, benign lesions have been described.

The other main neuroendocrine tumour type of the duodenum is the somatostatin (D cell)-rich type, sometimes termed glandular carcinoid. These epithelial tumours have been described as having a typical glandular or acinar histological pattern, with frequent psammoma bodies in the lumina of the glandular structures (Fig. 59.3), and

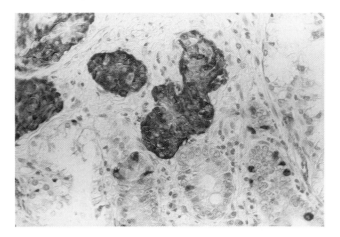

Fig. 59.2 Section of human duodenum immunostained for gastrin. Immunoreactivity can be seen in an infiltrating G cell tumour (gastrinoma) and in scattered endocrine cells in the mucosal epithelium. (Haematoxylin counterstain, × 350.)

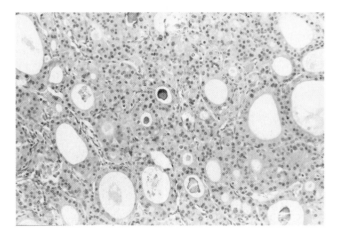

Fig. 59.3 Section of a duodenal somatostatin-rich neuroendocrine tumour showing characteristic acinar arrangement of cells and psammomatous bodies. (Haematoxylin and eosin stain, × 175.)

abundant somatostatin immunoactivity. These tumours are not associated with the so-called somatostatinoma syndrome described for some pancreatic D cell tumours, although there have been occasional reports of diabetes or gall stone formation. Most of these tumours arise in the peri-ampullary region of the duodenum and, thus, are frequently associated with obstructive biliary disease. These duodenal D cell tumours often occur as part of von Recklinghausen's syndrome and, in some cases, in association with a phaeochromocytoma in MEN-2a.

Gangliocytic paragangliomas are rare neuroendocrine lesions of the duodenum, and are benign tumours which are composed of fully differentiated ganglion cells, epithelial, endocrine cells and spindle cells. Immunoreactivity

for somatostatin has been detected in both neural and endocrine cell types and for pancreatic polypeptide in the endocrine cells. The exact histogenesis of gangliocytic paragangliomas is not known but a possible relationship between the epithelial, glandular D cell tumour and the paraganglioma has been suggested, with the former representing a purely epithelial form of the latter. Indeed, a few cases of von Recklinghausen's syndrome have been found to show both tumour types. However, most of the glandular tumours lack any gangliocytic paraganglioma components and ultrastructural studies show no evidence of common histogenesis.

The most frequent neuroendocrine tumour found in the lower small intestine is the argentaffin (EC cell; serotonin-producing) carcinoid. The majority arise in the ileum where most are malignant, or appendix, where most are benign. The first recognition of this tumour type is attributed generally to Lurbasch, who described a patient with multiple 'carcinomata' of the ileum. In 1909, Obendorfer coined the name carcinoid for these tumours, emphasizing their benign behaviour. In 1953, Lembeck reported a high content of the bioactive amine serotonin in the tumours. The term carcinoid is often used to describe all neuroendocrine tumours but it is preferable to restrict its usage to these argentaffin tumours. The typical syndrome associated with carcinoid tumours consists of episodes of flushing, hypertension, diarrhoea, cough, wheezing and telangiectasis. These symptoms become particularly prominent once the tumour has metastasized to the liver, allowing the tumour products to enter the systemic circulation. Unlike most other neuroendocrine neoplasms, the size of the tumour may be considered a prognostic factor. When a tumour measures more than 2 cm in diameter it is considered malignant and it is likely that metastases are already present. Carcinoid tumours are often multiple and sometimes associated with other malignant neoplasms. Histologically, the tumours are composed of polygonal, sometimes spindle-shaped cells, with a finely granulated cytoplasm arranged mainly in nests. Ultrastructurally, the tumour cells contain pleomorphic, often biconcave granules as seen in EC cells. In addition to serotonin, argentaffin carcinoids have been shown to contain the β-preprotachykinin-derived peptides, substance P and neurokinin A, which may contribute to the clinical syndrome. The behavioural differences of ileal and appendiceal carcinoid tumours may reflect their histogenesis in that ileal tumours are thought to arise from intra-epithelial EC cells, whereas appendiceal are considered to be derived from extra-epithelial neuroendocrine (Kultchitsky) cells. There is an appendiceal variant of this tumour type which contains goblet cells. These tumours are more malignant than pure carcinoids and ultrastructural analysis shows that they have features of both exocrine and endocrine differentiation.

Large intestine

Within the large intestine, the most frequent site for neuroendocrine tumours is the rectum. Tumours at this site are usually benign, but the rarer colonic forms tend to follow a more malignant course. The histological appearance is fairly variable, with cells arranged in trabeculae, tubulo-acinar formations or solid nests. Immunoreactivity for glucagon/glicentin is found in most of the hindgut neuroendocrine tumours, revealing that the L cell is the predominant tumour component. Despite this prevalence of glucagon in the tumours, no definite clinical syndrome has been associated with them. An enteroglucagon-producing tumour of the kidney, however, was found to consist of L cells and was associated with reduced intestinal absorption and motility, as well as with hypertrophy of the intestinal mucosa. The carcinoid syndrome has only rarely been associated with a hindgut tumour. Rare, mixed neuroendocrine and mucinous tumours have been described in the colon as in appendix.

Pancreas

The current classification of pancreatic neuroendocrine tumours is shown in Table 59.4. The most common of these is the β cell tumour or insulinoma. These are usually benign and confined to the pancreas, although they have been described at other sites, including the duodenum. Insulinomas represent one of the many causes of hypoglycaemia. They constitute 70–75% of all pancreatic endocrine tumours and are about equally common in both sexes. The highest incidence of insulinomas is found between the ages of 30 and 61 years, but insulinomas have been described in patients up to 82 years old and infants with nesidioblastosis may present with β cell hyperplasia, focal adenomatosis and/or clearcut β cell adenoma.

The diameter of the tumours is generally less than 3 cm and their weight less than 10 g, but the size of the tumours varies considerably and is unrelated to the severity of the symptoms. The ratio of malignant tumours varies between 4 and 16%. Histologically, a solid or trabecular (Fig. 59.4) growth pattern is most often found. This pattern varies from region to region of the same tumour. Amyloid with a characteristic fibrillary appearance at the electron microscopical level is frequently found in insulinomas. A 37 amino acid peptide called amylin has been isolated from this amyloid, which is also a feature of the type 2 diabetic pancreas. It is also found in normal β cells and is

Table 59.4 Classification of pancreatic neuroendocrine tumours (after [3])

Islet cell tumours
Mostly adenomas
 clinically silent A, B, D, PP, EC and P cell tumours
 insulinoma: β cells (with or without other islet cells)

Mostly low-grade carcinomas
 glucagonoma: A cells (with or without other islet cells)
 somatostatinomas: D cells (with or without other islet cells)
 non-functioning A, B, D, PP, EC and P cell tumours with local effects

Inappropriate tumours
Mostly low-grade carcinomas
 gastrinomas: G cells (with or without other cells)
 VIPoma: VIP cells (with or without other cells)
 others with syndromes (e.g. ACTH, calcitonin, PTH, etc.) (with or without other cells)

Other tumours
Highly malignant
 poorly differentiated (small-cell carcinomas)

The suffix -oma denotes a functioning tumour with a clinically defined syndrome.
ACTH, adrenocorticotrophic hormone; PTH, parathyroid hormone; VIP, vasoactive intestinal polypeptide.

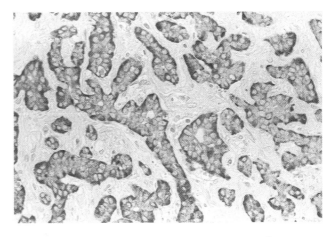

Fig. 59.4 Insulin immunostained in cells of a typical β cell tumour (insulinoma) arranged in trabeculae. (Haematoxylin counterstain, $\times 350$.)

thought to contribute to insulin resistance. Secretory granules may sometimes resemble the classic β cells of the pancreas with a crystalline core, but frequently the granules are round and small, many of them demonstrated to be immunostained by antibodies to proinsulin. Cells containing small D_1 type secretory granules have been shown to contain and store pancreatic polypeptide. Insulinomas are also often mixed and again pancreatic polypeptide is one of the frequent contaminants of this class of tumours.

A cell tumours or glucagonomas form about 1% of pancreatic neuroendocrine tumours and are associated with a clearcut clinical syndrome characterized by necrolytic erythema and diabetes. The disease occurs most often between 40 and 70 years of age and appears to be slightly more common in women than in men. More than 60% of glucagonomas causing the symptoms are malignant. This percentage is even higher if one considers tumours inducing hyperglucagonaemia but not causing the complete syndrome. The tumours associated with the syndrome are typically large, 3–5 cm, and generally malignant. Histologically glucagonomas show no remarkable features other than general endocrine morphology. These tumours can produce other derivatives of preproglucagon, in addition to pancreatic glucagon. Glucagonomas are often mixed; most often they contain pancreatic polypeptide-containing cells, but insulin or somatostatin cells may also be found. Ultrastructurally, typical A cell granules are found mainly in clinically silent tumours, with atypical granules occurring in functional tumours.

As mentioned earlier, gastrin-producing tumours occur rarely in the antrum, the major repository of G cells, but are the most common duodenal neuroendocrine tumour and comprise about 20% of all pancreatic neuroendocrine tumours. Pancreatic gastrinomas were long thought to be ectopic tumours but it seems that they may arise from cells which express the gastrin gene but show attenuated processing of progastrin in the adult pancreas. Pancreatic gastrinomas give rise to the Zollinger–Ellison syndrome, like those of the antrum and duodenum, and show a malignancy rate of around 60%. Most of these tumours can be immunostained for gastrin and about half contain pancreatic polypeptide, insulin and/or somatostatin cells. Secretory granules show morphological heterogeneity; some tumours have typical G cell granules, others have intestinal gastrin (IG) granules but there is a proportion of cases with few, non-diagnostic granules. Although pancreatic gastrinomas can produce both G17 and G34, there appears to be little correlation between ultrastructure and secretion.

Vasoactive intestinal polypeptide (VIP)-secreting tumours represent 3–5% of all pancreatic endocrine tumours and are associated with a clinical syndrome characterized by watery diarrhoea and achlorhydria. This VIPoma syndrome is also associated with ganglioneuroblastomas in about 20% of cases. The tumours are often quite large (2–7 cm) and 50–75% are malignant. Histologically, VIPomas tend to show a poorly differentiated morphology with flattened cells in a mainly trabecular arrangement.

Like G cells, VIP cells cannot be found in the normal human pancreas. In fact, VIP has not been demonstrated convincingly in any normal endocrine cell, although it is a highly abundant neuropeptide. Immunocytochemical detection of VIP is often difficult as little is stored by the tumours. Ultrastructurally, VIPoma granules tend to be small and haloed, similar to PP cells.

Comparatively rare pancreatic neuroendocrine tumours consisting mainly of somatostatin (D) cells have been reported but their association with a specific clinical syndrome remains in dispute. A syndrome of diabetes mellitus, steatorrhoea, hypochlorhydria and, in some cases, gall stones has been described. Most pancreatic D cell tumours are solitary and malignant.

Oversecretion of pancreatic polypeptide (PP) is one of the most frequent associations noted with well defined functioning pancreatic endocrine tumours, and, therefore, immunostaining of PP in a metastasis of an endocrine tumour of unknown origin points to the possibility of the primary being present in the pancreas. Where PP is the main hormonal product of a tumour, the term PPoma has been used but, unlike 'somatostatinomas', no clearcut clinical syndrome has been defined.

Some rare functioning neuroendocrine tumours of the pancreas produce ectopic hormones and have associated clinical syndromes. Tumours associated with acromegaly have been described and the symptoms appear to be due to growth hormone-releasing factor (GHRF). Cushing's syndrome can result from production of ACTH by pancreatic tumours. Parathyroid hormone (PTH) can also be produced and is associated with paraneoplastic hypercalcaemia. All of these tumours are usually malignant and form large masses in the pancreas.

Neuroendocrine tumours of the pancreas which show no clinical association with a syndrome are termed non-functioning. Almost all are malignant. PP is probably the most frequent peptide found in these tumours.

Although endocrine cell proliferation can sometimes be observed in non-endocrine cancer, true, mixed endocrine–exocrine tumours of the pancreas are rare. Klöppel and colleagues have stipulated that to be classified as mixed, such tumours should contain both types of cells in metastases, in addition to the primary tumour, as well as amphicrine cells which contain both secretory granules and zymogen or mucin vesicles.

Pancreatic neuroendocrine tumours occur in MEN-1, and it is becoming increasingly clear that the multifocal, neoplastic transformation can occur in this syndrome in part or all of the pancreas. It should be borne in mind, therefore, that removal of a single, macroscopically detectable lesion of the pancreas may not resolve all the patient's symptoms. Microadenomas, more commonly producing PP and/or glucagon rather than the other pancreatic peptides, are likely to be present. In addition, as described previously, Zollinger–Ellison syndrome in MEN-1 may be the result of a very small, possibly multicentric, lesion in the duodenum and so careful examination of this area is necessary during surgery.

Respiratory tract

Endocrine cells are known to occur in the human fetal and adult lung, both as single cells and part of neuro-epithelial bodies. The respiratory tract is a common site for neuroendocrine tumours and these have been divided into three main groups.
1 The so-called carcinoids, comprising mostly benign non-functioning tumours, tumours that are associated with a clinical syndrome which are mostly malignant, but of a low degree, and atypical carcinoids, of which about 70% are malignant.
2 Small- or intermediate-cell carcinomas, which are all highly malignant.
3 Paragangliomas, consisting of type I cells which are usually benign.
The highest incidence of bronchial carcinoids occurs in the 31–40-year age group with a slight preponderance for females (62%). The tumour usually arises in the main bronchi but may be located in the lung periphery. Multicentric growth has been described and carcinoids may be part of a pluriglandular syndrome. Carcinoids of the lung consist of small, regular cells with vesicular nuclei and eosinophilic granular cytoplasm (Fig. 59.5). The cells are arranged in mosaic, trabecular or adenopapillary patterns. Necrosis and mitotic figures are usually minimal or absent, but a typical variant characterized by cellular pleomorphism, nuclear atypia and mitotic figures has

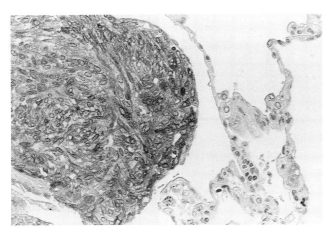

Fig. 59.5 The growth-promoting peptide bombesin (or gastrin-releasing peptide) immunostained in cells of a lung carcinoid tumour. (Haematoxylin counterstain, × 350.)

been described. Like other endocrine tumours, bronchial carcinoids grow slowly and have low malignancy potential, atypical carcinoids having a worse prognosis. Carcinoids may possess areas of glandular differentiation with mucus secretion. Small-cell carcinoma of the lung is the malignant counterpart of lung neuroendocrine tumours. It is one of the most frequent tumours and comprises 20% of all bronchial carcinomas. Small-cell carcinomas of the lung are aggressive neoplasms, having the poorest prognosis of all lung tumours with an overall 5-year survival rate of only 2%. The tumour is generally extremely sensitive to combination chemotherapy and radiotherapy, whereas other lung tumours are more amenable to surgery. It is therefore of paramount importance to classify lung tumours correctly and, in particular, to separate small-cell carcinomas from other types of lung tumour.

One of the most commonly found peptides in neuro-endocrine tumours of the respiratory tract is bombesin or gastrin-releasing peptide. Bombesin released from tumour cells acts in a paracrine (autocrine) manner to stimulate growth of the tumour. Immunocytochemistry of preprobombesin-derived peptides in these tumours has shown that the well differentiated carcinoids are strongly immunoreactive for bombesin, whereas the highly malignant small-cell carcinomas show dense immunoreactivity for the C-flanking peptide of human bombesin. Thus, it appears that the pattern of expression of a peptide precursor can provide prognostic information. Some lung carcinoids produce serotonin and tachykinins but are infrequently associated with the clinical carcinoid syndrome.

Skin

Neuroendocrine neoplasms of the skin are comparatively rare lesions and their histogenesis is disputed. However, the only well characterized skin neuroendocrine cell, the Merkel cell, is a major source of these tumours. These Merkel cell tumours, or Merkelomas, show variable histology, from small-cell types to trabecular forms composed of cells with well defined cytoplasm. Immunocytochemistry for the general neuroendocrine marker neurone-specific enolase (NSE), is a useful means to differentiate Merkel cell tumours from histologically similar skin lesions (e.g. lymphomas). Distinction from melanomas or from metastatic skin tumours (e.g. small cell carcinoma) is more difficult as they may also show NSE immunoreactivity. ACTH, calcitonin and bombesin have been detected in a few of these tumours. Electron microscopy reveals that they possess round, neurosecretory type granules and intermediate filaments.

Breast

Although neuroendocrine differentiation can occur in breast carcinomas, no neuroendocrine cell has been identified in normal breast. Around 30% of breast carcinomas have been reported, on the basis of NSE immunoreactivity, to show some degree of neuroendocrine differentiation. Ductal, mucinous and small-cell carcinomas show immunoreactivity, as well as tumours with a carcinoid appearance. Immunoreactivity for a variety of peptides has been detected in breast carcinomas, including ACTH, VIP, encephalin and prolactin, but only very few cases have had related clinical symptoms. Ultrastructural analysis of breast carcinomas with neuroendocrine differentiation has revealed the existence of five different cell types, based on the appearance of their secretory granules.

Urogenital tract

Ovarian neuroendocrine (often described as carcinoid) tumours have been observed and show a pattern of cell types seen in rectal neuroendocrine tumours.

Neuroendocrine cells have also been identified in adenocarcinomas of the cervix and, less rarely, endometrium. Pure prostatic carcinoid tumours are rare, although 10% of adenocarcinomas contain neuroendocrine cells. Secretion of ACTH and an associated Cushing's syndrome has been reported in some cases. In addition, an undifferentiated small-cell carcinoma of the prostate secreting ACTH has been described. Neuroendocrine cells are frequently found in testicular teratomas.

Conclusion

The advent of modern morphological techniques has allowed detailed classification of neuroendocrine neoplasia and provided further insight into their biology.

References

1. Polak JM. *Diagnostic Histopathology of Neuroendocrine Tumours.* Edinburgh: Churchill Livingstone, 1993.
2. Polak JM, Van Noorden S. *Immunocytochemistry: Modern Methods and Applications*, 2nd edn. Bristol: John Wright, 1986.
3. Solcia E, Bordi C, Creutzfeldt W *et al*. Histopathological classification of nonantral gastric endocrine growths in man. *Digestion* 1988;**41**:185–200.
4. Johannesson JV, Gould VE, Nesland JM. Diagnostic seminars: neuroendocrine tumours. *Pathol. Res. Pract.* 1988;**183**(2).

60

Tumour Markers

FRANK R.E. NOBELS AND STEVEN W.J. LAMBERTS

Introduction

The neuroendocrine cells of the gastroenteropancreatic (GEP) axis belong to the APUD (amine precursor uptake and decarboxylation) system, because they are capable of amine precursor uptake and decarboxylation, leading to the production of amines or small peptides. Currently, over 50 peptides have been identified, secreted by more than 15 different types of neuroendocrine cells scattered throughout the gut [1]. Tumours of these cells are generally characterized by an excessive production of one or several of these peptides. The presence of peptides in tumour tissue can usually be easily identified by immunohistochemical methods, or by demonstrating their mRNA with *in situ* hybridization techniques. The peptides are also frequently released into the circulation, where they can exert their endocrine effects on various targets, often inducing a typical clinical syndrome of hormonal overproduction. These tumours can be called *clinically functioning neuroendocrine tumours*. The circulating peptides can usually be measured by radioimmunological methods, allowing them to be used as tumour markers [2]. One tumour generally releases several amines or peptides in the circulation. Therefore the choice of possible tumour markers is much wider than in the case of non-endocrine tumours. The situation is much more difficult in so-called *clinically non-functioning neuroendocrine tumours*, not inducing symptoms or signs relating to hormonal hypersecretion. Sometimes these tumours remain hormonally active, producing peptides without clinical effect, which still can be used as tumour markers. When the tumour has lost all abilities to produce hormonally active substances one has to resort to the use of non-endocrine secretion markers, such as certain enzymes or other contents of secretory granules.

In the choice of an adequate tumour marker, the following criteria should be taken into account [3]. The marker must be useful:

1 to screen populations for the presence of a tumour;
2 to differentiate between the different types of neuro-endocrine tumours;
3 to distinguish between benign, intermediate or malignant tumour types;
4 to provide an estimate of the tumour load;
5 to follow the course of a particular tumour over time, in order to be able to evaluate the response to therapeutic interventions, and to rapidly detect an eventual relapse;
6 to assess the prognosis.

Unfortunately none of the current tumour markers can fulfil all these goals. Therefore, the search for better markers still goes on, and is at present one of the main activities of neuroendocrine research. In addition to the use of the circulating peptides themselves, the receptors for some peptides have recently been shown to be very valuable markers. Their presence on tumour tissue can be demonstrated *in vivo* by radioisotopic techniques, using radionucleotide labelled peptide, which specifically binds to a specific receptor.

Serum markers

Clinically functioning neuroendocrine tumours

Table 60.1 provides an overview of endocrine syndromes, with the most important peptides being responsible for the clinical expression. Most of these peptides can serve as excellent tumour markers, that can be used both in the diagnosis as well as in the follow-up of these neoplasms. In the interpretation of the data one should take into account the feedback system involved. The demonstration of inappropriate secretion is often an important clue to the presence of a tumour: high insulin levels in the presence of hypoglycaemia in insulinomas, high gastrin levels in the presence of gastric acid hypersecretion in gastrinomas, and high glucagon levels in the absence of hypoglycaemia in glucagonomas.

the GEP system. The serum levels are usually much lower than in trophoblastic neoplasms, requiring the application of highly sensitive detection methods. The prevalences reported in the literature vary considerably for similar neuroendocrine tumours, probably due to differences in patient selection and assay characteristics (sensitivity, crossreaction with other glycoprotein subunits, etc.). High levels occur frequently in patients with endocrine pancreatic tumours and in patients with carcinoids. Elevated levels are also frequently encountered in non-functioning neuroendocrine neoplasms, in the absence of other hormonal markers. Both subunits should be measured, since several tumours only secrete α subunit and no β subunit and vice versa. By analogy with other forms of ectopic hormonal secretion, it is postulated that elevated levels of hCG subunits are markers of malignant behaviour. This has not been proven yet, however. Rarely, hCG-α and -β can also be produced by tumours that are not of trophoblastic or neuroendocrine origin (e.g. craniopharyngioma). Thus, they are not entirely specific markers.

Non-endocrine markers

Neurone-specific enolase

Neurone-specific enolase (NSE) is a neurone-specific isomer of the ubiquitous glycolytic enzyme 2-phospho-D-glycerate hydrolyase or enolase. This isomer is only present in neurones and neuroendocrine cells, and can serve as an excellent immunohistochemical marker for tumours derived from these cells. Elevated serum concentrations of NSE can be detected in all kinds of neuroendocrine neoplasms, regardless of the original cell types or the secreted peptides. The levels are closely correlated with the tumour load, and can be used to estimate the prognosis of the neoplasm. Unfortunately, NSE has a poor sensitivity in patients with limited disease. Thus, it cannot be used as a screening marker for early diagnosis of neuroendocrine tumours (e.g. in multiple endocrine neoplasia), or for early detection of relapse after successful treatment. It is less sensitive than the classic hormonal markers of functioning neuroendocrine neoplasms. So, its interest is obviously limited to neuro-endocrine tumours without hormonal production, or with secretion products that are difficult to quantify (as is the case in carcinoids or phaeochromocytomas). In clinical practice, NSE is one of the most widely used tumour markers in small-cell lung cancer (SCLC), where it has been shown to be a reliable tool in the differentiation from non-SCLC and in the monitoring of the evolution of the disease.

Chromogranin A

CgA, a protein originally discovered in the chromaffin cells of the adrenal medulla, is widely distributed throughout the neuroendocrine system [4]. Inside the cells it is localized in the electron-dense core secretory granules, where it is co-stored and co-secreted with the local neuropeptides. Although its biological role has not yet been established, several functions have been postulated. It might fulfil regulatory activities in the packaging and processing of peptide hormones and in the modulation of neuroendocrine secretion. CgA is a well-established immunohistochemical marker of normal and neoplastic neuroendocrine tissues. During the last years several immunoassays have been developed to measure serum concentrations of CgA, allowing it to be used also as a serum marker of neuroendocrine tumours. Even less well-differentiated tumours, that have lost their ability to secrete neuropeptides, usually retain the capacity to synthesize and secrete CgA. Therefore, serum levels of CgA could be useful in diagnosing and monitoring clinically non-functioning neuroendocrine neoplasms. Unfortunately, it is again not a very sensitive marker. CgA is produced by nearly all normal neuroendocrine tissues throughout the body, resulting in a large circulating plasma pool. Therefore, only extensive tumours are able to induce significant increases in serum concentrations. Extreme elevations can occur in patients with metastatic carcinoids, with values in some patients exceeding 1000 times the upper limit of normal. High levels can also be encountered in large phaeochromocytomas, clinically functioning and non-functioning endocrine pancreatic tumours and medullary thyroid cancers. CgA is a more stable and thus more easily manageable marker for carcinoids and phaeochromocytomas than the existing determinations of, respectively, serotonin and catecholamines or their urinary metabolites. In the interpretation of the data one should take into account that hepatic and especially renal failure result in increased serum CgA levels, with severe renal failure (creatinine clearance lower than 25 ml/min) leading to concentrations otherwise only seen in patients with neuroendocrine neoplasia.

Peptide receptors as markers for neuroendocrine tumours

The synthesis and secretion of peptide hormones by most human neuroendocrine tumours allows the measurement of circulating hormone concentrations as a marker of tumour presence, size and/or activity (see above). In recent years it has become evident that virtually all tumours with neuroendocrine characteristics also express membrane receptors for small peptides like somato-statin, VIP, bombesin and substance P. The demonstration of peptide receptors on tumours by ligand binding studies or autoradiography has extended the number of 'neuroendocrine markers' that can be used in the pathological examination of tumours. However, apart from these *in vitro* investigations, peptide receptor expression by neuroendocrine tumours can also be studied *in vivo* after the administration of tracer amounts of peptides coupled to radionucleotides. This technique of peptide receptor scintigraphy has been developed successfully for the visualization of somatostatin receptors on (neuro)endocrine tumours. After the intravenous administration of [111In]-diethylenetriamine penta-acetic acid (DTPA)-octreotide (Octreoscan) the primary tumours, but also the previously unrecognized metastases of most carcinoids, islet cell tumours, paragangliomas, phaeo-chromocytomas, medullary thyroid cancers and SCLC can be visualized (Fig. 60.1). Also other tumour types containing neuroendocrine cells are often positive on the scan (see Table 60.2). The technique of peptide receptor scintigraphy is a new addition to the armament of circulating tumour markers, which gives information about the spread of the disease, but often also predicts a beneficial effect of therapy with somatostatin analogues.

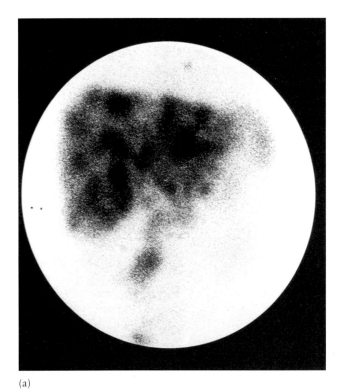

(a)

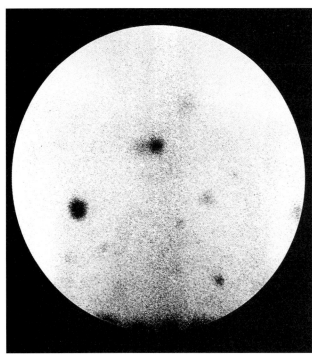

(b)

Fig. 60.1 (a) Anterior view of the abdomen, showing multiple somatostatin receptor-positive metastases in an enlarged liver, as well as the primary carcinoid tumour in the wall of the jejunum of a patient with severe attacks of flushing and diarrhoea. Pictures made 24 hours after [111In]-DTPA-octreotide administration. (b) Posterior view of the chest and neck of this same patient showing a metastasis in a lymph node on the left side of the neck (top), as well as multiple metastases in ribs and pleura. (Reproduced from [5] with permission.)

Table 60.2 Incidence of somatostatin receptors on human tumours (after [5])

Tumour type	Prevalence observed at scintigraphy
Pituitary adenomas:	
growth hormone	4/4 (100%)
TSH	2/2 (100%)
inactive	6/8 (75%)
Endocrine pancreatic tumours	18/21 (86%)
Carcinoids	37/39 (95%)
Paragangliomas	29/31 (94%)
Phaeochromocytomas	2/5 (40%)
Medullary thyroid carcinomas	7/12 (58%)
Lung tumours:	
SCLC	5/8 (63%)
non-SCLC	3/4 (75%)
Neuroblastomas	5/5 (100%)
Meningiomas	11/11 (100%)
Merkel cell tumours	4/5 (80%)
Breast cancers	39/52 (75%)
Adenocarcinomas:	
unknown origin	5/9 (56%)
pancreatic	0/20 (0%)
Lymphomas	10/10 (100%)

SCLC, small-cell lung cancer; TSH, thyroid-stimulating hormone.

References

1. Green DW, Gomez G, Greeley GH Jr. Gastrointestinal peptides. *Gastroenterol. Clin. North Am.* 1989;**18**(4):695–733.
2. Reubi J-C. The role of peptides and their receptors as tumor markers. *Endocrinol. Metab. Clin. North Am.* 1993;**22**(4):917–39.
3. Modlin IM, Basson MD. Clinical applications of gastrointestinal hor-mones. *Endocrinol. Metab. Clin. North Am.* 1993;**22**(4):823–44.
4. Deftos LJ. Chromogranin A: its role in endocrine function and as an endocrine and neuroendocrine tumor marker. *Endocr. Rev.* 1991;**12**:181–7.
5. Lamberts SWJ, Krenning EP, Reubi J-C. The role of somatostatin and its analogs in the diagnosis and treatment of tumors. *Endocr. Rev.* 1991;**12**:450–82.

61

Insulinomas and Hypoglycaemia

VINCENT MARKS

Prevalence

Insulinoma is the name given to any tumour of the endocrine pancreas that secretes insulin and manifests itself by producing fasting hypoglycaemia regardless of its histology [1–3]. Collectively, insulinomas are the most common of the endocrine tumours of the pancreas (60% of islet cell tumours) but nevertheless they are still rare. The best estimates indicate an incidence of about one new case for every 1 million persons per year, although estimates putting the rate at four times as high have also been made. They occur predominantly in patients over the age of 50 years. Unlike all other endocrine tumours of the pancreas, where malignancy is the rule, insulinomas are usually benign: less than 15% of them metastasize to distant organs, the only criterion of malignancy that is acceptable for these tumours.

Insulinomas are almost always confined to the pancreas, occurring in the head, body and tail with equal frequency, although exceptionally they may be ectopic in the duodenal wall.

More than 90% of insulinomas are between 10 and 20 mm in diameter at the time of diagnosis, but can be as small as 5 mm and still produce symptoms, or as large as 150 mm in diameter. More than 80% of benign insulinomas are solitary, but between 7 and 10% are multiple, either simultaneously or consecutively. When multiple tumours occur it is most often as part of the multiple endocrine neoplasia (MEN)-1 syndrome but is sometimes a singular finding. The possibility of MEN-1 must, therefore, always be borne in mind when a diagnosis of insulinoma is made and appropriate investigations undertaken to confirm or refute it.

Insulinomas are evenly distributed throughout the pancreas and benign, though not malignant, tumours are more common in women than in men, in the ratio of 6 : 4. Although no age is completely exempt, insulinomas are rare before the age of 5 years and unusual in persons over the age of 70; possibly, in the latter instance [4], because of underdiagnosis: the symptoms of chronic neuroglycopenia, to which they give rise, being attributed to dementia.

Symptoms

Patients in whom a diagnosis of insulinoma is made invariably present with symptoms attributable to hypoglycaemia, which can be defined, in persons under the age of 60, as a capillary or arterialized venous blood glucose concentration of 2.2 mmol/l or less; or of 3.0 mmol/l in older persons. The symptoms are almost always intermittent and generally neuroglycopenic, rather than adrenergic, in origin. Strange behaviour, inability to concentrate, forgetfulness, difficulty in waking in the morning and sleepiness in the afternoon are all common, but non-specific pointers to the diagnosis.

The duration of symptoms before diagnosis can be as short as a few days, or as long as 30 years, but nowadays is usually counted in months. Symptoms seldom bear any obvious relationship to feeding, meals or activity but can be brought on by unusually long abstinence from food, especially when accompanied by unaccustomed or vigorous exercise. Weight gain occurs in about 30% of patients and adherence to a strict diet in order to reduce it may provoke symptoms in a previously asymptomatic subject.

Diagnosis

Once suspicion of hypoglycaemia has been aroused, diagnosis proceeds in three sequential stages.
1 Confirmation of hypoglycaemia as the cause of the patient's symptoms.
2 Confirmation of inappropriate insulin secretion as the cause of hypoglycaemia.
3 Localization of the tumour responsible for it.

Confirmation of hypoglycaemia as the cause of the patient's illness

Confirmation of hypoglycaemia is achieved, preferably, by measuring the blood glucose concentration during a spontaneous symptomatic episode at home or wherever it occurs. It is comparatively simple to teach patients or their relatives how to collect free-flowing capillary blood on to specially prepared filter paper (or into capillary tubes containing anticoagulant and sodium fluoride as a preservative) when they feel unwell, and to send the samples to the laboratory for analysis. Alternatively the patient can be investigated as an out-patient; only very rarely is it necessary to admit the patient to hospital in order to establish a diagnosis of hypoglycaemia, thus making the 72-hour fast, the gold standard, now almost obsolete. It is both expensive and difficult to interpret, relying as it does on extensive laboratory testing.

Measurement of an overnight fasting blood glucose concentration on at least three occasions rarely fails to reveal hypoglycaemia, at least once, in patients with proven insulinomas. If these measurements are negative and the symptoms are still suggestive, then either exercising to exhaustion or a 72-hour fast will be necessary. The finding of inappropriately high plasma insulin (> 30 pmol/l), C peptide (> 300 pmol/l) and proinsulin (> 20 pmol/l) levels, in the presence of a blood glucose concentration of 2.2 mmol/l, is virtually diagnostic of insulinoma: the only conditions with which it may be confused being factitious self-administration of sulphonylureas or, the even more uncommon disorder referred to as adult nesidioblastosis, in which a diffuse rather than localized abnormality of B-cell functions is responsible. Attempts have been made by many authors to reduce the expression of 'inappropriateness' of insulin secretion to a simple numeric formula by dividing the plasma insulin concentration by the blood glucose concentration, but this can lead to erroneous diagnosis and is not encouraged.

In rare cases in which simple overnight fasting fails to reveal hypoglycaemia, coupling fasting with rigorous exercise in the clinic is usually successful in so doing. The patient, having had nothing to eat from 18.00 h the night before, is exercised on a stationary bicycle or treadmill for 30 minutes or until exhaustion. Blood is collected at 5-minute intervals and assayed for glucose (in the clinic in the first instance) and plasma hormones. In healthy subjects the blood glucose concentration usually rises or remains stationary (or exceptionally may fall) but plasma insulin and C-peptide levels generally fall to below 30 and 300 pmol/l, respectively. This does not happen in patients with hyperinsulinism due to insulinoma, in whom there is generally no discernible change in plasma insulin or C-peptide levels, but such a rapid and profound fall in blood glucose concentration that the test has to be terminated prematurely.

Many other procedures for the diagnosis of insulinoma have been advocated over the years and include the 72-hour fast test (still looked upon as the gold standard), the intravenous tolbutamide, the intravenous glucagon, the oral L-leucine, the calcium infusion, the glucose-clamp, the 5-hour glucose load, and the C-peptide suppression test. Rarely, however, do they contribute anything to the diagnosis that is not made by measurements of plasma insulin, C peptide and proinsulin in fasting blood samples, and none removes the absolute necessity of demonstrating fasting hypoglycaemia with inappropriate insulin (or proinsulin) and C-peptide secretion before a final diagnosis of insulinoma is made.

Differential diagnosis of fasting hypoglycaemia

Insulinoma is only one of the many causes of 'fasting' hypoglycaemia [5]. It is however distinguished from all other causes (Table 61.1) by the presence of inappropriately high plasma C peptide, insulin, and usually proinsulin, in the presence of hypoglycaemia and the absence of sulphonylureas. In about 5% of insulinomas all, or almost all, of the circulating plasma immunoreactive insulin is proinsulin or its partially cleaved products, rather than native insulin. Certain very rare forms of autoimmune disease can closely mimic the biochemical features of insulinoma but other features of the disease are generally present and enable the diagnosis to be made. This is true also of most, though not all, insulin-like growth factor (IGF)-2-secreting tumours, some of which simulate insulinoma very closely.

Localization

The diagnosis of insulinoma depends exclusively and absolutely upon the demonstration of inappropriate insulin secretion in the presence of fasting hypoglycaemia. Only after the diagnosis of insulinoma has been made by chemical means, and the decision taken to attempt curative therapy by surgical ablation, does the question of attempting to localize the lesion within the pancreas by imaging techniques become worthy even of consideration.

Virtually every imaging technique has been advocated, usually shortly after their first introduction, as an aid to localizing insulinomas. None has proved sufficiently reliable to enable them to be used to dismiss a diagnosis of insulinoma made on sound clinical and biochemical

Table 61.1 Differential diagnosis of the most important causes of fasting hypoglycaemia

Plasma levels of different substances during hypoglycaemia	Insulinoma (days–decades)	NICTH (days–weeks)	Factitious		Autoimmune (days-months)
			Sulphonylurea (days–months)	Insulin (days–months)	
Glucose	↓	↓	↓	↓	↓
NEFA	↓	↓	↓	↓	↓
β-Hydroxybutyrate	↓	↓	↓	↓	↓
Insulin	0–↑↑↑	↓	↑–↑↑	↑↑–↑↑↑	↑–↑↑
C-peptide	↑–↑↑↑	↓	↑–↑↑	↓↓	↑
Proinsulin	↑–↑↑↑	↓	0–↑	↓ : 1	1
Cortisol	0–↑	0–↑	↑–↑↑	↑–↑↑	↑–↑↑
hGH	0–↑	0–↑	↑–↑↑	↑–↑↑	↑–↑↑
Glucagon	0–↑	↓	0–↑	↑–↑↑	↑
IGF-1	0–↑	↓↓↓	0	0	0
IGF-2	0	0–↑	0	0	0
Anti-insulin antibodies	0	0	0	0–↑↑↑	↑↑↑
HbA1c	0–↓	0	0	0–↑↑	0

0, within reference range; ↑, ↑↑, ↑↑↑, increased; ↓, ↓↓, ↓↓↓, decreased.
HbA, adult haemoglobin; hGH, human growth hormone; IGF, insulin-like growth factor; NEFA, non-esterified fatty acid; NICTH, non-islet cell tumour hypoglycaemia.

grounds, and the best that can be achieved is a rough guide to localization. Since tumours are almost invariably within the pancreas, and because the risk of multiple tumours makes thorough examination of the whole pancreas by palpation at operation essential, the value of preoperative localization has been seriously questioned. Usually pancreatic ultrasound and computed tomography (CT) will be carried out. The former has a sensitivity range of 30–61%, the latter 42–78% (see Chapter 58). Evidently these rates vary according to the operator and his/her experience. Octreotide scanning and coeliac axis arteriography can also provide useful data (see Chapter 58).

Of the preoperative localizing techniques available, percutaneous transhepatic pancreatic venous catheterization with sampling and subsequent hormone assay is the only one with a more than 70% chance of being correct. Even this, however, is indicated only if, and when, a second laparotomy becomes necessary, either because no tumour was found at the first operation or because there has been a recurrence.

In contrast to preoperative imaging, especially when used incorrectly for confirmation of the diagnosis rather than as an aid to localization, intra-operative ultrasound has proved extremely useful for the localization of small, occult insulinomas with a better than 90% predictive value, occasionally revealing a tumour that had escaped detection by palpation.

Treatment

The treatment of choice for insulinoma is ablation in

all but the very elderly. When undertaken by a skilled pancreatic surgeon the perioperative mortality rate is under 1%, although in less experienced hands deaths are far from rare. Of the 111 operative deaths recorded in the older, pre-1970, literature and reviewed by Stefanini and colleagues [6], 37% were associated with acute pancreatitis and 23% with peritonitis. In 16% of the 1012 patients reviewed by Stefanini and colleagues, hypoglycaemia persisted after the operation. In 40% of these it was due to non-resectability of the lesion, either because of metastatic spread or involvement of the whole pancreas by multiple endocrine adenomatosis, but in most it was due to failure to localize a small, solitary, benign tumour which was removed at a later operation.

Following successful removal of a solitary insulinoma life expectancy is restored to normal. There does, however, appear to be an increased propensity for treated patients to develop diabetes, peptic ulcer disease and/or neuropsychiatric aberrations. Long-term follow-up studies are, however, limited to very few and these have yielded conflicting evidence.

Although only very rarely does a skilled pancreatic surgeon fail to find and remove an insulinoma if this has been diagnosed on sound clinical and biochemical grounds, it does occasionally happen, even today. Formerly it was quite common to do a 'blind' hemipancreatectomy in the hope that an occult tumour would be found in the part of the pancreas that was removed. The low success rate of this procedure, coupled with the fact that a second operation on someone who has already undergone hemi-pancreatectomy carries an unacceptably high mortality risk, has made blind hemi-pancreatectomy more or less obsolete. Instead one can either resort to intra-operative retrograde pancreatic venous catheterization with frequent sampling for urgent insulin and C-peptide analysis or, if these facilities are not available, the abdominal wound can be closed and reliance placed upon medical treatment with diazoxide and chlorothiazide to alleviate the hyperinsulinism for an indefinite period. Octreotide has been used with benefit in some cases of insulinoma, but in a small proportion — especially in patients with predominantly proinsulin-secreting tumours — it may exacerbate symptoms and increase the severity of the hypoglycaemia.

Histology and prognosis

Neither clinical nor biochemical techniques permit pre-operative differentiation of benign from malignant insulinomas, nor do traditional, or even the most modern and sophisticated, histopathological methods performed on the resected tumour enable the distinction to be made. Only if the tumour has already metastasized, usually to the liver, can an insulinoma be classified as malignant.

Malignant insulinomas are usually slow growing, with a natural history of years rather than months, and produce their adverse effects almost exclusively through their propensity to cause hypoglycaemia. As a result, many years of full and enjoyable life can be achieved providing hypoglycaemia is prevented. This can sometimes be achieved merely by removing the primary tumour surgically, as well as any large metastases in the liver but, more commonly, by the use of specific diabetogenic agents.

A combination of diazoxide and chlorothiazide is far more effective than either given alone and often prevents hypoglycaemia for many years after diagnosis of metastatic insulinoma is made. Specific antitumour therapy, most notably with streptozotocin, is often effective in restoring sensitivity to diazoxide/chlorothiazide therapy, once it has been lost, and substantially improves life-expectancy. Other cytotoxic agents that have been used with beneficial effect include 5-fluorouracil (especially in combination with streptozotocin), Adriamycin and chlorozotocin. Radiotherapy has little or no part to play in the treatment of malignant insulinoma.

Long-acting somatostatin preparations are less predictable in relieving symptoms produced by insulinomas than those of many other endocrine tumours of the pancreas. They are however worthy of a try when all else has failed.

References

1. Marks V, Teale JD. Tumours producing hypoglycaemia. *Diabetes Metab. Rev.* 1991;7:79–91.
2. Nauck M, Creutzfeldt W. Insulin-producing tumors and the insulinoma syndrome. In Dayal Y (ed.). *Endocrine Pathology of the Gut and Pancreas.* Boca Raton: CRC Press, 1991:195–225.
3. Service FJ, McMahon MM, O'Brien PC, Ballard DJ. Functioning insulinoma — incidence, recurrence, and long-term survival of patients: a 60-year study. *Mayo Clin. Proc.* 1991;66:711–19.
4. Mori S, Ito H. Hypoglycemia in the elderly. *Jpn J. Med.* 1988;27:160–5.
5. Marks V, Teale JD. Hypoglycaemia in the adult. In Gregory JW, Aynsley-Green A (eds). *Clinical Endocrinology and Metabolism, Vol. 7. Hypoglycaemia.* London: Baillière Tindall, 1993:705–29.
6. Stefanini P, Carboni M, Patrassi N, Basoli A. Beta-islet cell tumors of the pancreas: results of a study on 1067 cases. *Surgery* 1974;75:597–609.

62

Glucagonomas

PETER HAMMOND

Introduction

Glucagonomas are neuroendocrine tumours, almost always of pancreatic origin, synthesizing and usually secreting glucagon and other peptides derived from the preproglucagon gene (Fig. 62.1). They are associated with a characteristic syndrome [1], whose pathophysiology remains largely unexplained. The annual incidence of the syndrome is estimated at one in 20 million, and patients usually present between the ages of 40 and 60 years with a reported age range of 19 to 72 years. Over 70% of glucagonomas are malignant, but they are usually very indolent tumours and in many of these cases the diagnosis has been overlooked for many years, even up to two decades, in patients with an unexplained rash or diabetes. Indeed, data from autopsy studies suggest the incidence of glucagonomas in association with maturity-onset diabetes may be as high as 1%.

Clinical features

Necrolytic migratory erythema

The characteristic feature of the glucagonoma syndrome is the rash, necrolytic migratory erythema [2]. It occurs in over 90% of cases and is usually the presenting feature. The initial manifestation of the rash is well demarcated areas of erythema, usually in the groins, which migrate principally to the limbs, buttocks and perineum. These lesions may become vesicopustular or bullous and co-alesce, before eroding and encrusting occur (see Plate 62.1, between pp. 272 and 273). The rash may be mildly pruritic and occasionally painful. Mucous membrane involvement is common. Angular stomatitis, cheilitis and atrophic glossitis with a beefy red tongue occur almost invariably, and vulvovaginitis and urethritis accompanied by dysuria are frequent features. Nail and scalp involvement may result in onycholysis and alopecia. Healing commences after 10–15 days, lesions clearing centripetally to leave indurated and hyperpigmented areas, which are usually permanent (see Plate 62.2, between pp. 272 and 273). The rash remits and relapses unpredictably and this has made it difficult to assess treatment efficacy.

Skin biopsies are non-diagnostic. Typical histological findings include epidermal necrosis, parakeratotic hyperkeratosis, irregular epidermal hyperplasia, papillary dermal angiodysplasia, subcorneal pustules and suppurative folliculitis. None of these findings indicate a likely aetiology for this dermatosis, although histologically and clinically it is similar to the zinc-deficiency rash, acrodermatitis enteropathica. Topical application or oral supplementation of zinc have been reported to improve the rash, although circulating zinc levels are normal in patients with glucagonoma.

Amino acid deficiency is a frequent finding in the glucagonoma syndrome. Glucagon stimulates sustained gluconeogenesis, which depletes the glycogenic amino acids, particularly alanine, serine and glycine, and hepatic proteolysis with conversion of amino acid nitrogen to urea nitrogen, which depletes all amino acids. It has been postulated that this results in an increase in protein degradation, depleting epidermal protein and ultimately resulting in skin necrosis. Intravenous amino acid infusion, although not correcting hypoaminoacidaemia, has been reported to ameliorate the rash, but oral amino acid supplementation is ineffective. Similarly a high protein diet, despite normalizing plasma amino acids and nitrogen balance, may have no effect on the rash. The occurrence of the rash in patients without suppressed amino acid levels casts further doubt on a causal association.

Glucagon itself may act directly on the skin to cause the rash, perhaps by increasing arachidonic acid levels, which it does in human keratinocyte cultures. The rapid response of the rash to octreotide, before changes in circulating amino acids or glucagon, suggests a direct action on the skin, consistent with inhibition of hormone

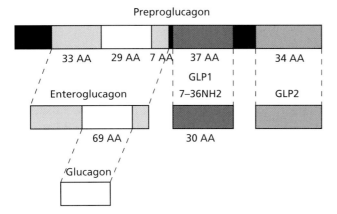

Fig. 62.1 Post-translational processing of preproglucagon. GLP, glucagon-like peptide.

action. Further evidence for the role of preproglucagon-derived peptides in the pathogenesis of necrolytic migratory erythema comes from its rare association with other diseases, notably hepatic cirrhosis and coeliac disease. The patient with coeliac disease had marked elevation of circulating enteroglucagon levels. In those patients with cirrhosis glucagon levels were not invariably elevated, but hepatocellular dysfunction may result in increased levels of other preproglucagon-derived peptides, such as enteroglucagon. In one case of cirrhosis the rash was successfully treated with fatty acid and zinc supplementation. However, in dogs, who can develop an identical dermatosis in association with cirrhosis or diabetes, not necessarily secondary to a glucagonoma, zinc and fatty acid supplementation is ineffective.

Other features

Glucose intolerance, and occasionally mild, non-ketotic, diabetes mellitus, occurs in about 90% of cases. Glucagon antagonizes the effects of insulin, principally by stimulating hepatic glucose production via glycogenolysis and gluconeogenesis. However there is little correlation between the plasma glucagon levels and the degree of glucose intolerance. This probably reflects variability in β cell insulin secretion, which may be influenced by loss of β cells as a result of tumour growth, but other factors may include insulin gene expression in glucagonoma cells, secretion of biologically inactive forms of immunoreactive glucagon by the tumour, depletion of glycogen stores, and down-regulation of glucagon receptors.

Unrelenting weight loss affects the majority of patients, usually despite a good appetite. The main cause is probably the organ protein catabolism, which occurs in response to the depletion in amino acids. If the body weight reduction exceeds 50%, it can be fatal.

A normochromic normocytic anaemia affects almost all patients, possibly as a result of a direct suppressive effect of glucagon on the bone marrow. The anaemia is usually mild, but occasionally the haemoglobin may fall as low as 4 g/dl.

Neuropsychiatric sysmptoms are probably under-diagnosed. Mental slowing is common and a few patients may suffer from severe depression or other psychoses. The demonstration of glucagon gene expression in the central nervous system may provide an explanation for these manifestations of the syndrome. Paraneoplastic syndromes, notably optic atrophy, have also been attributed to the syndrome.

The elevation in preproglucagon-derived peptides would be anticipated to affect gastrointestinal function. Enteroglucagon has been proposed as a humoral mediator of intestinal adaptation in response to injury. It appears to have a trophic action on intestinal mucosa, elevated levels causing villous hypertrophy. Three patients have been described with an enteroglucagonoma, in whom the principal clinical finding was of giant villous hypertrophy. Large molecular weight forms of glucagon inhibit gastrointestinal smooth muscle, resulting in constipation in the majority of patients. However a small proportion develop diarrhoea, the mechanism for which is unclear. Rarely, abdominal pain, nausea and vomiting occur, possibly as a result of local tumour effects.

A late feature of the disease is widespread venous thrombosis. This is resistant to conventional anticoagulant therapy and pulmonary embolism is a frequent cause of death. Secretion of factor X, which is synthesized in α cells and is found at high concentrations in glucagonomas, may explain this complication.

Glucagonomas rarely occur in association with multiple endocrine neoplasia type 1 (MEN-1), despite pancreatic endocrine tumours often containing as many as 30% of cells staining for glucagon. In those patients with a glucagonoma, the characteristic syndrome associated with sporadic tumours is often absent, and in particular necrolytic migratory erythema rarely occurs.

Diagnosis

Recognition of necrolytic migratory erythema is the most crucial part of diagnosis. Once the syndrome has been recognized the diagnosis is easily made by demonstrating increased plasma glucagon levels. These are usually elevated 10–20-fold, although up to 70% of immunoreactive glucagon may be biologically inactive. Other causes of elevated plasma glucagon rarely cause such a marked rise and are unlikely to cause diagnostic confusion. They include renal and hepatic failure, which reduce clearance, stress, burns, ketoacidosis, prolonged fasting and use of danazol or oral contraceptives. There has been one case of familial hyperglucagonaemia, with autosomal dominant inheritance, in which there were no sequelae attributable to the elevated circulating glucagon levels.

Provocative testing using tolbutamide or arginine are of little additional value in the evaluation of patients with suspected glucagonoma. Other biochemical abnormalities associated with the syndrome are the impaired glucose tolerance and hypoaminoacidaemia. Other circulating neuroendocrine tumour markers, such as pancreatic polypeptide and chromogranin, are frequently elevated. Radiological abnormalities of the small bowel, such as thickening of mucosal folds, villous hypertrophy and delayed gastric emptying may be demonstrated on abdominal computed tomography (CT) scanning or barium examination.

Histological specimens show the characteristic features of neuroendocrine tumours and immunocytochemistry can confirm the presence of immunoreactive glucagon.

Tumour localization

At the time of diagnosis over 50% of glucagonomas will have metastasized, and most primary tumours will be greater than 3 cm in diameter, with tumours up to 35 cm in diameter reported. Only two extrapancreatic glucagonomas, in the duodenum and in the kidney, have been reported. Thus localization of these tumours rarely presents a problem and abdominal ultrasonography or

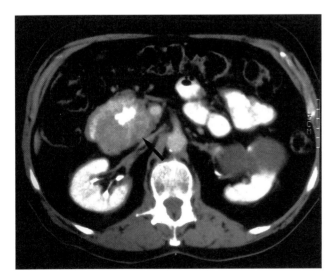

Fig. 62.2 Abdominal CT scan showing calcified glucagonoma in the head of pancreas (arrow).

CT scanning are usually adequate for this purpose. CT is particularly useful for assessing local spread. The indolence of these tumours is reflected in the frequent finding of tumour calcification (Fig. 62.2) and cystic degeneration may also occur.

The indications for other localization techniques are limited. Small benign tumours may not be imaged by ultrasound or CT, and then angiography or endoscopic ultrasonography should be employed, depending on the expertise of the institution. Somatostatin receptor scintigraphy using the indium-111 labelled somatostatin analogue, pentetreotide, is the best method for evaluating the extent of metastatic disease, and, to date, all glucagonomas have been somatostatin-receptor positive. Such an evaluation is most crucial in patients being considered for hepatic transplantation, but may also be of value in deciding on therapeutic modalities and assessing the response to treatment.

Therapeutic options

Surgery is the only curative therapeutic option, but the potential for cure is as low as 5% [3]. Cure can be achieved for malignant disease if tumour metastases can be enucleated or if metastases are confined to the liver and the patient is a candidate for hepatic transplantation.

Cytoreductive surgery may be appropriate as palliative therapy to reduce hyperglucagonaemia if there are a few well-circumscribed metastases amenable to enucleation. However surgery is complicated by the potential for venous thrombosis, the hypercatabolic state and anaemia. Total parenteral nutrition and blood transfusion are often required preoperatively, and prophylactic anticoagulation is usually instituted postoperatively. As a result of these factors, medical options are usually preferred for palliative therapy.

The morbidity associated with glucagonomas results principally from the hormonal syndrome, with the effects of tumour bulk rarely becoming apparent until the patient is in a terminal condition. Thus palliative medical therapy aims to reduce hormone levels either by reducing tumour bulk or by inhibiting the release of hormone. Cytotoxic chemotherapy or hepatic embolization may be used to reduce tumour bulk, while the somatostatin analogue, octreotide, both inhibits hormone release and antagonizes hormone action.

The conventional chemotherapy for glucagonomas and other pancreatic endocrine tumours is 5-fluorouracil 400 mg/m^2 and streptozotocin 500 mg/m^2 given on alternate days for 10 days and repeated at three monthly intervals. Administering the drugs at 18.00 h in combination with lorazepam 2 mg intravenously, dexamethasone

4 mg intravenously and metoclopramide 1 mg/kg intravenously over 15 minutes virtually overcomes the side-effects of nausea, vomiting, anorexia and general malaise. Patients need monitoring for evidence of nephrotoxicity, indicated by proteinuria and reduced creatinine clearance, and occasionally hepatotoxicity from streptozotocin, and myelosuppression from 5-fluorouracil. For patients with a glucagonoma, the response rate, measured by a 50% reduction in plasma glucagon levels, is about 70–80%, with remissions often lasting over a year, although no effect on survival has been observed. A recent report by Moertel [4] has suggested that the combination of streptozotocin 500 mg/m^2 on 5 consecutive days every 6 weeks and doxorubicin 50 mg/m^2 on days 1 and 22, up to a maximum total dose of 500 mg/m^2, is superior and may prolong survival, although the indolent nature of many of these tumours makes such claims difficult to substantiate. An alternative chemotherapeutic agent is dacarbazine which has been reported to be particularly successful in patients with glucagonoma, with a biochemical response sustained for over a year in all patients.

Hepatic artery embolization involves occlusion of hepatic artery collaterals to glucagonoma metastases in the liver, the portal vein maintaining supply to the normal liver. There is usually dramatic symptomatic relief following embolization and the procedure can be repeated at 6–9 month intervals [5]. However in frail patients the necrotic tumour load resulting from this procedure may be poorly tolerated.

Octreotide is now the first-line treatment for the glucagonoma syndrome, doses ranging from 150 to 1500 µg daily. It is particularly effective against the necrolytic migratory erythema, with resolution usually occurring within a week, independently of changes in plasma amino acids or glucagon. The effect is prolonged with remission for at least 6 months and reduced frequency of recurrence thereafter [6]. Octreotide is less effective at reversing the weight loss and has an inconsistent effect on diabetic control, perhaps reflecting inhibition of secretion of other hormones, such as insulin. It is not known whether octreotide has any effect on the tendency to venous thrombosis. The combination of chemotherapy or hepatic embolization with octreotide may delay the development of octreotide resistance, which usually develops after a mean of 2 years' therapy.

Simple measures to ameliorate the necrolytic migratory erythema such as topical and oral zinc and a high-protein diet, although unproven, are worth trying. Aspirin may be useful in preventing thrombo-embolic disease, but conventional anticoagulation is ineffective. If diabetic control cannot be achieved with diet alone, insulin should be used.

Prognosis and follow-up

The prognosis for patients with a glucagonoma is unpredictable. Most tumours are indolent but most patients present late in the course of the disease. The median survival from diagnosis is about 3 years, but ranges from a few months to 20 years. Patient follow-up is usually determined by exacerbations of the rash. Those patients in remission should be seen at least yearly, when a gut hormone screen should be performed, since up to 10% of tumours will be associated with secondary hormone syndromes.

References

1. Bloom SR, Polak JM. Glucagonoma syndrome. *Am. J. Med.* 1987;**82**:25–36.
2. Mallinson CN, Bloom SR, Warin AP *et al.* A glucagonoma syndrome. *Lancet* 1974;**2**:1–3.
3. Prinz RA, Badrinth K, Bunerji M *et al.* Operative and chemotherapeutic management of malignant glucagon-producing tumours. *Surgery* 1981;**90**:713–19.
4. Moertel CG, Lefkopoulo M, Lipstiz S, Hahn RG, Klaassen D. Streptozotocin–doxorubicin, streptozotocin–flourouracil or chlorozotocin in the treatment of advanced islet-cell carcinoma. *N. Engl. J. Med.* 1992;**326**:519–23.
5. Assaad SN, Carrasco CH, Vassilopoulou-Sellin R *et al.* Glucagonoma syndrome. Rapid response following arterial embolization of glucagonoma metastatic to the liver. *Am. J. Med.* 1987;**82**:533–5.
6. Altimari AF, Bhoopalam N, O'Dorisio T *et al.* Use of a somatostatin analog (SMS 201–995) in the glucagonoma syndrome. *Surgery* 1986;**100**:989–96.

63

Gastrinoma

STEPHEN G. GILBEY

Gastrin

Gastrin is the principal gut hormone stimulant of gastric acid production. Gastrin exists in both hG17 and hG34 ('big' gastrin) forms, and is synthesized by G cells situated predominantly in the antrum of the stomach. Gastrin released into circulation stimulates antral parietal cell gastrin acid production, both directly by its action on gastrin receptors, and indirectly through its stimulation of histamine release by neighbouring cells. Gastrin shares the same C terminal pentapeptide as cholecystokinin (CCK), and binds to receptors that are similar to the gastrointestinal CCK receptor. The gastrin gene is expressed in normal pancreatic islet cells in fetal life but not after birth.

Gastrin has other putative roles, in addition to its effect on acid secretion. An effect on gastric motility has been described, but is probably of little practical importance. Gastrin appears to have a trophic effect on gastric mucosa which is probably of physiological importance. The role of gastrin in carcinogenesis is controversial and topical, because the use of increasingly effective antisecretory drugs in the management of peptic ulcer patients has led to concern that the resulting hypergastrinaemia might increase the incidence of gastric neoplasms. There seems to be little doubt that hypergastrinaemia (as in pernicious anaemia patients) can lead to an increased incidence of gastric carcinoid tumours from enterochromaffin-like (ECL) cells. A possible effect of gastrin on chemical carcinogenesis and on the development of gastric or colonic adenocarcinoma remains unproven. The relevance of gastrin in the context of the influence of *Helicobacter pylori* infection on gastric ulceration is also unclear. The major effect of this organism seems to be on mucosal defences rather than acid production, although there is some evidence that *H. pylori* increases the sensitivity of G cells to the gastrin-releasing effect of gastrin-releasing peptide (GRP, or bombesin), and may diminish the concentration of somatostatin-secreting gastric D cells.

The release of gastrin and its net effect on acid secretion are, predictably, regulated by a complex network of endocrine, paracrine and neural influences, illustrated in Figs 63.1 and 63.2.

Gastrinoma syndrome

The gastrinoma syndrome is due to the excessive and autonomous release of gastrin by endocrine tumours in the gastrointestinal tract. Ninety percent of the tumours causing the gastrinoma syndrome are sited in the 'gastrinoma triangle', bounded by the junction of the cystic and common bile ducts superiorly, the junction of the second and third parts of the duodenum inferiorly, and the junction of the neck and body of the pancreas medially. Forty per cent of the tumours are less than 1 cm in diameter, and therefore difficult to locate.

Gastrinomas are the second most commonly diagnosed pancreatic islet cell tumours after insulinoma, with a prevalence of about one per million. Approximately 60% have metastasized (or are multicentric) at the time of diagnosis, and one-third of gastrinoma patients have type 1 multiple endocrine neoplasias (MEN-1) [1,2].

The clinical features of the gastrinoma (or Zollinger–Ellison syndrome) are due to the overproduction of gastrin, and are:

1 a relatively short (< 2 year) history of peptic ulceration;
2 ulcers that are multiple and atypical in site and refractory to standard medical or surgical treatment;
3 a high prevalence of complications include perforation, pyloric stenosis, haemorrhage and gastrojejunocolic fistulas;
4 diarrhoea and malabsorption due to acid-related inactivation of enzymes and mucosal damage in the upper small bowel may be the main clinical problem.

The recognition of one or more of these features may enable the differentiation of gastrinoma patients from the

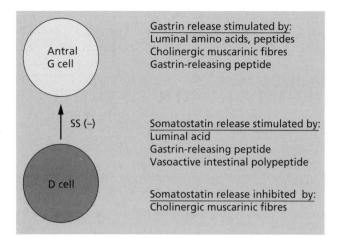

Fig. 63.1 Control of gastrin production by G cells. Somatostatin released by neighbouring D cells acts in a paracrine fashion to inhibit gastrin release into the local circulation.

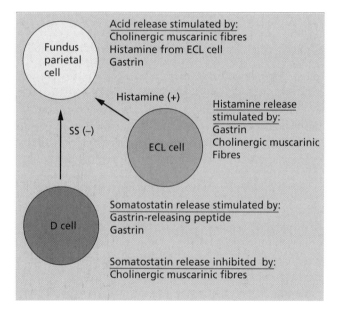

Fig. 63.2 Control of acid production by parietal cells in the gastric fundus. Circulating gastrin acts on local enterochromaffin-like (ECL) cells to cause histamine release which stimulates parietal cell acid release. In addition gastrin has a direct effect on parietal cells, and somatostatin released by neighbouring D cells inhibits parietal cell function.

mass of peptic ulcer sufferers. Suspicion should be heightened by a family history of peptic ulcer or endocrine disorders.

Diagnosis

Raised fasting plasma gastrin

A biochemical diagnosis is essential, and rests on the dem-

onstration of an inappropriately elevated fasting plasma gastrin in the presence of increased gastric acid secretion. A normal fasting plasma gastrin on one or more samples effectively excludes the diagnosis. Elevated circulating concentrations of pancreatic polypeptide (PP), other gut hormones such as glucagon, or non-specific neuro-endocrine tumour products such as chromogranins provide valuable additional evidence for the possible presence of a tumour. Demonstration of the presence of circulating gastrin precursors ('progastrin') or abnormally processed gastrin may also prove useful in distinguishing between tumours and other causes of a raised plasma gastrin.

Increased gastric acid secretion

A raised plasma gastrin is only significant in the presence of increased gastric acid secretion. Any cause of achlorhydria or hypochlorhydria may lead to an appropriate elevation of plasma gastrin (Table 63.1); this may be obvious from the clinical history but reinforces the importance of a formal estimation of gastric acid output. Patients should have antisecretory treatment stopped before the test (3 days for histamine H2 blockers, 2 weeks for omeprazole or similar compounds). A 1-hour basal acid output (BAO) is sufficient and should exceed 10 mmol/ h. If the patient has had a previous gastric surgical procedure, the diagnosis should be considered when the BAO exceeds 5 mmol/h. Low normal or diminished acid production in a patient not on antacid or antisecretory therapy excludes the diagnosis of gastrinoma. Some patients with duodenal ulcers may have borderline elevations of gastric acidity of over 15 mmol/h.

Provocative test for gastrin release

Provocative tests for gastrin release may be of value where plasma gastrin elevation is borderline. Intravenous

Table 63.1 Causes of hypergastrinaemia

With low gastric acid production
Vagotomy
Antisecretory treatment
Hypochlorhydria
Short gut syndrome
With normal/slightly elevated acid production
Renal failure
Hypercalcaemia
With elevated acid production
Excluded antrum syndrome
G cell hyperplasia
Zollinger–Ellison syndrome

secretin (2 u/kg) injection causes a characteristic rise in plasma gastrin within 10 minutes in gastrinoma patients which is not seen in normal subjects. However, false-positives may occur and routine use of this test is not justified except in cases where the diagnosis is still in question after the measurement of plasma gastrin and BAO. A number of other tests such as the gastrin response to a test meal, or to a calcium infusion have been suggested but have not been shown to be of discriminatory value.

Duodenal ulcer patients may be distinguishable from gastrinoma patients by having a more marked response to intravenous pentagastrin (gastrinoma patients are said to have BAO equal to or greater than 60% of the pentagastrin-stimulated peak output). However, up to 50% of gastrinoma patients fail to show this pattern, therefore the pentagastrin stimulation test is of little real value for diagnostic purposes.

Differential diagnosis

There are other conditions in which gastrin is elevated in the presence of high gastric acid output. G cell hyperplasia is of unknown origin and is diagnosed histologically on a gastric biopsy. The excluded antrum syndrome occurs after surgery when a portion of antrum is left isolated from the gastric lumen, feedback inhibition of gastrin production by luminal acidity is lost and hypergastrin-aemia and hyperacidity ensue.

Tumour localization

In patients with gastrinomas over 1 cm in size, with or without hepatic metastases, identification of the tumour by conventional scanning techniques (ultrasound or computed tomography) (CT) may present few practical difficulties. In many patients with the clinical and bio-chemical syndrome, however, tumour localization can be a major clinical problem. Up to 40% of tumours are duodenal; these duodenal tumours may be very small (< 5 mm), less likely than pancreatic tumours to have metastasized to the liver, yet frequently (up to 70%) associated with local lymph node spread.

Selective arterial angiography, in combination with CT scanning, is the most effective preoperative investigation, with a sensitivity of up to 86%. Intra-arterial secretin infusion may be a means of localizing small tumours: during selective arteriography secretin (30 u) is injected, and blood taken within 1 min from hepatic and peripheral veins. Injection of secretin into the region of the gastrino-ma leads to a rapid rise in gastrin levels [3]. This procedure may prove to be of value in localizing tumours in difficult cases, and, where rapid gastrin assay is available, may be of value intra-operatively, as confirmation that all tumour has been removed. Portal venous sampling is of limited value, but may help to identify the extent of tumour spread around the duodenum.

Despite these investigations many tumours remain elusive. In this event the choice lies between surgical exploration or medical treatment with repetition of CT scanning and angiography at a later date to try and find the tumour. Alternative techniques such as nuclear magnetic resonance (NMR) scanning and endoscopic ultrasonography have not so far proved superior methods for identifying small tumours.

Patients already on antisecretory treatment

Most patients in whom a gastrinoma is suspected will already be on antisecretory treatment and stopping this treatment in order to obtain a fasting plasma gastrin and acid output may be dangerous, even with careful monitoring. Each case has to be judged on its merits. It is probably safer in some cases to leave the patient on treatment but arrange imaging with or without angio-graphy to exclude an obvious lesion, than to expose the patient to unnecessary risks in order to clinch the bio-chemical diagnosis.

Treatment

The aims of treatment are to control hypersecretion of acid, and to remove the tumour(s) if this will effect a cure or at least alter the natural history of the condition.

Medical treatment

High-dose histamine H2 receptor blockers, and more recently the Na/K adenosine triphosphatase (ATPase) inhibitors such as omeprazole, have revolutionized the management of gastrinoma. The symptoms of gastrinoma can be alleviated and its complications avoided with antisecretory treatment while the location of a resectable tumour is sought.

Acid production should be formally monitored, par-ticularly during the initiation of treatment, the aim being to decrease BAO to a peak of 10 mmol/h. Higher doses of H2 blockers are usually required than for the treatment of peptic ulcer disease, and periodic increases in dosage are often necessary. A variety of H2 blockers are available and have been used for gastrinoma patients. Failure of therapy varies between series but may relate to inadequate dosage rather than variations between H2-blocking drugs.

Omeprazole and related compounds suppress acid production by inhibiting parietal cell Na/K ATPase. Compared to H2 blockers, these drugs are more potent acid suppressants, with longer duration of actions. Omeprazole, at doses of 80–120 mg daily, effectively produces a medical gastrectomy, reducing BAO to less than 5 mmol/h after 2 days of treatment and healing 98% of ulcers within 2 weeks and 100% within 1 month of therapy. Ulcers do not appear to recur if treatment is maintained.

Somatostatin is produced by cells within the gastric antrum, where it probably acts as a paracrine inhibitor of gastrin production. Treatment with the synthetic somatostatin analogue octreotide suppresses gastrin production in gastrinoma patients. However octreotide is no more effective than H2 blockers or omeprazole at relieving symptoms, and has not been shown to alter the natural history of islet cell tumours or their metastases. Its value in patients with tumours secreting only gastrin therefore seems limited.

Palliative treatment

Distant metastases generally involve the liver but may be found further afield. Patients with metastatic disease can lead a normal life on antisecretory treatment and so further therapeutic intervention should only be considered if clinical improvement is likely; for example, if metastatic tumour bulk is causing symptoms due to compression or infiltration. The major options for palliation are cytotoxic chemotherapy and hepatic embolization.

Chemotherapeutic regimens have proven less useful in gastrinoma patients than in other hormone syndromes: only 20% of gastrinomas respond to chemotherapy, as compared to 80% for the vasoactive intestinal polypeptide (VIP)oma syndrome. The most commonly used regimen is a combination of the islet cell toxin streptozotocin and 5-fluorouracil.

Hepatic artery embolization is directed at the relief of local symptoms and the reduction of hormone output by liver metastases, and may provide effective palliation if all other measures fail.

Surgical treatment

The major decision to be taken in all patients is whether to operate in order to locate and remove the primary tumour. In patients with good clinical and biochemical evidence for the gastrinoma syndrome, with no family history to suggest the possibility of MEN-1, and where a pancreatic or duodenal tumour(s) is identified preoperatively, operation and tumour resection has a good chance of effecting a complete cure even where affected lymph nodes are discovered at laparotomy [4]. Operation is rarely justified in patients who are known to have hepatic metastases, although some authors have claimed a beneficial effect from tumour debulking. Hepatic transplantation following the removal of the primary is a possible strategy where available. Total gastrectomy does not prolong survival and is not justified unless all other treatment options have failed.

The main clinical problems occur in patients in whom no tumour can be demonstrated preoperatively, in particular where there are clinical grounds to suspect MEN-1. Up to one-third of such patients have been found to have resectable pancreatic or extrapancreatic gastrinomas at operation. These include small duodenal tumours, which are difficult to detect preoperatively and yet potentially curable if resected, thus the duodenum should always be carefully explored. If a tumour is not identified at surgery, blind resection of the tail of the pancreas is not justified, since the great majority of pancreatic tumours are in the head of pancreas. Neither should patients be routinely exposed to the morbidity and mortality of pancreatoduodenectomy (Whipple's procedure).

A strong case can be made for not undertaking exploratory surgery in patients in whom tumours cannot be located: CT scanning and arteriography may be repeated at intervals while the patient is maintained on antisecretory treatment.

MEN-1 syndrome

Patients with MEN-1 are likely to present with multiple tumours, frequently microscopic and difficult to detect at operation, and may be particularly prone to multiple small gastrinomas in the duodenum. The policy in most centres is to investigate MEN-1 patients in the same manner as other gastrinoma patients and operate where well-defined pancreatic or duodenal tumours are positively identified. Hyperparathyroidism and hypercalcaemia may give rise to hypergastrinaemia and peptic ulceration and should be treated before a possible gastrinoma is investigated in a patient with MEN-1.

Conclusion

Management of patients with the gastrinoma syndrome has been greatly improved by increased clinical awareness, the ready availability of gastrin radioimmunoassay and effective medical treatment. The optimal surgical management of gastrinoma patients, particularly those whose tumours cannot be located preoperatively or who may have the MEN-1 syndrome, remains controversial.

References

1. Maton PN, Gardner JD, Jensen RT. Diagnosis and management of Zollinger–Ellison syndrome. *Endocrinol. Metab. Clin. North Am.* 1989;**18**:519–43.
2. Pipeleers-Marichal M, Somers G, Willems G *et al.* Gastrinomas in the duodenums of patients with multiple endocrine neoplasia type 1 and the Zollinger–Ellison syndrome. *N. Engl. J. Med.* 1990;**322**:723–7.
3. Doppman JL, Miller DL, Chang R *et al.* Gastrinomas: localization by means of selective intra-arterial injection of secretin. *Radiology* 1990;**174**:25–9.
4. Howard TJ, Zinner MJ, Stabile BE, Passaro E. Gastrinoma excision for cure. A prospective analysis. *Ann. Surg.* 1990;**211**:9–14.

VIPomas and Verner–Morrison Syndrome

ROGER R. PERRY AND AARON I. VINIK

Introduction

In 1958, Verner and Morrison first described the syndrome consisting of refractory watery diarrhoea and hypokalaemia associated with non-insulin secreting tumours of the pancreatic islets. This syndrome was later termed 'pancreatic cholera' because of the resemblance of the severe diarrhoea to *Vibrio cholera* disease. The agent that has been implicated in this syndrome is vasoactive intestinal polypeptide (VIP), and tumours that secrete VIP are known as VIPomas. The massive secretory diarrhoea associated with VIPomas results in profound hypokalaemia, hypochlorhydria (rarely achlorhydria), bicarbonate wasting and hyperchloraemic metabolic acidosis (Table 64.1) [1]. The commonly observed hypochlorhydria is due to the gastric acid inhibitory effect of VIP, a property shared with other members of the secretin and glucagon family: secretin, glucagon, gastric inhibitory peptide (GIP) and polypeptide histidine and isoleucine (PPHI). Although the acronym WDHA (watery diarrhoea, hypokalaemia and achlorhydria) has been used, a more appropriate acronym is WDHHA for watery diarrhoea, hypokalemia, hypochlorhydria and acidosis.

The most prominent symptom in most patients is a profuse cholera-like diarrhoea, often present for 3 or 4 years prior to diagnosis. Early in the clinical course the diarrhoea tends to be episodic and intermittent. As the VIP tumour enlarges, the diarrhoea becomes continuous and the ensuing electrolyte abnormalities are life-threatening. Increased intestinal motility as well as secretion contribute to the diarrhoea. The stools have the appearance of dilute tea, with volumes usually exceeding 6–8 l of stool/24 h. The stools are rich in electrolytes, with an average secretion of 300 mmol of potassium/24 h.

Diarrhoea in VIPoma syndrome is always secretory in nature, and will not disappear with fasting for 48 hours. The nature of the diarrhoea may be confused with other causes of secretory diarrhoea (Table 64.2)

including the Zollinger–Ellison syndrome (Table 64.3). Diarrhoea that is not secretory is always due to causes other than endocrine tumours [2]. Stool electrolytes should account for the osmolarity if the condition is due to an endocrine tumour. An osmolarity that is higher than expected from the concentration of electrolytes usually reflects laxative abuse which must be carefully excluded (Table 64.2).

Other clinical features in patients with VIPomas include hypercalcaemia, flushing and stimulation of glycogenolysis (Table 64.1) [1]. A large distended gall bladder is often noted, suggesting that VIP causes gall bladder relaxation. The mechanism whereby VIP causes hypercalcaemia in nearly 50% of patients with the syndrome is unknown, but may be related to dehydration and electrolyte disturbances from the diarrhoea, coincidental multiple endocrine neoplasia (MEN) including hyperparathyroidism, or the secretion by the tumour of a calcitropic peptide. Hypomagnesaemia has also been noted, and may be responsible for the tetany reported in several patients. Facial flushing occurs in approximately 8% of patients, and consists of patchy, erythematous and sometimes urticarial flush. The cause of the flushing is unknown but has been attributed to the secretion of VIP or prostaglandins. Hyperglycaemia is often noted and is felt to be secondary to the profound glycogenolytic effects of high portal vein concentrations of VIP.

Diagnostic evaluation

VIP is synthesized in the form of a 170 amino acid precursor known as preproVIP, which is posttranslationally modified to yield the 28 amino acid VIP, peptide histidine methionine (PHM) and other peptide fragments [3]. By definition, elevated levels of VIP are present in all patients with the VIPoma syndrome. Some of the other prepro VIP peptide products are secreted at higher levels than VIP, but assays to perform such measurements are

Table 64.1 Clinical features of the VIPoma syndrome

Watery diarrhoea
Hypokalaemia
Hypochlorhydria
Metabolic acidosis
Hypercalcaemia
Hyperglycaemia
Facial flushing
Hypomagnesaemia

Table 64.2 Aetiology of secretory diarrhoea

Infectious (i.e. cholera or *Escherichia coli* toxin)
Neuroendocrine tumours (VIPoma, carcinoid, medullary carcinoma
   of thyroid, PPoma, gastrinoma)
Villous adenoma
Laxative abuse
Infantile causes (congenital dysautonomia, congenital
   chloridorrhoea, enteric structural anomalies)
Immunodeficiency (i.e. immunoglobulin A deficiency)
Miscellaneous (i.e. basophilic leukaemia, systemic mastocytosis)
Idiopathic

PP, pancreatic polypeptide; VIP, vasoactive intestinal polypeptide.

Table 64.3 Differentiation of gastrinoma and VIPoma

Feature	Gastrinoma	VIPoma
Diarrhoea	Acid	Alkaline (HCO_3 loss)
Gastric acid	Increased	Decreased
Gastric volume	Increased	Normal or decreased
H2 blockers	Symptoms improve	Symptoms persist
Nasogastric suction	Diarrhoea improves	Diarrhoea unchanged
Motility	Increased*	Increased slightly†
Abdominal pain	Marked	Rare (initially)
Stool K^+ loss	Slight	Marked
Steatorrhoea	Common	Rare
Metabolic acidosis	No (alkalosis with gastric suction)	Yes
Lesion location	Primary pancreas (also liver, wall of stomach, duodenum)	Primary pancreas, ganglioneuroblastoma
Mediator	Gastrin	VIP/other

* Motility enhanced secondary to gastric acid stimulation.
† Motility may be slightly increased secondary to direct effects of either intra-arterial or intraluminal VIP.
VIP, vasoactive intestinal polypeptide.

not generally available, and their clinical usefulness is unknown.

Detection of VIP-secreting tumours requires a highly sensitive and specific VIP radioimmunoassay. The normal VIP concentration ranges from 0 to 190 pg/ml. The diagnosis of VIPoma in a patient with a good clinical history should not be excluded on the basis of a single normal VIP level because of vagaries in the assay procedure. It should also be noted that false-positive elevations of VIP can occur, particularly in patients with small-bowel ischaemia or severe low flow states and dehydration caused by diarrhoea due to non-VIP-producing tumours (Table 64.2).

VIP is not the only agent implicated in the diarrhoea syndrome. Gastrin, glucagon, pancreatic polypeptide (PP), thyrocalcitonin, prostaglandins, PHM or other peptide fragments from preproVIP, or any number of combinations have been identified as possible aetiological agents. In a comprehensive report of 1000 patients with various forms of diarrhoea, 39 patients (3.9%) had markedly elevated levels of VIP [4]. In each of these cases, a VIP-producing tumour was found; 53 other patients had diarrhoea secondary to non-VIP-producing tumours. Of these 53 patients, 12 had thyrocalcitonin-producing thyroid tumours, 13 had carcinoma of the lung, four had a villous adenoma of the rectum and 24 had carcinoid tumours. Eleven other patients had classic clinical features of the VIPoma syndrome, but VIP levels were normal and no tumour was found. This suggests these patients may have been secreting an unidentified humoral substance with the biological properties of VIP.

Tumour localization

Tumours secreting VIP usually originate in the pancreas or along the sympathetic chain. In a series of 62 patients, 52 (84%) had pancreatic tumours and 10 (16%) had ganglioneuroblastomas [5]. Of the 10 patients with ganglioneuroblastomas, seven were children. Catecholamines are frequently elevated in children, and may be responsible for the flushing, increased sweating and hypertension which have been observed. Hyperglycaemia and hypercalcaemia have not been noted in children, but priapism has, presumably due to the increased blood flow to the corpora cavernosa induced by VIP.

There have been occasional case reports of elevated plasma levels of VIP associated with other retroperitoneal neurogenic tumours including ganglioneuroma, neurofibroma and phaeochromocytoma. Primary VIP-secreting tumours have, rarely, been reported in other sites including colon, lung, oesophagus, jejunum and liver, and we have seen eventual emergence of these tumours in the kidney and skin [6].

It was hoped that PP levels would distinguish between pancreatic and non-pancreatic sources of VIP. Plasma levels of PP are nearly always elevated if the tumour is in the pancreas. PP levels are normal in VIP-producing ganglioneuroblastomas. However, in our experience three adults with neurogenic tumours and one adult with a VIPoma of the inferior left kidney had high serum levels of PP.

Most patients with VIPomas have large solitary tumours, usually 8 cm or more in diameter [5]. Most of these tumours are demonstrable using ultrasound or computed tomography (CT) scanning, but occasionally angiography or percutaneous transhepatic venous sampling are required. Somatostatin receptor scintigraphy may be useful in identifying extrapancreatic VIPomas, particularly those in the sympathetic chain, or metastases [7].

Treatment

The first step in the treatment of these patients is prompt replacement of fluid and electrolyte losses. Symptoms of severe electrolyte imbalance include cardiac arrhythmias, neuromuscular deficits, profound shock and cardiovascular collapse. The fluid of choice is an isotonic electrolyte solution containing adequate sodium, potassium and base.

Most VIPomas are malignant and due to their large size are usually detectable before operation as described in the previous section. If a tumour has been identified, complete surgical excision is the primary form of treatment. If the tumour cannot be completely removed, surgical debulking may be of palliative benefit. In one series, surgical excision of the primary pancreatic tumour relieved all symptoms in 17 of the 52 patients (27%) [5]. Surgical removal of the ganglioneuroblastoma was successful in seven of 10 patients. In patients in whom no tumour is demonstrated, we do not advocate blind total pancreatectomy. Spontaneous remission of the watery diarrhoea syndrome without establishing a cause has been observed.

In patients who have diarrhoea in whom no tumour is localized, a variety of medications have provided some symptomatic relief. The clinical usefulness of native somatostatin was limited because of its short half-life, necessitating continuous intravenous infusion. The long-acting analogue of somatostatin, octreotide, has obviated these difficulties and has been used successfully in managing the diarrhoea from gastroenteropancreatic tumours including VIPomas. Somatostatin has a direct effect on the gut and may improve diarrhoea by multiple mechanisms. Native somatostatin delays gut motility, stimulates sodium and potassium absorption in rabbit ileum *in vitro*, inhibits secretion induced by prostaglandin E and theophylline in rat jejunum *in vivo*, and inhibits the effect of VIP on water movement in rat colon *in vitro*

[2]. The diarrhoea of both cholera and VIPoma is due to increased cyclic adenosine monophosphate (cAMP) production. Recent evidence suggests that somatostatin binds to and activates the inhibitor subunit of the guanine nucleotide protein, thus decreasing formation. The effectiveness of somatostatin in other diarrhoea syndromes of diverse aetiology may reside in its additional ability to inhibit cellular calcium translocation as well as phosphoinositide turnover. Long-term octreotide not only helps to control diarrhoea in VIPoma patients, but in occasional cases has caused regression of the tumour (Fig. 64.1). An initial response is sometimes followed by a rebound effect with a recurrence of the diarrhoea and a rise in plasma VIP levels after a few days. The cause for this tachyphylaxis to octreotide is unknown, but may be due to increased enzymatic degradation of octreotide and/or down-regulation of somatostatin receptors.

Other medications are useful in the management of these patients. Glucocorticoids in large doses have been shown to stimulate Na^+/K^+ adenosine triphosphate

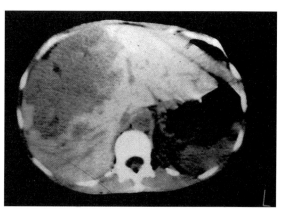

(a)

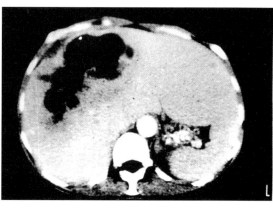

(b)

Fig. 64.1 VIPoma metastatic to the liver before (a) and after (b) 6 months of treatment with octreotide. The tumour appears to have undergone infarction.

(ATP)ase activity and electrolyte and fluid absorption in the intestine of rats. Glucocorticoids have been used clinically (prednisolone, usually 1 mg/kg/day), with some improvement of symptoms. A trial of inhibitors of prostaglandin synthesis (e.g. indomethacin), phenothiazines and lithium, may be warranted. The mechanism by which phenothiazines reduce endocrine secretory diarrhoea without affecting plasma VIP levels is not clear, although binding to calmodulin and inhibition of adenylate cyclase activity have been postulated. Lithium helps to control diarrhoea in VIPoma without significantly affecting VIP levels. We have successfully used lithium alone or in combination with octreotide in endocrine secretory diarrhoeas. Lithium may control diarrhoea by inhibiting cAMP synthesis or by blocking phosphoinositide turnover. Because of the relative rarity of gastroenteropancreatic neoplasms, chemotherapy trials have generally included several tumour subtypes. Although data are limited, streptozotocin alone or in combination with 5-fluorouracil is extremely effective against most VIPomas [7]. Response rates to streptozotocin alone or combined with other agents can exceed 50%. Streptozotocin alone is fairly toxic, and when combined with 5-fluorouracil is associated with a high prevalence of moderately severe gastrointestinal, haematopoietic and renal toxicity. The use of other agents, including monoclonal antibodies directed against VIP, remains a matter for investigation.

Conclusion

In a patient with severe chronic diarrhoea, it must be established that the diarrhoea is secretory by fasting the patient for 48 hours and measuring stool volume. If the diarrhoea persists with fasting, plasma samples should be analysed for VIP, and if elevated, a VIPoma should be strongly suspected. If the tumour is located in the pancreas, PP levels will almost invariably be elevated. In children, catecholamine levels should also be obtained, since tumours may reside in the adrenal medulla. Tumour localization should include CT scanning, and, if required, selective angiography or percutaneous transhepatic venous sampling. If a localized tumour is found, surgical excision should be performed. In patients with unresectable or metastatic disease, treatment with medications including octreotide, glucocorticoids or chemotherapy should be considered. Even hepatic artery embolization can give temporary respite from severe diarrhoea. In the absence of finding a tumour, symptomatic therapy is warranted, not empiric surgery.

If VIP levels are normal, other causes of secretory diarrhoea should be considered and appropriate screening for other potential causative agents should be performed.

Acknowledgement

These studies were supported by NCI grant No. RO1 CA54641.

References

1. Verner V, Morrison AB. Endocrine pancreatic islet disease with diarrhea: report on a case due to diffuse hyperplasia of nonbeta islet tissue with a review of 54 additional cases. *Arch. Intern. Med.* 1974;**133**(3):492–9.
2. Vinik AI, Moattari AR. Neuroendocrine tumors, secretory diarrhea, and responses to somatostatin. In Lebenthal E, Duffey M (eds). *Textbook of Secretory Diarrhea.* New York: Raven Press, Ltd., 1990:309–24.
3. Itoh N, Obata K, Yanaihara N, Okamoto H. Human preprovasoactive intestinal polypeptide contains a novel PHI 27-like peptide PHM-27. *Nature* 1983;**304**:547–9.
4. Bloom SR, Polak J M. Glucagonomas, VIPomas and somatostatinomas. *Clin. Endocrinol. Metab.* 1980;**9**(2):285–97.
5. Long RG, Byrant MG, Mitchell S, Adrian TE, Polak M, Bloom SR. Clinicopathological study of pancreatic and ganglioneuroblastoma tumors secreting vasoactive intestinal polypeptide (vipomas). *Br. Med. J.* 1981;**282**:1767–71.
6. Wesley JR, Vinik AI, O'Dorisio TM, Glaser B, Fink A. A new syndrome of symptomatic cutaneous mastocytoma producing vasoactive intestinal polypeptide. *Gastroenterology* 1982;**82**:963–7.
7. Mekhjian HS, O'Dorisio TM. VIPoma syndrome. *Semin. Oncol.* 1987;**14**:282–91.

65

Somatostatinoma

JOHN A.H. WASS

Introduction

Somatostatin was isolated in 1973 by Paul Brazeau in Roger Guillemin's laboratory. It was found to have a widespread distribution, not only in the hypothalamus and brain but also in the gastrointestinal tract. Sixty-five percent of the body's somatostatin is in the gut, mostly in the D cells of the gastric and intestinal epithelium. It is also present in the myometric and submucosal plexuses. The highest concentration is in the antrum of the stomach and there is a gradual decrease of concentrations down the gastrointestinal tract. Five percent of the body's somatostatin is in the pancreas.

Infused somatostatin, which has a short half-life of 3 minutes, has a large number of actions on the pituitary gland, the endocrine and exocrine pancreas, gastrointestinal tract, other hormones and on the nervous system (Table 65.1). Of importance in the gastrointestinal tract, gastrin and cholecystokinin (CCK) are inhibited. In the pancreas, insulin and glucagon are inhibited. Non-endocrine actions include inhibition of gastric acid secretion, pancreatic exocrine function, gall bladder contraction and intestinal motility. Intestinal absorption of nutrients including glucose, triglycerides and amino acids is also inhibited [1].

Somatostatin exists in two main forms, as a 14-amino-acid peptide (SMS 14) present mainly in the pancreas and the stomach, and as a 28-amino-acid peptide present mainly in the intestine. Somatostatin 14 is the peptide present in enteric neurones.

Somatostatin receptors are present on many cell types including parietal cells of the stomach, G cells, D cells themselves and cells of the exocrine and endocrine pancreas. A large number of tumours also have somatostatin receptors and these include pituitary adenomas, endocrine pancreatic tumours, carcinoid tumours, paraganglioma, phaeochromocytomas, small-cell lung carcinomas, lymphoma and meningiomas. Five different somatostatin receptors have been cloned (SSTR1 to SSTR5). These

have a varying affinity for somatostatin 14 and somatostatin 28 and varying tissue distribution.

Somatostatin can act either as an endocrine hormone or in a paracrine or autocrine way. It probably also has luminal effects in the gastrointestinal tract. Lastly, it can act as a neurotransmitter [2].

Somatostatinoma

Somatostatinomas are rare tumours with an incidence of about 1 : 40 000 000. Two main types exist, pancreatic somatostatinoma, which are large tumours often associated with features of somatostatin excess, and duodenal tumours, which are usually small and more amenable to surgical resection [3].

Pancreatic somatostatinoma

Somatostatinoma syndrome was first described in 1979. Fifty such cases have been reported with features as in Table 65.2. The syndrome consists of cholelithiasis due to inhibition of CCK production. Almost certainly the decline in gastrointestinal motility allows increased biliary cholesterol to develop which is probably another factor. This has been demonstrated with octreotide therapy but not with somatostatinoma syndrome. Mild diabetes occurs and has often been present for many years before diagnosis. It is probably due to suppression of insulin secretion. Diarrhoea and steatorrhoea also occur and relate to the inhibition of pancreatic exocrine function. Hypochlorhydria relates to the inhibition of gastric acid secretion and gastrin. Anaemia, abdominal pain and weight loss are also present and are non-specific. They are probably related to the size of the tumour which is usually large and also to the fact that it is malignant. Those tumours are often diagnosed late and distant metastases may be present in lymph nodes, liver or bone.

Table 65.1 Actions of exogenously administered somatostatin on endocrine and exocrine secretion

Endocrine secretion	Exocrine secretion
Inhibits the secretion of:	Inhibition of:
Pituitary	Gastric acid secretion
Growth hormone	Gastric emptying rate
Thyroid-stimulating hormone	Pancreatic exocrine function:
	volume, electrolytes and enzyme
Gastrointestinal tract	content
Gastrin	Gall bladder contraction
Cholecystokinin	Intestinal motility
Secretin	Intestinal absorption of nutrients
Vasoactive intestinal polypeptide	Splanchnic blood flow
Gastrin-inhibiting peptide	Renal water re-absorption
Motilin	Activity of some central nervous system neurones
Enteroglucagon	
Pancreatic polypeptide	*Excitation of:*
Insulin	Activity of some neurones
Glucagon	
Somatostatin	
Other peptides	
Renin	
Growth hormone-releasing hormone	

Table 65.2 Features of pancreatic somatostatinoma

Hyperglycaemia
Cholelithiasis
Steatorrhoea
Hypochlorhydria
Diarrhoea
Abdominal pain
Weight loss
Anaemia
Elevated plasma and tissue somatostatin
Histologically malignant, may be associated with ACTH, calcitonin and insulin secretion

ACTH, adrenocorticotrophic hormone.

Plasma and tissue levels of somatostatin are elevated. These somatostatin-secreting cells often also secrete adrenocorticotrophic hormone (ACTH), calcitonin, insulin or some other peptides. This means that Cushing's syndrome, flushing or hypoglycaemia (if there is co-secretion of insulin, Fig. 65.1) may be present [4].

Duodenal somatostatinoma

Duodenal somatostatinomas tend to be smaller and present earlier. The vast majority occur near the ampulla of Vater, where they tend to cause obstructive biliary disease. Some are associated with neurofibromatosis type 1. At presentation paraduodenal lymph nodes are involved because there is a high malignancy rate, although this is low grade. None of the duodenal somatostatinoma patients have developed the full-blown somatostatinoma syndrome but diabetes and gall stones have been noted in some cases.

Histologically these are psammomatous tumours. Treatment is with surgery if this is feasible, chemotherapy and if necessary hepatic embolization.

Table 66.1 Properties of neuroendocrine cells

Morphological	Ultrastructural	Histochemical	Immunohistochemical
Cell and nuclear uniformity Eosinophilic cytoplasm Secretory vesicles	Dense core vesicles	Enzymes: 　decarboxylases 　esterases Amines: 　argentaffin reaction Dense core vesicles: 　argyrophil reaction 　masked metachromasia 　lead haematoxylin	NE markers: 　neurone-specific enolase 　synaptophysin 　chromogranin A 　secretogranins 　Leu 7 　neural cell adhesion molecule Secretory products: 　amines, peptides, hormones

Table 66.2 Neuroendocrine cells: nomenclature

Term	Synonym
Clear cell	APUD cell
Feyrter cell	Neuroendocrine cell
Kultschitzky cell	Dense-core granulated cell
Neuroepithelial body (lung only)	Paracrine cell
Enterochromaffin-like cell (ECL)	Neurosecretory cell
Argyrophil cell	Argentaffin cell

APUD, amine precursor uptake and decarboxylation.

Table 66.3 Cell populations in the dispersed neuroendocrine system

Bronchopulmonary tract	Pancreas and biliary tree
Anterior pituitary gland	Gastrointestinal tract
Thymus	Adrenal gland/extra-adrenal chromaffin cells
Thyroid (C cells)	Breast/cervix/prostate/ovary
Parathyroids	Skin (Merkel cells)

The age-adjusted incidence rate is estimated at 0.2 : 100 000. Peak incidence is in the fifth decade. It is slightly more common in women (55%) and in Caucasians compared to Negroes [10].

No aetiological associations other than multiple endocrine neoplasia, usually type 1, have been found. In this syndrome, over 75% of women with carcinoids have bronchial primaries whereas thymic tumours are the commonest type (66%) of carcinoid in men.

Pathology

BCs were once classified as bronchial adenomas on the mistaken assumption that they were benign. However, they are now regarded as prototypical NE tumours. On both pathological and clinical grounds there seems little doubt about their heterogeneity. The term atypical, dated to Arrigoni's description in 1972, refers to a subset of BC with morphological evidence of malignancy including mitosis, nuclear pleomorphism and necrosis [11]. The clinical phenotype is correspondingly more malig-

nant as suggested by an incidence of metastases of 70%, compared to 5–15% in typical cases, and reduced survival.

Eighty to ninety percent of BCs are found in the proximal bronchial tree and, of these, three-quarters occur in the lobar bronchi. Atypical tumours may be more common in the periphery. Most of them grow as solitary, well-circumscribed, endobronchial polyps (explaining why bronchial obstruction is such a frequent problem). They may also expand extraluminally but are rarely intra-parenchymal. The mucosa tends to remain intact and the cut surface is usually buff-coloured and homogeneous. Metastases to lymph nodes are found in about 15% of cases; distant sites, notably liver, bone and adrenal glands, are less often affected. Atypical lesions are prone to metastasize to the brain.

The classic light microscopic findings are of a well-preserved, insular architecture containing dense masses of uniform cells with pale eosinophilic cytoplasm. Foci of ossification are not unusual, and amyloid too may be found. Diagnostic hallmarks are architectural organization and nuclear uniformity.

Clinical features

The great majority of BCs come to light because of symptoms, and signs of bronchial obstruction (typically cough, haemoptysis (50%), wheeze and recurrent distal infection) and, especially in the case of peripheral tumours, abnormal chest radiology. Ectopic hormone syndromes due to BCs are the classic clinical association (Fig. 66.1) [12].

Ectopic hormone syndromes

Ectopic (paraneoplastic) endocrine syndromes are an uncommon presenting feature except when the tumour is occult. The most common of these is Cushing's syndrome followed by, in decreasing order of frequency, acromegaly and syndrome of inappropriate antidiuretic hormone (ADH) secretion (SIADH).

Table 66.4 Classification schemes of pulmonary neuroendocrine tumours (approximate relationships). (Reproduced by courtesy of Butterworth Heinemann and author from [1])

WHO 1967 [4]	WHO 1982 [5]	WHO with IASLC modifications [6]	Paladugu *et al.* 1985 [7]	Mosca *et al.* 1986 [8]	Gould *et al.* 1983 [3]
Carcinoid tumour	Carcinoid tumour	Carcinoid tumour	KCC I	NEC of carcinoid type	Carcinoid tumour
Atypical carcinoid tumour*	Atypical carcinoid tumour*	Atypical carcinoid tumour*	KCC II	Well-differentiated NEC	Well-differentiated NEC
Lymphocyte-like type of SCLC	Oat-cell type of SCLC }	SCLC	Small-cell type of KCC III	NEC of small-cell (microcytoma) type	NEC of small-cell type
Polygonal/fusiform type of SCLC	Intermediate type of SCLC		Intermediate type of KCC III		
		Small-cell/large-cell carcinoma†		NEC of intermediate (poorly differentiated) type‡	NEC of intermediate type‡
Other types of SCLC	Combined type of SCLC	Combined type of SCLC	Combined type of KCC III	Combined type of NEC	NEC of combined type

* The World Health Organization (WHO) schemes do not classify typical and atypical carcinoid tumours separately.
† A category without an equivalent in the 1967 and unmodified 1982 WHO schemes.
‡ Do not correspond to the intermediate category of the 1982 WHO scheme.
IASLC, International Association for the Study of Lung Cancer; KCC, Kultschitzky cell carcinoma; NEC, neuroendocrine cancer; SCLC, small-cell lung carcinoma.

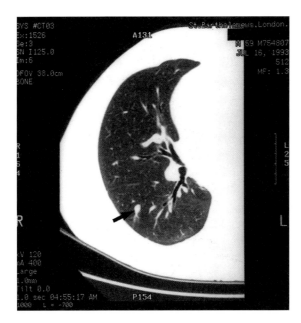

Fig. 66.1 Computed tomography of the chest in a patient with a bronchial carcinoid (arrow) and ectopic adrenocorticotrophic hormone secretion causing Cushing's syndrome.

In strict terms carcinoid syndrome (CS) is viewed as a separate entity. The clinical, biochemical and pathological features of CS are well known. These and the standard management of CS are dealt with in Chapters 30, 51 and 79. When due to BCs it is similar to CS produced by primaries at other sites except for a few important points. It manifests, in up to 5% of cases, almost invariably in the presence of hepatic metastases, despite a commonly held view that BCs differ from extrapulmonary carcinoids in this respect. In contrast to midgut (e.g. ileal) carcinoids, BCs cause a more intense, protracted, purplish flush often leaving the face disfigured (leontine) and with telangiectasia. Urinary 5-hydroxyindoleacetic acid (5-HIAA) is not as elevated, presumably because foregut tumours lack aromatic acid decarboxylase and fail to decarboxylate 5-hydroxytryptophan to serotonin.

Cushing's syndrome. BC is the most common cause of ectopic adrenocorticotrophic hormone (ACTH) syndrome. It accounts for 28–38% of cases in some series, and 1% of all cases of Cushing's syndrome. Less than 100 published cases have been reported since this association was found in 1962 [13]. This clinical scenario may be difficult to distinguish from pituitary-dependent Cushing's disease when BC is inapparent at presentation. As a result many patients have experienced prolonged morbidity and undergone unnecessary treatments including hypophysectomy. Diagnosis is elusive because these tumours occasionally suppress with high-dose dexamethasone, they may function cyclically, and can occasionally secrete corticotrophin-releasing factor (CRF) all in addition to being occult.

Management requires aggressive evaluation and close follow-up if the tumour is not located at the outset. Helpful investigations include venous sampling for ACTH/CRF at multiple sites and high-resolution contrast-enhanced computed tomography (CT). Magnetic resonance imaging (MRI) may be superior to CT in localizing BC. Indium-labelled octreotide scanning has proven useful. Metaiodobenzylguanidine (MIBG) scintigraphy, perhaps in conjunction with octreotide, has also been advocated.

Acromegaly. This is a rare complication. By 1991, less than 20 cases had been published. Interestingly, a number of BCs contain significant quantities of growth hormone-releasing hormone (GHRH) as judged by bio- or immuno-assay but only a few reports have demonstrated unequivocally that excess circulating GHRH is the underlying cause. Ectopic GHRH production as a whole only accounts for less than 1% of all cases of acromegaly.

Diagnosis

Investigative techniques, including octreotide scintigraphy [14], are non-specific. Chest X-rays are abnormal in more than 60% of patients, although the lesion is often missed initially in the case of 'occult' hormonally active tumours. CT and MRI are of value as noted. Tissue specimens can generally be obtained by bronchoscopic biopsy, but there is a risk that any ensuing haemorrhage may be uncontrollable if a fibreoptic instrument is used. It is, nevertheless, generally considered safe to do so nowadays even when the diagnosis is suspected [15].

Treatment

Total excision of the tumour is the treatment of choice. Experience has shown that the extent of resection need not be radical unless there are lymph node metastases. The most common procedures are lobectomy, segmentectomy and bronchotomy plus tumour enucleation. Bronchoscopic resection is considered unsatisfactory as a primary treatment since it is mostly incomplete and so leads to a high recurrence rate.

As most carcinoids progress slowly, attempts at resecting metastases, with curative or palliative intent, are certainly worthwhile. Liver and even cluster (organ) transplantation have been tried. Limited results are available and most are unfavourable. Palliation of hepatic metastases by arterial embolization is a well established and comparatively safe procedure; the risk of a carcinoid crisis can be lessened by prophylactic octreotide.

Chemotherapy may be indicated in selected patients.

Many of the large series examining its utility, as with other therapeutic modalities, have involved patients with metastatic midgut carcinoids and it is, therefore, difficult to extrapolate to BCs. With this reservation in mind, there appears to be a role for using a combination of 5-fluorouracil and streptozotocin [16] or, as with SCLC, etoposide and cisplatin in the treatment of tumours that are atypical and/or have metastasized [17]. Radiotherapy is mainly useful for relieving symptoms from metastases and of bronchial obstruction in inoperable subjects.

Other treatments for metastatic carcinoid include the use of octreotide (a somatostatin analogue), which produces significant but usually temporary tumour shrinkage in many cases. It is particularly effective in treating the diarrhoea and bronchospasm of malignant carcinoid syndrome. A more recent derivative called lanreotide (to be licensed) has been formulated as a slow-release preparation, somatuline SR, and consists of lyophilized microspheres which can be given, by intramuscular injection, every 1 or 2 weeks. Recent characterization of five somatostatin receptor subtypes suggests that tumour responsiveness to octreotide is a function of the presence of receptor subtypes 2 and 5. Antagonists specific for other subtypes have yet to be developed for clinical use. Another palliative therapy in future may be radiolabelled octreotide. ^{131}I-MIBG and interferon α are sometimes useful.

Prognosis

The indolent growth of BCs is manifested in an extremely good prognosis. Taken as a whole, the 5-year survival exceeds 90% following thoracic surgery. If lymph nodes have been metastasized, the 5-year survival drops to 71%. At 30 years, survival is about 50% [15]. Atypical tumours can be associated with a much poorer outlook, with a 5-year survival of less than 60%. This was estimated prior to the availability of modern NE markers, and may also have been confounded by the inclusion of some cases of SCLC.

Small-cell lung carcinoma

Tumour cell biology

Major advances in unravelling SCLC biology have occurred over the past decade or so, although this has not been translated into significant therapeutic success. Most of the progress stems directly from the ability to establish permanent SCLC (and NSCLC) cell lines. This has helped to identify autocrine growth factors (e.g.

bombesin/gastrin-releasing peptide), develop serum-free cell culture techniques, delineate genetic abnormalities, and to develop NE markers [18].

Tumour cell lines have also been used for *in vitro* chemosensitivity testing, and the development of panels of monoclonal antibodies to identify tumour antigens. Even though none of the antibodies is entirely specific for SCLC, those directed against major cluster 1 have revealed a useful NE marker called neural cell adhesion molecule (NCAM). Most of the numerous peptides secreted by cell lines are clinically silent.

Epidemiology

SCLC accounts for 20–25% of all cases of lung cancer, and possibly a greater fraction in patients younger than 40. The annual incidence varies geographically, and is currently highest in Scotland. Peak incidence is in the seventh and eighth decades; the age-adjusted incidence in 1978 in Britain was 112 : 100 000 and 27 : 100 000 in males and females, respectively.

Of all types of lung cancer, SCLC has the strongest correlation with cigarette smoking, accounting for the predominance in men. Apart from genetic factors, as yet incompletely understood, other aetiological agents, e.g. ionizing radiation, asbestos and aromatic hydrocarbons, are well documented but numerically less important.

Pathology

SCLC is typically an invasive endobronchial, greyish, semi-necrotic mass. Metastases, usually to bone (35% of cases), liver (25%), bone marrow (20%), brain (10%), extrathoracic lymph nodes (5%) and to various subcutaneous sites (5%), are often apparent at presentation. Adrenal (44%) and lymph node metastases (85%) are more often detected at autopsy [19].

Morphologically, the classical oat-cell tumour consists of sheets of densely packed cells exhibiting plenty of mitotic activity, necrosis, a high nuclear : cytoplasmic ratio and smudged/crushed nuclei; this last feature, due to fragility, makes the diagnosis difficult. Haemotoxyphilic impregnation of blood vessel walls, secondary to DNA deposition, is another typical finding. Most SCLC has this morphology. Other subtypes are distinguished on the basis of subpopulations composed of large or neoplastic adeno/squamous cells. Table 66.4 summarizes the classifications and overlapping terminologies. The main diagnostic difficulty is the distinction between SCLC with a major NSCLC (large/squamous/adeno) component and NSCLC with a significant NE component (NE-NSCLC).

Clinical features

This highly aggressive tumour usually presents because of cough, dyspnoea and constitutional upset; up to two-thirds of patients will have clinically detectable metastases at this point.

Ectopic hormone syndromes

SCLC is the tumour par excellence associated with paraneoplastic manifestations, and of these endocrine abnormalities are the most common [20]. A specific humoral profile has been postulated but not substantiated. The exact incidence of ectopic syndromes is difficult to quantify since it depends on the varying criteria that have been used for their definition. The issue is complicated by the recognition that, in the vast majority of cases, so-called 'ectopic' hormone production does not cause gross clinical disturbance. One clinical survey [21] documented a rate of 14%, whereas the incidence is understandably higher (21%) when laboratory tests are applied in addition.

Cushing's syndrome. The reported clinical incidence of Cushing's syndrome ranges between 2.8 and 19%; more realistically it is 3–8% [22]. Interestingly, abnormalities of the hypothalamus–pituitary–adrenal axis, such as loss of diurnal variation and aberrant dexamethasone suppression, have been found in about 50% of individuals who are asymptomatic. Nearly one-third of subclinical cases have a raised plasma ACTH, virtually always accompanied by an elevated 24-hour urinary free cortisol [23]. Pro-opiomelanocortin processing in SCLC and, indeed, many other tumours is abnormal, often resulting in ACTH-like products with altered bioactivity. This and the rapidly fatal course of SCLC probably underlies the infrequency of the typical signs of Cushing's syndrome.

In the absence of confounders like medication, the usual metabolic derangements (hypokalaemic alkalosis and glucose intolerance) and clinical features (muscle weakness, oedema, pigmentation, hypertension and, sometimes, psychosis) should prove sufficient to suggest the diagnosis. SCLC can secrete CRF, and this may explain why high-dose dexamethasone sometimes 'suppresses' in a manner suggesting pituitary-dependent disease; this phenomenon is much more commonly seen with BC. Other findings characteristic of primary ectopic ACTH syndrome are : hypokalaemia, plasmacortisol > 1000 nmol/l, a high plasma ACTH (> 36 pmol/l), and greatly raised urinary 17-ketosteroids or plasma dehydroepiandrosterone sulphate.

Primary treatment is obviously directed towards the

tumour; this can result in endocrine improvement. Metyrapone, ketoconazole and op'DDD can all be used to ameliorate symptoms prior to antineoplastic therapy.

Ectopic ADH syndrome (SIADH). First described in 1957, in relation to lung cancer, SIADH is the most common humoral syndrome due to SCLC. It manifests clinically in 8% of patients but is diagnosable using routine investigations in 5–22% [24]. More detailed testing reveals water-handling defects in as many as two-thirds of cases. Generally, raised plasma arginine vasopressin (AVP) is unaccompanied by hyponatraemia, possibly implying that coexistent abnormalities of thirst are necessary for its genesis. There is also some evidence that tumour-derived atrial natriuretic peptide/factor plays an aetiological role.

SIADH may, of course, be due to non-tumour factors. Notable in the context of cancer are antineoplastic drugs (cisplatin, cyclophosphamide, vincristine), morphine, chest infections, and intracranial metastases. The therapeutic approach (drug withdrawal, fluid restriction, demeclocycline and, rarely, hypertonic saline in conjunction with diuretics and central venous pressure monitoring and controlled rate of correction) is the same whatever the underlying cause. Antitumour therapy may itself correct the low sodium, but biochemical recurrence is not usually tied to tumour relapse.

Other hormonal syndromes and metabolic abnormalities. A vast array of other glycoprotein hormones, peptides and amines have been described in relation to SCLC, either in the tumour and/or in plasma; examples include luteinizing hormone (LH) and follicle-stimulating hormone (FSH), melanocyte-stimulating hormone (MSH), growth hormone (GH) and renin. As mentioned earlier, clinical sequelae are comparatively unusual. This may be due to reduced bioactivity. None of them have proven sufficiently useful as universal NE markers. Hypercalcitonaemia is yet another paraneoplastic phenomenon first discovered in relation to SCLC. It too is a subclinical finding in over 50% of individuals studied. Hypercalcaemia is not a characteristic feature, and is usually due to widespread metastases rather than being endocrine in origin. A surprisingly high proportion (29%) of patients have been found to have paradoxical GH responses to glucose challenge and abnormal glucose tolerance (50%) [20].

Reports of carcinoid syndrome are sparse and it is possible that the tumours implicated have, in fact, been atypical BCs. There is one documented case of SCLC presenting with the somatostatinoma syndrome.

Management and prognosis

Chemotherapy and surgery are significantly better than primary radiotherapy in improving survival.

The significance of clinical endocrine dysfunction is unclear since the available evidence is inconsistent. An example is Cushing's syndrome in BC compared with SCLC. SIADH seems to be correlated with tumour extent, perhaps explaining why hyponatraemia is an adverse prognostic factor. Another study has shown that patients with a clinically evident ectopic hormone syndrome may be more likely to develop metastases to the liver and brain and have a shorter survival [21].

Plasma cortisol levels are known to correlate with chemoresistance and consequently predict prognosis but ACTH and calcitonin show no such connection. Other circulating tumour markers, such as chromogranin A, gastrin-releasing peptide (GRP), NSE and CK-BB, have been advocated for diagnosis, monitoring and therapeutic targets, but none have found a place in routine clinical practice. The gamma-gamma isoenzyme of NSE is, at present, probably the most sensitive and specific of them as an indicator of SCLC activity.

Attempts are underway to both detect and therapeutically target marrow metastases using monoclonal antibodies directed against NE markers like NCAM. Immunodetection uncovers micrometastases in 30–50% of patients who would otherwise be labelled as having disease confined to one hemithorax [18].

A number of studies using SCLC biopsies have confirmed *in vitro* findings showing that *myc* oncogene (C-, N- and L-types) overexpression/amplification is correlated with resistance to chemotherapy and radiotherapy and poor survival.

The clinical significance of histopathological subtypes of SCLC, showing differing degrees of NE differentiation, is contentious. The evidence so far suggests that the presence of a 'large-cell' component (< 10% of all cases) is associated with a poorer response to chemotherapy and decreased median survival. It is noteworthy that as many as 35% of patients who relapse with SCLC have developed a substantial large-cell component in the repeat biopsy as compared to the first, and are also more resistant to chemotherapy and radiotherapy. This finding is associated with a reduction in survival from 280 to 168 days [25]. Whether loss of the NE phenotype is the primary event in malignant evolution, or simply an epiphenomenon, is presently unclear.

NSCLC with features of NE differentiation

Similar considerations to those just discussed also apply

to the substantial proportion of NSCLC (approximately 75% of all lung cancer) that exhibit a notable degree of NE differentiation. Depending on the criteria chosen, as many as 4–30% of NSCLC conform to this description. In an analysis of 141 biopsies, adenocarcinoma demonstrated this property more often than large-cell and squamous varieties. An even greater fraction harbour smaller numbers of cells with NE features, presumably reflecting those present in health [26].

Clinical characterization of this subgroup of tumours has demonstrated that NE features may be correlated with greater metastatic potential and chemoresponsiveness but not survival [27].

Thymic neuroendocrine tumours

Like the bronchopulmonary tract, the thymus is the seat of a population of NE cells of foregut origin, first described in 1906 [28]. Endocrine disturbances occurring in association with thymic tumours have also long been recognized but were commonly misascribed to thymomas, until the delineation of thymic carcinoids (TCs) in 1972 by Rosai and Higa [29]. Excepting histological variants, these are, for practical purposes, synonymous with the term thymic NE tumour. The other main categories of thymic tumours are: lymphoma, germ cell (seminoma, teratoma and mixed germ cell), thymolipoma, myoid tumours and myosarcoma, and metastatic tumours (extremely rare).

Pathology

TCs are nearly always located in the anterior mediastinum, with rare reports describing posterior and middle mediastinal tumours. Invasion of surrounding structures is commonly seen. However, at least 90% of anterior mediastinal tumours are thymomas. The average size is 5–6 cm, with a range of between less than 1 and 19 cm. Hormonally silent tumours are understandably the largest. Fewer than 50% are encapsulated. In contrast to thymomas, the cut section (often gritty) lacks lobulation and fibrous septae and has a homogeneous, grey-tan-coloured appearance with foci of haemorrhage and necrosis. Metastases (up to 75% of cases) may affect the lung, lymph nodes, liver, adrenal glands, skin and even optic nerves [30].

The main histological patterns of TC are 'classic', spindle, pigmented and diffuse. In addition, an atypical form with its greater degree of anaplasia, and a subtype resembling medullary thyroid carcinoma are recognized. Central necrotic balls detached from the surrounding stroma are a characteristic morphological finding.

Morphology is otherwise similar to that of NE tumours in general. A completely distinct subcategory of thymic NE tumour is the oat cell form, although this behaves essentially the same as other varieties.

As a group they exhibit varying degrees of typical NE characteristics such as argyrophilia, dense core vesicles, and positive immunocytochemistry for markers like NSE, chromogranin A, and Leu 7. Interestingly, somatostatin immunoreactivity has been found in more than 50% of tumours associated with Cushing's syndrome, although the significance of this is unknown [30].

Clinical features

TC is an extremely rare tumour with only about 100 cases reported in the world literature. Males have a three-fold higher incidence, and it presents most commonly in the third and fourth decades [28]. Presentation is quite often due to non-endocrine effects of the tumour (50%), with symptoms and signs of intrathoracic/mediastinal compression (although superior vena caval obstruction is unusual) and constitutional disturbance (fever, night sweats, fatigue). Ectopic ACTH syndrome is the commonest associated endocrinopathy and, as is true of BC, often mimics pituitary-dependent Cushing's disease, particularly since the tumour is likely to be occult. By analogy with classic Nelson's syndrome, massive and rapid tumour expansion plus cutaneous hyperpigmentation has been observed following bilateral adrenalectomy. SIADH has been reported, equivocally and rarely, to complicate TC. There are no undisputed reports of carcinoid syndrome even though raised urinary 5-HIAA has been found. Five per cent of patients with TC develop it in the context of a MEN syndrome, more often type 1 [31,32]. Affected individuals have all been male with particularly aggressive tumours. Other reported associations of TC are pericarditis, polyarthropathy, clubbing and myositis.

Management and outcome

Hormonally active tumours are often difficult to find when they are otherwise occult, even with the aid of CT scanning. Tumours that present for other reasons are, almost by definition, nearly always detectable on a routine chest X-ray. They appear as lobulated, uniformly radio-dense masses, occasionally with fine internal calcification and are often misdiagnosed as thymomas. Metastases are generally osteoblastic. In addition to mediastinoscopic sampling and Tru-cut biopsy, preoperative diagnosis can be achieved by fine-needle aspiration cytology with a low reported risk of track implantation by malignant cells; ultrasound guidance has been advocated to avoid sampling necrotic tissue.

Complete surgical excision is the treatment of choice. Chemotherapy (e.g. streptozotocin, 5-fluorouracil and BCNU (1,3-bis(2-chloroethyl)-1-nitrosourea)) and radiotherapy have been used both as adjuvants and for the treatment of recurrences. Given the rarity of TCs there is no clinical trial data to support this widespread practice. It is perhaps understandable when recurrence rates, estimated to be as high as 70–80%, are taken into consideration. Postoperative prophylactic irradiation of the tumour bed has been advocated. Local and distant recurrence is initially managed with surgery.

Overall, the outlook is considered poor despite the protracted course of relapsed disease witnessed in some patients. Coexisting endocrinopathy is generally regarded as an adverse prognostic factor. Mortality rate at 10 years follow-up has been calculated to lie between 30 and 60% [33].

References

1. Gosney, JR. *Pulmonary Endocrine Pathology. Endocrine Cells and Endocrine Tumours of the Lung.* Oxford: Butterworth Heinemann, 1992.
2. Brown WH. A case of pluriglandular syndrome: diabetes of bearded women. *Lancet* 1928;**2**:1022–3.
3. Gould VE, Linnoila RI, Memoli VA, Warren WH. Neuroendocrine components of the bronchopulmonary tract: hyperplasias, dysplasias, and neoplasms. *Lab. Invest.* 1983;**49**:519–37.
4. Kreyberg L, Liebow AA, Uehlinger EA. Histological typing of lung tumours. In *International Histological Classification of Tumours*, No. 3. Geneva: World Health Organization, 1967.
5. World Health Organization. Histological typing of lung tumours. *Am. J. Clin. Pathol.* 1982; **77**: 123–36.
6. Hirsch FR, Matthews MJ, Aisner S *et al.* Histopathologic classification of small cell lung cancer. *Cancer* 1988; **62**:973–7.
7. Paladugu RR, Benfield JR, Pak HY *et al.* Bronchopulmonary Kulchitsky cell carcinomas. A new classification scheme for typical and atypical carcinoids. *Cancer* 1985;**55**:1303–11.
8. Mosca L, Ceresoli A, Anzanello E *et al.* Neuroendocrine structures in normal and diseased human lung. *Appl. Pathol.* 1986;**4**:147–61.
9. Vinik AI, Renar IP. Neuroendocrine tumors of carcinoid variety. In De Groot L (ed.). *Endocrinology*, 3rd edn. Philadelphia: W.B. Saunders, 1995:2803–14.
10. Godwin JD, Brown CC. Comparative epidemiology of carcinoid and oat-cell tumors of the lung. *Cancer* 1977;**40**:1671–3.
11. Arrigoni MA, Woolner LB, Bernatz PE. Atypical carcinoid tumors of the lung. *J. Thorac. Cardiovasc. Surg.* 1972;**64**:413–21.
12. Davila DG, Dunn WF, Tazelaar HD, Pairolero PC. Bronchial carcinoid tumors. *Mayo Clin. Proc.* 1993;**68**:795–803.
13. Hofland J, Schneider AJ, Cuesta MA, Meijer S. Bronchopulmonary carcinoids associated with Cushing's syndrome—report of a case and an overview of the literature. *Acta Oncol.* 1993;**32**:571–3.
14. Breeman WA, Kooij PP, Oei HY *et al.* Somatostatin receptor scintigraphy with [111 In-DTPA-D-Phe]- and [123 I-Tyr3]-octreotide: the Rotterdam experience with more than 1000 patients. *Eur. J. Nucl. Med.* 1993;**20**:716–31.
15. Hurt R, Bates M. Carcinoid tumours of the bronchus: a 33 year experience. *Thorax* 1989;**39**:617–23.
16. Oberg K. The use of chemotherapy in the management of tumours. *Endocrinol. Metab. Clin. North Am.* 1993;**22**:941–52.
17. Moertel CG, Kvols LK, O'Connell MJ, Rubin J. Treatment of neuroendocrine carcinomas with combined etoposide and cisplatin. Evidence of major therapeutic activity in the anaplastic variants of these neoplasms. *Cancer* 1991;**68**:227–32.
18. Weynants P, Humblet Y, Canon JL, Symann M. Biology of small cell lung cancer: an overview. *Eur. Respir. J.* 1990;**3**:699–714.
19. Johnson BE. Management of small-cell lung cancer. *Clin. Chest Med.* 1993;**14**:173–87.
20. Bondy PK, Gilby ED. Endocrine function in small cell undifferentiated carcinoma of the lung. *Cancer* 1982;**50**:2147–53.
21. Lokich JJ. The frequency and clinical biology of the ectopic hormone syndromes of small cell carcinoma. *Cancer* 1982;**50**:2111–14.
22. Odell WD, Scott Appleton W. Humoral manifestations of cancer. In Wilson JD, Foster DW (eds). *Williams Textbook of Endocrinology*, 8th edn. New York: W.B. Saunders, 1992:1599–617.
23. Hansen M, Hansen HH, Hirsch FR *et al.* Hormonal polypeptides and amine metabolites in small cell carcinoma of the lung, with special reference to stage and subtypes. *Cancer* 1980;**45**:1432–7.
24. Seaton A, Seaton D, Leitch AG. Cancer of the lung. In Seaton A, Seaton D, Leitch AG. *Crofton and Douglas's Respiratory Diseases*, 4th edn. Oxford: Blackwell Scientific Publications, 1989:912–74.
25. Hirsch FR, Osterlind K, Hansen HH. The prognostic significance of histopathologic subtyping of small cell carcinoma of the lung according to the classification of the World Health Organization. A study of 375 consecutive patients. *Cancer* 1983;**52**:2144–50.
26. Linnoila RI, Mulshine JL, Steinberg SM *et al.* Neuroendocine differentiation in endocrine and nonendocrine lung carcinomas. *Am. J. Clin. Pathol.* 1988;**90**:641–52.
27. Sundaresan V, Reeve JG, Stenning S, Stewart S, Bleehen NM. Neuroendocrine differentiation and clinical behaviour in non-small cell lung tumours. *Br. J. Cancer* 1991;**64**:333–8.
28. Wick MR, Rosai J. Neuroendocrine neoplasms of the mediastinum. *Semin. Diagn. Pathol.* 1991;**8**:35–51.
29. Rosai J, Higa E. Mediastinal endocrine neoplasm of probable thymic origin, related to carcinoid tumour: clinico-pathological study of 8 cases. *Cancer* 1972;**29**:1061–74.
30. Wick, MR, Rosai J. The endocrine thymus. In Kovacs K, Asa SL (eds). *Functional Endocrine Pathology*. Oxford: Blackwell Scientific Publications, 1991:790–813.
31. Rosai J, Higa E, Davie J. Mediastinal endocrine neoplasm in patients with multiple endocrine adenomatosis: a previously unrecognized association. *Cancer* 1972;**29**:1075–83.
32. Marchevsky AM, Dikman SH. Mediastinal carcinoid with an incomplete Sipple's syndrome. *Cancer* 1979;**42**:2497–501.
33. Economopoulos GC, Lewis JW Jr, Lee MW, Silverman NA. Carcinoid tumors of the thymus [see comments]. *Ann. Thorac. Surg.* 1990;**50**:58–61.

Carcinoid Syndrome

KJELL ÖBERG

Introduction

The first clinical and histopathological description of carcinoid tumours was made by Otto Lubarsch in 1888. He described the multicentric origin of carcinoid tumours of the gastrointestinal tract. Two years later Ranson reported on a patient with ileal carcinoma with liver metastases who experienced diarrhoea and dyspnoea induced by eating. The term 'karzinoid' was introduced in 1907 by Oberndorfer to describe intestinal tumours with a less aggressive course than more common intestinal adenocarcinomas.

The argentaffin properties of carcinoid tumours were demonstrated in 1914 by Gosset and Masson and the tumours were named argentaffinomas. In 1953 Lembeck demonstrated the presence of serotonin in carcinoid tumours and 1 year later Thorson and co-workers first described a series of patients with small intestinal carcinoids and hepatic metastases producing serotonin and causing the typical symptoms of diarrhoea, flushing, asthma, cyanosis and right heart failure, the so called 'carcinoid syndrome'.

Definitions, classifications and incidence

Williams and Sandler [1] introduced a new classification of gastrointestinal carcinoid tumours into foregut, midgut and hindgut tumours on the basis of their topographical location. This classification has an embryological basis and its aim is to gather tumours with common features into distinct groups. The foregut carcinoids include tumours arising in the thymus, lung, stomach, duodenum and pancreas, and midgut tumours arise in jejunum, ileum and ascending colon, whereas the hindgut tumours originate in distal colon and rectum. Such properties of carcinoid tumours as an argentaffin reaction and an ability to produce the carcinoid syndrome are almost exclusively attributable to midgut carcinoids and these tumours are therefore frequently designated 'classic' carcinoids, while foregut and hindgut carcinoids are called 'non-classic' or 'atypical'. However, it is also well known that foregut carcinoids not infrequently present with the carcinoid syndrome (Table 67.1) [2].

The so-called enterochromaffin cells (EC) are said to be the origin of carcinoid tumours of midgut origin. The appendiceal carcinoids develop from another cell type which is more related to the peripheral nervous system. This might also explain the benign clinical feature of this type of carcinoid.

About 85% of carcinoid tumours develop in the gastrointestinal tract, 10% in the lung and the rest in various organs such as thymus, kidney, ovary and prostate. The most frequent location in the gastrointestinal tract is the appendix, followed by small intestine and rectum (Table 67.2) [3]. Carcinoids constitute about 34% of all tumours in the small intestine but only 1% of all neoplasms in the stomach, colon or rectum [4]. In total, carcinoids constitute about 2% of all malignant tumours in the annual report to the National Cancer Registry in Sweden. The incidence of malignant carcinoid tumours found at autopsy was 2.1 : 100 000 inhabitants but the incidence based on clinically significant carcinoids varies between 0.3 : 100 000 and 0.7 : 100 000 inhabitants. The incidence of the carcinoid syndrome has been reported to be 0.5 : 100 000 inhabitants [5].

Carcinoid tumours may be found at all ages, even in children. In young patients the appendix is the most common location and the tumours are frequently found incidentally during operations for acute appendicitis. Carcinoid tumours of the ileum and jejunum are diagnosed at an average age of 50–60 years and with equal frequency in males and females.

Table 67.1 Classification of carcinoid tumours

Origin	Organ	Silver staining	Hormone production*	Clinical symptoms
Foregut†	Thymus	Argyrophil	CRH, ACTH, GHRH (serotonin)	Cushing's syndrome Acromegaly
	Lung	Argyrophil Sevier–Munger (argentaffin)	CRH, ACTH, GHRH PP, hCG-α, neurotensin, serotonin, histamine	Cushing's syndrome Acromegaly Carcinoid syndrome
	Stomach	Argyrophil	CRH, ACTH, GHRH	Cushing's syndrome
	Stomach (ECLoma)	Argyrophil	Histamine, gastrin, somatostatin	Flushes, pernicious anaemia, Zollinger–Ellison syndrome
	Duodenum	Sevier–Munger Argyrophil	Gastrin, somatostatin Neurotensin, serotonin	Zollinger–Ellison syndrome, somatostatinoma Carcinoid syndrome
Midgut ('classic carcinoid')	Ileum Jejunum Proximal colon Appendix	Argyrophil Argentaffin Argyrophil	Tachykinins, bradykinins CGRP Serotonin (Tachykinins, serotonin)	Carcinoid syndrome Not hormone-related
Hindgut	Distal colon Rectum	Argyrophil Sevier–Munger	PP, hCG-α, PYY Somatostatin	Not hormone-related

* All carcinoids produce peptides from the chromogranin family (A, B, C).

† Endocrine pancreatic tumours are not included among carcinoids.

ACTH, adrenocorticotrophic hormone; CGRP, calcitonin gene-related peptide; CRH, corticotrophin-releasing hormone; ECL, enterochromaffin-like; GHRH, growth hormone-releasing hormone; hCG, human chorionic gonadotrophin; PP, pancreatic polypeptide; PYY, peptide YY.

Table 67.2 Percentage distribution of 1867 carcinoids by site* (from [3])

Site	Distribution (%)
Lung and bronchi	10
Stomach	2
Duodenum	2
Jejunum	1
Ileum	11
Small intestine (not specified)	5
Caecum	3
Appendix	44
Colon	5
Rectum	15

* Only frequencies of at least 1% are listed.

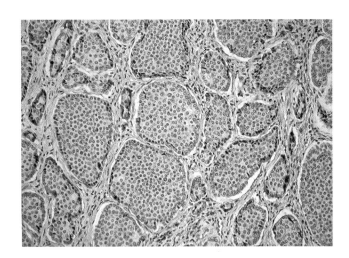

Fig. 67.1 Section through a classic midgut carcinoid with insular growth pattern.

Histological appearance and pathological features

By light microscopy carcinoid tumours are easily identified with their uniform round cell nuclei and regular
growth pattern (insular, trabecular or glandular or a
mixture of these three types; Fig. 67.1). These growth
patterns are not related to the site of origin but are found
in foregut, midgut or hindgut tumours. Foregut carcinoids
exhibit an argyrophil reaction with the Grimelius silver
staining method and are often positive with the Sevier–
Munger staining technique. Almost all midgut carcinoids
are Grimelius positive but also show argentaffin reaction
(Masson staining) indicating their content of serotonin
(see Table 67.1). Serotonin-positive cells can also be
demonstrated by immunohistochemical methods. Hindgut tumours demonstrate mainly positive reactions with
Grimelius and Sevier–Munger silver staining [6].

Neuroendocrine properties of carcinoid tumours can
further be shown by immunohistochemical stainings using
antibodies against chromogranin A and B, synaptophysin

or neurone-specific enolase (NSE). Extensive immuno-histochemical investigations have revealed that particular foregut and hindgut tumours are multihormonal, whereas midgut carcinoids demonstrate more uniform patterns of hormone production, predominantly tachykinins and serotonin. Electron microscopy has demonstrated the presence of both amines and peptides within the same tumour cells, for example serotonin and substance P.

Recently, studies of expression of growth factors and receptors in carcinoid tumours demonstrate the capacity of these tumours to express most of the well known growth factors such as platelet-derived growth factor (PDGF), transforming growth factor (TGF)-β family, fibroblast growth factor (FGF), epidermal growth factor (EGF), TGF-α and their related receptors. The clinical relevance of the expression of these growth factors has to be evaluated. The expression of the adhesion molecule CD44 is related to more malignant behaviour and larger molecular forms are expressed in carcinoids with metastatic potential (particularly gastrin producing) but are not found in tested primary tumours of midgut type.

The neurosecretory granules within tumour cells are dependent on the origin of the primary tumour; foregut carcinoid tumours have small, round, regular cytoplasmic granules, whereas midgut carcinoids contain large, pleomorphic granules and hindgut tumours contain large, round, neurosecretory granules. Macroscopically the gastrointestinal carcinoids, particularly midgut carcinoids present as small primary tumours (0.5–1.0 cm), being multiple in one-third of the patients. Lymph node and liver metastases, being the most common, metastatic sites may be fairly large, 10–15 cm, despite small primary tumours. The distribution of metastases is indicated in Table 67.3 [7].

Several factors should be considered when evaluating carcinoid tumours for metastatic behaviour.

1 The location of the primary tumour: colonic and ileal carcinoids are considered to be more prone to produce metastases. About 70% of all colonic carcinoids give rise to metastases, compared to 30–60% of ileal tumours. Metastases are found in about 18% of patients with rectal carcinoids but only in 2–5% with appendiceal carcinoids.
2 The size of the primary tumour: this has an impact on the development of metastases. The risk increases as the tumour becomes larger. In patients with primary tumours with a diameter of less than 1 cm metastases were found in 6% but among those with primary tumours measuring more than 2 cm, 70% developed metastases.
3 The depth of tumour penetration into the bowel wall is important for the development of metastases. Among patients whose tumours invaded the serosa, metastases were found in 69% but no metastases were observed when the tumour was limited to the submucosa.
4 The histological growth pattern has also been claimed to be of importance for the development of metastases. The five main growth patterns are insular, trabecular, glandular, undifferentiated and mixed type. The most favourable growth patterns are insular and glandular giving an almost 10 times longer median survival compared with undifferentiated tumours.

Simultaneous occurrence of other malignant tumours in patients with carcinoid tumours is fairly frequent. The presence of accessory malignant neoplasm has ranged from 5 to 53% in various studies. Most commonly the second tumour is a colonic carcinoma and this is important to keep in mind in the follow-up of carcinoid patients, as many symptoms may mimic those of the carcinoid tumour. Other accessory malignancies have been breast cancer, prostatic carcinoma, myeloma and chronic myelogenic leukaemia [5].

Biochemistry

Serotonin (5-hydroxytryptamine, 5-HT) was isolated from a carcinoid tumour by Lembeck in 1953 and has been shown to be increased in circulation in patients with the carcinoid syndrome. 5-HT is synthesized in the carcinoid tumour by two enzymatic steps, first tryptophan is 5-hydroxylated to form 5-hydroxytryptophan (5-HTP) which is then decarboxylated to form 5-HT. Tumours arising from the lung, pancreas and stomach may have relative lack of 5-HTP decarboxylase whereby the tumour fails to decarboxylate all the 5-HTP. The tumour then excretes 5-HTP, 5-HT and 5-hydroxyindoleacetic acid (5-HIAA) in the urine. Measurement of urinary 5-HIAA is still one of the most important tumour markers for carcinoid patients with the carcinoid syndrome. The high 5-HT levels in blood are mainly due to increased amounts

Table 67.3 Percentage distribution of metastases from carcinoid tumours (*n* = 301) (from [7])

Site	Distribution (%)
Lymph nodes	27
Liver	74
Peritoneum	8
Bone	4
Pancreas	2
Ovary	2
Skin	2
Brain	2
Spleen	1
Adrenal	1
Breast	1

of 5-HT bound to blood platelets rather than to a marked rise in plasma 5-HT itself. The 5-HT released is oxidatively deaminated to 5-HIAA, which is excreted in the urine. However, 5-HIAA may also be produced within the tumour, thus urinary 5-HIAA reflects not only circulating 5-HT oxidatively deaminated but also 5-HIAA produced and released from the tumour.

Oats and colleagues some 20 years ago [2] provided evidence that kinins are released in patients with the carcinoid syndrome. Carcinoid tumours contain the enzyme kallikrein, which after incubation with purified human kininogen produces lysyl-bradykinin, which is converted within the circulation to bradykinin. Several investigations have found increased histamine and histamine metabolites in the urine, particularly in patients with gastric and pulmonary carcinoid tumours.

Blood levels of prostaglandin E and F have also been found to be elevated in some patients with the carcinoid syndrome. However, no correlation between clinical symptoms and blood levels has been demonstrated.

Several members of the tachykinin peptide family have been demonstrated in carcinoid tumours and are secreted *in vivo* and *in vitro* from carcinoid tumour cells. The mRNA for β-preprotachykinin, the precursor of substance P, neuropeptide K and neurokinin A, can be demonstrated by *in situ* hybridization technique to be present in carcinoid tumour cells. The tachykinins represent a peptide family which shares an identical C-terminal amino acid sequence and is widely distributed from vertebrate to invertebrate animals. The most well known member of the family is substance P which was isolated from the mammalian gastrointestinal tract and brain in 1931. The presence of substance P in carcinoid tumours was first demonstrated by Håkansson and co-workers in 1977 [5]. Ten years later we were able to demonstrate production and secretion of several members of the tachykinin family from carcinoid tumours, including neuropeptide K (NPK) and neurokinins A and B (NKA, NKB). The β-preprotachykinin is the larger molecular form and contains substance P, neuropeptide K and neurokinin A and these peptides can be cleaved off at specific cleavage sites. This might explain the ability of carcinoid tumours to secrete different molecular forms of tachykinins [5].

Members of the tachykinin peptide family are not the only peptides produced by carcinoid tumours. All types of carcinoid tumours contain and release members of the chromogranin family, namely A, B (secretogranin I), and some of them also chromogranin C (secretogranin II). These glycoproteins are important tumour markers with a long half-life in plasma and therefore easy to measure by radioimmunoassays. The physiological role of the chromogranin family of peptides is still unknown but the

Table 67.4 Tumour markers in carcinoids

Marker	Gastrointestinal carcinoids		
	Foregut	Midgut	Hindgut
p-Chromogranin A	+++	+++	+++
Urinary 5-HIAA	+	+++	–
p-NPK	(+)	++	–
s-PP	+	+	+
s-hCG-α	++	+	+
s-hCG-β	+	+	(+)
s-Gastrin	++	–	–
u-Histamine metabolites	++	–	–
p-Somatostatin	+	–	(+)
p-Neurotensin	+	–	–

+++, very useful; ++, useful; +, may be useful; –, useless.
hCG, human chorionic gonadotrophin; 5-HIAA, 5-hydroxyindoleacetic acid; NPK, neuropeptide K; PP, pancreatic polypeptide.

proteins might increase the storage capacity for amines and peptides in the neuroendocrine cells and might also act as precursor molecules for active peptides as they contain cleavage sites for enzymes. As an example the sequence for the peptide pancreastatin is found within chromogranin A. Other peptide hormones secreted by carcinoids are pancreatic polypeptide (PP), human chorionic gonadotrophin α and β subunits (hCG-α/β), calcitonin gene-related peptide (CGRP), calcitonin, gastrin, somatostatin, neurotensin, corticotrophin-releasing hormone (CRH) and growth hormone-releasing hormone (GHRH). Clinically relevant tumour markers are summarized in Table 67.4.

Clinical presentation

A majority of all carcinoids demonstrated in various necropsy series have not been clinically diagnosed before death and did not give rise to any significant clinical symptoms. The reason for this is obviously that the majority of these carcinoids are appendiceal tumours, which normally do not give any hormone-related clinical symptoms. On the other hand studies of patients with known gastrointestinal carcinoids who are referred for medical treatment present with a large amount of hormone-related clinical symptoms; these are summarized in Table 67.5. In our own series [5] 84% of the patients presented with diarrhoea, 75% with flushing and 44% of the patients with intestinal obstruction. Altogether 67% presented with the carcinoid syndrome. The initial symptoms in a patient with midgut carcinoid tumours may be diffuse abdominal pain which can delay diagnosis. We found that the median duration of delay between the first

Table 67.5 Clinical characteristics in patients with carcinoid tumours (after [4])

	At presentation		During course of disease		
	Davis *et al.* 1973 [8]	Norheim *et al.* 1987 [5]	Thorson 1958 [9]	Feldman 1987 [10]	Norheim *et al.* 1987 [5]
Number of patients	91	91	79	111	91
Sex (% males)	59	46	61	NR	46
Mean age years	57	59	52	NR	NR
range	25–79	NR	18–80		
Tumour location (%)					
Foregut	5	9	2	NR	9
Midgut	78	87	75	NR	87
Hindgut	5	1	8	NR	1
Unknown	11	2	15	NR	2
Symptom (%)					
Diarrhoea	73	32	68	73	84
Flushing	65	23	74	63	75
Ileus/subileus	NR	44	NR	NR	NR
Asthma/wheezing	8	4	18	3	15
Pellagra	2	NR	5	NR	NR
None	12	NR	NR	22	NR
Carcinoid heart disease present	11	NR	41	14	33

NR, not reported.

symptoms until the diagnosis was verified to be one year. Tumours causing intestinal obstruction showed the shortest delay from onset of first symptoms until diagnosis (median 0.6 years), whereas patients with diarrhoea and flushing had a delay of 1.5 and 2.0 years respectively [5].

Distinct clinical syndromes have been described in patients with carcinoid tumours. The most common is the carcinoid syndrome which is predominantly found in patients with ileal and jejunal carcinoids with liver metastases. Other syndromes related to foregut carcinoids include the Zollinger–Ellison syndrome due to gastrin production, somatostatinoma syndrome, Cushing's syndrome due to production of adrenocorticotrophic hormone (ACTH) and/or CRH and acromegaly due to tumour secreting GHRH. Patients with so-called enterochromaffin-like (ECL)oma of the stomach might present with bright red flushes which are mainly histamine mediated. Patients with carcinoids of the hindgut area, distal colon and rectum present with gastrointestinal bleeding, obstruction and/or an abdominal mass. All these tumours are known to contain several peptides such as PP, peptide YY (PYY) or chromogranin A, none of which are known to cause any definite clinical symptoms.

Carcinoid syndrome

Almost all patients with the carcinoid syndrome and

gastrointestinal carcinoids have metastatic disease, mainly liver metastases. Some bronchial carcinoids may present with a syndrome without recognized metastases which might depend on the liberation of causative agents directly into the systemic circulation. A small proportion of patients with midgut carcinoid tumours did not have liver metastases but still present with the carcinoid syndrome. These patients may have metastases in the retroperitoneal space. The blood flow from these metastases might then be drained directly into systemic circulation via prevertebral veins. The original description of the carcinoid syndrome includes flushing, diarrhoea, asthma, oedema, right heart valvular lesions, pellagra-like skin lesions and occasionally also peptic ulcers and arthralgia. The term malignant carcinoid syndrome was introduced later to denominate patients with these symptoms but also liver metastases and elevated urinary 5-HIAA levels [2,5,9].

Flush

The mechanism of flush reactions are pharmacologically and physiologically heterogeneous. Precipitating factors of the carcinoid flush include eating, especially spicy food, hot drinks, exercise, alcohol, excitement, sexual intercourse, defaecation and postural changes. The most spontaneous flush attacks occur in the morning when the patient is standing upright, washing or having breakfast. Surgery and infections can provoke severe life-threatening attacks; for example, carcinoid crisis including severe vasodilatation, hypermetabolism and hypotension. Carcinoid tumour cells are known to express adrenoreceptors on their surface. The alcohol-induced flush can be blocked by α-adrenergic blockade, indicating that alcohol might act via release of catecholamines. Pentagastrin, an agent used for flush provocation, is thought to act in a similar way via release of catecholamines acting on the carcinoid tumour cells causing a release of vasoactive substances such as 5-HT, tachykinins, kallikrein and CGRP. Initially it was thought that serotonin was the main mediator but no correlation between flushes and the excretion of urinary 5-HIAA has been found. Another proposed mediator has been bradykinin but several studies have failed to demonstrate any increase in bradykinin after spontaneous or stimulated flush. We have been able to demonstrate release of the tachykinins, neuropeptide K, neurokinin A and substance P during spontaneous, alcohol-induced and pentagastrin-stimulated flush in patients with malignant carcinoid tumours. The pentagastrin-induced flush cannot be blocked by pretreatment with the 5-HT$_2$ receptor-blocking agents but can be reduced or abolished by somatostatin analogues [5].

Four different clinical types of flushing have been described: a diffuse erythematous flush which affects the normal flushing area (face and upper part of the thorax) (see Plate 67.1, between pp. 272 and 273) and is paroxysmal, usually lasting for 2–5 minutes. Another more violaceous flush associated with dilated cutaneous facial veins and telangiectases is very often seen in patients with long-standing carcinoid syndrome. A bright red, patchy flush associated with gastric carcinoids (ECLomas) with an excess of histamine release is the third type. Bronchial carcinoids are sometimes associated with bluish-red flushes lasting for hours with facial skin swelling, lacrimation, swelling of the salivary glands and hypotension. This is the most severe type of flush reaction and it may be part of a carcinoid crisis. It is important to realize that patients with chronic flushes sometimes do not feel them because they get used to the symptoms [2,5].

Diarrhoea

Diarrhoea is almost as common as flushing and it may not be completely associated with a flushing attack, suggesting that the mediators are different. Watery stools, accompanied by colicky abdominal pain and urgency of defaecation is common. 5-HT stimulates small bowel motility and secretion and 5-HT$_2$ receptor blockers might abolish the diarrhoea without affecting the flushing.

Steatorrhoea occurs more rarely but signs of malabsorption can be found in patients with carcinoid tumours. The malabsorption might be due to obstruction of the lymphatics. Other causes of diarrhoea might be bacterial overgrowth and sometimes it might be part of a small bowel resection and bile salt malabsorption [2,5].

Abdominal pain

Abdominal pain is a common clinical symptom associated with carcinoid tumours of the gastrointestinal tract. About 40% of patients with midgut carcinoids are referred to hospital due to symptoms of gastrointestinal obstruction. This obstruction may be due to the primary tumour, although in most situations it is very small. On the other hand intestinal obstruction might also depend on tumour-associated fibrosis causing entrapment of the intestine and mesenteric blood supply. Pain related to intestinal infarction is very rare but in patients with long-standing disease intestinal entrapment is quite common. Pain arising from hepatic metastases is uncommon and is predominantly noticed in patients with large metastases and grossly enlarged livers. Tension of the liver capsule might lead to tenderness and pain. Some patients experience periods of metastatic infarction with fever and abdominal pain, which is quite common in patients with large liver metastases [2,5].

Respiratory symptoms

Symptoms of bronchoconstriction are less common than other features of the carcinoid syndrome, constituting about 4–18%. Asthma-like episodes, which are associated with flushing attacks, might be related to the same mediators, tachykinins and/or bradykinin. Bronchospasm is rather rare and in most situations lung symptoms might depend on hyperventilation, which is observed during flushing episodes. Bronchoconstriction can be seen during anaesthesia and catecholamines should not be given systemically because they may worsen the symptomatology. Nowadays treatment with somatostatin analogues has solved most of the anaesthetic problems.

Carcinoid heart disease

It is unique for a malignant tumour to be associated with a pathognomonic cardiac disease which is also of great importance in the morbidity and mortality of the carcinoid syndrome. The frequency of carcinoid heart disease based on autopsy diagnosis in patients with carcinoid syndrome has been reported as 35–50%. However, in a recent study we were able to demonstrate (by means of echocardiography) that about 70% of consecutively referred patients with the carcinoid syndrome presented with signs of carcinoid heart disease. The most frequent pathological findings were morphological and functional abnormalities of the tricuspid valve. The carcinoid heart lesions are plaque-like or diffuse, pearly grey endocardial thickening. They are almost invariably found on the right side of the heart. The tricuspid leaflets as well as the pulmonary cups are frequently retracted by a fibrotic process [2,5].

Microscopically the lesions are mainly composed of elastine-deficient stroma rich in acid mucopolysaccharides and collagen intermingled with a moderate number of cells. The aetiology of carcinoid heart disease remains obscure. The tumours release vasoactive substances which might be involved in the pathogenesis and there exists a correlation between the degree of heart involvement and circulating levels of tachykinins and serotonin. Very recently we also found increased expression of the TGF-β family of growth factors within these carcinoid heart plaques and these growth factors are well known to be involved in stromal formation and in stimulating matrix production in tumours. However, the link between the locally increased expression of TGF-β and circulating hormones is still missing.

Miscellaneous manifestations

Pellagra-like skin lesions are found in a small number of patients with carcinoid syndrome and long-standing advanced disease. These occur because of the excessive and disturbed metabolic degradation of tryptophan, which results in nicotinic acid and protein deficiency. The symptoms may be reversed by administration of vitamin B6. Paraneoplastic polyneuropathy has also been described in rare cases, as has myopathy. Hypoglycaemia has been reported in single cases and has been found to be related to production of insulin-like growth factor (IGF)-1 and IGF-2 in the tumours. Retroperitoneal fibrosis is found in patients with lymph node metastases located to the retroperitoneal space and might occasionally cause ureteric obstruction and renal failure. Similar to the fibrosis in the right heart, fibrosis of great veins and large abdominal arteries can be seen and may cause abdominal pain, discomfort and even intestinal infarction. Gastrointestinal bleeding may occur from carcinoid tumours throughout the gastrointestinal tract. Foregut carcinoid tumours might produce gastrin and give rise to the Zollinger–Ellison syndrome. The occurrence of psychiatric disturbances in the carcinoid syndrome is disputed. There are few observations of patients who develop severe

mental depression concomitant with a discovery of a carcinoid tumour. Treatment with oral tryptophan reverses mental depression suggesting a tryptophan deficiency which might perhaps have been causing brain serotonin deficiency. Carcinoids of foregut origin may sometimes be associated with multiple endocrine neoplasia type 1 syndrome (MEN-1). Duodenal carcinoids and carcinoids of the ampulla of Vater have been reported to be associated with von Recklinghausen's disease.

Diagnosis

Biochemical

The diagnosis of a carcinoid tumour may be suspected by clinical symptoms suggestive of a carcinoid syndrome or by the presence of other clinical symptoms such as abdominal pain. Attempts are being made to identify specific and sensitive serum or urine markers for carcinoid tumours that allow earlier diagnosis (see Table 67.4). Urinary 5-HIAA has been reported to have a sensitivity of around 70% and a specificity of 100% in patients with the carcinoid syndrome, whereas plasma substance P has been reported to have a sensitivity of about 30% and a specificity of 85%. In our study [5] of 103 patients with metastasizing carcinoid tumours (87% of midgut origin), urinary 5-HIAA was increased in 88%, plasma neuropeptide K in 66%, serum pancreatic polypeptide in 43% and α-hCG in 28%. The most sensitive marker was plasma chromogranin A, which was increased in 100% of the patients. The specificity of chromogranin A is less than urinary 5-HIAA in carcinoid tumours because almost all tumours with neuroendocrine differentiation present with increased levels of plasma chromogranin A and patients with neuroendocrine cell hyperplasia without adenomas or tumours may also show increased circulating levels of chromogranin A. In patients with carcinoid syndrome but normal urinary 5-HIAA levels, measurements of 5-HT in platelets can be of value. When analysing urinary 5-HIAA or 5-HT it is important to give the patient a specific diet excluding bananas, avocado, pineapple, walnuts, chocolate and coffee and avoiding medications such as chlorpromazine, salicylates and L-dopa [2,5].

Sometimes measurements of urinary 5-HIAA and plasma levels of amines or peptides are unable to identify all patients with carcinoid tumours. Therefore, provocative tests have been proposed. Pentagastrin given as a bolus injection i.v. of 0.6 μg/kg body weight may give a flushing reaction similar to spontaneous flushes, and measurements of neuropeptide K at –1.5, 0, 1, 3, 5, 15 and 30 minutes can demonstrate release of tachykinins. In our hands plasma neuropeptide K has been more sensitive as a marker than substance P [5].

Histology and immunocytochemistry

Specimens obtained from tumour tissue either at surgery or by coarse needle biopsies from liver or lymph node metastases should be screened for neuroendocrine properties on histology. Staining with both the argyrophil (Grimelius) and argentaffin staining (Masson) not only confirms the diagnosis of a gastrointestinal carcinoid but a positive argentaffin reaction also suggests a midgut offspring. Other useful neuroendocrine markers are immunohistochemical staining with antibodies against chromogranin A, synaptophysin and NSE [6].

Localization

Many techniques have been used to determine the location of a primary tumour and metastases including gastrointestinal endoscopy, barium enema, chest X-ray, ultrasound, computed tomography (CT), magnetic resonance imaging (MRI), angiography, selective venous sampling for hormones, radionucleotide scanning (radiolabelled octreotide, iodinated metaiodobenzylguanidine (MIBG) and most recently positron emission tomography (PET)). The main problem is in localizing midgut carcinoids, which may be small and frequently are missed by barium enema. Some of these tumours can be localized by angiography. Sometimes local lymph node metastases adjacent to the primary intestinal carcinoid may be seen by CT scan or abdominal ultrasound investigation. Liver metastases are usually detected by CT scan or ultrasound investigation. MRI spectroscopy can give additional information during treatment and follow-up.

Recently radionucleotide scanning has become very popular starting with ^{125}I-MIBG, which has today been replaced by indium-labelled octreotide (^{111}In-diethylenetriame penta-acetic acid (DTPA)-octreotide). Five subtypes of somatostatin receptors (SSTR) have been cloned and carcinoid tumours are known to express at least two subtypes of the receptor, SSTR-1 and -2. The somatostatin analogue octreotide binds SSTR-2 and about 85% of carcinoid tumours have somatostatin receptors. Somatostatin receptor scintigraphy is particularly useful for localization of metastases outside the abdomen, for example, in the skeleton and lymph nodes outside the abdomen (see Plate 67.2, between pp. 272 and 273). The detection limit is 0.5–1.0 cm in diameter. Therefore by using somatostatin receptor scintigraphy, a more reliable staging of the disease can be obtained [7]. PET has come into clinical use in some centres. This method uses short-lived isotopes generated by a cyclotron with a very short half-life (20–30 minutes). ^{11}C-labelled 5-HTP, the precursor of serotonin synthesis, has been particularly useful (see Plate 67.3, between pp. 272 and 273). This isotope is concentrated and taken up in carcinoid tumours and gives, not only the topographical location of primary tumours and metastases, but also information about the metabolism and can be used to follow the treatment. The detection limit is 0.5–1.0 cm in diameter.

Echocardiography is also essential to assess the degree of carcinoid heart disease.

Treatment

Surgical treatment should be considered in every patient with a carcinoid tumour. In cases with local disease, primary tumour and only local metastases, surgery can be curative. However, even in patients with bulky disease and liver and mesenteric metastases an aggressive surgical approach may be of clinical benefit. The reduction of tumour mass by surgical intervention enhances a favourable outcome for forthcoming medical treatment. Intestinal obstruction may occur during medical treatment and conservative resections of the intestine and fibrotic areas may also alleviate clinical symptoms.

The majority of patients with midgut carcinoid tumours presenting with a carcinoid syndrome have multiple liver metastases and cannot be cured surgically. In these situations hepatic artery occlusion has been attempted with palliation of clinical symptoms for a median of 6–12 months. Due to development of collateral blood supply this treatment is very rarely curative but the procedure can be repeated several times. The effect of embolization, however, diminishes with the number of performed occlusions. The procedure can be performed with gelfoam powder alone or combined with chemotherapy, so-called chemoembolization. Chemoembolization has been used in patients with advanced stages of carcinoid tumours not responding to systemic medical treatment. Doxorubicin, cisplatin or mitomycin C is mixed with contrast medium and injected into the hepatic artery followed by plugging with gelfoam powder.

Radiotherapy has been attempted in a number of patients with metastatic gastrointestinal carcinoids. The results have so far been poor and radiotherapy is nowadays mostly utilized for treatment of bone metastases in order to obtain pain relief. High doses of ^{111}In-DTPA-octreotide can be used as 'internal' radiation and is now used in clinical trials.

Medical therapy

Medical treatment includes mainly chemotherapy, interferon and somatostatin analogues (Table 67.6).

Table 67.6 Medical treatment of carcinoid tumours
(a) Chemotherapy

Agent	Number of patients	Objective response		Reference
		Number of patients	Rate (%)	
STZ+5-FU	43	14	33	11
	80	18	23	12
	24	2	8	13
	10	4	40	14
STZ+CTX	47	12	26	15
STZ+DOX	10	4	40	14
STZ+CTX+DOX	20	7	35	16
STZ+DOX+DPP+5-FU	15	2	14	16
ETP+DPP	13	0	0	17
STZ+DOX+IFN	11	0	0	18

(b) Somatostatin analogue (octreotide)

Number of patients	Dose	Biochemical response (%) (number objective tumour regression)	Reference
	150 µg × 3/day	72 (4)	19
	50 µg × 2/day	28 (9)	20
14	100 µg × 3/day	63	21

(c) Alpha-interferon therapy

Number of patients	Dose	Biochemical response (%)	Tumour response (%)	Reference
	IFN-2a 24 Mu/m^2 × 3/week s.c.	39	20	22
21	IFN-2b 3 Mu/m^2 × 3/week s.c.	56	10	23
19	IFN-2b 5 Mu × 6/week s.c. alone or with embolization	40;86	10;86	24
18	rIFN-2c 2 Mu/m^2 × 7/week s.c.	44	0	25
8	nIFN-α 3 Mu × 7/week s.c.	50	12.5	26
37	nIFN-α 6 Mu × 7/week i.m.	49	11	27
21	rIFN-2b 5 Mu × 3/week s.c.	53	0	28
20	nIFN-α 6 Mu × 7/week s.c.	50	11	29
	STZ+5-FU	0	0	
111	nIFN-α × 7/week or s.c. rIFN-2b 5 Mu × 3/week	42	15	30
22	rIFN-2a 3 Mu/m^2 × 3/week	25	17	18
	rIFN-α2 3 Mu/m^2 × 3/week+STZ+DOX	0	0	
	rIFN-α2b 2.5 Mu × 7/week s.c.	60	18	31

CTX, cyclophosphamide; DOX, doxorubicin; DPP, cisplatinum; ETP, etoposide (VP16); 5-FU, fluorouracil; IFN, α-interferon; STZ, streptozotocin.

Chemotherapy in different combinations has been attempted for the last two decades in the treatment of malignant carcinoid tumours and the carcinoid syndrome striking a rather low response rate in most series. The most promising combination of cytostatic drugs has so far been streptozotocin and 5-fluorouracil giving rather short-lasting responses in 10–30% of patients with a median duration of 3–9 months. The results of chemotherapy in carcinoid tumours are in contrast to the results obtained in the closely related, endocrine pancreatic tumours, where 50–65% of these tumours demonstrate objective biochemical responses. The adverse reactions to streptozotocin include mainly vomiting and impaired renal function [32,33].

In 1982 we introduced the treatment with α-interferon (IFN-α) and today more than 300 patients have been treated and reported in the literature [27,33]. The most widely applied dosages are 3–9 Mu s.c. 3–5 times per week and individual dosing is mandatory. The biochemical response rate has been a median of 45% with a significant tumour shrinkage in around 12% of the patients. Clinical improvement of the carcinoid syndrome is noticed in a median of 70% of the patients. IFN-α exerts a direct effect on the tumour cells and causes a block in cell division in G0 phase. It also stimulates differentiation of the tumour cells and increases apoptosis. Furthermore, it is immuno-modulatory and increases the expression of class I antigens on the tumour cells. In a historical study at our institution the median survival for patients with the carcinoid syndrome and liver metastases was 80+ months on IFN-α to be compared with only 8 months for the combination of streptozotocin and 5-fluorouracil. The side-effects of IFN-α therapy are mainly dose dependent and include influenza-like symptoms, fatigue and sometimes mental depression [27,33].

During the last decade treatment with somatostatin analogues has been developed. Today at least three different somatostatin analogues are clinically available, octreotide, octatstatin (RC-160) and somatuline. All these somatostatin analogues are octapeptides and bind to SSTR-2 and -4. Octreotide is the most widely used and, at doses of 50–150 μg s.c. 2–3 times per day, biochemical responses have been obtained in 30–70% of the patients and control of the clinical symptoms in around 70% of the patients. We have recently been able to demonstrate that somatostatin analogues can stimulate apoptosis and this might cause a reduction of tumour size. The most recent medical treatment is a combination of IFN-α and somatostatin analogues, giving biochemical responses in around 70% of patients previously resistant to either octreotide or IFN-α alone [19,33].

Octreotide has been most effective in cases of carcinoid crisis. The carcinoid crisis is usually reported in patients with foregut carcinoids and is frequently precipitated by stressful situations such as infections, chemotherapy, tumour biopsies or anaesthesia. The use of octreotide may be life saving and in these situations given as i.v. infusion 50–100 μg/h over 24–72 hours. The main long-term side-effects of octreotide include gall stone formation.

Symptomatic therapy

Most of the previous drugs for symptomatic treatment have nowadays been replaced by somatostatin analogues. However, diarrhoea may be treated with loperamide in selected patients. Histamine receptor antagonists may sometimes be of value in foregut carcinoid patients to control flushing.

Prognosis

The carcinoid syndrome is generally a manifestation of advanced disease. Carcinoid tumours are reported to be very benign, and liver metastases grow very slowly and patients have been reported to live for 10–15 years after occurrence of metastatic disease. While it is true that single patients can live for more than 30 years with a carcinoid syndrome, a critical review of the literature demonstrates that the 5-year survival rate when liver metastases are present is about 18–38% in different patient groups [3,5,7,32,34]. The median survival time has been calculated to be about 23 months in patients with liver metastases and increased urinary 5-HIAA levels. In our series of 103 carcinoid patients, median survival from histological diagnosis was only 24 months. It is also important to notice that 33% of the patients do not die from tumour progression but from the carcinoid heart disease and nowadays heart valve replacement is important. This is particularly true when the median survival by more active and aggressive therapy seems to improve survival time, being 60–80 months from start of therapy, for patients with the carcinoid syndrome [33]. Not only has survival been improved but also the quality of life after introduction of somatostatin analogues and interferon in the therapy. Many patients are working full time despite metastatic liver disease.

References

1. Williams ED, Sandler M. The classification of carcinoid tumours. *Lancet* 1963;1:238–9.
2. Grahame-Smith DG. The carcinoid syndrome. In de Groot LJ (ed.). *Endocrinology*, Vol. 3. New York: Grune and Stratton, 1979:1721–31.
3. Goodwin DJ. Carcinoid tumours; an analysis of 2837 cases. *Cancer* 1975;36:560–9.
4. Norton JA, Doppman JL, Jensen RT. Cancer of the endocrine system. In De Vita VT Jr, Hellman S, Rosenberg SA (eds). *Cancer: Principles and Practice of Oncology*, 4th edn. Pennslyvania: J.B. Lippincott, 1993; 1333–435.
5. Norheim I, Öberg K, Theodorsson-Norheim E *et al.* Malignant carcinoid tumors: an analysis of 103 patients with regard to tumour localization, hormone production and survival. *Ann. Surg.* 1987;206:115–25.
6. Wilander E, Lundquist ML, Öberg K. Gastrointestinal carcinoid tumours. *Prog. Histochem. Cytochem.* 1989;12:2.
7. Tiensuu Janson E. Carcinoid tumors: clinical aspects and the use of somatostatin analogues for characterization and treatment. Thesis, Uppsala University, 1995.
8. Davis Z, Moertel CG, McIlrath DC. The malignant carcinoid syndrome. *Surg. Gynecol. Obstet.* 1973;13:637–44.
9. Thorson AH. Studies on carcinoid disease. *Acta Med. Scand.* 1958;334:81.

10. Feldman JM. Carcinoid tumours and syndrome. *Sem. Oncol.* 1982;**17**:237.

11. Moertel CG, Hanley JA, Johnsson LA. Streptozocin alone compared with streptozocin plus fluorouracil in the treatment of advanced islet cell carcinoma. *N. Engl. J. Med.* 1980;**303**:1189–94.

12. Moertel CG, Hanley JA. Combination chemotherapy trials in metastatic carcinoid syndrome. *Cancer Clin. Trials* 1979;**2**:327–34.

13. Murray-Lyon IM, Eddelston ALWF, Williams R *et al.* Treatment of multiple hormone-producing malignant islet cell tumors with streptozotocin. *Lancet* 1968;**2**:895–8.

14. Kelsen DP, Cheng E, Kemeny N *et al.* Streptozotocin and Adriamycin in the treatment of apud tumors (carcinoid, islet cell and medullary carcinomas of the thyroid). *Proc. Am. Assoc. Cancer Res.* 1982;**23**:433.

15. Bukowski RM, Johnsson KG, Peterson RF *et al.* A phase II trial combination chemotherapy in patients with metastatic carcinoid tumors: a Southwest Oncology Group study. *Cancer* 1987;**60**:2891.

16. Bukowski RM, Stephens R, Oishi N *et al.* Phase II trial of 5-FU, Adriamycin, cyclophosphamide, and streptozotocin (FAC-S) in metastatic carcinoid. *Proc. Am. Soc. Clin. Oncol.* 1983;**2**:130.

17. Moertel CG, Kvols LK, O'Connell MJ *et al.* Treatment of neuroendocrine carcinomas with combined etoposide and cisplatin. Evidence of major therapeutic activity in the anaplastic variants of these neoplasms. *Cancer* 1991;**68**:227–32.

18. Tiensuu Janson E, Rönnblom L, Ahlström H *et al.* Treatment with alpha-interferon versus alpha-interferon in combination with streptozocin and doxorubicin in patients with malignant carcinoid tumors: a randomized trial. *Ann. Oncol.* 1992;**3**:635–8.

19. Kvols LK, Moertel CG, O'Connell MJ *et al.* Treatment of the malignant carcinoid syndrome: evaluation of a long acting somatostatin analogue. *N. Engl. J. Med.* 1986;**315**:663–6.

20. Öberg K, Norheim I, Theodorsson E. Treatment of malignant midgut carcinoid tumors with a long-acting somatostatin analog octreotid. *Acta Oncol.* 1991;**4**:503–7.

21. Vinik AL, Moattari AR. Use of somatostatin analog in management of carcinoid syndrome. *Dig. Dis. Sci.* 1989;**34**:14–27S.

22. Moertel CG, Rubin J, Kvols LK. Therapy of metastatic carcinoid tumor and the malignant carcinoid syndrome with recombinant leukocyte A interferon. *J. Clin. Oncol.* 1989;**7**:865–8.

23. Schober C, Schuppert F, Schmoll E *et al.* Interferon-alpha-2b in patients with advanced carcinoids and apudoma. *Blut* (Abstr. 34th Ann. Cong. German Soc. Hematol. Oncol.) 1989;**59**:331.

24. Hanssen LE, Schrumpf E, Kolbenstvedt AN *et al.* Treatment of malignant metastatic midgut carcinoid tumours with recombinant human alpha-2b interferon with or without prior hepatic artery embolization. *Scand. J. Gastroenterol.* 1989;**24**:787–95.

25. Bartsch HH, Stockmann F, Arnold R *et al.* Treatment of patient with metastatic carcinoid tumours by recombinant human interferon—alpha results from a phase II study. *J. Cancer Res. Clin. Oncol.* 1990;**116**:305.

26. Välimäki M, Jarvinen H, Salmela P *et al.* Is the treatment of metastatic carcinoid tumor with interferon not as successful as suggested? *Cancer* 1991;**67**:547–9.

27. Öberg K, Norheim I, Lind E *et al.* Treatment of malignant carcinoid tumours with human leukocyte interferon. Long-term results. *Cancer Treat. Rep.* 1986;**70**:1297–304.

28. Öberg K, Alm G, Magnusson A *et al.* Treatment of malignant carcinoid tumors with recombinant interferon alpha-2b (Intron-A); development of neutralizing interferon antibodies and possible loss of antitumor activity. *J. Natl. Cancer Inst.* 1989;**81**:531–5.

29. Norheim I, Öberg K, Alm G. Treatment of malignant carcinoid tumors; a randomized controlled study of streptozocin plus 5-FU and human leucocyte interferon. *Eur. J. Cancer Clin. Oncol.* 1989;**25**:1475–9.

30. Öberg K, Eriksson B. The role of interferons in the management of carcinoid tumors. *Acta Oncol.* 1991;**30**:519–22.

31. Biesma B, Willemse PHB, Mulder NH *et al.* Recombinant interferon alpha 2b in patients with metastatic apudomas. *Br. J. Cancer* 1992;**66**:880–5.

32. Moertel CG. An odyssey in the land of small tumors. *J. Clin. Oncol.* 1987;**5**:1503–22.

33. Öberg K. Treatment of neuroendocrine tumors. *Cancer Treat. Rev.* 1994;**20**:331–55.

34. Moertel CG, Sauer WG, Dockerty MB, Baggentoss AH. The life history of the carcinoid tumor of the small intestine. *Cancer* 1961;**14**:901–12.

Appendiceal tumours are, in general, insular; rectal are trabecular, insular or glandular. In the colon and rectum, confusion can occur because the cells become admixed with colonic or rectal crypts, giving a misleading appearance of malignancy, or mimicking the appearances of colitis cystica profunda. Marked desmoplasia was noted in 7% of rectal carcinoids in one series [6].

Of colorectal (predominantly rectal) carcinoids, a minority (but in one series 28%) are reported as argentaffin. Many more (55–75%) are argyrophilic; the majority stain positively for neurone-specific enolase (e.g. 87%) and chromogranin (58%) [8] (Fig. 68.1b). Many specific products are identified: for example, serotonin 4–45%, pancreatic polypeptide 45%, glucagon 10%, gastrin 3%, somatostatin 3%, adrenocorticotrophic hormone (ACTH) 1%. Substance P, insulin, encephalin and β-endorphin are occasionally recognized, and, in the majority of tumours, more than one product is present. Cholecystokinin (CCK), motilin, neurotensin and calcitonin have been stated to be absent. Carcino-embryonic antigen and prostatic acid phosphatase are relatively commonly identified (24 and 82%, respectively); this raises an important consideration, as carcinoids may be misdiagnosed as carcinomas by inexperienced pathologists.

The composite adenocarcinoid may also cause diagnostic confusion: a tumour predominantly of the appendix with malignant epithelial as well as neuroendocrine elements (Fig. 68.2). Now it is appreciated that clonal specialization can occur in carcinomas, these are generally interpreted as primarily carcinomas rather than carcinoids.

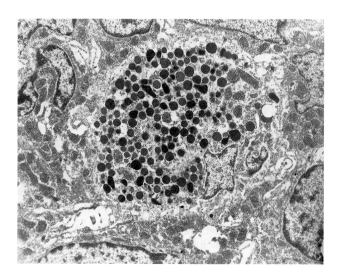

Fig. 68.2 Electron micrograph of a hindgut carcinoid tumour showing a typical L cell packed with large secretory granules with variable electron density. (Courtesy of Dr A. Bishop and Professor J. Polak.)

Clinical features and management

Appendiceal carcinoids

Most appendiceal carcinoids are identified histologically when appendicectomy has been performed for other reasons. As most of the tumours are at the tip, they are unlikely to induce obstructive appendicitis. Local infiltration into the mesoappendix may occur, or marked desmoplasia, and these may predispose to appendicitis by reducing motility of the organ.

What needs to be done when an appendiceal carcinoid has been detected, either at operation or subsequently by the histopathologist? The Mayo Clinic series emphasized the prognostic importance of size of the tumour. Most are < 1 cm, with only 15% > 2 cm, and in that series no metastases were identified in tumours < 2 cm followed for over 25 years [9]. For a large (> 2 cm) tumour, or one with a marked local desmoplastic reaction identified surgically, the appropriate surgical manoeuvre is to perform a right hemicolectomy as for caecal carcinomas. If a small tumour is found only at histopathological examination after appendicectomy, usually nothing needs to be done, but a second-look hemicolectomy has been recommended if there is tumour infiltration into the meso-appendix or lymphatic invasion. With reported 5-year survival rates of over 99%, clinicians and patients can indeed be optimistic about appendiceal carcinoid tumours.

Colonic carcinoids

Unless presenting with metastatic disease, the characteristic presentation of colonic carcinoid tumours is with pain or obstruction, or with bleeding. Those in the proximal colon, of midgut origin, are more likely to have an associated desmoplastic reaction. Perhaps reflecting the lesser likelihood of incidental diagnosis compared with either appendiceal or rectal carcinoids, they tend to be larger and have a higher incidence of metastasis than tumours in those locations. Treatment of symptomatic lesions is clearly by surgical resection with a cancer-type operation. There is little reported experience of endoscopic resection of small tumours with fulguration of the base as used for rectal carcinoids (see below); this technique is less applicable to submucosal lesions in the colon than in the rectum due to the risk of colonic perforation.

Rectal carcinoids

As already mentioned, more recent series indicate that rectal carcinoids are relatively common, and may indeed be more common than appendiceal carcinoids [1,6]. They are likely to be recognized clinically as incidentals at proctosigmoidoscopy. Despite their submucosal location, endoscopic biopsies are almost always diagnostic. The majority will be small, less than 1 cm, and metastasis at that stage is extremely rare. Endoscopic biopsy, with fulguration of the base, appears curative [1], although more sophisticated centres may wish to apply endoscopic ultrasound or magnetic resonance to define the lack of transmural spread of the tumour before proceeding. Between 1 and 2 cm in size, the incidence of metastasis is again very low, perhaps 5%, but at this size a more formal operating room transanal approach may be appropriate. Over 4 cm in size, the chances of metastatic disease are very high, so formal cancer operations are indicated for all tumours over 2 cm, or if imaging suggests local spread of smaller tumours [6].

References

1. Matsui K, Iwasa T, Kitagawa M. Small, polypoid-appearing carcinoid tumors of the rectum: clinicopathologic study of 16 cases and effectiveness of endoscopic treatment. *Am. J. Gastroenterol.* 1993;**88**:1949–53.
2. Sjoblom S-M. Clinical presentation and prognosis of gastrointestinal carcinoid tumours. *Scand. J. Gastroenterol.* 1988;**23**:799–87.
3. Marshall JB, Bodnarchuk G. Carcinoid tumors of the gut: our experience over three decades and review of the literature. *J. Clin. Gastroenterol.* 1993;**16**(2):123–9.
4. Lluis F, Thompson JC. Neuroendocrine potential of the colon and rectum. *Gastroenterology* 1988;**94**:832–44.
5. Hodgson HJF. Carcinoid tumours and the carcinoid syndrome. In Bouchier IAD, Allan RN, Hodgson HJF, Keighley MRB (eds). *Gastroenterology: Clinical Science and Practice*, 2nd edn, vol. 1. London: W. B. Saunders, 1994:643–58.
6. Jemore AB, Ray JE, Gathright JB *et al*. Rectal carcinoids: the most frequent carcinoid tumour. *Dis. Colon. Rectum* 1992;**35**:717–25.
7. Dayal Y. Neuroendocrine cells and their proliferative lesions. In Norris TH (ed.). *Pathology of the Colon, Small Intestine and Anus*, 2nd edn. Edinburgh: Churchill Livingstone, 1991:305–65.
8. Federspiel BH, Burke AP, Sobin LE, Shekitka KM. Rectal and colonic carcinoids: a clinicopathological study of 84 cases. *Cancer* 1990;**65**:135–40.
9. Moertel CG, Weiland LH, Nagorney DM, Dockerty MB. Carcinoid tumour of the appendix: treatment and prognosis. *N. Engl. J. Med.* 1987;**317**:901–12.

69

Chemotherapy for Malignant Neuroendocrine Tumours

MATTHEW T. SEYMOUR AND MAURICE L. SLEVIN

Introduction

Currently, surgery is the only potentially curative treatment for neuroendocrine cancers. As yet we have no data to support the use of drug treatment as a means of increasing the surgical cure rate (surgical adjuvant therapy), although this is a potential role to be explored. The current role of medical treatments, therefore, is to maximize the quality and duration of life for those patients whose disease is not completely resectable.

However, in contrast to many other solid cancers, where the duration of such 'palliative' treatment is usually measured in months, patients with neuroendocrine cancers may frequently coexist with their disease for several years. This, along with the wide variety of clinical problems faced and the wide range of treatments which may be considered, makes their medical management particularly challenging.

For patients with unresectable disease, a number of medical treatment approaches are considered. These include:
1 expectancy;
2 symptomatic treatments and hormone antagonists;
3 somatostatin analogues (which inhibit hormone secretion);
4 interferon-α (IFN-α) (cytostatic; may also reduce hormone secretion);
5 cytotoxic chemotherapy;
6 interventional tumour debulking (hepatic artery embolization; laser, etc.).
It is common for patients with neuroendocrine cancer to receive several sequential modalities of treatment over a protracted disease course. An important aspect of the specialist's role is to select treatments at appropriate times to maximize the overall benefit to the patient in terms of the duration and quality of survival. This requires careful assessment of the pace of disease progression and the relative contributions of hormonal secretion and tumour bulk to the patient's symptoms. The usual approach is to use the least interventional and least toxic treatment which, at any particular stage of the disease, can suppress symptoms to an acceptable level. Treatments with significant side-effects, such as IFN and chemotherapy, are therefore only introduced when less complicated, purely symptomatic approaches are failing. However, this cannot be assumed to be the best policy: randomized trials of palliative chemotherapy in more common cancers (such as metastatic colorectal cancer) are teaching us that the patient's longer term benefit, in terms of both quality and duration of life, might be better served by using chemotherapy earlier, when general fitness and organ function allow adequate doses to be given with tolerable side-effects.

Chemotherapy

Well-differentiated neuroendocrine tumours are not highly chemosensitive [1–4]. This may be due to their generally low rate of mitosis, the target of many cytotoxic drugs, but also to other biological properties; for example, they show constitutively high levels of expression of mRNA for the multidrug-resistance gene *MDR-1*, which encodes the transmembrane efflux pump P-glycoprotein. This pump, which is believed to play a role in the efflux of hormones from endocrine cells, is also able to extrude a variety of anticancer drugs, resulting in resistance to them.

The rarity of neuroendocrine tumours and paucity of good preclinical models have all but precluded the methodical process of preclinical screening followed by adequate phase II and large phase III clinical trials, which have been used to establish chemotherapy treatments for more common cancers. Many reports in the literature are retrospective and involve too few patients, or too diverse a population, to draw statistically valid conclusions. The majority of our knowledge comes from a North American programme of multi-institutional clinical trials in malignant carcinoid and islet cell carcinomas conducted under the direction of the late Charles Moertel [5–8].

Overall patterns of chemosensitivity

In general, islet cell carcinomas are more chemosensitive than carcinoid tumours. This is partly due to the particular specificity of one agent, streptozotocin, for pancreatic tumours, although other drugs including dacarbazine and doxorubicin also produce higher response rates in islet cell carcinoma than in carcinoid tumours. Among carcinoid tumours, those of foregut origin (thymus, bronchus, stomach, duodenum) have proven less chemosensitive than the midgut carcinoids (jejunum, ileum, caecum, appendix). Other neuroendocrine cancers have generally been included in protocols for carcinoid and islet cell cancers.

Differentiation

The histological differentiation of neuroendocrine tumours, and hence their proliferative rate, is an important determinant of chemosensitivity. Anaplastic neuroendocrine tumours are an increasingly recognized group, which show histological similarity to small-cell lung cancer (SCLC). Like SCLC, these tumours behave aggressively, with rapid growth and early metastasis, and they also demonstrate a relatively high response rate to chemotherapy. In a phase II study of etoposide and cisplatin (both agents with high activity in SCLC), only two of 27 (7%) patients with well-differentiated carcinoid or islet cell cancers had objective responses, while 12 of 18 (67%) patients with anaplastic neuroendocrine cancer responded [5].

Chemotherapy drugs

The chief cytotoxic drugs currently used in neuroendocrine cancer treatment are streptozotocin, 5-fluorouracil (5-FU), dacarbazine and doxorubicin.

Streptozotocin

Streptozotocin is a nitrosourea alkylating agent isolated from *Streptomyces* with specific toxicity towards normal pancreatic beta cells, making it an obvious choice for treatment of islet cell tumours. It is not myelosuppressive, but unfortunately it carries significant renal toxicity and is highly emetogenic, although the latter problem is largely alleviated by the modern generation of 5-hydroxytryptamine (5-HT$_3$)-receptor antagonist anti-emetics. Streptozotocin has little toxicity towards bone marrow, making it a good candidate for inclusion in combination chemotherapy regimens. A promising analogue of streptozotocin, chlorozotocin, was developed in the anticipation of having reduced toxicity, but unfortunately it has shown no advantages over the parent compound in clinical trials to date.

5-Fluorouracil

5-FU is the mainstay of drug treatment for the common gastrointestinal adenocarcinomas. It is a pyrimidine antimetabolite with complex effects upon DNA and RNA synthesis and function. One of its activities, inhibition of thymidylate synthase, requires a reduced folate cofactor. 5-FU's cytotoxicity is in part phase-specific, principally affecting cells exposed during the DNA-synthesis phase (S-phase) of the cell cycle, and for this reason its effects, both *in vitro* and *in vivo*, are affected by the schedule of administration as well as by the total dose administered. Intense research in 5-FU treatment of common gastro-intestinal cancers over the past decade has led to significant improvements in activity, through continuous infusional schedules and/or co-administration of reduced folate (calcium leucovorin; folinic acid). These approaches are only recently being applied to neuroendocrine cancer, but it is hoped that here too they will eventually lead to improved therapeutic results.

Dacarbazine

Dacarbazine (dimethyltriazeno-imidazole-carboxamide, DTIC) also has useful activity in neuroendocrine cancers. Like streptozotocin, it is associated with particularly severe emesis, which had limited its value in what is essentially palliative therapy until the advent of potent new anti-emetic drugs.

Other drugs

Cisplatin, carboplatin, etoposide and actinomycin-D have shown little or no activity in neuroendocrine cancers, except anaplastic tumours (see above). New drugs currently undergoing phase II assessment include taxol, a derivative of the western yew (*Taxus brevifolia*), which exerts its cytotoxicity by stabilizing tubulin.

Goals and endpoints of treatment

Response to chemotherapy in clinical trials is usually reported using the World Health Organization (WHO) criteria, in which an objective tumour response is defined as a reduction of at least 50% in the product of the longest measurable tumour diameter and its greatest perpendicular, in all marker lesions, confirmed by two assessments at least four weeks apart. Provided these stringent criteria are carefully and impartially applied, the 'objective response rate' is a useful endpoint for comparing the efficacy of different treatments in a randomized trial and, to a lesser extent, for comparing the results of different trials.

However, it must be stressed that the objective response rate is not a measure of the proportion of patients benefiting from treatment; many patients whose tumours fail to satisfy the WHO response criteria nonetheless obtain obvious and sustained relief of symptoms with chemotherapy, while others who have a WHO objective response may find that any benefit this affords is offset by treatment side-effects. In general, the objective response rate is an underestimate of the proportion of patients who feel that they have benefited from chemotherapy.

Patients with neuroendocrine hormonal secretion and its symptoms may sometimes obtain reduction of hormone levels, and relief of symptoms, with little or no reduction of tumour size. Some investigators therefore report an 'endocrine' or 'biological' response rate. This is a valid endpoint, but should not be confused with WHO tumour response when comparing results of different trials.

Chemotherapy for islet cell carcinoma

Chemotherapy agents and combinations with activity in metastatic islet cell carcinoma are shown in Table 69.1. The rarity of these tumours has required investigators to combine all islet cell tumours in their studies, and numbers of individual tumour subtypes have generally not allowed comparisons to be made; however, it has been suggested that differences in the pattern of chemosensitivity may exist; for example, streptozotocin may be more effective against vasoactive intestinal polypeptide (VIP)omas than glucagonomas, with the converse pattern for dacarbazine. Such observations should be regarded as anecdotal.

Table 69.1 Chemotherapy for islet cell carcinoma

Drug or combination	Response rate (%)
Streptozotocin	30–40
Chlorozotocin	30–40
Dacarbazine	25–50
Doxorubicin	20
Streptozotocin + 5-fluorouracil	45–65
Chlorozotocin + 5-fluorouracil	32
Streptozotocin + doxorubicin	69

The combination of streptozotocin and 5-FU came to be regarded as a standard therapy for islet cell carcinomas after a multi-institutional randomized study which showed the two drugs together to be superior to streptozotocin alone in terms of response rate, response duration and survival [6]. In their subsequent randomized trial, the same collaborative group compared streptozotocin/5-FU with streptozotocin/doxorubicin and with single-agent chlorozotocin. This study showed a statistically significant advantage for streptozotocin/doxorubicin over the other two treatments in terms of response rate and survival, although interestingly the results in the streptozotocin/5-FU 'control' arm were inferior to those obtained in the previous study [7]. There are as yet no reports of the obvious next step, a three-drug combination of streptozotocin, 5-FU and doxorubicin.

When used as a single agent, DTIC has produced objective responses in around 50% of patients in the small phase II trials reported to date, but this has not been tested in larger controlled trials.

The reported median duration of response to chemotherapy has varied widely, but is usually between 6 and 18 months. Thus for most patients who respond to initial chemotherapy the question will eventually arise whether to attempt retreatment. The general experience is that patients who benefited from first-line chemotherapy are likely to do well with repeated or second-line chemotherapy on relapse, while those with primarily resistant disease are unlikely to benefit from a change to different drugs [7].

Chemotherapy for carcinoid tumours

Although the drugs and combinations used for advanced carcinoid are similar to those for islet cell carcinomas, the response rates are generally lower. For this reason, systemic chemotherapy is still regarded as experimental treatment for this disease, and is often turned to only after exhausting other modalities such as interferon, iodine-131 labelled metaiodobenzylguanidine (^{131}I-MIBG) or hepatic artery embolization.

The reported objective response rates for single agent and combination chemotherapy schedules are shown in Table 69.2. Streptozotocin as a single agent is less effective than in islet cell tumours. A recent series of collaborative trials has established that the true objective response rate for combination chemotherapy in this disease is around 15–25%. At this point there seems little justification for using the more toxic doxorubicin- or cisplatin-containing regimens. If any regimen could be regarded as 'standard' in this disease, it would be streptozotocin/5-FU (see Table 69.3), although clearly there is much room

Table 69.2 Chemotherapy schedules used in islet cell carcinoma and carcinoid tumours

Streptozotocin + 5-fluorouracil
  Streptozotocin 500 mg/m² i.v. days 1–5
  5-FU 400 mg/m² i.v. days 1–5
    repeated on a 6-week cycle

Streptozotocin + doxorubicin
  Streptozotocin 500 mg/m² i.v. days 1–5
  Doxorubicin 50 mg/m² i.v. days 1 and 22
    repeated on a 6-week cycle

Single-agent dacarbazine (DTIC)
  DTIC 250 mg/m² i.v. days 1–5
    repeated on a 3- or 4-week cycle

Table 69.3 Chemotherapy for carcinoids

Drug or combination	Approximate response rate (%)
Streptozotocin	10
Dacarbazine (DTIC)	15
Doxorubicin	20
5-Fluorouracil (5-FU)	25
Streptozotocin/5-FU	15–33
Streptozotocin/cyclophosphamide	25
5-FU/doxorubicin	15
5-FU/doxorubicin/cisplatin	15
Streptozotocin/5-FU/doxorubicin Cyclophosphamide	30

for improvement, and in particular the role of streptozotocin in this disease is not certain.

Chemotherapy and interferon

There is laboratory evidence of synergistic interaction between IFN-α and a number of cytotoxic drugs, especially 5-FU, against a variety of tumour models. Accordingly, some groups have looked at the simultaneous use of chemotherapy and IFN-α in patients with carcinoid. In two small studies to date, patients received IFN-α along with 5-FU or 5-FU/streptozotocin/doxorubicin; neither suggested any advantage for combined treatment. Recent large randomized studies in colorectal cancer have suggested that the synergistic interactions observed in the laboratory are not reproduced in the clinic with tolerable schedules of IFN-α. For the time being, combined IFN-α and chemotherapy cannot be recommended for carcinoid, and sequential use of the two treatment modalities would seem the more sensible option.

Chemotherapy and hepatic artery embolization

Selective hepatic arterial embolization using gelfoam or polyvinyl alcohol sponge is described in Chapter 10. This treatment relies on the relative dependence of hepatic metastases upon their hepatic arterial supply, and on the high capacity of normal liver for regeneration following vascular compromise. Hepatic artery ligation or embolization alone produce a high response rate in patients with slow-growing tumours predominantly confined to the liver; however the responses tend to be short-lived.

The combination of hepatic artery embolization with regional or systemic chemotherapy has been suggested as a means of increasing the duration of response, although clearly patients must be carefully selected. In a recent report of patients with islet cell and carcinoid tumours metastatic to the liver, 111 underwent hepatic artery ligation or embolization, and 71 were then selected for four-drug alternating chemotherapy doxorubicin/DTIC/streptozotocin/5-FU). This approach produced a high objective response rate of 80%, with a median response duration of 18 months, but involved significant side-effects [8].

Conclusion

Chemotherapy has an established role in the treatment of advanced islet cell carcinoma. For patients with advanced carcinoid tumours, where response rates are lower, a trial of chemotherapy should also be considered, preferably in the context of a collaborative clinical trials programme. Useful drugs for neuroendocrine cancers include 5-FU, streptozotocin, doxorubicin and DTIC. It is important that new drugs and schedules are assessed in controlled clinical trials. In particular, recent advances in the use of 5-FU in colorectal cancer deserve assessment in neuroendocrine cancer. Hepatic arterial therapy in combination with arterial embolization techniques may produce excellent results in suitable patients, and this approach deserves further development.

Anaplastic neuroendocrine cancers are a separate disease entity with patterns of clinical growth and chemosensitivity more akin to SCLC than to the well-differentiated neuroendocrine cancers.

References

1. Haller DG. Carcinoid and islet cell tumours of the gastrointestinal tract. In Ahlgren JD, MacDonald JS (eds). *Gastrointestinal Oncology* Pennsylvania: J.B. Lippincott, 1992:449–60.
2. Norton JA, Doppman JL, Jensen RT. Cancer of the endocrine system.

In De Vita VT, Hellman S, Rosenberg SA (eds). *Cancer – Principles and Practice of Oncology*, 4th edn. Pennsylvania: J.B. Lippincott, 1993:1371–95.

3. Oberg K. The use of chemotherapy in the management of neuroendocrine tumours. *Endocrinol. Metab. Clinic North Am.* 1993;**22**:941–52.

4. Vinik AI, Thompson NW, Averbuch SD. Neoplasms of the gastroenteropancreatic endocrine system. In Holland JF, Frei E (eds). *Cancer Medicine*, 3rd edn. Philadelphia: Lea and Febiger, 1994:1180–209.

5. Moertel CG, Kvols LK, O'Connel MJ, Rubin J. Treatment of neuroendocrine carcinomas with combined etoposide and cisplatin. Evidence of major therapeutic activity in the anaplastic variants of these neoplasms. *Cancer* 1991;**68**:227–32.

6. Moertel CG, Hanley JA, Johnson LA. Streptozotocin alone compared with streptozotocin plus fluorouracil in the treatment of advanced islet-cell carcinoma. *N. Engl. J. Med.* 1980;**303**:1189–94.

7. Moertel CG, Lefkopoulo M, Lipsitz S, Hahn RG, Klaassen D. Streptozocin-doxorubicin, streptozocin-fluorouracil or cholozotocin in the treatment of advanced islet-cell carcinoma. *N. Engl. J. Med.* 1992;**326**:519–23.

8. Moertel CG, Johnson CM, McKusick MA *et al.* The management of patients with advanced carcinoid tumours and islet cell carcinomas. *Ann. Intern. Med.* 1994;**120**:302–9.

6

MEDICAL SYNDROMES
AND ENDOCRINE NEOPLASIA

Multiple Endocrine Neoplasia Type 1

RAJESH V. THAKKER

Introduction

Multiple endocrine neoplasia type 1 (MEN-1), which has also been referred to as Wermer's syndrome, is characterized by the combined occurrence of tumours of the parathyroid glands, the pancreatic islet cells and the anterior pituitary gland [1]. In addition to these tumours which constitute the major components of MEN-1, adrenal cortical, carcinoid and lipomatous tumours have also been described (reviewed in [2]). These MEN-1 tumours may either be inherited in an autosomal dominant manner or they may occur sporadically, that is, without a family history. However, this distinction between sporadic and familial cases may sometimes be difficult; in some sporadic cases the family history may be absent because the parent with the disease may have died before developing symptoms. In addition, the combinations of the affected glands and their pathological features, for example hyperplasia or single or multiple adenomas of the parathyroid glands, have been reported to differ in members of the same family [3]. The manifestations of MEN-1 that are related to the sites of the tumours and to their products of secretion are summarized in Table 70.1. The treatment and management of each of these is reviewed separately in the individual chapters describing each endocrine tumour. The focus of this chapter will be to review the clinical applications of molecular genetics in MEN-1.

Molecular genetics of neoplasia

The development of tumours may be associated with mutations or inappropriate expression of specific normal cellular genes, which are referred to as oncogenes (reviewed in [4]). Two types of oncogenes referred to as dominant and recessive oncogenes have been described. An activation of *dominant* oncogenes leads to transformation of the cells containing them, and the genetic changes which cause this activation have recently been elucidated; for example, chromosomal translocations affecting such dominant oncogenes are associated with the occurrence of chronic myeloid leukaemia and Burkitt's lymphoma. In these conditions, the mutations that lead to activation of the oncogene are dominant at the cellular level, and therefore only one copy of the mutated gene is required for the phenotypic effect. Such dominantly acting oncogenes may be assayed in cell culture by first transferring them into recipient cells and then scoring the numbers of transformed colonies, and this is referred to as the transfection assay.

However, in some inherited neoplasms which may also arise sporadically, such as retinoblastoma, tumour development is associated with two recessive mutations which inactivate oncogenes, and these are referred to as recessive oncogenes. In the inherited tumours, the first of the two recessive mutations is inherited via the germ-cell line and is present in all the cells. This recessive mutation is not expressed until a second mutation, within a somatic cell, causes loss of the normal dominant allele (Fig. 70.1). The mutations causing the inherited and sporadic tumours are similar but the cell types in which they occur are different. In the inherited tumours the first mutation occurs in the germ cell, whereas in the sporadic tumours both mutations occur in the somatic cell. Thus, the risk of tumour development in an individual who has not inherited the first germ-line mutation is much smaller, as both mutational events must coincide in the same somatic cell. In addition, the apparent paradox that the inherited cancer syndromes are due to recessive mutations but dominantly inherited at the level of the family is explained because, in individuals who have inherited the first recessive mutation, a loss of a single remaining wild-type allele is almost certain to occur in at least one of the large number of cells in the target tissue. This cell will be detected because it forms a tumour, and almost all individuals who have inherited the germ-line mutation

markers in linkage studies of affected families to localize the gene causing MEN-1.

Tumour deletion mapping studies in MEN-1

A two-stage genetic mutational model has been proposed for the development of tumours in MEN-1, and this is analogous to that reported for retinoblastoma. A comparison of the alleles obtained from leucocyte DNA and tumour DNA using either RFLPs or microsatellite polymorphisms can facilitate the detection of the chromosomal abnormalities associated with the 'second hit' in tumour DNA, and this is illustrated in Fig. 70.2. A restriction enzyme is used to cleave leucocyte and tumour DNA, and the resulting DNA fragments are separated according to size by agarose gel electrophoresis and transferred by Southern blotting to a nylon membrane, which is hybridized with a single-stranded radiolabelled DNA probe. The labelled DNA probe will anneal to any fragments which have a complementary sequence, and these restricted fragments of varying lengths (RFLPs) are revealed by autoradiography. The exact number and size of RFLPs will vary in relation to the number of recognition sites for the restriction enzyme, as shown in Fig. 70.2.

In this example, the two chromosomes from the leucocytes differ in the number of restriction enzyme cleavage sites; one chromosome has three cleavage sites and the other has two cleavage sites. Following digestion and hybridization, two fragments will be revealed at autoradiography. The chromosome bearing the recessive oncogenic mutation has three cleavage sites, and although two fragments of 4 kilobases (kb) and 1 kb will result from the enzymatic cleavage, only the 4 kb fragment will be visualized at autoradiography as it contains the complementary sequence to the radiolabelled DNA probe. However, the normal chromosome, that is the one not containing the recessive oncogenic mutation, has a loss of one restriction enzyme cleavage site, due to a change in the DNA sequence, and following digestion only restriction fragments of 5 kb in size will result. A single 5 kb RFLP is observed at autoradiography. Alleles can be designated to these RFLPs; for example, the larger, 5 kb RFLP is designated allele 1 and the smaller, 4 kb RFLP, is designated allele 2. Thus, the leucocytes in this example are heterozygous (alleles 1,2) and the chromosome bearing the recessive oncogenic mutation has allele 2, whilst the normal chromosome with the dominant allele has allele 1. A partial loss of the normal chromosome, that is the 'second hit' (see Fig. 70.1), associated with the development of the tumour, would be detected by the loss of the 5 kb RFLP (allele 1). Thus, the tumour cells would be hemizygous (allele –,2) as illustrated in Fig.

70.2, or they may be homozygous (allele 2,2) if a reduplication of the chromosome bearing the recessive oncogenic mutation had occurred (see Fig. 70.1).

This type of analysis, involving paired leucocyte and tumour DNA, which has been referred to as the detection of a loss of alleles, or allelic deletions, or a loss of heterozygosity in tumours, has been used in localizing the tumour-suppressor gene causing MEN-1. Microsatellite polymorphisms can also be used in a similar way to detect loss of heterozygosity in tumour DNA, and this is illustrated in Fig. 70.4. A loss of alleles involving the whole of chromosome 11 is observed in the parathyroid tumour of a patient with familial MEN-1. This loss of alleles in the tumour results from the loss of chromosomal regions containing the marker loci; the complete absence of alleles suggests that this abnormality has occurred within all the tumour cells studied and indicates a monoclonal origin of the tumour. In addition, combined pedigree and tumour studies have demonstrated that such tumour-related allelic deletions of chromosome 11 occur on the chromosome inherited from the normal parent and not the one from the affected parent [3,7]. Thus, the second mutation involves the normal dominant allele and these studies provided additional evidence for the proposed two-stage recessive mutation model for the development of tumours in MEN-1.

Studies of MEN-1 and non-MEN-1 parathyroid tumours, insulinomas and anterior pituitary tumours have revealed that allelic deletions on chromosome 11 are also involved in the monoclonal development of these tumours. A detailed examination of such tumours has revealed allele loss within tumours involving smaller regions of chromosome 11, and these studies have mapped the MEN-1 locus to the region within chromosome band 11q13 (reviewed in [2]). These results indicate that the MEN-1 gene is telomeric to the PYGM locus, which encodes human muscle glycogen phosphorylase, and centromeric to the locus D11S146. In addition, these studies have demonstrated that allelic deletions of chromosome 11 are involved in the development of sporadic non-MEN-1 parathyroid tumours, gastrinomas, prolactinomas and somatotrophinomas, and thus, the region 11q13 appears to be involved in the development of non-MEN-1 and MEN-1 endocrine tumours [8].

Family linkage studies in MEN-1

In order to localize the gene causing MEN-1, family linkage studies were used as a parallel and complementary approach to the deletion mapping studies. This investigation of the tumour-suppressor gene involved in the MEN-1 syndrome was facilitated by the use of RFLPs

Locus

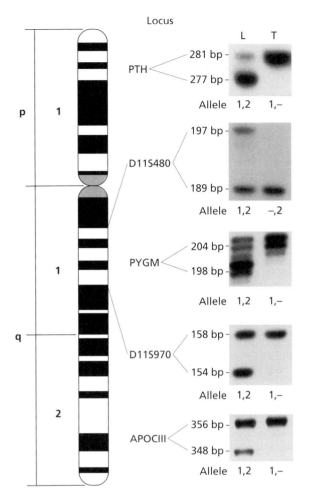

Fig. 70.4 Loss of alleles on chromosome 11 in a parathyroid tumour from a patient with familial MEN-1. The microsatellite polymorphisms obtained from the patient's leucocyte (L) and parathyroid tumour (T) DNA at the PTH, D11S480, PYGM, D11S970 and APOCIII loci are shown. These microsatellite polymorphisms have been identified using specific primers or sequence tagged sites for each of the loci which have been localized to chromosome 11, and are shown juxtaposed to their region of origin on the short (p) and long (q) arms of chromosome 11. The microsatellite polymorphisms are assigned alleles (see Fig. 70.3); for example, D11S480 yielded a 197 bp product (allele 1) and a 189 bp product (allele 2) following PCR amplification of leucocyte DNA, but the tumour cells have lost the 197 bp product (allele 1) and are hemizygous (alleles –,2). Similar losses of alleles are detected using the other DNA markers, and an extensive loss of alleles involving the whole of chromosome 11 is observed in the parathyroid tumour of this patient with MEN-1. In addition, the complete absence of bands suggests that this abnormality has occurred within all the tumour cells studied, and indicates a monoclonal origin for this MEN-1 parathyroid tumour. (From [6] with permission.)

and microsatellite polymorphisms as genetic markers in studies of affected families. These polymorphisms are inherited in a Mendelian manner and their inheritance can be followed together with a disease in an affected family. The consistent inheritance of a polymorphic allele with the disease indicates that the two genetic loci are close together, that is, *linked*. Genes that are far apart do not consistently co-segregate but show recombination because of the crossing-over during meiosis. By studying recombination events in family studies, the distance between two genes and the probability that they are linked can be ascertained [4]. The distance between two genes is expressed as the recombination fraction (θ), which is equal to the number of recombinants divided by the total number of offspring resulting from informative meioses within a family. The value of the recombination fraction (θ) can range from 0 to 0.5. A value of zero indicates that the genes are very closely linked, while a value of 0.5 indicates that the genes are far apart and not linked. The probability that the two loci are linked at these distances is expressed as a LOD score, which is $\log_{10}$ of the odds ratio favouring linkage. The odds ratio favouring linkage is defined as the likelihood that two loci are linked at a specified recombination (θ) versus the likelihood that the two loci are not linked. A LOD score of +3, which indicates a probability in favour of linkage of 1000 to 1, establishes linkage between two loci, and a LOD score of –2, indicating a probability against linkage of 100 to 1, is taken to exclude linkage between two loci. LOD scores are usually evaluated over a range of recombination fractions (θ), thereby enabling the genetic distance and the maximum (or peak) probability favouring linkage between two loci to be ascertained. This is illustrated in Fig. 70.5 for family 16/91 which suffers from MEN-1.

In family 16/91, shown in Fig. 70.5, the disease and INT2 loci are co-segregating in nine out of the ten children, but in one individual (III.6), assuming a 100% penetrance (see below) in early childhood, recombination is observed. Thus, MEN-1 and INT2 are co-segregating in 9/10 of the meioses and not segregating in 1/10 meioses, and the likelihood that the two loci are linked at $\theta = 0.10$ is $(9/10)^9 \times (1/10)^1$. If the disease and the INT2 loci were not linked, then the disease would be associated with allele 1 in one-half (1/2) of the children and with allele 2 in the remaining half (1/2) of the children, and the likelihood that the two loci are not linked is $(1/2)^{10}$. Thus, the odds ratio in favour of linkage between the MEN-1 and INT2 loci at $\theta = 0.10$, in this family, is therefore $(9/10)^9 \times (1/10)^1 \div (1/2)^{10} = 39.67 : 1$, and the LOD score = 1.60 (i.e. $\log_{10} 39.67$). Additional studies from other families have also demonstrated positive LOD scores between MEN-1 and the INT2 locus. LOD scores from individual families can be summed, and the peak LOD score between MEN-1 and the INT2 locus has exceeded +3, thereby establishing linkage between MEN-1 and INT2 loci.

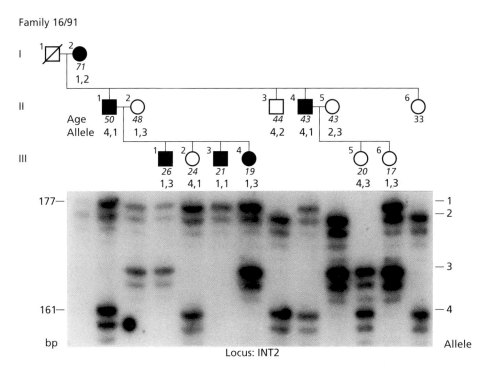

Fig. 70.5 Segregation of INT2 and MEN-1 in family 16/91. Genomic DNA from the family members (upper panel) was used with $\gamma^{32}P$ adenosine triphosphate for PCR amplification of the polymorphic repetitive element $(TG)_n$ at this locus. The PCR amplification products were detected by autoradiography on a polyacrylamide gel (lower panel). PCR products were detected from the DNA of each individual; these ranged in size from 161 to 177 bp. Alleles were designated for each PCR product and are indicated on the right; for example, individuals II.1 and II.4 reveal two pairs of bands on autoradiography. The upper pair of bands is designated allele 1 and the lower pair of bands is designated allele 4; and these two individuals are therefore heterozygous (alleles 1,4). A pair of bands for each allele is frequently observed in the PCR detection of microsatellite repeats. The upper band in the pair is the 'true' allele and the lower band in the pair is its associated 'shadow' which results from slipped-strand mispairing during the PCR. The segregation of these bands and their respective alleles together with the disease can be studied in the family members whose alleles and ages are shown. In some individuals, the inheritance of paternal and maternal alleles can be ascertained; the paternal allele is shown on the left. Individuals are represented as unaffected males (□), affected males (■), unaffected females (○) and affected females (●). The MEN-1 phenotypes in this family were determined by biochemical screening and the age-related penetrance values derived from Fig. 70.6 were used in linkage analysis, as described in the text. Individual II.1 is affected and heterozygous (alleles 4,1) and an examination of his affected children (III.1, III.3 and III.4) and his mother (I.2) and sibling (II.4) reveals inheritance of allele 1 with the disease. The unaffected individuals II.3, II.6, III.2 and III.5 have not inherited this allele 1. However, the daughter (III.6) of individual II.4 has inherited allele 1, but remains unaffected at the age of 17 years; this may either be a representation of age-related penetrance, or a recombination between the disease and INT2 loci. (From [9] with permission.)

This segregation analysis relies on an accurate assignment of the MEN-1 phenotype (i.e. affected or unaffected) and this depends on the methods used to detect MEN-1 and the age of the individual (Fig. 70.6). The age-related onset, which helps in the estimation of the penetrance of MEN-1 and is detailed below in screening studies, was used in the phenotypic assessment of individuals in MEN-1 families, and linkage was established (i.e. LOD score > +3) between MEN-1 and the 11q13 loci, PYGM and INT2 [3,7]. Recombinants between INT2 and MEN-1 have been observed, and this indicates that the oncogene INT2 is not the MEN-1 gene itself. No recombinants between MEN-1 and PYGM have been observed in affected individuals from two large studies of six and 27 [10] families with MEN-1. The genetic map of this region (11q13) has been defined with polymorphic markers to be 11pter-D11S288-D11S149-11cen-PGA-PYGM-D11S97-D11S146-INT2-11qter, and linkage between MEN-1 and 6 of these markers has been established (Table 70.2). In addition, the MEN-1 gene has been located to a region telomeric to PGA and centromeric to D11S97 and in the vicinity of PYGM. The region containing the MEN-1 gene has been identified by genetic and physical mapping studies using pulsed field gel electrophoresis to be approximately 2–3 centiMorgans (cM) in size, which is equivalent to 2–3 Mbp (reviewed in [5]). The genetic markers defining this small region around the MEN-1 locus are proving useful in further

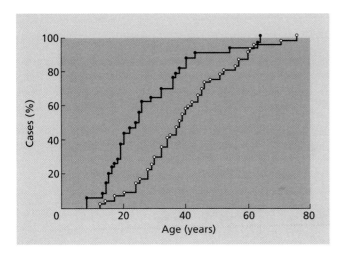

Fig. 70.6 Age-related onset of familial MEN-1. The ages for diagnosis in 87 patients with familial MEN-1 were found to range from 8 to 76 years. The patients were subdivided, depending on the method used to detect MEN-1, into two groups. The symptomatic group (○—) consisted of 53 patients and the age-related onset for MEN-1 in these members at 20, 35 and 50 years of age was 9, 43 and 75%, respectively. In another 34 asymptomatic patients (●—●), MEN-1 had been detected by biochemical screening and the respective age-related onset for MEN-1 in these members increased to 44, 74 and 91%. Thus, biochemical screening detected an earlier onset of MEN-1 in all age groups. (From [5] with permission.)

Table 70.2 LOD scores for linkage of chromosome 11 markers and MEN-1 (from [10] with permission)

Locus	Peak LOD score	Recombination fraction (θ)
D11S149	6.29	0.032
PGA	7.78	0.023
PYGM	13.71	0.047
D11S97	13.76	0.076
D11S146	8.27	0.000
INT2	7.04	0.059

studies of cloning the gene and in identifying individuals within a family who are at risk of developing the disorder.

Family screening in MEN-1

The detection by biochemical screening for the development of MEN-1 tumours in asymptomatic members of families with MEN-1 is of great importance, as earlier diagnosis and treatment of these tumours reduces morbidity and mortality. The attempts to screen for the development of MEN-1 tumours in the asymptomatic relatives of an affected individual have depended largely on measuring the serum concentrations of calcium, gastrointestinal hormones and prolactin (reviewed in [2]). Parathyroid overactivity causing hypercalcaemia is in-

variably the first manifestation of the disorder and this has become a useful and easy screening investigation. Pancreatic involvement in asymptomatic individuals has previously been detected by estimating the fasting plasma concentrations of gastrin and PP. However, one recent study has reported that a stimulatory meal test is a better method for detecting pancreatic disease in individuals who have no demonstrable pancreatic tumours by computerized tomography (CT). An exaggerated increase in serum gastrin and/or PP proved to be a reliable early indicator for the development of pancreatic tumours in these individuals. Some asymptomatic pituitary tumours may be detected by demonstration of hyperprolactinaemia.

Screening in MEN-1 is difficult because the clinical and biochemical manifestations in members of any one family are not uniformly similar and because the age-related penetrance (i.e. the proportion of gene carriers manifesting symptoms or signs of the disease by a given age) has not been established. The proportion of affected individuals who have been detected at a certain age by clinical symptoms or biochemical screening in different series has ranged from 11 to 47% at 20 years of age, 52 to 94% at 35 years and 83 to 100% at 50 years; biochemical screening, which detects asymptomatic patients, increased the proportion of affected individuals at all ages [2]. Thus, the likelihood of wrongly attributing an 'unaffected' status to an individual with no manifestations of the disease at the age of 35 years may be as high as one in two, or approaching one in 20 and depends on whether clinical symptoms alone or biochemical screening methods are used to detect the disease. In order to improve this situation, further biochemical screening and systematic family studies have been undertaken. Results from two studies in which 87 patients with familial MEN-1 were investigated are shown in Fig. 70.6. This reveals that the age-related onset for MEN-1 detected by clinical manifestations (symptomatic group), at 20, 35 and 50 years of age is 9, 43 and 75%, respectively. The respective age-related onset for MEN-1 detected by biochemical screening is markedly improved to 44, 74 and 91%. However, the identification of individuals at risk in an affected family can still be difficult (Fig. 70.7) and the recent availability of DNA markers for MEN-1 has helped to reduce these problems [9].

The use of DNA markers, which may enable carriers of the mutant MEN-1 gene to be detected within a family, may help to identify those individuals who need to undergo repeated screening tests for the development of tumours. This is illustrated in Fig. 70.5 for a family suffering from MEN-1. The alleles of each individual at the INT2 locus which reveals a < 6% recombination rate with MEN-1 (Table 70.2) are shown. Individual I.2 is an

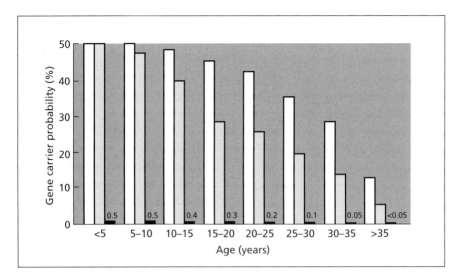

Fig. 70.7 Probabilities for gene carriers of MEN-1. The probabilities for a child of an affected MEN-1 parent being a gene carrier following negative screening results using clinical history (□), biochemical screening (▨), that is, serum calcium, prolactin and gastrointestinal hormone concentrations,and/or DNA marker studies (■) (see Fig. 70.5) are shown for eight age groups. The risk, assessed clinically at birth, of having inherited this autosomal dominant disorder is 50%, and biochemical estimations are not useful in reducing this risk further. In contrast, DNA marker studies using flanking DNA probes can markedly reduce the risk of being a carrier to 0.5%. With increasing age, the clinically assessed risk for the unaffected child of an affected parent declines gradually from 50% to only 28% at the age of 35 years. However, the risk as assessed by biochemical tests declines more rapidly from 50% at birth to 25% by age 25 years, and to 12.5% by age 35 years. These risks can be further decreased by the combined use of flanking DNA markers and the significantly lower 0.5% risk of being a gene carrier at birth is reduced to 0.05% at the age of 35 years. Thus, the use of DNA markers can help considerably in reassuring those individuals who are not gene carriers for MEN-1 and in identifying those individuals who are MEN-1 gene carriers and who therefore require regular screening. (From [2] with permission.)

affected female who is heterozygous (allele 1,2) and is the mother of four children; her affected children, II.1 and II.4, indicate segregation of allele 1 and the disease. Her other children II.3 and II.6, who are 44 and 33 years old, respectively, are biochemically normal and this indicates that they have a low probability (5 and 13%, respectively) of being gene carriers (Fig. 70.7). In addition, the results of genetic marker analysis reveal that II.3 and II.6 have inherited allele 2 which is not associated with the disease in this family, and this indicates a low probability (< 6%) for these being gene carriers. The use of a closer flanking marker, for example PYGM, would help to reduce this probability to < 1% and the combined use of flanking DNA markers and biochemical screening in this age group helps to reduce further the risk for these individuals being carriers to < 0.05%. The two daughters (III.5 and III.6) of the affected male II.4 who is heterozygous (alleles 4,1) are in a younger age group (17–20 years) and have not developed the disease. The finding of normal serum biochemistry in these individuals still indicates a residual 40% risk of their being gene carriers. However, individual III.5 has inherited allele 4 from her affected father II.4, and this indicates a low probability (< 6%) of her being a gene carrier. The combined use of flanking DNA markers and biochemical screening in this individual, who is 20 years old, reduces this risk to 0.3%. In contrast, individual III.6 has inherited allele 1 from her affected father and is at high risk of developing the disease, as the probability of being a gene carrier exceeds 94%. The use of a closer flanking marker such as PYGM (see Table 70.2) would help to confirm and increase this probability to 99.5%. This individual should undergo regular biochemical screening. Thus, the application of DNA markers has helped to determine the carrier risk status of many individuals, and this has substantially altered the screening strategy (see Fig. 70.7) and clinical management of these patients. It is suggested that DNA analysis should now be introduced in the screening programme of MEN-1 families [2].

The advantages of DNA analysis are that it requires a single blood sample and does not need to be repeated, unlike the biochemical screening tests [4]. This is because the analysis is independent of the age of the individual and provides an objective result. The limitations of DNA analysis are that blood samples for DNA analysis must be available from two or more affected family members to conclude which allele of the marker is inherited with the MEN-1 gene. In addition, DNA analysis may be subject to a small but significant error rate because of recombination between the marker and the gene. This error rate can be minimized by the use of flanking DNA markers. The ultimate cloning of the gene itself will help to identify mutations directly and thereby remove this limited uncertainty. At present, an integrated programme of both DNA screening, to identify gene carriers, and biochemical screening, to detect the development of tumours, is recommended [9]. Thus, a DNA test identifying an individual as a mutant gene carrier is likely to lead not to immediate medical or surgical treatment but to earlier and more frequent biochemical screening, whereas a DNA result that leaves an individual with a residual carrier risk of less than 1% will lead to a decision for either infrequent or no screening.

At present it is suggested that individuals at high risk of developing MEN-1 should be screened once per annum. Screening should commence in early childhood, as the disease has developed in some individuals by the age of 5 years, and should continue for life as some individuals have not developed the disease until the eighth decade. Screening history and physical examination should be directed towards eliciting the symptoms and signs of hypercalcaemia, nephrolithiasis, peptic ulcer disease, neuroglycopenia, hypopituitarism, galactorrhoea and amenorrhoea in women, acromegaly, Cushing's disease, visual field loss and the presence of subcutaneous lipomata [2]. Biochemical screening should include serum calcium and prolactin estimations in all individuals, and measurement of gastrointestinal hormones and more specific endocrine function tests should be reserved for individuals who have symptoms or signs suggestive of a clinical syndrome [2]. Thus, the recent advances in molecular biology, which have enabled the localization of the gene causing MEN-1, have helped in the clinical management of patients and their families with this disorder.

Role of other oncogenes in MEN-1-associated tumours

$G_s\alpha$ and GSP mutations

The molecular genetic abnormalities associated with growth hormone-secreting pituitary tumours, which are also referred to as somatotrophinomas, have been investigated and dominantly and recessively acting genes identified. The dominantly acting oncogene involves the $G_s\alpha$ protein, and the recessively acting oncogene involves the MEN-1 locus on chromosome 11q13. The G proteins are a family of guanine nucleotide (guanine triphosphate (GTP))-binding proteins that mediate signal transduction across cell membranes. These proteins couple cell-surface receptors to their second messenger signal-generation systems and thereby regulate the activity of intracellular effector enzymes, for example adenylate cyclase and ion channels. The G proteins share a heterotrimeric structure composed of α, β and γ subunits. The β and γ subunits are tightly associated with each other as a $\beta\gamma$ complex and appear to be functionally interchangeable among some of the G proteins. The α subunits are the most diverse and are unique to each G protein. The α subunit which contains the guanine nucleotide-binding site and has intrinsic GTPase activity is thought to confer specificity on each G protein, and thereby allow it to discriminate among multiple receptors and effectors; for example, the hormone-sensitive adenylate cyclase system is regulated by at least two G proteins, one of which stimulates ($G_s\alpha$) and another which inhibits ($G_i\alpha$), the activity of the membrane-bound enzyme that catalyses the formation of the intracellular second messenger cyclic adenosine monophosphate (cAMP). The role of these G proteins in the development of growth hormone (GH)-secreting tumours has been studied [11–13]. Growth hormone-releasing hormone (GHRH) acts via cAMP to stimulate GH secretion and proliferation of somatotrophs, and a subset of somatotrophinomas is associated with an elevation in basal adenylyl cyclase activity which is unresponsive to further stimulation by GHRH and GTP analogues. This alteration in the hormone-sensitive adenylyl cyclase system has been further investigated and a constitutive activation of $G_s\alpha$, which was associated with an inhibition of GTPase activity, was demonstrated in these somatotrophinomas. An analysis of the gene encoding $G_s\alpha$, which is located on chromosome 20, has revealed four mutations at two codons in 40% of somatotrophinomas. These tumour-specific missense mutations of $G_s\alpha$ occurred either in codon 201, which is in exon 8, or in codon 227, which is in exon 9 and were detected by the method of allele-specific oligonucleotide (ASO) hybridization as illustrated in Figs 70.8 and 70.9. At codon 201 the mutation led to a replacement of arginine (R), wild type codon CGT, with either cysteine (C) mutant codon TGT, or histidine (H) mutant codon CAT, and at codon 227 the mutation led to a replacement of glutamine (Q) wild-type codon CAG with either arginine (R) mutant codon CGG, or with leucine (L) mutant codon CTG [11–13]. The mutation in the G_s protein α-chain, which is referred to as a *gsp* mutation, occurred in only one copy of the gene and thus appeared to act as a dominant oncogene.

Some of these somatotrophinomas from one study [13] have also been investigated for inactivation of the MEN-1 tumour-suppressor gene located on chromosome 11q13.

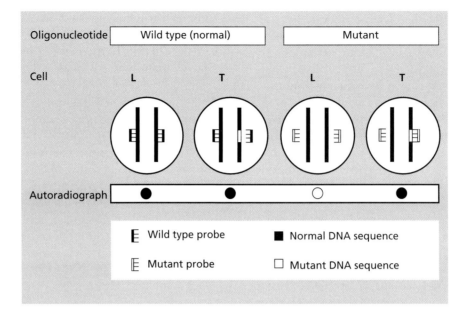

Fig. 70.8 Schematic representation of the use of allele-specific oligonucleotide hybridization to detect mutations of $G_s\alpha$ at codons 201 and 227. Leucocyte (L) and tumour (T) DNA (250 ng) from a patient were utilized for PCR amplification of the genomic segment containing exons 8 and 9 of the $G_s\alpha$ gene and dot blotted onto nylon filters [13]. The filters were then hybridized with radiolabelled oligonucleotide probes which were 20 bases in length and which differed by only one base pair and thereby contained either the wild-type (normal) sequences of arginine or glutamine or the mutant sequences. The resulting signals were visualized by autoradiography. Thus, the wild-type probe would yield a hybridization signal from the leucocyte DNA and tumour DNA as these would contain two copies and one copy respectively of the complementary normal DNA sequence. In contrast, the mutant probe would not yield a hybridization signal from leucocyte DNA as this does not contain a complementary sequence. However, the mutant probe would yield a hybridization signal from tumour DNA which contained a complementary mutant sequence. Thus, the absence of mutant sequences in the leucocyte DNA and the presence of wild-type and mutant sequences in the tumour would be revealed (see Fig. 70.9) and thereby indicate the dominant nature of the mutation (From [8] with permission.)

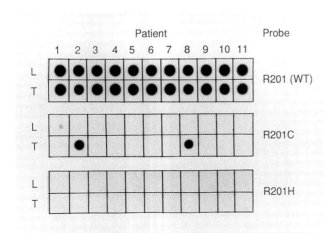

Fig. 70.9 Analysis of *gsp* mutations in the somatotrophinomas from 11 patients. The results obtained by utilizing the allele-specific oligonucleotide probes R201 (WT), R201C and R201H and the patients' leucocyte (L) and tumour (T) DNA are shown, and an analysis revealed the presence of the R201C mutation in the tumour DNA from patients 2 and 8. (From [13] with permission.)

One somatotrophinoma was also associated with allelic deletions on chromosome 11 and these combined results may help to elucidate further the roles of these two mutations. A genetic model for the development of somatotrophinomas involving the following possibilities has been proposed [13]:

1 tumorigenesis may be associated with either an allelic deletion on chromosone 11 or a mutation of $G_s\alpha$;

2 an early mutation of $G_s\alpha$ may initiate a clonal proliferation during which a mitotic disjunction involving an allele loss of chromosome 11 occurs;

3 an allelic deletion of chromosome 11 precedes a $G_s\alpha$ mutation, which would then convert a small adenoma to a larger proliferative one by enhancing clonal expansion of the cell with the allelic deletion;

4 the order in which these mutations occur may not be invariant, and the accumulation of these genetic abnormalities may be more important in the development and progression of the tumour.

Further detailed analysis of these proposed models for the development of somatotrophinomas, which are similar to those reported for colorectal tumours, will help to elucidate the roles of the dominant and recessive onco-genes associated with these growth hormone-secreting pituitary tumours.

PRADI

The molecular basis of non-MEN-1 parathyroid tumours has been investigated and a structural defect within the parathyroid hormone (PTH) gene itself identified. The human PTH gene has been localized to the short arm of chromosome 11 by using rodent–human hybrid cell lines and its nucleotide sequence determined. Further analysis of the organization of the pre-pro-PTH gene revealed that it consists of three exons and two intervening sequences (introns). The first exon, at the 5′ end, encodes an un-translated regulatory domain, the second exon encodes the signal peptide and part of the 'prohormone' sequence, and the third exon encodes the remainder of the 'pro-hormone' sequence, together with the PTH peptide and the 3′ untranslated region (reviewed in [4]). Structural abnormalities within the organization of the PTH gene have been identified in two non-MEN-1 parathyroid adenomas. These abnormalities involved a separation of the first exon from the fragment containing the second and third exons, together with a rearrangement in which the PTH regulatory elements became juxtaposed with 'new' non-PTH DNA, which was referred to as D11S287. Investigation of D11S287 localized it to the long arm of chromosome 11, band 11q13, a region which contains the MEN-1 gene. Detailed analysis revealed that D11S287 contained a sequence that was highly conserved in differ-ent species and that was expressed in normal parathyroids and in parathyroid adenomas. This expressed sequence from D11S287 was designated PRADI and further map-ping studies revealed that the PRADI gene was not the MEN-1 gene. However, the combination of the clonal rearrangement of one copy of the PRADI gene and the altered gene expression indicated that PRADI is a domi-nant oncogene whose activation is associated with the development of parathyroid tumours. Similar activation of cellular oncogenes through analogous rearrangements (reviewed in [4]) has been implicated in the pathogenesis of several tumours, for example Burkitt's lymphoma and chronic myeloid leukaemia. The PRADI cDNA was isolated from a human placental cDNA library, and an analysis revealed that this cDNA encoded a protein of 295 amino acids which had similarities to the cyclin family of proteins [14].

Cyclins were first identified in the dividing cells of clams and sea urchins, in which they were associated with a cell cycle-regulated proteolysis in the immediate period preceding the onset of anaphase. Cyclins have also been

identified in humans, in whom they also have an im-portant role in regulating progress through the cell cycle (reviewed in [6]). Thus, PRADI, which appears to encode a novel cyclin, referred to as cyclin D1 (CCND-1) may also be a regulator of the cell cycle, and an overexpression of PRADI may be an important event in the develop-ment of parathyroid tumours. In addition, studies of lymphomas have revealed that PRADI is likely to be the B-cell lymphoma type 1 (BCL-1) oncogene and to be involved in breast carcinomas and squamous cell carcinomas of the head and neck (reviewed in [8]). A further characterization of the role of the PRADI gene in regulating the cell cycle and in mitosis will help to elucidate the aetiology of these and parathyroid tumours.

Retinoblastoma gene

The proliferation of parathyroid cells in the aetiology of tumours is likely to involve regulators of the cell cycle, for example, PRADI [14]. Another such gene regula-ting the cell cycle is the retinoblastoma (RB) tumour-suppressor gene, whose protein product normally inhibits cell growth by a possible interaction with cyclin D1, which itself is a product of the PRADI gene. An analysis of the RB gene in parathyroid carcinomas, by examining for allelic deletions in these tumours, revealed that inactivation of the RB gene was common in parathyroid carcinomas [15] and that this was likely to be an im-portant component in the progression to these malignant tumours.

Conclusion

Molecular genetic studies have localized the gene causing MEN-1 to a 2–3 cM region within 11q13 and have revealed the MEN-1 gene to be a tumour-suppressor gene. The establishment of genetic markers flanking the disease locus has helped in further studies aimed at cloning this gene, and also in identifying those family members who are at a high risk of developing the disease. In the future, a greater understanding of the pathogenesis of endocrine tumours will result from the cloning and characterization of the gene causing MEN-1.

Acknowledgements

I am grateful to the Medical Research Council for support, to the clinical and scientific colleagues who have provided valuable resources for these studies, to Ms Carol Wooding and Ms Joanna Pang and Dr Mark Pook for help in preparation of some of the figures, and to Ms Lesley Sargeant for typing the manuscript.

References

1. Wermer P. Genetic aspects of adenomatosis of endocrine glands. *Am. J. Med.* 1954;**16**:363–71.

2. Thakker RV. Multiple endocrine neoplasia type 1 (MEN1). In DeGroot LJ, Besser GM, Burger HG, Jameson JL, Loriaux DL, Marshall JC, Odell WD, Potts JT, Rubinstein AH (eds). *Endocrinology.* Philadelphia: W.B. Saunders, 1995:2815–31.

3. Thakker RV, Bouloux P, Wooding C *et al.* Association of parathyroid tumors in multiple endocrine neoplasia type 1 with loss of alleles on chromosome 11. *N. Engl. J. Med.* 1989;**321**:218–24.

4. Thakker RV, Ponder BAJ. Multiple endocrine neoplasia. In Sheppard MC (ed.). *Clinical Endocrinology and Metabolism. Vol. 2, No. 4. Molecular Biology and Endocrinology.* London: Baillière Tindall, 1988:1031–67.

5. Thakker RV. The molecular genetics of the multiple endocrine neoplasia syndromes. *Clin. Endocrinol.* 1993;**38**:1–14.

6. Pang JT, Thakker RV. Multiple endocrine neoplasia type 1. *Eur. J. Cancer* 1994;**30A**:1961–8.

7. Larsson C, Skogseid B, Oberg K, Nakamura Y, Nordenskjold MC. Multiple endocrine neoplasia type I gene maps to chromosome 11 and is lost in insulinoma. *Nature* 1988;**332**:85–7.

8. Thakker RV. Endocrine tumours. In Kurzrock R, Talpaz M (eds). *Molecular Biology in Cancer Medicine.* London: Martin Dunitz, 1995:359–83.

9. Thakker RV. Molecular mechanisms of tumor formation in hereditary and sporadic tumors of the MEN1 type: the impact of genetic screening in the management of MEN1. *Endocrinol. Metab. Clin. North Am.* 1994;**23**:117–35.

10. Thakker RV, Wooding C, Pang J, Farren B and the MEN1 Collaborative Group. Linkage analysis of 7 polymorphic markers at chromosome 11p11.2-11q13 in 27 multiple endocrine neoplasia type 1 families. *Ann. Hum. Genet.* 1993;**57**:17–25.

11. Landis CA, Masters SB, Spada A *et al.* GTPase inhibiting mutations activate the chain of Gs and stimulate adenyl cyclase in human pituitary tumours. *Nature* 1989;**340**:692–6.

12. Lyons J, Landis CA, Harsh G *et al.* Two G protein oncogenes in human endocrine tumors. *Science* 1990;**249**:655–9.

13. Thakker RV, Pook MA, Wooding C *et al.* Association of somatotrophinomas with loss of alleles on chromosome 11 and with *gsp* mutations. *J. Clin. Invest.* 1993;**91**:2815–21.

14. Motokura T, Bloom T, Kim HG *et al.* A novel cyclin encoded by a *bcl1*-linked candidate oncogene. *Nature* 1991;**350**:512–15.

15. Cryns VL, Thor A, Xu H-J *et al.* Loss of the retinoblastoma tumor-suppressor gene in parathyroid carcinoma. *N. Engl. J. Med.* 1994;**330**:757–61.

Multiple Endocrine Neoplasia Type 2 and Medullary Thyroid Carcinoma

FRIEDHELM RAUE

Classification and incidence

Medullary thyroid carcinoma (MTC) is a rare calcitonin-secreting tumour of the parafollicular or C cells of the thyroid. It accounts for 8–12% of all thyroid carcinomas and occurs in both sporadic and hereditary forms [1]. The familial variety of MTC is inherited as an autosomal dominant trait with a high degree of penetrance and is associated with multiple endocrine neoplasia (MEN) type 2 syndrome. Three hereditary varieties of MTC are known:

1 the MEN-2a syndrome, characterized by MTC in combination with phaeochromocytoma and tumours of the parathyroids;

2 the MEN-2b syndrome, consisting of MTC, phaeochromocytoma, ganglioneuromatosis, and Marfanoid habitus;

3 familial MTC (FMTC), without any other endocrinopathies (Table 71.1) [2]. Many patients with MEN-2b do not have a family history of the disease. Their tumours and characteristic appearance are therefore due to new mutations, which present as sporadic cases of potentially hereditable disease. About 30% of the MEN-2a gene carriers never manifest clinically significant disease.

These four varieties of MTC, three heritable and one sporadic, are clinically distinct with respect to incidence, genetics, age of onset, associations with other diseases, histopathology of the tumour, and prognosis. The majority of patients have sporadic MTC (75%), while 25% suffer from hereditary MTC, mostly MEN-2a (17%), followed by FMTC (5%), and MEN-2b (3%) [3]. A family history is often inadequate in establishing familial disease and more thorough evaluation by biochemical and genetic screening often reveals a family history of MTC in a patient originally thought to have the sporadic form of the disease.

The sex ratio in sporadic MTC is 1 : 1.4 (male : female), while both sexes are nearly equally affected in the familial variety. The highest incidence of sporadic disease occurs in the fifth decade of life, while hereditary disease can be diagnosed earlier, depending on the possibility of genetic and biochemical screening.

Pathology and biochemical markers

The histological appearance of MTC is enormously variable with regard to cytoarchitecture (solid, trabecular or insular) and cell shape (spindle, polyhedral, angular or round) [4]. MTC is most commonly confused with anaplastic carcinoma, Hürthle cell tumours, or papillary thyroid carcinoma. Characteristic is the presence of stromal amyloid in about 50–80% of MTC patients. This feature had been an auxiliary diagnostic criterion for MTC before the use of calcitonin immunocytochemistry. Hereditary MTC characteristically presents as a multifocal process, mostly in the superior portions of both lobes of the gland and with C-cell hyperplasia in areas distinct from the primary tumour. Bilateral C-cell hyperplasia is a precursor lesion to hereditary MTC. The earliest reported finding of C-cell hyperplasia in MEN-2a is at 20 months of age, and children with MEN-2b may have this lesion at birth. The time frame of the progression from C-cell hyperplasia to microscopic carcinoma remains unclear but may take years. Metastasis may be found in central and lateral, cervical and mediastinal lymph nodes of the neck or more distantly in the lung, liver and bone.

The primary secretory product of MTC is calcitonin, a peptide hormone consisting of 32 amino acids and with a molecular mass of 3400. Calcitonin serves as a tumour marker, and measurement of monomeric calcitonin remains the definitive test for prospective diagnosis of MTC. The test is widely available, accurate, reproducible, and cost-effective. Either basal or stimulated plasma calcitonin levels are elevated in virtually all patients with MTC. Similarly, elevated plasma calcitonin levels following surgery to remove the tumour are indicative of persistent

Table 71.1 Classification of medullary thyroid carcinoma (MTC)

Variety of MTC	Incidence (%)	Age at onset	Sex ratio (M : F)	Associated endocrinopathies
Sporadic MTC	75	5th decade	1 : 1.4	None
Hereditary MTC	25		1 : 1.0	
FMTC	5	4th decade		None
MEN-2a	17	3rd decade		Phaeochromocytoma
				Parathyroid hyperplasia/adenoma
MEN-2b	3	1st decade		Phaeochromocytoma
				Marfanoid habitus, mucosal neuromas

FMTC, familial MTC; MEN, multiple endocrine neoplasia.

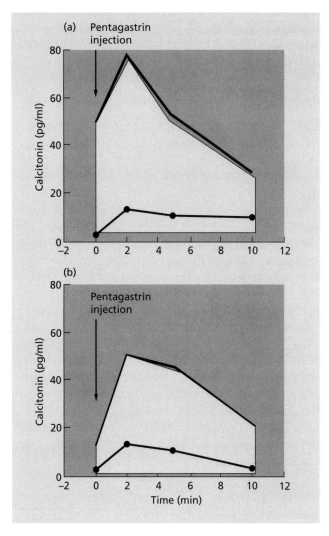

Fig. 71.1 Pentagastrin stimulation in normals: (a) men (*n* = 17); (b) women (*n* = 12). The 95th percentile (light grey) and the median (●—●) are given. Data were evaluated with a commercial two-site immunoassay for calcitonin (Medgenix).

or recurrent disease. Therefore the preferred biochemical screening method for MTC in hereditary varieties of the disease is provocative stimulation of calcitonin release using pentagastrin; abnormal elevations of calcitonin are a reliable predictor of C-cell hyperplasia. The test is administered by giving 0.5 μg pentagastrin/kg body weight as an intravenous bolus over 5–10 seconds. Calcitonin measurements are made at 2 and 5 minutes (Fig. 71.1). In order to interpret the calcitonin values obtained from this test, it is necessary to define the precise upper limit for stimulated calcitonin concentrations. Basal plasma calcitonin can also be elevated during normal childhood and pregnancy, in small-cell lung cancers (SCLCs), breast cancers, hepatomas, pancreatic tumours, gastrinomas, pernicious anaemia, thyroiditis and chronic renal failure.

Table 71.2 Bioactive substances produced by medullary thyroid carcinomas

Peptides derived from the calcitonin gene
Calcitonin
Katacalcin (PDN-21, C-pro-calcitonin)
PAS-57 (N-pro-calcitonin)
Calcitonin gene-related peptide (CGRP)

Neuroendocrine markers
Chromogranin A (CgA)
Neurone-specific enolase (NSE)
DOPA-decarboxylase

Peptide hormones and releasing factors
Somatostatin
Gastrin-releasing peptide
Adrenocorticotrophic hormone (ACTH)
β-endorphin
β-melanocyte-stimulating hormones
Substance P
Neurotensin
Serotonin

Others
Carcino-embryonic antigen (CEA)

Patients with these conditions, however, usually have blunted or absent stimulatory responses to calcitonin secretagogues. Provocative calcitonin stimulation tests thus help to sort out these false-negative and false-positive conditions. Commonly experienced side-effects following pentagastrin administration include nausea, flushing and substernal tightness. These symptoms are transient and usually resolve within 2–3 minutes.

There are a number of other substances, including carcino-embryonic antigen (CEA), that are produced by MTC and which may help to differentiate it from other tumours (Table 71.2) [5]. Most of these substances, however, are probably of no clinical significance, except for the occasional patient who has developed Cushing's syndrome due to production of excessive quantities of adrenocorticotrophic hormone (ACTH).

Clinical syndromes

Sporadic medullary thyroid carcinoma

The most common clinical presentation of sporadic MTC is a single nodule or thyroid mass found incidentally during routine examination. The presentation does not differ from that observed in papillary or follicular thyroid carcinoma. Metastases to cervical and mediastinal lymph nodes are found in one-half of the patients at the time of initial presentation. Distant metastases to lung, liver and bone occur late in the course of the disease. A thyroid nodule identified by physical examination is generally evaluated by ultrasonography and radioisotopic scanning. An ultrasound examination of a palpable MTC shows hypo-echogenic regions, sometimes with calcifications, and a thyroid scan almost always shows no trapping of radioactive iodine or technetium ('cold nodule') (Fig. 71.2). Cytologic examinations of the cold, hypo-echogenic nodule will lead to a strong suspicion, or a correct diagnosis in most cases of sporadic MTC. A plasma calcitonin measurement can clarify the diagnosis, since, in the presence of a palpable MTC, the plasma calcitonin concentration will usually be greater than 1000 pg/ml (normal range below 50 pg/ml) and the CEA level will be clearly elevated. Although calcitonin is produced in large quantities by MTC and has profound biological effects when given acutely (hypocalcaemia and inhibition of bone resorption), there appears to be no biological effects following chronic exposure of the usual target organs, bone and kidney. Diarrhoea is the most prominent of the hormone-mediated clinical features of MTC. Severe diarrhoea is relatively common (30%) in patients with widespread tumours and can be effectively controlled with tinctura of opium, codeine or loperamide.

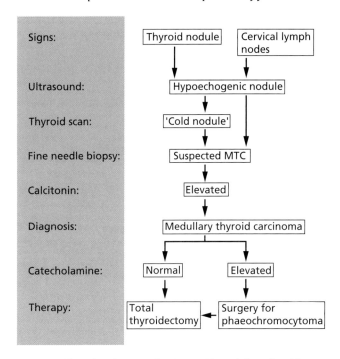

Fig. 71.2 Clinical evaluation of patients with medullary thyroid carcinoma (MTC).

Multiple endocrine neoplasia type 2

Only 70% of all genetically determined MEN-2a patients develop clinically apparent MTC by the age of 70 years. The clinical presentation of familial MTC in index cases does not appear to differ from that in patients with sporadic MTC. MTC is often the initial manifestation of the MEN-2 syndrome, as the other manifestations, phaeochromocytoma and hyperparathyroidism, develop later in the disease. The diagnosis of familial MTC is often made postoperatively when pathohistological examination may show multifocal bilateral MTC accompanied by diffuse or nodular C-cell hyperplasia. MTC/C-cell hyperplasia in other family members is detected at early ages by genetic and biochemical screening and the clinical presentation is silent. C-cell hyperplasia is the first abnormality observed in the thyroid gland of MEN-2 patients, but it is not specific for MEN-2. Nodular C-cell hyperplasia can be detected occasionally adjacent to benign or malignant follicular cell tumours of the thyroid and in Hashimoto's thyroiditis. This C-cell hyperplasia can cause a false-positive pentagastrin test. A positive pentagastrin test in conjunction with an identification of a missense mutation on *ret* proto-oncogene (see below) are sufficient evidence to make the diagnosis of hereditary C-cell hyperplasia or microcarcinoma of the C-cells.

In some MEN-2a families, a skin disorder known as cutaneous lichen amyloidosis is observed. It is characterized by bilateral or unilateral pruritic and lichenoid

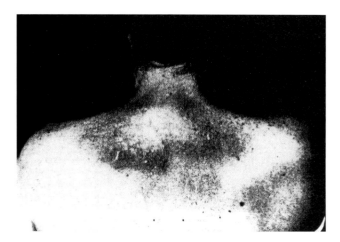

Fig. 71.3 The characteristic clinical picture of cutaneous lichen amyloidosis associated with MEN-2a. The pruritic skin lesions may cover a small area of the entire, right or left upper back, as shown in this patient (from [2] with permission).

skin lesions located over the upper portion of the back and often appears before development of MTC (Fig. 71.3). Skin biopsy specimens show deposition of amyloid at the dermal–epidermal junction. In most patients, the diagnosis of cutaneous lichen amyloidosis precedes diagnosis of MEN-2a, thereby serving as a phenotypic marker of MEN-2a [6].

Phaeochromocytoma

Phaeochromocytoma is usually found later than MTC in MEN-2a, and only 20–50% of the affected individuals develop a unilateral or bilateral adrenal tumour. As with MTC, the phaeochromocytomas of MEN-2 are also multicentric (diffuse adrenomedullary hyperplasia). Approximately half of the phaeochromocytomas are bilateral; malignant phaeochromocytoma is rare, with an incidence between 0 and 8%. In index cases, the clinical manifestation of phaeochromocytoma associated with MEN-2a is similar to that in sporadic phaeochromocytoma with signs and symptoms such as palpitations, nervousness and hypertension. However, phaeochromocytomas are usually identified early as a result of regular biochemical screening in genetically disease-prone family members and clinical manifestations are thus subtle or absent. The presence of phaeochromocytoma must be ruled out prior to any surgical procedure.

Hyperparathyroidism

Primary hyperparathyroidism, with hypercalcaemia and an elevated serum parathyroid hormone (PTH) level,

occurs in 10–25% of individuals with the mature form of MEN-2a. MTC postpones the occurrence of primary hyperparathyroidism in most cases. In patients with primary hyperparathyroidism in MEN-2 the mild clinical characteristics often do not differ from those in patients with sporadic primary hyperparathyroidism. The usual pathological findings are those of chief cell hyperplasia involving multiple glands. MEN-2 patients detected early by screening often manifest little clinical evidence of hyperparathyroidism, although hyperplasia of parathyroid glandular tissue may be observed during the removal of one or two parathyroid glands from patients undergoing thyroidectomy for the C-cell disease.

Multiple endocrine neoplasia type 2b

MEN-2b is clinically characterized by the presence of mucosal neuromas located on the distal tongue and subconjunctival areas, thickened lips, a Marfanoid habitus (long, thin extremities, an altered upper–lower body ratio, slipped femoral epiphysis, pectus excavatum) and mucosal neuromas throughout the gastrointestinal tract [7]. The mucosal neuromas are a pathognomonic clinical feature present during childhood which make it possible to diagnose MTC (see Plate 71.1, between pp. 272 and 273). Other features of this syndrome occurring in childhood include gastrointestinal colic or obstruction and abnormal cramping or diarrhoea. In general, MEN-2b is a more aggressive form of the syndrome, with an earlier clinical presentation of MTC. Phaeochromocytoma occurs as often as in MEN-2a, but hyperparathyroidism is rare in MEN-2b.

Diagnostic procedure

MEN-2 gene and genetic testing

The MEN-2 gene was localized to a small region of the long arm of chromosome 10, near the centromere (10q 11.2). This region included the proto-oncogene *ret*, a transmembrane receptor containing an intracellular tyrosine kinase domain (Fig. 71.4) [8]. The ligand for this receptor is unknown. Recently, in MEN-2a and FMTC kindreds, mutations have been identified at the *ret* locus within regions coding for the proposed cysteine-rich extracellular domain of the protein. Mutations involving four cysteine residues in exon 10 and one cysteine residue in exon 11, codon 634 are found in the germline. In MEN-2b there is a different germline mutation which is the same in almost every case: a substitution of the methionine by threonine at codon 918 in the heart of the catalytic region of the tyrosine kinase domain of the protein [9].

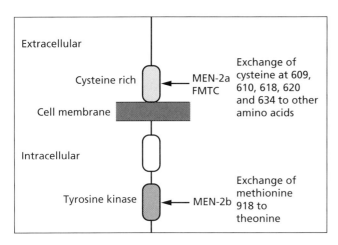

Fig. 71.4 Mutations in the ret protein in multiple endocrine neoplasia (MEN) type 2a, type 2b and familial medullary thyroid carcinoma (FMTC).

How the mutation affects the function of the ret protein and how this is linked to tumorigenesis have not yet been answered. It might be that the mutations result in abnormal activation of the *ret* tyrosine kinase, leading to uncontrolled proliferation of the various endocrine tissues. Consistent with this, the other allele of the *ret* gene is normal and is not lost by the tumour. In addition, the typical MEN-2b mutation is found in about 30% of truly sporadic cases of MTC as a somatic mutation rather than in the germline, further suggesting that it is involved in tumour formation.

Using DNA testing, it is now possible in the great majority of families to predict which individuals have inherited the MEN-2 gene. Those who are negative can be reassured and require no further biochemical screening. Those who are positive should undergo regular biochemical screening. A definitive diagnosis based on demonstration of a specific gene mutation should be made as early as possible, at the age of 3 years. This allows the concentration of biochemical screening on those who need it and will reduce the possibility of false-positive interpretations of biochemical tests, for example, a false-positive pentagastrin test in C-cell hyperplasia associated with, for instance, Hashimoto's thyroiditis. Testing for a mutation may also be helpful in apparently sporadic cases of MTC, since, if a mutation is found, it will imply that the disease is hereditary and that the family should be screened. The failure to find a mutation does not, however, rule out familial MTC, because not all MEN-2 mutations have been identified yet [10].

Biochemical testing

Biochemical screening for C-cell hyperplasia and for early

phaeochromocytoma is effective in preventing morbidity and mortality in individuals who have inherited the MEN-2 gene [11]. The clinical situation most affected by genetic testing is the management of MTC. More than 90% of MEN-2a gene carriers will develop C-cell abnormalities by the age of 31 years and C-cell abnormalities have been demonstrated at very young ages using the biochemical screening programme.

Exactly when early thyroidectomy should be performed remains unclear, as the data for a risk/benefit analysis are not yet available [12]. In a child with a MEN-2 gene mutation and a negative pentagastrin test, total thyroidectomy can be postponed until the results of the calcitonin stimulation test become positive or until the age of 5–6 years when local metastases have been observed in some cases. Guidelines pertaining to screening for the other components of the MEN syndrome, for example phaeochromocytoma and hyperparathyroidism, remain unchanged, except that it is now recommended that only affected family members be tested.

Annual biochemical screening for phaeochromocytoma should be performed, beginning at the age of 6 years, by urine and plasma catecholamine determination. Once the diagnosis of phaeochromocytoma is made by laboratory testing, the tumour should be localized by imaging techniques, that is, sonography, computerized tomography (CT) or magnetic resonance imaging (MRI). [131]Metaiodobenzylguanidine (MIBG) scintigraphy provides a non-invasive and specific technique for localization of a catecholamine-producing tumour. In most MEN-2 families parathyroid disease is an uncommon manifestation. Periodic measurements of serum calcium concentration is probably adequate for screening purposes.

Management

Surgery

The definitive treatment for MTC is surgery. Several studies have shown that survival in patients with MTC is dependent upon the adequacy of the initial surgical procedure. The appropriate surgery for MTC is total thyroidectomy and careful lymph node dissection of the central compartment of the neck. The latter is necessary for tumour staging and prevention of later midline complications related to local metastatic disease. If there is no evidence of local lymph node metastases during the primary surgical procedure, a surgical cure is likely and further neck dissection is probably unnecessary. Total thyroidectomy is absolutely necessary in hereditary cases because of the bilateral and multifocal nature of MTC. If the initial surgical procedure was inadequate then reoperation with an appropriate surgical procedure is indicated. In contrast, unilateral lobectomy is sufficient in a patient with sporadic MTC showing a single, unilateral tumour focus and normal postoperative plasma calcitonin levels after provocative testing. All patients should receive adequate L-thyroxine replacement therapy after total thyroidectomy.

Perhaps the most difficult problem associated with management of MTC is what to do with the patient who has persistently elevated serum calcitonin levels after an adequate surgical procedure. In almost all cases, persistent elevation of serum calcitonin implies the presence of tumour. A thorough evaluation should be undertaken to define the extent of local and distant metastatic disease. Localization of metastases can be done by ultrasound of the neck and abdomen, CT of the neck, mediastinum, lung and liver or MRI technique. Selective venous catheterization with blood sampling for calcitonin determination is helpful in detecting liver metastases at a very early stage and in identifying a particular region of the neck or mediastinum that the surgeon should focus upon. Octreotide scanning may also be helpful, especially in identifying lung metastases at a very early stage of MTC. At the conclusion of these diagnostic procedures, a decision regarding reoperation must be made. If the primary operation was inadequate, if there is no evidence of distant metastases and if local disease is found in the neck and/or mediastinum, reoperation is advocated. A successful cure, even long after primary thyroidectomy, is possible by meticulous lymph node dissection of all compartments of the neck and mediastinum, with the complete removal of the lymphatic and fatty tissue between important anatomical structures [13]. This surgical technique has produced a cure rate of 25% in such patients.

Surgery for phaeochromocytoma in MEN-2 should precede surgery for MTC. Prophylactic removal of the contralateral adrenal gland is not indicated unless there is evidence of excess catecholamine secretion or a visible radiological abnormality on CT. Approximately one-third of patients who undergo a unilateral adrenalectomy will eventually require a second operation for a contralateral phaeochromocytoma, but this may not occur for many years, during which time the patient will not be steroid dependent. Patients with bilateral phaeochromocytomas should be treated with total bilateral adrenalectomy.

The parathyroid glands in MEN-2 patients are frequently found to be enlarged at thyroidectomy for MTC and should therefore be carefully evaluated. The goal in MEN-2 patients with primary hyperparathyroidism is to excise the enlarged glands and to leave at least one normal

parathyroid gland intact. If they are all enlarged, a subtotal parathyroidectomy should be performed.

Postsurgical follow-up and management

All patients with MTC should undergo calcitonin determination at regular intervals after total thyroidectomy (Fig. 71.5). Normal basal and pentagastrin-stimulated calcitonin levels suggest a tumour-free state and thus patients require no further treatment. They can be followed-up at half yearly intervals with physical examination and calcitonin determination; every 2 or 3 years a pentagastrin-stimulation test must be done.

Patients with persistent elevation of serum calcitonin after total thyroidectomy should be thoroughly evaluated to define the extent of local and distant disease (see above). If there is no evidence of distant metastases and if local disease is found in the neck, reoperation is advocated using meticulous dissection and microsurgical techniques.

In patients remaining calcitonin-positive with evidence of non-curable and non-operable disease (distant metastases) or occult disease (no local recurrence is found), close observation of the changes in serum calcitonin concentration is required. Many patients may exhibit a remarkably stable course and no further treatment is recommended; a 'wait and see' approach is advocated,

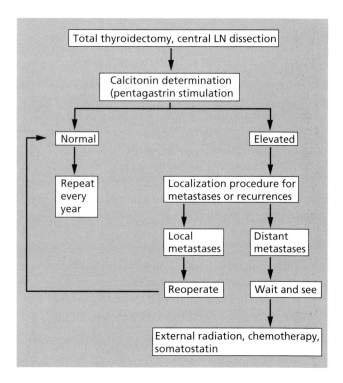

Fig. 71.5 Recommended postoperative management of patients with medullary thyroid carcinoma. LN, lymph node.

as experience with non-surgical therapy in the management of metastatic MTC has been disappointing. In those patients whose disease shows rapid and steady progress, intervention with chemotherapy, radiotherapy, or somatostatin can be considered as a palliative therapeutic modality [14]. Since the C cells and MTC do not concentrate iodine or generally respond to thyroid hormone, therefore, the administration of ^{131}I is not recommended postoperatively nor in the treatment of metastatic MTC.

The role of regional external radiotherapy in the treatment of MTC continues to be controversial. In patients with inoperable tumour, radiotherapy can offer prolonged palliation and achieve local tumour control. Radiotherapy may be helpful for patients with expanding final-stage lesions or for painful osseous metastases, but the response is poor.

As MTC is relatively insensitive to chemotherapy and the results are correspondingly poor, chemotherapy cannot be recommended for patients with asymptomatic disease which persists after surgery as tumour mass and plasma calcitonin and CEA levels may remain stable for years. Such treatment might be indicated when the tumour mass seems to have escaped local control and entered a more aggressive growth phase. Monotherapy with Adriamycin (60 mg/m^2 every 3 weeks) or a combination of Adriamycin and cisplatin has been used in some trials but with a response rate below 30%. Life quality, toxic side-effects and survival have to be taken into account when chemotherapy is recommended. Therefore chemotherapy in advanced MTC must be individualized based on clinical grounds. The stable analogue of somatostatin, octreotide, has been used in a limited number of patients with advanced metastatic MTC. A transient reduction of calcitonin and CEA levels and a transient improvement of symptomatic diarrhoea and flushing in some patients, but no real effect on tumour mass, have been reported but not yet confirmed [14].

Prognostic factors

The natural history of sporadic MTC is variable. The spectrum ranges from years of dormant residual disease after surgery to rapidly progressive disseminated disease and death related to either metastatic thyroid tumour or complications of phaeochromocytoma in MEN-2. The 10-year survival rates for all MTC patients range from approximately 61 to 67%. The overall prognosis is intermediate between that of differentiated papillary and follicular carcinoma and the more aggressive anaplastic thyroid cancer. There is general agreement that surgical management has a favourable influence on the clinical course of the disease. Early detection and treatment of

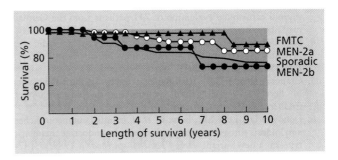

Fig. 71.6 Survival curves of patients with medullary thyroid carcinoma (MTC) comparing different varieties of MTC from the German MTC Register (1994; *n* = 1048). FMTC, familial MTC; MEN, multiple endocrine neoplasia.

MTC is likely to be curative, more than 95% of patients detected at an early stage of disease remain disease-free (normal or undetectable calcitonin values). The main factors that influence survival are the stage of disease at the time of diagnosis (size of the tumour and lymph node involvement), the type of MTC (sporadic, familial), and the age and sex of the patient: Stage I disease, familial MTC, age less than 40 years, and female gender are favourable prognostic factors. Patients with MEN-2a have a better survival rate than those with sporadic disease (Fig. 71.6); however, the difference may be more related to the tumour stage at the time the disease is detected than to an inherent difference in the biological behaviour of the tumours. In a multivariate analysis adjusted for tumour stage, the significant difference in survival advantage between patients with sporadic and familial disease disappears [3]. Patients with familial MTC detected by screening are younger and thus diagnosed at an earlier stage of disease. Nonetheless, the survival rate for patients with MEN-2b is significantly worse than that of patients with MEN-2a or familial MTC, but does not differ from that of patients with sporadic disease.

The excellent prognosis associated with identification of MTC at its earliest stage underscores the importance of prospective screening and early diagnosis followed by adequate therapy. Detection of the specific mutations of the *ret* proto-oncogene in MEN-2a, MEN-2b and familial MTC will change screening and treatment methods and thereby hopefully improve the prognosis.

References

1. Saad MF, Ordonez NG, Rashid RK *et al*. Medullary carcinoma of the thyroid: a study of the clinical features and prognostic factors in 161 patients. *Medicine* 1984;63:319–42.
2. Raue F, Frank-Raue K, Grauer A. Multiple endocrine neoplasia type 2, clinical features and screening. *Endocrinol. Metab. Clin. North Am.* 1994;23:137–56.
3. Raue F, Kotzerke J, Reinwein D *et al*. Prognostic factors in medullary

Table 72.1 Lesions associated with von Hippel–Lindau disease (after [1])

	% affected	Mean age at diagnosis (years)
Major lesions		
Central nervous system		
Retinal haemangioblastoma	60	25
Cerebellar haemangioblastoma	60	29
Spinal cord haemangioblastoma	13	33
Visceral		
Renal cell carcinoma and cysts	25	44
Phaeochromocytoma	20	20
Pancreatic cysts, adenoma and carcinoma	?	?
Epididymal cystadenoma	15	?
Rare lesions		
Central nervous system		
Syringomyelia		
Meningioma		
Visceral		
Liver adenoma, haemangioblastoma and cysts		
Lung angioma and cysts		
Splenic angioma		

fluoroscein angioscopy may be needed. Untreated they tend to grow. The high flow rate of blood through these malformations leads to fluid leakage and exudates. Bleeding may occur, with retinal detachment and scarring as complications. Treatment is with laser or cryotherapy, and the treatment of small lesions is more successful than larger tumours.

Cerebellar and other central nervous system haemangioblastomas

About 75% of the haemangioblastomas in VHL occur in the cerebellum; the rest occur in the spinal cord, with rare cases having supratentorial localizations (Fig. 72.2). Cerebellar haemangioblastomas occur as the first manifestation in about 40% of VHL patients. Overall 59% of patients will have a cerebellar haemangioblastoma diagnosed. This tumour was the most common reason for death in the earlier series [2,11]. Cerebellar lesions are now rarely fatal, probably because of easier and earlier detection (due to computed tomography (CT)) and improvements in anaesthetic and surgical technique. The patient usually presents with symptoms of a mass lesion (morning headaches, vomiting) as well as ataxia and incoordination. CT may show a solid or cystic lesion, and magnetic resonance imaging (MRI) or angiography may be needed to show the vascular nature of the lesion (Fig. 72.3). One precaution is that a phaeochromocytoma should be excluded in all patients before invasive procedures or angiography are done. Treatment is by surgical excision, with radiotherapy a possible second-line therapy.

Renal cell carcinoma and cysts

Renal cell carcinoma is now the most common cause of death in VHL patients. The renal carcinomas occur at a later mean age (44 years) than some of the other VHL manifestations. However they occur at a younger age in the VHL patients compared to sporadic, non-familial renal carcinomas (mean 60 years). Renal cell carcinomas in VHL also tend to be multifocal. The probability that a VHL patient will develop a renal cell carcinoma by the age of 60 has been estimated to be 70%.

Renal cysts occur at a younger age in VHL patients and the cyst epithelium is frequently dysplastic. The relation-

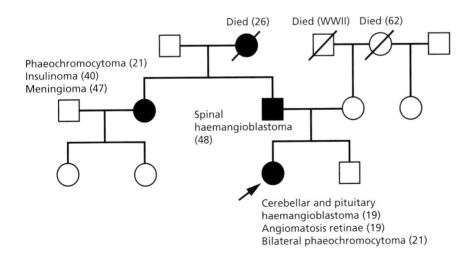

Fig. 72.1 Partial family tree of a family with von Hippel–Lindau disease. Filled in symbols indicate phenotypically affected members and the numbers the age of the patient (years) at the time of the event. Arrow, index case; circles, females; squares, males. (Courtesy of Dr Gareth Evans, St Mary's Hospital, Manchester.)

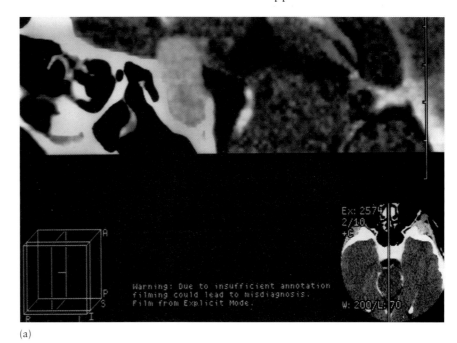

(a)

ship between cysts and carcinoma is unclear. Although carcinomas can have cystic elements, carcinomas sometimes develop in the absence of cysts. Repeated CT scanning suggests that most simple cysts are benign, but complex cysts or solid lesions will enlarge and contain tumour.

Diagnosis is best made by a combination of ultrasound scanning, CT and MRI. Percutaneous aspiration cytology of suspicious cysts or lesions may help in deciding whether surgical exploration is required. The definitive treatment is by conservative surgical excision of the tumour. Lesions are often recurrent and multifocal and repeat operations are frequently required. In most cases as much normal kidney as possible should be spared at each operation, but even so some patients may eventually require renal replacement therapy.

Phaeochromocytoma and other adrenal lesions

Phaeochromocytomas occur in approximately 10% of VHL cases, but the prevalence within an affected family can range from 0 to 92% [9]. Bilateral tumours are found in up to 40% of those with phaeochromocytomas [12,13] (Fig. 72.4). Looked at from another point of view, recent data suggest that up to 23% of patients presenting with phaeochromocytomas had either VHL or multiple endocrine neoplasia (MEN) when fully investigated [12].

Surveillance programmes should detect most phaeochromocytomas before patients develop symptoms. Establishing the diagnosis of a phaeochromocytoma is complicated by the fact that VHL patients have been

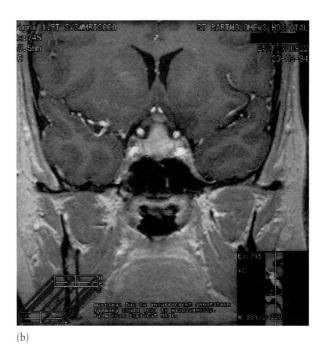

(b)

Fig. 72.2 (a) Pituitary haemangioblastoma from a patient with von Hippel–Lindau disease. Sagittal reconstruction of a CT scan showing a mass in the fossa with suprasellar extension. The mass enhances densely with contrast. (b) Pituitary haemangioblastoma from the same patient. MRI in coronal slice.

reported with a variety of adrenal pathologies including cortical adenomas, haemangioblastomas and hyperplasia. High-resolution CT and ultrasound scanning by a radiologist with an interest in adrenal radiology will detect most lesions. The function and nature of an adrenal lesion is

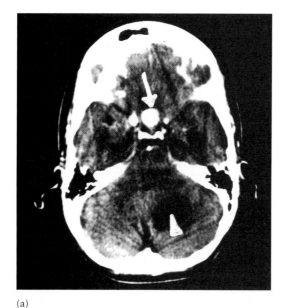

(a)

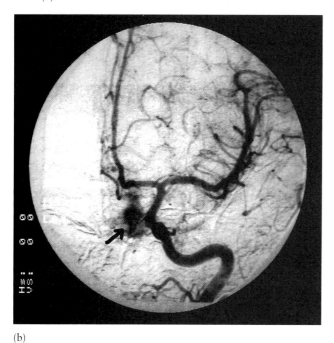

(b)

Fig. 72.3 (a) Left cerebellar cyst (white arrowhead) and a pituitary haemangioblastoma shown by CT (white arrow). (b) The vascular nature of the pituitary lesion (black arrow) is confirmed by a left carotid angiogram. (Courtesy of Dr C.G.D. Beardwell, Christie Hospital, Manchester.)

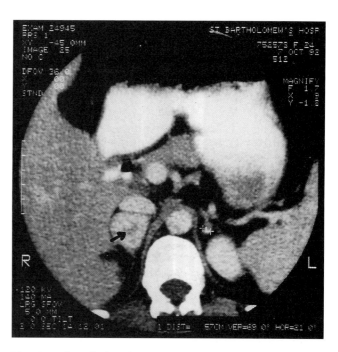

Fig. 72.4 Bilateral adrenal tumours shown by CT and both confirmed to be phaeochromocytomas by histology. The right-sided lesion (black arrow) is larger (25 mm), while the left adrenal contains a 5 mm nodule (white crosses).

best assessed by a combination of several 24-hour urinary free catecholamine levels, MRI and metaiodobenzyl-guanidine (MIBG) isotope scanning. However, when the phaeochromocytomas are small in size, MRI may fail to show the characteristic high T_2-weighted signal. Radio-labelled MIBG may be taken up by up to 20% of normal adrenal medullas, again giving rise to uncertainty when lesions are small. If these tests are equivocal or negative, adrenal vein catheterization and catecholamine sampling (by an experienced operator) may help in confirming the presence of a small intra-adrenal phaeochromocytoma.

Initial treatment consists of α- and β-adrenoreceptor blockade, especially before any invasive test or procedure. Before any procedure we would treat any VHL patient harbouring an adrenal lesion with phenoxybenzamine, even if catecholamine secretion was apparently normal. This is because paroxysmal surges of blood pressure and catecholamines may occur only when a patient is stressed by a procedure or operation.

Definitive treatment is by adrenalectomy. Great care must be taken not to miss bilateral disease. Some of these tumours are small and may not be seen or felt macro-scopically. Missing these may result in unnecessary repeat adrenalectomies. Conversely, over aggressive removal of non-phaeochromocytoma adrenal masses will result in unnecessary lifelong adrenal replacement therapy. Thus as much data as possible should be gathered about any adrenal lesion in a VHL patient before surgical treatment is undertaken. Non-phaeochromocytoma and non-functioning adrenal lesions can be observed by scanning and 24-hour urinary free catecholamine estimation at yearly intervals.

Other visceral manifestations

The other lesions associated with VHL are listed in Table 72.1. In general most cystic lesions can be observed clinically and by yearly ultrasound and CT scanning. Solid lesions may be biopsied or aspirated for a tissue diagnosis. Pancreatic tumours are not rare in VHL, but are often asymptomatic and detected on routine scanning. Most are islet cell tumours and approximately 50% are malignant. Hence solid pancreatic lesions will usually require surgical excision. Most of the pancreatic islet cell tumours are clinically non-functioning but secretion of vasoactive intestinal polypeptide (VIP), insulin, glucagon and calcitonin has been reported [14].

Diagnostic work-up and disease surveillance

The approaches we recommend are listed in Tables 72.2 and 3. Early diagnosis remains fundamental to the well-being of VHL patients. Genetic testing may allow surveillance programmes to focus on abnormal gene carriers, and all affected subjects should have a blood sample taken for DNA banking so that their relatives can be offered presymptomatic DNA diagnosis. Molecular genetic diagnosis by characterization of the VHL mutation not only allows precise carrier testing but can also identify those individuals who are likely to develop phaeochro-

mocytoma. Substitution of an arginine at codon 167 by a glutamine or tryptophan is associated with a high risk of phaeochromocytoma [6].

References

1. Maher ER, Yates JR, Harries R *et al.* Clinical features and natural history of von Hippel–Lindau disease. *Q. J. Med.* 1990;**77**:1151–63.
2. Melmon KL, Rosen SW. Lindau's disease. *Am. J. Med.* 1964;**36**:595–617.
3. Seizinger BR, Rouleau GA, Ozelius LJ *et al.* Von Hippel–Lindau disease maps to the region of chromosome 3 associated with renal cell carcinoma. *Nature* 1988;**332**:268–9.
4. Latif F, Tory K, Gnarra J *et al.* Identification of the von Hippel–Lindau disease tumor suppressor gene. *Science* 1993;**260**:1317–20.
5. Knudson AG. Antioncogenes and human cancer. *Proc. Natl. Acad. Sci. USA* 1993;**90**:10914–21.
6. Crossey PA, Richards FM, Foster K *et al.* Identification of intragenic mutations in the von Hippel–Lindau disease tumour suppressor gene and correlation with disease phenotype. *Hum. Mol. Genet.* 1994;**3**:1303–8.
7. Duan DR, Pause A, Burgess WH *et al.* Inhibition of transcription elongation by the VHL tumor suppressor protein. *Science* 1995;**269**:1402–6.
8. Kibel L, Iliopoulos O, DeCaprio JA, Kaelin WG Jr. Binding of the von Hippel–Lindau tumor suppressor protein to Elongin A and B. *Science* 1995;**269**:1444–6.
9. Neumann HPH, Wiestler OD. Clustering of features of von Hippel–Lindau syndrome: evidence for a complex genetic locus. *Lancet* 1991;**337**:1052–4.
10. Maher ER, Iselius L, Yates JR *et al.* Von Hippel–Lindau disease: a genetic study. *J. Med. Genet.* 1991;**28**:443–7.
11. Horton WA, Wong V, Eldridge R. Von Hippel–Lindau disease. *Arch. Intern. Med.* 1976;**136**:769–77.
12. Neumann HPH, Berger DP, Sigmund G *et al.* Pheochromocytomas, multiple endocrine neoplasia type 2, and von Hippel–Lindau disease. *N. Engl. J. Med.* 1993;**329**:1531–8.
13. Chew SL, Dacie JE, Reznek RH *et al.* Bilateral phaeochromocytomas in von Hippel–Lindau disease: diagnosis by adrenal vein sampling and catecholamine assay. *Q. J. Med.* 1994;**87**:49–54.
14. Binkovitz LA, Johnson CD, Stephens DH. Islet cell tumors in von Hippel–Lindau disease: increased prevalence and relationship to the multiple endocrine neoplasias. *Am. J. Roentgenol.* 1990;**155**:501–5.

Table 72.2 Testing for von Hippel–Lindau disease

Palpate for renal and epididymal lesions
Urinalysis
24-hour urine collection for adrenaline, noradrenaline and dopamine
Fundoscopy and fluorescein angioscopy
Brain computed tomography (CT)
Renal and adrenal ultrasound and CT

Table 72.3 Surveillance programme for von Hippel–Lindau disease (from [1])

Affected patient	At risk relative
Examination and urinalysis, yearly	Examination and urinalysis, yearly
24-hour urinary free catecholamines, yearly	24-hour urinary free catecholamines, yearly
Fundoscopy and fluorescein angioscopy, yearly	Fundoscopy and fluorescein angioscopy, yearly from age 10 to 60
Renal ultrasound, yearly	Renal ultrasound, yearly from age 15
Abdominal CT scan, 3-yearly	Abdominal CT scan, 3-yearly from age 20 to 65
Brain scan (CT/MRI), 3-to age 50 then 5-yearly	Brain scan (CT/MRI), 3-yearly from age 15 to 40 then 5-yearly to age 60

CT, computed tomography; MRI, magnetic resonance imaging.

Neurofibromatosis

VINCENT M. RICCARDI

Introduction

There are two universally recognized forms of neuro-fibromatosis (NF). The current names of both are based upon the classification I proposed in 1982 and which was formally adopted by the NIH in 1987: NF-1, or von Recklinghausen disease [1], and NF-2, or bilateral acoustic neurofibromatosis [2]. The latter, NF-2, has virtually no associated endocrine abnormalities. The situation for NF-1 is more complex; in general, the frequency of endocrine problems is relatively low, while the range is rather broad.

Neurofibromatosis 1

Overview

The NF-1 gene locus is on chromosome 17; it comprises over 300 kilobases (kb) of genomic DNA, arranged in approximately 50 exons that are transcribed into a mRNA molecule of about 13 kb [3]. This transcript has at least two alternative splice sites, allowing for the gene product, *neurofibromin*, to have at least three different forms. The unmodified protein has 2818 amino acid residues and a molecular mass of 327 kDa. Neurofibromin has at least one specifically defined function, namely that of a guanine triphosphate (GTP)ase-activating protein (GAP). The GAP element presumably accounts for neurofibromas and other tumours by influencing the interaction of guanosine nucleotides with ras oncoproteins. GTP is required for an 'active' ras protein; wild-type neurofibromin promotes the cleavage of a phosphate group from GTP to form guanosine diphosphate (GDP), diminishing the growth-promoting activities of ras. The GAP function of neuro-fibromin has generated much interest in a medicinal approach to treating NF-1 tumour growth, specifically, obviating the NF-1 mutation by an opposite effect on the ras control system.

Confirming the diagnosis of NF-1 using a molecular (i.e. DNA) marker has little use. By 1 year of age the diagnosis is always readily apparent to the trained professional. Moreover, currently, less than 70% of all NF-1 mutations can be identified at the molecular level. For families with at least two generations of affected or at-risk persons, molecular diagnosis using genetic linkage strategies is possible for prenatal diagnosis.

Defining features

Every person with NF-1 eventually will have café-au-lait spots, iris Lisch nodules and multiple neurofibromas. The café-au-lait spots (Fig. 73.1) are apparent at or shortly after birth. The Lisch nodules (Fig. 73.2) become apparent sometime after 5 years of age. Neurofibromas (Fig. 73.3) become obvious both as a function of age and of the type of neurofibroma. Cutaneous and subcutaneous neuro-fibromas usually appear at or around the time of puberty. Nodular plexiform neurofibromas tend to become apparent in the late teen years. Diffuse plexiform neurofibromas are congenital lesions, although they might not be readily obvious until they grow larger or until the appropriate diagnostic studies are done (e.g. radiography). A corollary to this congenital nature of diffuse plexiform neuro-fibromas is that if a person with NF-1 does not manifest such a tumour (and it has been realistically looked for), that person will not develop one subsequently. That is, for such a person there is not a continuing risk of such a development. This is a source of solace to many parents.

Although each of these defining features will be present eventually in each patient there is tremendous variation in the number and severity of the lesions, and severity thus is not predictable from one generation to another, even in a single family. A minimally affected parent can have a child that is severely affected, for example, with very numerous cutaneous neurofibromas.

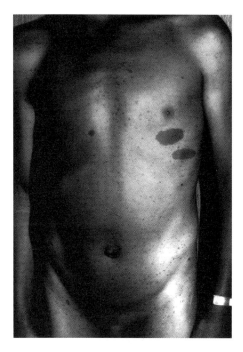

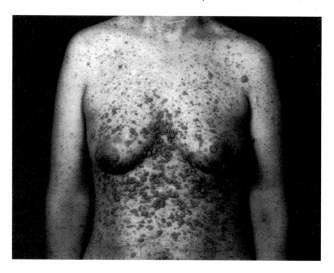

Fig. 73.3 Cutaneous neurofibromas clustered in a manner typical of NF-1 on the chest of a woman with that disorder. Notice the prominent involvement of the nipples and areolae.

Fig. 73.1 Multiple café-au-lait spots and freckling in a young boy, who died from his metastatic neurofibrosarcoma just before his eleventh birthday shortly after this photo was taken.

The frequencies of variable features range from somewhere around 0.1% for juvenile chronic myelogenous leukaemia, through about 0.5% for phaeochromocytoma and 15% for optic pathway gliomas to as high as 60% for learning disabilities. Many features have a frequency of about 5%, as for example with sphenoid wing dysplasia. The sum of these estimated average frequencies make an important clinical point: it is very unusual for a patient with NF-1 to avoid all of the variable features. As a practical matter it is usual for a patient to have at least two or three of such variable features. This is among the reasons why I tend to see NF-1 as a relatively serious disorder, not as a disorder that is more often mild than serious.

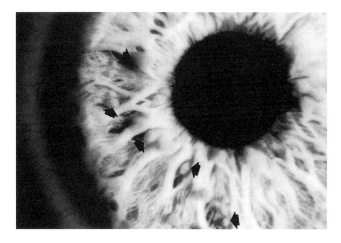

Fig. 73.2 Iris Lisch nodules (arrows).

Variable features

All the other features of NF-1 are variable: not only in terms of their respective levels of severity, but also in terms of their frequencies. I will not try to itemize all of the variable features, though I will pick several to make some broad, general points. For a complete review the reader is referred to my monograph [1]. Endocrine features will be discussed later in this chapter.

Optic pathway gliomas

Optic pathway gliomas are symptomatic in no less than 5% of patients with NF-1, although the total number of patients with NF-1 that have this form of tumour is 15% or more. The symptoms include visual deficits, hypothalamic/pituitary impingement (discussed below), and less specific consequences of an intracranial space-occupying lesion (e.g. hydrocephalus). Several percent of patients with NF-1 have non-optic pathway gliomas, most often in the posterior fossa, but occasionally in a cerebral hemisphere. The issue of screening children for optic pathway gliomas prior to irreversible vision loss is controversial presently, although I personally encourage such screening as a realistic alternative to irreversible symptoms of the types described above in at least 5% of these at-risk youngsters.

Neurofibrosarcoma

This malignancy occurs in about 6% of patients with NF-1, almost, but not quite, always arising in a diffuse plexiform neurofibroma. If this observation is verified, then the 6% risk may not apply to all patients with NF-1, but rather be lower for those without diffuse plexiform neurofibromas and higher for those with such a lesion. This malignancy is nonetheless very rare in the first decade of life; most of the patients with this feature present in the second or third decades.

Skeletal dysplasias

Skeletal dysplasias include pseudarthrosis of the tibia (about 1%) or other tubular bones (less than 0.5%); sphenoid wing dysplasia (5%); dystrophic scoliosis (5%); and non-specific features including pectus excavatum, angulation deformities at the knees, ankle valgus and pes planus. A key aspect of acknowledging these features is the resultant emphasis on the embryonic and fetal onset of the disorder, as well as its protean nature: it is more than a skin pigmentation and tumour disorder.

Vascular dysplasias

A similar point can be made about the vascular dysplasias. The most frequent portion of the vascular tree to be involved is that feeding the kidneys. Renovascular hypertension afflicts at least 3% of patients with NF-1. Another somewhat smaller group of patients with NF-1 have involvement of the gastrointestinal or cerebral vascular systems.

Learning disabilities

School performance problems occur in at least 40%, and probably as high as 60%, of youngsters with NF-1. Although in some generic sense this is a type of 'learning disability' some experts object to applying that phrase in any strict sense to the problems seen in NF-1. However, the parents of affected youngsters understand the generic sense and it sums up the situation for them well. The precise basis for this performance abnormality is not known. Efforts to correlate its presence with other variable features of NF-1 have been unsuccessful, with particular regard to macrocephaly and to the hyperintense T_2-weighted signals seen on cranial magnetic resonance imaging (MRI) scans of patients with NF-1. Plain and simply, there is no correlation between learning problems and the MRI findings [4]. Early identification is helpful, as remedial intervention is quite salutary.

Seizures

I emphasize seizures here only because there is no specified anatomical basis to account for this feature, which is present in about 5% of patients with NF-1 (i.e. only slightly different from the general population). The types of seizures include all the usual ones, including infantile spasms as seen in tuberous sclerosis.

Short stature and macrocephaly

At least 16% of patients with NF-1 have short stature (height 2 or more standard deviations below the mean for age and sex) [1]. Similarly, at least 16% of patients with NF-1 have macrocephaly (head circumference 2 or more standard deviations above the mean for age and sex) [1]. In addition, there is probably another group with *relative* macrocephaly: less than 2 standard deviations above the mean, but excessively large with respect to the patient's short stature. The short stature is not explained by chiasm optic gliomas or by unequivocal deficiencies in human growth hormone (hGH), as discussed further below.

Endocrine features

Pregnancy

Puberty and pregnancy are both associated with a change in the rate of development and size of neurofibromas. In general the neurofibroma changes precede and accompany puberty, rather than necessarily being 'caused' by puberty and its defining physiological changes. Pregnancy tends to make neurofibromas more obvious, most likely on the basis of intercellular turgidity, which dissipates shortly after delivery [1]. There is no reliable evidence for an adverse affect of birth control pills in NF-1 [1]. The overall severity of NF-1 as determined by the number, nature and consequences of neurofibromas is the same for both men and women.

Hypothalamus–pituitary

Optic pathway gliomas involving the optic chiasm not infrequently impinge on the adjacent hypothalamus and/or pituitary gland. It is common in such situations for there to be either of three types of clinical problems. However, each of these problems as part of the NF-1 picture may be present without an apparent optic chiasm glioma.

Short stature

Short stature is frequent in NF-1, as noted above. It is much more common than tumours involving the optic chiasm or hypothalamus. Moreover, the role of deficient hGH secretion has yet to be defined. No publications have documented that such a deficiency actually accounts for the short stature, although endocrinology specialists in local facilities often interpret hGH (baseline and provocative-testing) data to provide a basis for hGH replacement therapy. Personally, I am sceptical, and my reservations go beyond the cost of the therapy and the vanity of the clinicians involved: the use of a growth-promoting substance in the setting of a disorder characterized by aberrant growth in multiple tissues is an experiment in nature that warrants thoughtfulness in the extreme.

Puberty disturbances

Premature puberty in NF-1 almost always indicates a chiasmal optic pathway glioma, although the hormonal details are usually unclear. Delayed puberty, on the other hand, may have no specified anatomical basis, or there may be a chiasmal glioma, or a less specific brain abnormality, such as ventricle dilation. In general, these cases have not been keenly studied and the 'exact' basis for the puberty disturbance is usually not apparent.

Russell diencephalic syndrome

Patients with NF-1 and an optic chiasm glioma may present with the Russell diencephalic syndrome (hypothalamic syndrome, skin pallor, visual loss). These patients are important for two reasons. First, they document the presence of avoidable symptoms attributable to NF-1 chiasmal gliomas. Second, they document how effective radiotherapy can be. I have seen patients with this syndrome reverse their downward courses within days of initiating radiotherapy. Optic pathway gliomas and their consequences are clearly amenable to treatment.

Phaeochromocytoma

Most commonly involving the adrenal medulla, phaeo-chromocytomas probably occur with a frequency of 0.5% among patients with NF-1. The involvement of other sites, including the aortic bifurcation (organ of Zuckerkandl), is well known in NF-1. I know of no patients in the first decade of life, and the frequency after that age is still about 0.5% (1 in 200), a relatively low likelihood. A phaeochromocytoma is a key part of NF-1 because it represents an avoidable lethal complication. It is essential to consider this diagnosis in all patients with this condition.

Neuroendocrine tumours of the gut

Neuroendocrine tumours of the gut probably occur with a frequency of about 1%, although no accurate numbers are known. It may be that the frequency is closer to 2 or 3%. Presentation is usually as a pancreatic mass. Serotonin-related symptoms are the exception.

Parathyroid

Although several groups have published on an excessive frequency of parathyroid adenomas among patients with NF-1, I am unconvinced that the frequency represents anything other than investigator bias.

Neurofibromatosis 2

Overview

The locus for NF-2 is on chromosome 22, identified originally by noting loss of heterozygosity in meningiomas and Schwannomas. Linkage studies later confirmed the 22q locus, leading to its cloning [5]. The gene product has been dubbed *merlin*, an acronym for other proteins structurally related to it: *moesin-ezrin-radixin-like protein*. The cDNA for one of the merlin clones has over 2200 base pairs (bp); the gene itself probably includes about 300 kb. Seventeen exons have been identified and the protein contains 595 amino acids. The gene is expressed ubiquitously and alternative splicing is important in gene transcription. Several different types of mutations have been identified, and in each instance the effect is loss of function of the protein. Presymptomatic molecular identification of a mutant NF-2 gene, including for prenatal diagnosis, is available only through the use of a genetic linkage approach presently.

NF-2 is a disorder primarily of the central nervous system. The main problems are cranial nerve and meningeal tumours. There may be cutaneous Schwannomas and neurofibromas, but these are not the main source of clinical problems. The central nervous system tumours include brain meningiomas, cranial nerve Schwannomas (especially vestibular Schwannomas), ependymomas and spinal cord meningiomas and gliomas. Optic gliomas are not seen. Deafness from bilateral acoustic neuromas, or, preferably, vestibular Schwannomas, is a very likely development for all patients with NF-2. Treatment is limited essentially to surgery or computer-assisted radiotherapy (e.g. the 'gamma knife').

In addition to the neural crest tumours just described, there are recently identified ocular features, including posterior subcapsular cataracts, retinal gliomas, a pigmentary retinopathy, and gaze palsies. The ocular features may be among the earliest features and may actually be the basis for clinical presentation.

There may be two or more forms of NF-2: a mild, later onset variety, and a relatively severe, earlier onset variety. Whether this apparent clinical heterogeneity can be explained by different types of mutations (i.e. allelism) is currently under investigation.

Endocrine features

Although technically there are no endocrine consequences of NF-2 mutations, it is worth noting that the course of the disease may be influenced by sex steroids. Presentation with a vestibular or cranial meningioma during pregnancy is relatively common, and for at least some patients with NF-2, birth control pills may aggravate the course of patients with these same tumours. It is unclear whether puberty marks a turning point in the natural history of NF-2.

References

1. Riccardi VM. *Neurofibromatosis: Phenotype, Natural History and Pathogenesis*, 2nd edn. Baltimore: Johns Hopkins University Press, 1992.
2. Martuza RL, Eldridge R. Neurofibromatosis 2 (bilateral acoustic neurofibromatosis). *N. Engl. J. Med.* 1988;318:684–8.
3. Gutmann DH, Collins FS. The neurofibromatosis type 1 gene and its protein product, neurofibromin. *Neuron* 1993;10:335–43.
4. Ferner RE, Chaudhuri R, Bingham J, Cox T, Hughes RAC. MRI in neurofibromatosis 1. The nature and evolution of increased intensity T_2-weighted lesions and their relationship to intellectual impairment. *J. Neurol. Neurosurg. Psychiatry* 1993;56:492–5.
5. Trofatter JA, MacCollin MM, Rutter JL *et al.* A novel moesin-, ezrin-, radixin-like gene is a candidate for the neurofibromatosis 2 tumour suppressor. *Cell* 1993;72:791–800.

McCune–Albright Syndrome

WILLIAM F. SCHWINDINGER AND MICHAEL A. LEVINE

Introduction

McCune–Albright syndrome (MAS) is characterized by the clinical triad of polyostotic fibrous dysplasia, café-au-lait pigmented skin lesions, and autonomous functioning of multiple endocrine glands [1,2]. Endocrinopathies that have been described in patients with MAS include precocious puberty, hyperthyroidism, growth hormone (GH) excess, hyperprolactinaemia, Cushing's syndrome, and hypophosphataemic osteomalacia [3]. MAS occurs as a sporadic condition and is not inherited. A mutation in the gene (*GNAS1*) that encodes the α chain of the stimulatory G protein of adenyl cyclase, $G_s\alpha$, has been identified in patients with MAS. This mutation is present in a mosaic distribution, consistent with the hypothesis that MAS results from a somatic mutation that occurs during early embryogenesis. The $G_s\alpha$ mutation results in constitutive activation of adenyl cyclase and may be the molecular basis for autonomous function and hyperplasia of the affected cells.

Clinical features

Café-au-lait pigmented skin lesions

Patients with MAS may have one or more flat, café-au-lait pigmented skin lesions with irregular borders (Fig. 74.1). Biopsy reveals that the pigment is melanin in both melanocytes and keratinocytes. The irregular border of these lesions distinguishes them from the pigmented lesions of neurofibromatosis which have a smooth border. The distribution of the café-au-lait skin lesions in MAS is also characteristic. Individual lesions on the torso or face rarely extend across the midline. The majority of the skin lesions tend to be on the same side as the most severe skeletal involvement. Pigmented lesions occur most frequently on the sacrum, buttocks and lumbar region, which may be related to the embryological origin

of melanoblasts from the neural crest. Happle [4] noted that the pattern of the cutaneous lesions follows the embryological lines of ectodermal migration described by Blashko, and first suggested that MAS might be a mosaic disorder.

Polyostotic fibrous dysplasia

Patients with MAS commonly develop expansile skeletal lesions that can cause fracture, deformities and nerve entrapment. These lesions typically develop before the age of 10 years, in contradistinction to the isolated lesions of mono-ostotic fibrous dysplasia that develop in the second or third decade. Enlarging lesions may cause progressive deformity, but few new lesions develop over time. Plain radiographs reveal thinning of the cortex and circumscribed lesions with a characteristic ground glass appearance (Fig. 74.2). The lesions may appear multilocular due to a scalloped pattern of endosteal erosion. Any bone may be affected, but radiographs of the femora and pelvis are the most useful in screening for bone involvement. Scintigraphy with ^{99m}Tc methylene diphosphonate is more sensitive than radiography in detecting early lesions. Histological sections reveal fibrous tissue with embedded bony trabeculae (Fig. 74.3).

Multiple endocrinopathies

Precocious puberty

Precocious puberty is a common initial manifestation of MAS in girls. Cyclical elevation of oestrogen levels, development and involution of ovarian cysts, menstrual bleeding, and development of secondary sexual characteristics typically begin between 1 and 9 years of age. The ovaries are hyperfunctional despite low circulating levels of gonadotrophins and prepubertal responses of gonadotrophins to gonadotrophin-releasing hormone

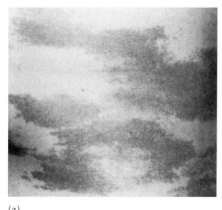

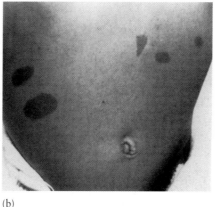

(a)   (b)

Fig. 74.1 Café-au-lait lesion of MAS (a) as compared to that of neurofibromatosis (b). Note the irregular border of the lesion in MAS ('coast of Maine') as compared to the smooth border in neurofibromatosis ('coast of California').

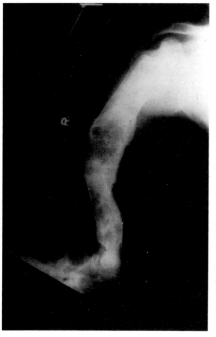

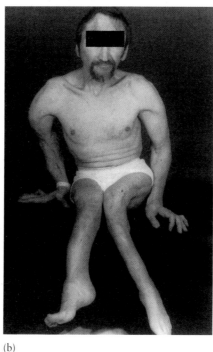

(a)   (b)

Fig. 74.2 Polyostotic fibrous dysplasia. Plain radiographs reveal expansile lesions that may appear scalloped (a). Recurrent fractures can lead to progressive deformity (b).

(GnRH). Physiological activation of the hypothalamic–pituitary–ovarian axis occurs as the child reaches maturity. Although some adult women may experience menstrual irregularities, they are usually fertile. Precocious puberty occurs less frequently in boys with MAS, and testicular biopsy reveals varying degrees of seminiferous tubule development.

Autonomous thyroid nodules

About 50% of patients with MAS develop excessive thyroid function that ranges from subclinical laboratory abnormalities to hyperthyroidism that is refractory to surgery or radioactive iodine ablation. MAS patients with hyperthyroidism do not develop orbitopathy or cutaneous features of Graves' disease, and do not have detectable serum levels of thyroid stimulating immunoglobulins. The hyperthyroidism in MAS is due to autonomous function of the thyroid gland. Clinically evident goitre is present in many MAS patients with hyperthyroidism, and nodules are detected by thyroid ultrasound in essentially all patients. Thyroid function testing reveals suppressed thyroid-stimulating hormone (TSH), a blunted response of TSH to thyrotrophin-releasing hormone (TRH), and failure of synthetic liothyronine (T_3) to suppress radioactive iodine uptake [5].

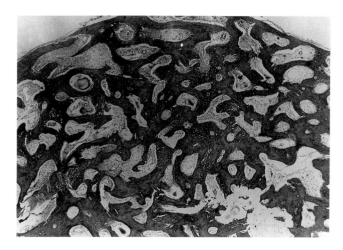

Fig. 74.3 Histology of polyostotic fibrous dysplasia demonstrating fibrous tissue with embedded boney trabeculae, collagen arranged in intersecting whorled bundles, and large osteocyte lacunae.

Growth hormone excess and hyperprolactinaemia

Patients with MAS may develop pituitary-dependent growth hormone (GH) excess. GH excess in MAS is indistinguishable biochemically from that which occurs in patients with isolated GH producing pituitary adenomas. GH secretion is stimulated by growth hormone releasing hormone (GHRH) and TRH, poorly inhibited by oral glucose, and increased by sleep. However, only 40% of patients with MAS and GH excess have radiological evidence of a pituitary tumour, and over 80% have associated hyperprolactinaemia. Pituitary pathology in MAS varies and includes adenoma, nodular hyperplasia or mammosomatotroph hyperplasia.

Hypercortisolism

Patients with MAS occasionally develop hypercortisolism. In most cases hypercortisolism appears to be due to autonomous activity of the adrenal gland. Cortisol levels show no diurnal variation and are not suppressible by dexamethasone. Plasma levels of ACTH are undetectable and adrenal biopsy reveals nodular adrenal hyperplasia or adrenal adenoma [6].

Hypophosphataemic rickets and osteomalacia

Some patients with MAS develop a generalized metabolic bone disease that is associated with low serum levels of phosphate, low or low-normal serum levels of 1,25-dihydroxy vitamin D, high levels of alkaline phosphatase, depressed renal tubular maximum reabsorption of phosphate (TMP/glomerular filtration rate (GFR)) and normal levels of serum calcium, 25-hydroxyvitamin D and parathyroid hormone (PTH). These biochemical abnormalities are similar to those that occur in patients with either X-linked hypophosphataemic rickets or tumour-associated hypophosphataemic osteomalacia (oncogenous osteomalacia). A circulating factor that inhibits renal phosphate transport and 1-α-hydroxylation of 25-hydroxyvitamin D appears to be the cause of hypophosphataemia in subjects with tumour-associated osteomalacia. These tumours can be benign or malignant, and commonly are composed of mesenchymal cells. Removal of the tumour results in normalization of phosphate and vitamin D metabolism. A similar factor has been proposed as the basis for the biochemical abnormalities present in patients with inherited forms of hypophosphataemic rickets. Hypophosphataemic osteomalacia has been described in patients with polyostotic fibrous dysplasia, and removal of virtually all the abnormal tissue in one case resulted in biochemical and radiological improvement. It is conceivable that a circulating factor is also secreted by fibrous dysplasia lesions in MAS.

Involvement of other organs

Patients with MAS may develop metabolic problems in additional tissues that can lead to hepatobiliary disease (neonatal jaundice, elevated transaminases, hepatomegaly, cholestasis, extramedullary haematopoiesis), cardiac disease (cardiomegaly, tachyarrhythmias, sudden death), gastrointestinal polyps, hyperplasia of the thymus and spleen, acute pancreatitis, failure to thrive, developmental delay, and microcephaly. These disorders may result from expression of the activated $G_s\alpha$ mutation in cells of the affected organ or may develop as a response to an underlying endocrinopathy. Hepatobiliary disease and cardiac disease are particularly common problems in patients with MAS, and are associated with the presence of activating $G_s\alpha$ mutations in the affected tissues. MAS may present as a severe neonatal disease with involvement of multiple endocrine glands and non-endocrine organs that leads to premature death [7].

Pathogenesis

Identification of mutations

Insight into the pathogenesis of MAS came with the identification of mutations in the gene encoding $G_s\alpha$ (*GNAS1*) in a subset of GH-secreting pituitary tumours with increased adenyl cyclase activity. Landis and colleagues [8] established that the molecular basis for this anomaly was a missense mutation that resulted in

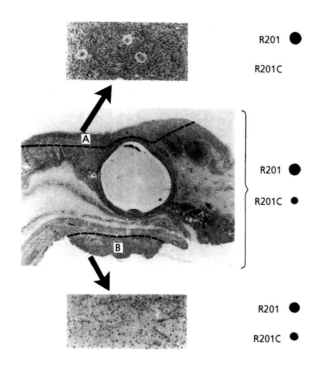

R201 ●
R201C

R201 ●
R201C ●

R201 ●
R201C ●

Fig. 74.4 Mosaic distribution of activating mutation of $G_s\alpha$ in the ovary of a patient with MAS. DNA prepared from a histologically normal area of the ovary (above) showed little of the mutant allele (R201C). While DNA prepared from the histologically abnormal area of the ovary (below) revealed almost 50% mutant allele. (From [9].)

replacement of either Arg201 or Gln227 in the $G_s\alpha$ protein. In $G_s\alpha$, Arg201 is the site for covalent modification by cholera toxin, while Gln227 is analogous to the Gln61 that is commonly replaced in the oncogene *p21ras*. Replacement of either Arg201 or Gln227 inhibits the intrinsic GTPase activity of $G_s\alpha$, and leads to constitutive activation of adenyl cyclase. Increased levels of intracellular cAMP may account for both autonomous function and proliferation of cells expressing the mutation. Thus, these activating mutations of the *GNAS1* gene have been proposed to function as oncogenes, termed *gsp*. Weinstein and colleagues [9] identified *GNAS1* gene mutations in DNA from surgical and autopsy specimens from four patients with MAS. These mutations were present in some but not all of tissues examined from each patient, and involved tissues were derived from each of the three embryological germ layers. Each patient had a single mutation in $G_s\alpha$, either Arg201→Cys or Arg201→His. In some cases, the mutation was present in abnormal portions of a tissue but not in histologically normal portions of the same tissue (Fig. 74.4). Schwindinger and colleagues [10] confirmed and extended these findings by identifying an Arg201→His mutation in DNA from the peripheral blood leucocytes and a café-au-lait pigmented skin lesion of a patient with MAS. Taken together these observations suggest that mutations in the *GNAS1* gene arise as a postzygotic event during early embryogenesis. Mutations in Arg201 of $G_s\alpha$ have also been identified in

Table 74.1 Role of mutations in the adenyl cyclase signal transduction system in human neoplasia

Disease	Neoplasm	G protein	Receptor
Hyperthyroidism	Thyroid adenoma	$G_s\alpha$ G227H G227K R201S	TSH D619G A623I
Acromegaly	Growth hormone-secreting pituitary adenoma	$G_s\alpha$ R201H R201C G227R G227L	
Female precocious puberty	Ovarian sex cord tumours	$G_i\alpha$ R179H R179C	
Cushing's syndrome	Adrenal cortical adenoma and adenocarcinoma	$G_i\alpha$ R179H R179C	
McCune–Albright syndrome	POFD; thyroid, pituitary, ovarian and adrenal adenomas	$G_s\alpha$ R201H R201C	
Male precocious puberty	Leydig cell hyperplasia		LH D578G

LH, luteinizing hormone; POFD, polyostotic fibrous dysplasia; TSH, thyroid-stimulating hormone.

fibrous dysplastic bone lesions and other organs of patients with MAS, including liver, heart, thymus and pancreas [7].

McCune–Albright syndrome as a paradigm for G-protein-related neoplasia

Activating mutations of $G_s\alpha$ are representative of a broader class of abnormalities of G-protein coupled signal transduction that have been identified in various neoplasms (Table 74.1). Activating mutations in $G_s\alpha$ have been identified in sporadic thyroid adenomas, as well as in pituitary tumours and MAS. GH excess, pituitary hyperplasia and gigantism have been produced in transgenic mice in which the GH gene promoter directs the cell-specific expression of the cholera toxin gene, resulting in adenosine diphosphate (ADP)-ribosylation of $G_s\alpha$ and constitutive activation of adenyl cyclase in somatotrophs. Missense mutations ($Arg^{179}\rightarrow Cys$ and $Arg^{179}\rightarrow His$) in the gene encoding the inhibitory G-protein of adenyl cyclase, $G\alpha_{i2}$, have been identified in a subset of ovarian and adrenal cortical tumours. These mutations in $G\alpha_{i2}$ have been termed *gip2*.

Our lack of complete understanding of the role of G proteins in cell growth and differentiation is underscored by the observation that neoplasia may be produced by activating mutations of $G_s\alpha$, which increase intracellular cAMP, and activating mutations of $G_i\alpha$, which decrease intracellular cAMP [11]. The role of intracellular cAMP in cellular proliferation differs by cell type even amongst endocrine cells; for example thyrotrophin stimulates proliferation of thyroid follicular cells, whereas corticotrophin induces G_1 arrest in adrenal cortical cells. It is also important to note that G_s and G_i each modulate distinct intracellular second messengers in addition to cAMP. G_s activates calcium channels, while G_i modulates potassium channels. Although *gip2* has been shown to increase proliferation of NIH 3T3 fibroblasts, it is unlikely that *gsp* produces malignant transformation of cells; for example, *gsp*-bearing tumours that arise sporadically or in patients with MAS are benign and do not undergo malignant transformation. Moreover, a *gsp* mutation, $Gln^{227}\rightarrow Leu$, has recently been shown to *suppress* transformation of NIH 3T3 cells by H-ras [12].

Mutations in several of the seven-transmembrane-spanning receptors that are coupled by G proteins leading to stimulation of adenyl cyclase have also been implicated as the basis for benign neoplasms in humans. Mutations of the thyrotrophin receptor have been identified in three of eleven sporadic thyroid adenomas. These mutations occurred in the third cytoplasmic loop and are postulated to release steric constraints, thereby producing the conformational changes typically brought about by agonist binding. These mutant TSH receptors result in constitutive activation of adenyl cyclase when expressed in COS cells [13]. Overexpression of the A2 adenosine receptor in thyroid cells of transgenic mice activated the cAMP cascade and produced hyperfunctioning thyroid adenomas. Inherited mutations in the luteinizing hormone (LH) receptor are responsible for male-limited precocious puberty, which is associated with Leydig cell hyperplasia. One form of autosomal dominant retinitis pigmentosa is caused by inherited mutations of rhodopsin. Substitution at the retinal binding site, $Lys^{296}\rightarrow Glu$, results in constitutive activation of the photoreceptor and stimulation of the cGMP phosphodiesterase through the G-protein transducin [14].

In vitro studies have suggested possible roles in tumorigenesis for other G proteins that regulate signal transduction pathways other than adenyl cyclase. Transformation of NIH 3T3 cells had been produced by a GTPase inhibiting mutation ($Gln^{209}\rightarrow Leu$) of $G_q\alpha$. Purified $G_o\alpha$ activated with GTPγS was shown to stimulate protein kinase C and induce oocyte maturation. A GTPase inhibiting mutation of $G_o\alpha$, $Gln^{205}\rightarrow Leu$, was shown to transform NIH 3T3 cells, but did not stimulate phospholipase C activity.

Underlying genetics

While MAS is not an inherited disease, it is a genetic disease. There are several other examples of human disease caused by somatic mosaicism occurring during embryogenesis [10]. Hypomelanosis of Ito has been attributed to trisomy 18 mosaicism. Survival beyond infancy in ornithine transcarbamoylase deficiency has been associated with a mosaic distribution of a deletion mutation. Somatic mosaicism has been described in the factor VIII gene in haemophilia A and in the factor IX gene in haemophilia B.

Patient management

Diagnosis

The diagnosis of MAS is confirmed clinically when a patient is found to have at least two features of the classical triad of polyostotic fibrous dysplasia, café-au-lait pigmented skin lesions, and multiple endocrinopathies [5]. Recent reports have suggested that the diagnosis should be considered in patients with any one of the three clinical manifestations of the full syndrome. Frisch and colleagues [15] discuss a case of a 4.5-year-old girl with recurrent ovarian cysts, vaginal bleeding and a single smooth bordered café-au-lait lesion, in whom the diagnosis of MAS was made when polyostotic fibrous dysplasia was disclosed by bone scan. Abs and colleagues [16] described a 36-year-old woman with a toxic multinodular goitre, acromegaly and a history of early menarche and menstrual irregularities in whom magnetic resonance imaging (MRI) of the pituitary sella revealed sphenoid bone dysplasia. The identification of specific activating mutations in the *GNAS1* gene in patients with suspected MAS can provide a laboratory confirmation of the diagnosis. However, these mutations are present in peripheral blood leucocytes of only a fraction of patients with MAS, and biopsy of affected tissues is only rarely indicated. Thus, in most cases the diagnosis of MAS will be made on clinical criteria.

Current therapy

The treatment of MAS must be individualized for each patient. Because of the mosaic nature of the disease, patients with MAS may vary significantly in the expression of endocrinopathies and skeletal lesions. Thus a history and physical examination should be directed to the signs and symptoms of precocious puberty, menstrual irregularities, hyperthyroidism, hyperprolactinaemia, acromegaly, Cushing's syndrome and skeletal deformity. An initial evaluation should include at a minimum: radiographs of affected bones; a ^{99m}Tc bone scan if bone lesions are not clinically evident; a chemistry panel, including liver function tests, calcium, phosphorus, and alkaline phosphatase; and assessment of thyroid function with a TSH level.

Bone disease

Polyostotic fibrous dysplasia may be asymptomatic or associated with pathological fractures or progressive deformities that require multiple orthopaedic procedures. Surgery may be complicated by heavy bleeding from affected bone. Radiation therapy to fibrous dysplastic lesions has been met with only limited success.

Endocrinopathies

Precocious puberty in girls with MAS does not respond to therapy with GnRH agonists. Therapy with testolactone or cyproterone acetate can reduce oestrogen levels and lead to cessation of menses but will have no effect on ultimate adult height achieved. Hyperthyroidism may be treated long term with antithyroid drugs, radioactive iodine ablation, or surgical resection. It is often refractory to treatment and may recur years after successful treatment. Pituitary surgery for GH excess or hyperprolactinaemia may be complicated by bleeding from dysplastic bone in the pituitary fossa. GH excess may respond to the long-acting somatostatin analogue octreotide. Treatment of Cushing's syndrome has usually required bilateral adrenalectomy. Hypophosphataemic osteomalacia or rickets is usually treated with calcitriol and inorganic phosphate supplements, but bone histology generally shows little improvement.

Prognosis

Because MAS is expressed in a mosaic distribution, the clinical manifestations extend over a wide spectrum. At one extreme, MAS may occur as a single endocrinopathy or an asymptomatic bone lesion, and a diagnosis of MAS may not be obvious. At the other extreme MAS may present at birth with jaundice, abnormal liver function tests, persistent tachycardia, hyperthyroidism, Cushing's syndrome, and crippling bone deformities, leading to death in early childhood. Most patients with MAS live beyond reproductive age. Crippling bone deformities may reduce life expectancy because of loss of mobility and attendant risks of thrombosis and infection. Sudden death is an uncommon feature of MAS and may be due to cardiac involvement.

Conclusion

Diagnosis still must be made on the basis of clinical evaluation. Specific *GNAS1* gene mutations are detectable in DNA from peripheral leucocytes of only a minority of patients. Polymerase chain reaction (PCR)-based techniques for detection of the mutation are not widely available, and surgical specimens of affected tissue may be required for DNA diagnosis.

Recognition of the molecular basis of MAS has led to the identification of other tissues that are involved in MAS, including liver, heart, pancreas and thymus. This has enabled recognition of a severe form of the disease that is fatal in infancy or early childhood. The full clinical spectrum of this disorder remains to be appreciated.

Acknowledgements

This work was supported by an NIH, NCRR, Osler 5 GCRC grant No. RR00035, and grants from the NIH (DK-34281) and March of Dimes (Basic Grant No. 1-1065).

References

1. Albright F, Butler AM, Hampton AO, Smith P. Syndrome characterized by osteitis fibrosa disseminata, areas of pigmentation and endocrine dysfunction, with precocious puberty in females. *N. Engl. J. Med.* 1937;**216**:727–41.

2. McCune DJ, Bruch H. Osteodystrophia fibrosa. *Am. J. Dis. Child.* 1937;**54**:806–48.

3. Schwindinger WF, Levine MA. McCune–Albright syndrome. *Trends Endocrinol. Metabol.* 1993;**4**:238–42.

4. Happle R. The McCune–Albright syndrome: a lethal gene surviving by mosaicism. *Clin. Genet.* 1986;**29**:321–4.

5. Lee PA, Van Dop C, Migeon CJ. McCune–Albright syndrome: long term follow-up. *JAMA* 1986;**2256**:2980–4.

6. Mauras N, Blizzard RM. The McCune–Albright syndrome. *Acta Endocrinol. Suppl. (Copenh.)* 1986;**279**:207–17.

7. Shenker A, Weinstein LS, Moran A *et al.* Severe endocrine and nonendocrine manifestations of the McCune–Albright syndrome associated with activating mutations of stimulatory G protein G$_s$. *J. Pediatr.* 1993;**123**:509–18.

8. Landis CA, Masters SB, Spada A *et al.* GTPase inhibiting mutations activate the α chain of G$_s$ and stimulate adenylyl cyclase in human pituitary tumors. *Nature* 1989;**340**:692–6.

9. Weinstein LS, Shenker A, Gejman PV *et al.* Activating mutations of the stimulatory G protein in the McCune–Albright syndrome. *N. Engl. J. Med.* 1991;**325**:1688–95.

10. Schwindinger WF, Francomano C, Levine MA. Identification of a mutation in the gene encoding the α subunit of the stimulatory G protein of adenylyl cyclase in McCune–Albright syndrome. *Proc. Natl Acad. Sci. USA* 1992;**89**:5152–56.

11. Lyons L, Landis CA, Harsh G *et al.* Two G protein oncogenes in human endocrine tumors. *Science* 1990;**249**:655–9.

12. Chen J, Iyengar R. Suppression of ras-induced transformation of NIH 3T3 cell by activated Gα$_s$. *Science* 1994;**263**:1278–81.

13. Parma J, Duprez L, Van Sande J *et al.* Somatic mutations in the thyrotropin receptor gene cause hyperfunctioning thyroid adenomas. *Nature* 1993;**365**:649–51.

14. Spiegel AM, Weinstein LS, Shenker A. Abnormalities in G protein-coupled signal transduction pathways in human disease. *J. Clin. Invest.* 1993;**92**:1119–25.

15. Frisch LS, Copeland KC, Boepple PA. Recurrent ovarian cysts in childhood: diagnosis of McCune–Albright syndrome by bone scan. *Pediatrics* 1992;**90**:102–4.

16. Abs R, Beckers A, Van de Vyer FL *et al.* Acromegaly, multinodular goiter and silent polyostotic fibrous dysplasia. A variant of the McCune–Albright syndrome. *J. Endocrinol. Invest.* 1990;**13**:671–5.

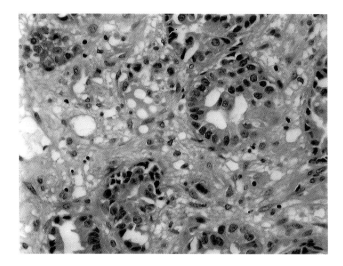

Fig. 75.3 Metastatic ductal carcinoma of the breast infiltrating posterior pituitary gland. The tumour is moderately differentiated, with recognizable glands in the finely fibrillary background of the neurohypophysis.

Table 75.2 Metastases in the pituitary gland

Site	Type of tumour
Relatively common	
Breast	Ductal carcinoma
Bronchus	Oat cell carcinoma
Kidney	Renal cell carcinoma
Prostate	Adenocarcinoma
Relatively rare	
Rectum	Adenocarcinoma
Colon	Adenocarcinoma
Breast	Lobular carcinoma
Endometrium	Adenocarcinoma
Skin	Melanoma
	Cylindroma
Ovary	Papillary serous carcinoma
Thyroid	Follicular carcinoma
Bladder	Transitional cell carcinoma
Bronchus	Carcinoid tumour
(Lymph nodes	Hodgkin's lymphoma
	Non-Hodgkin's lymphoma)

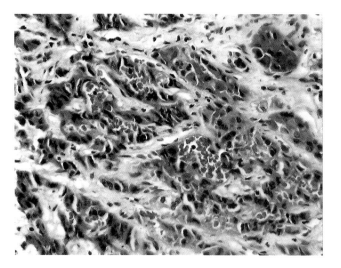

Fig. 75.4 Metastatic carcinoma of the bronchus of large cell undifferentiated type infiltrating the anterior pituitary gland. Surviving groups of basophil cells can be seen in the top right of the figure.

Leukaemic and lymphoma deposits can also affect the pituitary. The most common leukaemia type in the pituitary is acute lymphoblastic leukaemia (33% of cases) then acute myeloid leukaemia (21% of cases). Involvement by non-Hodgkin's lymphoma exceeds that by Hodgkin's lymphoma by three times, but both are rare. The area around the pituitary capsule is involved in 55% of cases of leukaemia and lymphoma of the pituitary: the anterior and posterior lobes together are involved in 21%

of cases; the posterior lobe alone in 16% of cases; and the anterior lobe alone in 8% of cases.

Tumour-to-tumour metastasis can occur in the pituitary. Metastasis of a gastric carcinoma into a prolactin-containing adenoma of the pituitary has been reported. Other primary tumours that have been reported to metastasize into pituitary adenomas include prostate adenocarcinoma (into a non-functioning chromophobe adenoma); melanoma (into an ACTH-containing adenoma); and breast carcinoma (into a prolactin-containing adenoma).

Metastatic carcinoma may involve the parasellar and suprasellar tissues, and be mistaken on imaging and clinically for an intrasellar lesion [6]. The primary tumours that have been found to involve these sites are listed in Table 75.3. There is an understandable overlap with the tumours listed in Table 75.2.

Table 75.3 Metastases in parasellar and suprasellar areas that can clinically mimic intrasellar metastases

Site	Type of tumour
Nasopharynx	Nasopharyngeal carcinoma
Bronchus	Oat cell carcinoma
Salivary gland	Undifferentiated carcinoma
Breast	Ductal carcinoma
Thyroid	Papillary carcinoma
Colon	Adenocarcinoma
Skin	Melanoma
(Lymph nodes	Non-Hodgkin's lymphoma)

Thyroid gland

The thyroid gland is more commonly involved by metastatic spread than is generally realized (Figs 75.5, 75.6). The reported incidence of thyroid metastases is listed in Table 75.4: it varied among series of patients with malignant disease at post-mortem examination from 1.9 to 26.4% [7]. The overall percentage involved, derived from meta-analysis of the reports studied, was 3.1% of 9858 cases. By far the most common metastatic tumour to the thyroid is renal cell carcinoma. As with the pituitary,

Table 75.4 Metastases in the thyroid gland

Site	Type of tumour
Relatively common	
Kidney	Renal cell carcinoma (by far the most common)
Breast	Ductal and lobular carcinoma
Bronchus	Oat cell carcinoma
Rectum	Adenocarcinoma
Relatively rare	
Oesophagus	Squamous cell carcinoma
Stomach	Adenocarcinoma
Colon	Adenocarcinoma
	Carcinoid tumour
Skin	Melanoma
	Squamous cell carcinoma
Nasopharynx	Nasopharyngeal carcinoma
Tonsil	Squamous cell carcinoma
Larynx	Squamous cell carcinoma
Trachea	Squamous cell carcinoma
Bone marrow	Leukaemia
	Multiple myeloma
Testis	Seminoma
Cervix	Squamous cell carcinoma
Uterus	Choriocarcinoma
	Adenocarcinoma
Bladder	Transitional cell carcinoma
Uvea	Melanoma
(Lymph nodes	Non-Hodgkin's lymphoma
	Hodgkin's disease)
Soft tissues	Malignant fibrous histiocytoma
	Rhabdomyosarcoma
	Leiomyosarcoma
	Fibrosarcoma
	Neurofibrocarcinoma
	Malignant Schwannoma
	Kaposi's sarcoma

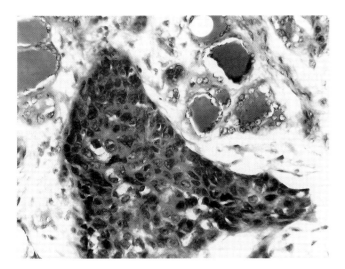

Fig. 75.5 Thyroid gland infiltrated by poorly differentiated metastatic adenocarcinoma of the endometrium. The patient had been treated for endometrial carcinoma 8 years previously and presented with a goitre.

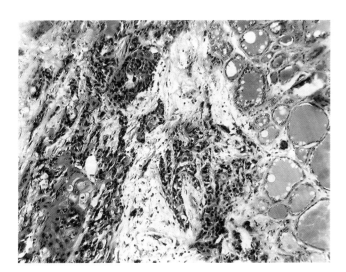

Fig. 75.6 Metastatic squamous cell carcinoma of oesophagus infiltrating the thyroid.

endocrine organ metastases can occur; adrenal carcinoma metastatic to the thyroid gland has been described.

Squamous cell carcinoma in the thyroid can be diagnostically very difficult to determine whether it is primary or metastatic. Squamous change in a papillary or follicular thyroid carcinoma can occur, and primary squamous cell carcinoma of the thyroid has been described after irradiation of the neck. Metastases of squamous cell carcinoma to the thyroid can arise from primaries in the oesophagus, skin, tonsil, larynx and trachea (Fig. 75.6). A diagnosis of primary squamous cell carcinoma of the thyroid cannot be regarded as definitive unless there has been direct inspection, clinical examination and careful imaging of these sites.

Calcispherites (psammoma bodies) in the thyroid are indicators of malignancy. They occur very rarely in non-neoplastic lesions or benign thyroid neoplasms, but when discovered on histology in an apparently innocent lesion

Table 76.1 Pathogenesis of paraneoplastic syndromes

Tumour production of protein hormones or their precursors
Metabolism of steroids by the tumour
Tumour production of enzymes or fetal proteins
Tumour production of cytokines
Tumour stimulation of antibody production
Other unknown causes

turally specific immunoradiometric assays demonstrates that in patients with cancers *and Cushing's syndrome*, both ACTH precursors, and ACTH itself, are increased [5]. Thus, specific endoprotease activity is increased in those cancers that result in the clinical Cushing's syndrome, and is largely lacking in the bulk of cancers that do not produce the clinical syndrome. In this context, the most common cancer to produce the paraneoplastic Cushing's syndrome is small-cell lung carcinoma (SCLC). However, only 1.6–2.8% of patients with SCLC have Cushing's syndrome [6].

Table 76.2 lists the protein hormones and related proteins that have been reported to be produced by cancers, most often carcinomas. Whereas each of these could now be discussed in terms of: (i) clinical symptoms; (ii) association with various tumour types; (iii) molecular pathogenesis; (iv) diagnosis; and (v) treatment, that task is far too extensive for this review. However, general comments may be summarized as follows: many normal, non-endocrine cells, appear to produce small amounts of protein hormones, or protein hormone precursors, that presumably act in paracrine or autocrine functions. Cancers often produce increased quantities of such protein

Table 76.2 Protein hormones and related proteins produced by cancers

Pro-opiomelanocortin products
Corticotrophic hormone
Human chorionic gonadotrophin and its subunits
Parathyroid-related hormone
Parathyroid hormone
Erythropoietin
Growth hormone
Growth hormone-releasing hormone
Prolactin
Gastrin
Gastrin-releasing peptide and bombesin
Secretin
Glucagon
Calcitonin
Endothelin
Renin
Somatostatin
Hypophosphataemia-producing factor
Atrial natriuretic factor
Eosinophilopoietin

hormone precursors, which have less biological activity than the most potent forms of the hormone. A small fraction of cancers either produce very large quantities of weakly bioactive protein hormone precursor or convert the precursor to a more potent product to produce the clinical syndrome. It is in this context that *ectopic hormone production is not ectopic* [2,3].

As indicated earlier, Chapter 78 reviews the syndrome of hypercalcaemia as caused by tumour production of excess parathyroid hormone related-peptide (PTHrP). The most common cause of tumour-associated hypercalcaemia is excess PTHrP production; however, other causes of hypercalcaemia may be associated with cancer. These other causes are:

1 increased hydroxylation of 25-hydroxyvitamin D by the neoplasm that produces vitamin D toxicity;

2 production of osteoclast-activating cytokines such as interleukin-1, transforming growth factor (TGF)-α and prostaglandins of the E series;

3 parathyroid hormone production by the cancer (rare) [7];

4 widespread bony metastatic disease.

The last may also be caused by cytokine-mediated increases in bone resorption.

Metabolism of steroids

Metabolism of normally produced precursor steroids by a neoplasm to produce biologically active products is rare. Two examples exist.

1 Increased aromatase activity of a neoplasm leading to increased oestrogen formation and gynaecomastia in male patients with hepatic cancers, and large sarcomas has been reported. These neoplasms metabolize androgen precursors such as dehydroepiandrosterone produced by the adrenal, or testosterone produced by the testes, to oestradiol. The increased oestradiol produces gynaecomastia.

2 Increased vitamin D hydroxylase activity may lead to increased 1,25-dihydroxyvitamin D formation and hypercalcaemia; for example, T-cell lymphomas may produce hypercalcaemia by hydroxylating circulating 25-hydroxyvitamin D to the more potent 1,25-dihydroxyvitamin D. Other haematological neoplasms, as well as granulomatous diseases such as sarcoidosis and tuberculosis, may produce hypercalcaemia by a similar mechanism.

Tumour production of enzymes or fetal proteins

A variety of fetal proteins may be produced by neoplasms.

Generally, these produce no clinical symptoms but may be useful as tumour markers. Examples include alpha feto protein (AFP), carcino-embryonic antigen (CEA), and alkaline phosphatase isoenzymes.

Tumour production of cytokines

Some paraneoplastic syndromes appear to be caused by tumour production of substances that, under normal circumstances, are locally acting paracrine or autocrine message proteins (i.e. cytokines). Table 76.3 lists some of these syndromes. These have not been as extensively studied or documented as are the paraneoplastic protein hormone syndromes. Yoneda and colleagues [8] reviewed 225 patients with oral cancers in order to evaluate the frequency of the paraneoplastic syndrome of hypercalcaemia and leukocytosis reported in some patients. Ten (4.4%) of the 225 patients had hypercalcaemia, 11 patients (4.9%) had leukocytosis and five patients (2.2%) had both hypercalcaemia and leukocytosis. The cause of the syndrome was not evaluated in this review, but Wetzler and colleagues [9] evaluated a patient with transitional cell carcinoma of the bladder and leukocytosis, and found that plasma granulocyte–macrophage colony-stimulating factor (GM-CSF) was elevated, but granulocyte-CSF and interleukin-3 (IL-3) were not elevated. They postulated that increased tumour production of GM-CSF caused the leukocytosis. Whether GM-CSF is the cytokine-causing leukocytosis in most or all patients with this paraneoplastic syndrome, is unknown.

As was discussed in the protein hormone section, local cytokine production with osteoclast-activated bone resorption appears to be the cause of hypercalcaemia in multiple myeloma and some additional haematological neoplasms that may cause hypercalcaemia.

Table 76.3 Possible cytokine-mediated paraneoplastic syndromes

Syndrome	Tumour	Possible cytokine
Neutrophilia	Lymphoma/leukaemia	Granulocyte colony-stimulating factor
Eosinophilia	Lymphoma/leukaemia	Eosinophilopoietin
Leukocytosis	Oral cancers	GM-CSF
Cachexia	Multiple neoplasms	Tumour necrosis factor
Hypercalcaemia	Multiple myeloma and rarely other haematological malignancies	Osteoclast-activating cytokines (e.g. interleukin I, prostaglandins E series, TGF-α)

GM-CSF, granulocyte–macrophage colony-stimulating factor; TGF, transforming growth factor.

Tumour stimulation of antibody production

Neoplasms may express immunoaccessible antigens that

Table 76.4 Paraneoplastic syndromes that may be caused by antibody production

Syndrome	Possible antigen	Comment
Stiff-man	Synaptic neural protein*	Symptoms are progressive rigidity of body musculature
Visual	Photoreceptor protein (recoverin)	Retinal degeneration
Subacute cerebellar degeneration	Purkinje cell proteins (e.g. Yo)	Progressive cerebellar symptoms
Eaton–Lambert	Voltage-operated calcium channel (VOCC) protein	Multifocal central nervous symptoms
Encephalomyelitis	Neuronal protein (homologous to *Drosophila* Elav and sex-lethal protein)	Multifocal central nervous symptoms
Intestinal pseudo-obstruction	Antineuronal nuclear protein	Degeneration of the myenteric plexus Gut dysmotility
Subacute sensory neuropathy	A pan-neuronal nuclear antigen	Painful sensory neuropathy
Opsoclonus-ataxia	DNA-binding protein (homologous to yeast splicing protein, MER 1)	Abnormal motor control of eyes, trunk and limbs
Glomerulonephritis	Multiple tumour antigens	Antigen–antibody complex deposition
Pemphigus	Desmoplakin I and II epithelial cell junction proteins	Acantholysis
Idiopathic thrombocytopenic purpura	Platelet antigens	Thrombocytopenia

* Most patients with stiff-man syndrome do not have cancer; 60% of these non-cancer-associated stiff-man patients have antibodies against the synaptic enzyme glutamic acid decarboxylase.

are not normally available to the immune system. Such antigens may lead to antibody production, which in turn may produce striking symptoms if the normal tissue expressing those antigens is damaged. Table 76.4 lists the syndromes that have been described to be associated with cancer and which may be caused by antibody production.

It is attractive to postulate that a particular antibody causes a particular clinical syndrome, but this is not proven. The most common cancer type associated with neurological syndromes is SCLC; however, other carcinomas are also associated with such neurological syndromes. As was true for the protein hormone-related syndromes, only a small percentage of patients with a given neoplasm develop a neurological syndrome. Thus, in a prospective study of 150 patients with SCLC, only two had Eaton–Lambert syndrome, and one had subacute sensory neuropathy [10]. When patients with specific neurological syndromes are studied, however, the incidence of cancer is high. About 60% of patients with Eaton–Lambert syndrome and 50% of patients with subacute cerebellar degeneration have an associated cancer. When cerebellar degeneration is associated with breast or ovarian cancer, an antibody directed against Purkinje cells is usually present. When cerebellar degeneration is associated with other cancers, anti-yo is usually absent. Patients with encephalomyelitis and SCLC almost always have antibodies against a neuronal nuclear antigen (anti-hu) [11].

Buchanovich and colleagues [12] recently reported that the circulating antibody in patients with breast and lung cancer, and the paraneoplastic opsoclonus-ataxia syndrome, is directed against a nuclear neuronal protein. The protein is highly homologous to the yeast splicing protein MER 1. Opsoclonus-ataxia is a dramatic disturbance characterized by abnormal or inability to control eyes, limbs and trunk, and occurs in women with breast or lung cancer.

Table 76.5 Miscellaneous paraneoplastic syndromes of unknown cause

Sweets syndrome (acute febrile neutrophilia dermatosis)
Acute necrotizing myopathy
Fever
Pulmonary osteoarthropathy

Miscellaneous syndromes

A number of other indirect effects of neoplasms have been described for which the pathogenesis remains unknown. Some of these are listed in Table 76.5.

References

1. Lipsett MB, Odell WD, Rosenberg LE, Waldmann TA. Humoral syndromes associated with non-endocrine tumors. *Ann. Intern. Med.* 1964;**61**(4):733–56.
2. Odell WD, Wolfsen A, Yoshimoto Y *et al.* Ectopic peptide synthesis: a universal concomitant of neoplasia. *Trans. Assoc. Am. Physicians* 1977;**90**:204–27.
3. Odell WD, Saito E. Protein hormonelike materials from normal and cancer cells — 'ectopic' hormone production. In Mirand EA, Hutchinson WB, Mihich E (eds). *13th International Cancer Congress, Part E, Cancer Management.* New York: Alan R. Liss, 1983:247–58.
4. Saito E, Iwasa S, Odell WD. Widespread presence of large molecular weight adrenocorticotropin-like substances in normal rat extrapituitary tissues. *Endocrinology* 1983;**113**(3):1010–19.
5. Stewart PM, Gibson S, Crosby SR *et al.* ACTH precursors characterized the ectopic ACTH syndrome. *Clin. Endocrinol.* 1994;**40**:199–204.
6. Delisle L, Boyer MJ, Warr D *et al.* Ectopic corticotropin syndrome and small-cell carcinoma of the lung. Clinical features, outcome, and complications. *Arch. Intern. Med.*1993;**153**:746–52.
7. Nussbaum SR, Gaz RD, Arnold A. Hypercalcemia and ectopic secretion of parathyroid hormone by an ovarian carcinoma with rearrangement of the gene for pocathormone. *N. Engl. J. Med.*1990;**323**:1324–8.
8. Yoneda T, Nishimura R, Kato I *et al.* Frequency of the hypercalcemia-leukocytosis syndrome in oral malignancies. *Cancer* 1991;**68**:617–22.
9. Wetzler M, Estrov Z, Talpaz M, Markowitz A, Gutterman JU. Granulocyte macrophage colony-stimulating factor as a cause of paraneoplastic leukemoid reaction in advanced transitional cell carcinoma. *J. Intern. Med.* 1993;**234**:417–20.
10. Elmington GM, Murray NM, Spiro SG. Neurological paraneoplastic syndromes in patients with small cell lung cancer. A prospective survey of 150 patients. *J. Neurol. Neurosurg. Psychiatry* 1991;**54**(9):764–7.
11. Graus F, Rene R. Clinical and pathological advances on central nervous paraneoplastic syndromes. *Rev. Neurol. (Paris)* 1992;**148**:496–501.
12. Buchanovich RJ, Posner JB, Darnell RB. Nova, the paraneoplastic Ri antigen, is homologous to an RNA-binding protein and is specifically expressed in the developing motor system. *Neuron* 1993;**11**:657–72.

77

Syndrome of Inappropriate Antidiuretic Hormone Secretion

PETER H. BAYLIS

Introduction

The syndrome of inappropriate antidiuretic hormone secretion (SIADH) was first described over half a century ago. A group of patients who mainly had pulmonary tuberculosis was characterized by persistent hypochloraemia and excessive urinary chloride excretion. The hypothesis generated to account for these observations was that water overload had occurred, probably due to continuous secretion of antidiuretic hormone (ADH; also known as vasopressin). Later, two patients with bronchogenic carcinoma were reported to show hyponatraemia, urinary salt wasting and impaired urinary dilution. Persistent ADH secretion was proposed as the underlying pathogenetic mechanism. A similar cluster of biochemical observations had already been made in a group of healthy volunteers given exogenous vasopressin injections over a number of days, which lent support to the original hypothesis. By 1967, Bartter and Schwartz had formally characterized the syndrome and defined the cardinal features (Table 77.1) [1]. During the past 25 years, extensive studies on man and animal models have expanded our knowledge of hypotonic hyponatraemia, its effects on cellular, brain and whole body physiology, and have started to clarify its management.

Diagnosis and differential diagnosis

SIADH is probably the most common cause of hyponatraemia, and certainly the most frequent cause of clinically euvolaemic hyponatraemia. It must be differentiated from other causes of hyponatraemia.

Hyponatraemia may be classified into three groups dependent on the status of the extracellular volume. In hypervolaemic hyponatraemia the extracellular compartment is expanded, and therefore recognized clinically by dependent oedema, raised jugular venous pressure and occasionally ascites. Severe cardiac failure, decompensated cirrhosis and acute renal failure are typical causes of this form of hyponatraemia. Hypovolaemic hyponatraemia is characterized by postural hypotension, poor skin turgor, increased thirst, tachycardia and other signs of extracellular dehydration. Salt and water losses due to profound vomiting and diarrhoea, excessive burns, renal or adrenal disorders (renal salt-wasting syndromes or mineralocorticoid deficiency) account for most conditions leading to hypovolaemic hyponatraemia.

In SIADH, although there are no clinical signs of extracellular volume disturbance, there is increase in total body water, which is distributed between intracellular and extracellular compartments, approximately in the ratio of 2 : 1. Therefore, there is some expansion of the extracellular volume, but not sufficient to be detected clinically. There is evidence that volume regulatory mechanisms do sense the slight expansion of the extracellular compartment to drive renovascular and endocrine reflexes to reduce the size of this compartment, principally by inducing a persistent natriuresis. Interestingly, this renal sodium loss is believed to contribute substantially to the degree of hyponatraemia in SIADH [2].

Since the management of hyponatraemia varies considerably depending on the volume status it is critical that a firm diagnosis of SIADH is made. Since the majority of causes of any type of hyponatraemia are associated with detectable or even elevated circulating concentrations of vasopressin, the measurement of this hormone is *not* central to establishing a diagnosis of SIADH [3]. The clinician must return to the original cardinal features of the syndrome that were described by Bartter and Schwartz almost 30 years ago (Table 77.1) [1].

There are five essential criteria which support the diagnosis (Table 77.1). Dilutional hyponatraemia (serum sodium < 135 mmol/l) with plasma osmolality < 275 mosmol/kg ensures that hyponatraemia is not spurious, due to a high circulating concentration of macromolecules (proteins or lipoproteins). Usually urinary osmolality is

Table 77.1 Criteria necessary to establish the diagnosis of SIADH

Essential

Dilutional hyponatraemia (low plasma osmolality < 275 mosmol/kg) with hyponatraemia (serum sodium < 135 mmol/l))

Inappropriate urinary concentration in face of hyponatraemia (usually urinary osmolality greater than plasma osmolality)

Normal extracellular fluid volume on clinical examination

Persistent urinary sodium excretion (> 20 mmol/24 h)

Absence of: oedema-forming states; hypovolaemia; other causes of euvolaemic hyponatraemia (e.g. hypothyroidism, ACTH deficiency, recent diuretic therapy)

Supportive

Abnormal water load test (inability to excrete at least 80% of a 20 ml/kg water load over 4 hours)

Detectable or elevated plasma vasopressin

ACTH, adrenocorticotrophic hormone.

greater than plasma osmolality. Occasionally urinary osmolality may drop below 300 mosmol/kg but is never maximally dilute. By definition, the extracellular volume appears to be clinically normal. There is persistent urinary sodium excretion if patients maintain normal regular salt and water intake. Supportive but not diagnostic features of SIADH are also given in Table 77.1.

Clinical features of hyponatraemia

The symptoms and signs of hyponatraemia caused by SIADH relate to the absolute value of serum sodium and to its rate of fall.

Moderate degrees of hyponatraemia, even with values of serum sodium falling to 120 mmol/l, may not cause any symptoms. Sudden reduction in serum sodium, often as a result of iatrogenic intervention, to levels of just 125 mmol/l can cause seizures. As serum sodium falls below 120 mmol/l there is an increasing likelihood of the development of clinical features, and it is most unusual for patients with serum sodium values less than 110 mmol/l to be free of symptoms. Clinical features and morbidity are more evident in children, the elderly and menstruant women [4].

The most significant signs and symptoms relate to the central nervous system, and are due to brain oedema [5]. Table 77.2 gives the important features of hyponatraemic encephalopathy divided into groups defined by order of severity, which may not be directly related to the absolute concentration of serum sodium.

By the time symptomatic hyponatraemia occurs there is cellular hypervolaemia which leads to brain oedema. Pressure of the swollen brain on the skull results in a decrease in cerebral blood flow and even pressure necrosis of brain tissue. Brain cells are able to adapt to hypotonicity to some extent. The initial effect of hypo-osmolality is

Table 77.2 Features of hyponatraemic encephalopathy

Mild
Headache
Nausea and vomiting
Weakness

Moderate
Confusion
Hallucinations
Incontinence

Severe
Seizure activity
Unresponsive
Hypoventilation
Extensor plantar response
Coma

an increase in cellular volume, which is minimized by the loss of intracellular solutes; first intracellular potassium is extruded, followed by a substantial decrease in a variety of brain organic osmolytes, including amino acids [6]. If cerebral adaptation is incomplete and symptomatic hyponatraemia is not corrected, then tentorial herniation may occur with consequent respiratory arrest, cerebral hypoxia and ischaemia leading to death. This dramatic sequence of events has now been verified by magnetic resonance imaging (MRI) and computed tomography (CT) images.

Causes of SIADH in malignant disease

It has been recognized for many years that malignant tumours cause SIADH (Table 77.3). Many tumours are capable of synthesizing a variety of endocrine peptides, of which vasopressin is only one. Bronchogenic carcinoma is probably the most common malignancy associated

Table 77.3 Some causes of SIADH associated with malignancy

Tumorous
Chest:
    bronchogenic carcinoma
    mesothelioma
    thymoma
    Hodgkin's lymphoma

Non-chest:
    pancreatic carcinoma
    duodenal carcinoma
    Ewing's sarcoma
    bladder, urethral carcinoma
    prostatic carcinoma
    leukaemia
    lymphoma

Drug-related
Chemotherapeutic agents:
    vincristine
    vinblastine
    cyclophosphamide

Analgesics:
    narcotics
    non-steroidal anti-inflammatory agents

Intercurrent illnesses
Chest:
    pneumonia
    lung abscess
    empyema

Central nervous system:
    brain abscess
    intracranial haemorrhage
    cavernous sinus thrombosis

with SIADH. Vasopressin, its precursor molecule and mRNA have all been isolated from tumours. Interestingly, some tumours appear to be capable of synthesizing vasopressin but do not cause SIADH. It is presumed that these tumours fail to release the peptide into the systemic circulation or do so at such a slow rate that the ectopic vasopressin is in insufficient circulating concentrations to influence water balance.

Although there is no doubt that ectopic production by tumours leads to SIADH, there are alternative mechanisms by which tumours cause this syndrome. It appears that tumours can influence the secretion of neurohypophysial vasopressin which results in SIADH. Details of these non-ectopic mechanisms are given below.

SIADH associated with malignant disease may not be due to the tumour itself, but can result from the administration of chemotherapeutic agents, analgesics (particularly narcotics), or drugs used to control associated neuropsychiatric complications (Table 77.3). Similarly, an intercurrent illness associated with malignancy could cause SIADH; for example, a respiratory infection related to a bronchogenic carcinoma not infrequently leads to hyponatraemia due to SIADH. Of particular importance is the recognition of hyponatraemia due to hypocortisolaemia, which can result from metastatic spread of tumours to both adrenal glands. Treatment with replacement steroids leads to rapid resolution of hyponatraemia, immensely improved quality of life, and the patient may survive for a number of years despite widespread disease.

After severe head injury, with or without fracture, hyponatraemia may develop, usually due to SIADH. Immediately after the trauma there is a short period of a few days of polyuria due to vasopressin deficiency followed by a variable length of time of antidiuresis, which is thought to be due to excessive leakage of vasopressin from the posterior pituitary stores. Complete recovery usually occurs but occasionally diabetes insipidus recurs. A small proportion of post-trauma patients develop hyponatraemia due to persistent renal sodium excretion for up to a week. This should not be confused with SIADH because treatment of cerebral salt wasting requires saline replacement, which is not appropriate for the management of SIADH.

Pathogenesis

Persistent secretion of vasopressin from a tumour or from the neurohypophysis which is inappropriate for the ambient hypo-osmolality is pivotal to the development of SIADH. Continued fluid intake, however, is also central to maintain hyponatraemia. Many acute animal models designed to mimic SIADH fail to do so because the animals regulate water intake. This does not happen in man who persists in drinking. The precise reason is unknown but it is suggested that the osmotic inhibitory mechanism for thirst is weaker in man.

A considerable advance in the understanding of osmoregulation of vasopressin secretion in SIADH came from the studies performed by Zerbe and colleagues [7]. At least four distinct patterns of vasopressin secretion emerged from the group of SIADH patients, each of whom was stimulated osmotically by infusion of hypertonic saline. The patterns of vasopressin response are represented in Fig. 77.1. Patients with malignant disease and SIADH were not confined to one particular response pattern but were represented in each of the four responses.

Type A is characterized by erratic fluctuations in plasma vasopressin which are completely independent of plasma osmolality. Random ectopic release of vasopressin from tumours is a ready explanation of this pattern of secretion.

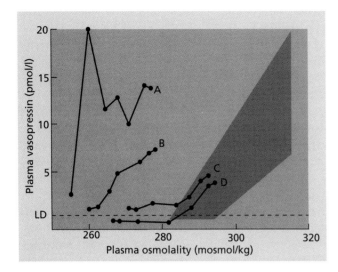

Fig. 77.1 Four patterns (Types A–D) of vasopressin response to osmotic stimulation in a group of patients all of whom have the syndrome of inappropriate antidiuretic hormone secretion. The darker shaded area represents the normal response. (Adapted from [7] with permission.)

However, as the erratic response is also observed in patients without tumorous disease, other mechanisms, possibly transient erratic non-osmotic stimulation of vasopressin release, must play a role.

A second group of patients (type B) demonstrate resetting of the 'vasopressin osmostat' to the left of normal, which is identified by a normal incremental increase in plasma vasopressin in response to graded rises in plasma osmolality but the osmotic threshold for vasopressin release is abnormally low. Although patients with malignant disease can show this type of vasopressin response, there is no evidence that vasopressin-secreting tumours are osmotically sensitive. Therefore, it is most probable that these patients have SIADH due to inappropriate neurohypophysial vasopressin release. A shift to the left of normal of the vasopressin osmoregulatory line could be accounted for by: (i) interruption of the normal afferent inhibitory baroregulatory pathways; (ii) loss of intracellular osmolytes; or (iii) hypotension and/or hypovolaemia. The latter, however, is untenable because SIADH patients are, by definition, euvolaemic.

A small number of patients with malignant disease had type C pattern, which is characterized by normal vasopressin osmoregulation except that secretion could not be switched off at low plasma osmolalities. This 'leak' of vasopressin could be due to: (i) loss of inhibitory osmoregulatory neurones; (ii) injury to the neurohypophysis; or, most likely, (iii) persistent ectopic vasopressin secretion from a tumour combined with normal osmoregulated neurohypophysial vasopressin.

Type D patients have entirely normal osmoregulated vasopressin release but fulfilled the essential criteria for SIADH and were unable to excrete a water load. It is a very unusual situation, identified in few patients with malignant disease. This combination of observations implies that either the kidney is peculiarly sensitive to normal circulating concentrations of vasopressin or there is another antidiuretic agent.

Although these studies are of considerable pathophysiological interest, establishing the pattern of vasopressin response to osmotic stimulation in SIADH is of no value in identifying its cause.

'Renal escape' from antidiuresis

Animal models of SIADH have clearly shown that when treated chronically with vasopressin they can reduce urine osmolality and increase urine volume despite continued administration of vasopressin. This phenomenon is described as 'renal escape' from antidiuresis, and is largely due to a pressure diuresis resulting from alterations in intrarenal haemodynamics and only partly to increases in systemic atrial natriuretic peptide. In humans, the 'renal escape' phenomenon is less pronounced than in the animal models [6]. 'Renal escape' from antidiuresis does offer a mechanism to limit further water retention and the development of more profound hyponatraemia.

Treatment

The management of hyponatraemia including SIADH, remains confused and controversial [4,8]. It is, however, generally accepted that asymptomatic patients are at no major risk of complications from hyponatraemia *per se*, and therefore do not require specific therapy. Thus, it is essential to assess patients for central nervous system symptoms and signs of hyponatraemia. There is substantial morbidity and mortality in severely hyponatraemic patients, with mortality rates approaching 50% in early studies. The development of acute hyponatraemia appears to be associated with more complications than chronic hyponatraemia since the brain has had less time to adapt to hypo-osmolality. Treatment of hyponatraemia itself, however, can also lead to significant mortality and morbidity, particularly if the correction rate of serum sodium is rapid [9].

The management of chronic SIADH has traditionally been total fluid restriction to 0.5–1 litre per 24 hours. Many patients can tolerate rigorous reductions in water intake, but others find it difficult. For these patients, a variety of alternative means of increasing renal water excretion have been devised. Partial nephrogenic diabetes insipidus can be induced with demeclocycline (1.2 g daily in divided doses) or with lithium, which is more toxic and less reliable than demeclocycline. An alternative approach is the administration of frusemide (40–80 mg daily) to induce a natriuresis but replace the sodium loss by giving salt 3 g daily. These methods have the advantage of slowly correcting serum sodium and are suitable mainly for patients with mild or, possibly, moderate degrees of symptomatic hyponatraemia (Table 77.2).

Severely symptomatic patients require more active therapy and consideration must be given to infusion of isotonic and, occasionally, hypertonic saline solutions. There are good data to suggest that serum sodium must not be corrected more rapidly than 0.5 mmol/l per hour, or 10 mmol/l per 24 hours [9]. It is probably unnecessary fully to correct hyponatraemia, and a target serum sodium of 125 mmol/l is quite satisfactory.

The development of an efficacious specific receptor antagonist to the antidiuretic actions of vasopressin (V_2-receptor antagonist) would increase renal water excretion effectively but has proved elusive. Although V_2-receptor agonists are readily available, V_2-receptor peptide antagonists based on modifications of the native vasopressin molecule have all failed to be effective in man to date. There are, however, promising preliminary data on linear V_2-receptor antagonists which may allow another class of drugs to be used in the management of both acute and chronic symptomatic hyponatraemia of SIADH.

Osmotic demyelination syndrome (central pontine myelinolysis)

During the past two decades, a few patients recovering from profound hyponatraemia have developed myelinolysis in pontine and extrapontine structures. Neurological sequelae were grave, with patients suffering from quadriparesis, bulbar palsy, coma or death, which tended to occur 2–4 days after normonatraemia had been achieved. Controversy surrounds all the factors responsible for the demyelination but one that appears to be important in man is the rapid correction of serum sodium [9]. Results from recent animal studies suggest that both rate and magnitude of correction of serum sodium are risk factors for brain demyelination.

To minimize the problems of overactive treatment a rational approach to therapy should consider the following points: (i) the patient must have symptomatic hyponatraemia; (ii) the rate of sodium correction should be no greater than 0.5 mmol/l per hour; (iii) active treatment should stop when serum sodium reaches 125 mmol/l; and (iv) magnitude of total correction should not exceed 25 mmol/l.

References

1. Bartter FC, Schwartz WB. The syndrome of inappropriate secretion of antidiuretic hormone. *Am. J. Med.* 1967;**42**:790–806.
2. Verbalis JG. Hyponatraemia. In Baylis PH (ed.). *Water and Salt Homeostasis in Health and Disease.* London: Baillière Tindall, 1989:499–530.
3. Anderson RJ, Chung H-M, Kluge R, Schrier RW. Hyponatraemia: a prospective analysis of its epidemiology and the pathogenetic role of vasopressin. *Ann. Intern. Med.* 1985;**102**:164–8.
4. Arieff AI. Management of hyponatraemia. *Br. Med. J.* 1993;**307**:305–8.
5. Arieff AI. Central nervous system manifestations of disordered sodium metabolism. *Clin. Endocrinol. Metab.* 1984;**13**:269–94.
6. Verbalis JG. Hyponatremia: answered and unanswered questions. *Am. J. Kidney Dis.* 1991;**18**:546–52.
7. Zerbe R, Stropes L, Robertson GL. Vasopressin function in the syndrome of inappropriate antidiuresis. *Annu. Rev. Med.* 1980;**31**:315–27.
8. Narins RG. Therapy of hyponatremia. Does haste make waste? *N. Engl. J. Med.* 1986;**314**:1573–5.
9. Sterns RH, Riggs JE, Schochet SS. Osmotic demyelination syndrome following correction of hyponatremia. *N. Engl. J. Med.* 1986;**314**:1535–42.

Hypercalcaemia of Malignancy

E. BARBARA MAWER

Normal calcium homeostasis

The human body contains 25–35 mol (1.0–1.4 kg) of calcium of which 99% is in the skeleton; only about 25 mmol (1 g) is present in the extracellular fluid and a further 25 mmol in soft tissues. The plasma calcium concentration is maintained within a narrow range, around 2.4 mmol/l, by means of complex homeostatic mechanisms. Inside cells cytoplasmic calcium concentration may be as low as 0.1 µmol/l, although it can be concentrated at millimolar concentrations in intracellular organelles. Many basic cellular processes require calcium ions and are controlled by the ionized fraction (about half the total) of the plasma calcium.

Processes in which calcium is intimately involved include controlling the excitability of nerve and muscle cells, muscular contraction, hormone secretion, blood clotting and intracellular signalling. A combination of non-hormonal mechanisms and a series of hormonal loops together control fluxes of calcium between the extracellular fluid and the three major organs or tissues involved, namely, bone, intestine and kidney, to achieve the appropriate ionized calcium concentration [1].

Calcium, present in the diet, enters the body from the intestinal lumen and is excreted primarily through the kidney, although some calcium is secreted into the intestine and excreted in the faeces together with unabsorbed dietary calcium. One of the major hormones involved is the active metabolite of vitamin D, 1,25-dihydroxyvitamin D (1,25(OH)$_2$D), whose primary function is to promote the intestinal absorption of calcium by receptor-mediated up-regulation of the synthesis of specific calcium-binding proteins.

Urinary excretion of calcium is increased when the filtered load is large, and renal tubular reabsorption increases when calcium needs to be conserved. Around 98% of the filtered load is usually reabsorbed; about 65% by an active mechanism linked to the reabsorption of

sodium in the proximal tubule, 20–25% in the ascending limb of the loop of Henle and about 10% in the distal convoluted tubule; the latter process is promoted by parathyroid hormone (PTH), which also acts as a trophic hormone for the synthesis of 1,25(OH)$_2$D in the cells of the proximal tubule.

In adults calcium is mobilized from the mineral phase of bone by the process of remodelling. Under the influence of PTH and 1,25(OH)$_2$D, bone matrix and mineral are removed by osteoclastic resorption and replaced in a linked sequence by osteoblast-mediated mineralization. When the two processes are synchronized there will be no net gain or loss of calcium, but the opportunity for exchange with the plasma pool arises. The remodelling sequence, which is measured in weeks, is too long to be important in normal short-term homeostasis but calcium can be exchanged rapidly between the extracellular fluid and the bone lining and periosteal cells. Calcitonin, a hormone produced by the C cells of the thyroid gland, causes calciuresis and has an inhibitory effect on osteoclastic resorption *in vitro*; there is little evidence that it is important in normal calcium homeostasis in adults but it is useful in controlling resorption in certain bone diseases. The components of normal homeostatic control of plasma calcium are shown in Fig. 78.1.

Hypercalcaemia

A tendency for plasma ionized calcium to rise is normally counteracted by homeostatic mechanisms coming into play. Even a small increase in ionized calcium can be detected by calcium receptors on the surface of parathyroid cells which respond by decreasing the release of PTH. The lowered PTH concentration permits increased renal excretion of calcium and also decreases the synthesis of 1,25(OH)$_2$D, resulting in less calcium absorption from the duodenum. In the longer term the decreased concentration of both hormones will lead to lower bone

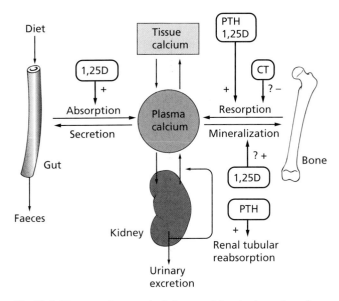

Fig. 78.1 Homeostatic control of plasma calcium in the region of 2.20–2.60 mmol/l is achieved largely through the actions of parathyroid hormone (PTH) and 1,25-dihydroxyvitamin D (1,25D) on bone, kidneys and gut. In an adult in calcium balance, the net absorption of calcium from the gut will equal the urinary excretion, and calcium released from bone by resorption will equal that deposited by mineralization. CT, calcitonin.

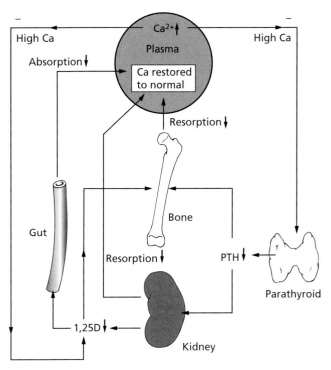

Fig. 78.2 The homeostatic response to a rise in plasma calcium (Ca) involves the inhibitory effects of calcium on parathyroid hormone (PTH) release and on renal synthesis of 1,25-dihydroxyvitamin D (1,25D). The resulting decreases in renal tubular reabsorption and intestinal absorption of calcium, together with reduced bone resorption, all contribute to the lowering of plasma calcium.

mineral turnover. The net result of all these actions is to lower the plasma calcium to normal (Fig. 78.2).

Hypercalcaemia, defined as a total serum calcium concentration above 2.60–2.65 mmol/l becomes symptomatic and potentially serious, when the level exceeds 3 mmol/l. Characteristic symptoms are shown in Table 78.1. Cardiac arrhythmias and acute renal failure may develop, with fatal results, if the calcium concentration exceeds about 4.0 mmol/l, and urgent treatment is required.

The major causes of hypercalcaemia are primary hyperparathyroidism and malignant disease, although other, rarer conditions may need to be considered in the differential diagnosis (Table 78.2).

In most cases hypercalcaemia complicating malignant disease is believed to occur by one of two mechanisms, either following metastasis to bone resulting in local osteolysis, or as a result of bone mobilizing factors produced by the tumour or its metastases, which act on bone, and possibly kidney, in a humoral fashion. Increasingly, however, there is evidence for overlap between these processes and the details are discussed below. It is appropriate here to consider biochemical measurements [2] which may help to distinguish hypercalcaemia secondary to malignant disease from other types, although in practice it is likely that the presence of a tumour will already be evident. Malignant disease may coexist with primary

Table 78.1 Signs and symptoms of hypercalcaemia

Anorexia, nausea, vomiting, constipation, acute pancreatitis

Thirst, polyuria, impaired glomerular filtration, dehydration, hypercalciuria, renal stones

Lethargy, confusion, depression, headache, irritability, sleep disturbance

Cardiac arrhythmias

Acute renal failure

Table 78.2 Differential diagnosis of hypercalcaemia

Primary hyperparathyroidism
Malignant disease with/without metastases
Granulomatous disease
Vitamin D or vitamin A intoxication
Thyrotoxicosis
Addison's disease
Familial hypocalciuric hypercalcaemia
Idiopathic hypercalcaemia of infancy (Williams' syndrome)
Milk alkali syndrome
Immobilization
Spurious, from abnormal proteins (macroglobulinaemia)

hyperparathyroidism, in which case PTH measurement is crucial to understanding the cause of the hypercalcaemia.

Hypercalcaemia is usually defined in terms of the total plasma calcium concentration, although it is the ionized or free fraction which is responsible for biological activity. Ionized calcium (normal range about 1.15–1.30 mmol/l) can be measured in suitably collected samples by using a calcium electrode but few routine laboratories have this facility. Instead, total calcium can be corrected for the plasma albumin concentration, which is the major determinant of plasma calcium binding. Various formulae are available, for example, corrected plasma calcium (mmol/l) = measured plasma calcium (mmol/l) + 0.02 (40-plasma albumin (g/l)). Correction is particularly necessary in malignant disease where plasma albumin levels may be low and an apparently normal total calcium may mask a raised ionized fraction.

Hypercalcaemia arising from a benign tumour of the parathyroids (primary hyperparathyroidism) will, by definition, be associated with a raised plasma PTH level. $1,25(OH)_2D$ tends to be high or at the upper end of the normal range and urinary calcium is usually raised because of the increased filtered load of calcium, despite the effects of PTH on renal tubular reabsorption. In contrast, in malignancy-associated hypercalcaemia the primary cause is usually increased mobilization of calcium from bone leading to suppression of PTH. The combination of hypercalcaemia and low PTH would be expected to result in suppressed levels of $1,25(OH)_2D$, as is indeed found in many cases; however, this is not an inevitable part of the biochemical picture (see below). The main humoral factor responsible for malignancy-associated hypercalcaemia, parathyroid hormone-related peptide (PTHrP), will be described in detail below, but it may be noted that this hormone can now be assayed reliably in plasma and its presence above control level will confirm a malignant origin of the hypercalcaemia, although its absence will not rule it out. Urinary calcium is usually raised provided the patient has been adequately rehydrated, but may be masked by the dehydration often present at initial diagnosis. It is more reliably expressed as urinary calcium excretion in µmol/l glomerular filtrate.

Hypercalcaemia associated with granulomatous disease, such as sarcoidosis, follows an increase in vitamin D, either in the diet or as a result of exposure to sunlight. The 25-hydroxyvitamin D produced provides substrate for uncontrolled 1α-hydroxylase activity induced in activated macrophages and produces high serum concentrations of $1,25(OH)_2D$. A similar mechanism in some types of haematological malignancy, for example Hodgkin's lymphoma, also causes raised $1,25(OH)_2D$ [3]. In these cases increased intestinal absorption of calcium contributes to the hypercalcaemia. Other potential causes of hypercalcaemia can be identified by the appropriate measurements, for example thyroid hormones in thyrotoxicosis, cortisol in Addison's disease or 25-hydroxyvitamin D in vitamin D intoxication.

Hypercalcaemia of malignancy

Hypercalcaemia is most commonly associated with cancers of the lung (squamous cell), breast, pancreas, urogenital organs and with haematological malignancies such as lymphoma and myeloma, although other types of cancer are not excluded [4]. Classically, tumours associated with hypercalcaemia have been divided into two categories, those releasing calcium directly by metastatic spread to bone and those producing humoral calcium-releasing factors which reach the bone through the systemic circulation. More recent evidence suggests that the differences may be less clearcut and that some tumours may produce their effects by more than one mechanism. Table 78.3, for convenience, classifies tumours into four types and summarizes the present state of knowledge on the agents responsible for hypercalcaemia of malignancy.

Solid tumours that readily metastasize to bone, such as breast and squamous cell lung cancers, may result in large lytic lesions. At one time it was thought that tumour cells could resorb bone directly, but there is little recent evidence for this and it is now generally thought that tumour cells, attracted to bone by a chemotactic mechanism, secrete factors that increase osteoclastic activity. These factors include the transforming growth factors, TGF-α and TGF-β which are present in conditioned medium from many breast cancer cells and cell lines. Prostaglandins produced by breast cancer cells have also been reported to cause bone resorption *in vitro*, and this resorption to be inhibited by aspirin or indomethacin. Treatment of hypercalcaemia with non-steroidal anti-inflammatory agents (NSAIDs) has, however, not been successful in patients (see below). It has also been suggested that breast cancer cells could stimulate cells of the immune system to produce cytokines such as lymphotoxin, interleukin-1 (IL-1) or tumour necrosis factor (TNF), which would then resorb bone.

Widespread bone destruction with osteolytic lesions is a common complication of myeloma, the haematological malignancy with the highest incidence of hypercalcaemia. Osteolysis is believed to be mediated by cytokines such as lymphotoxin, IL-1 or TNF; more recent evidence implicates IL-6 as another possible cause. The extent of the hypercalcaemia does not appear to relate directly to the amount of bone destruction, and its high incidence suggests that it may be precipitated by other factors.

Table 78.3 Causes of hypercalcaemia in different types of cancer

Type of tumour	Agents implicated	Effect
Tumours with bone metastases		
Solid tumours		
breast, lung, prostate	TGF-α/β, lymphotoxin, TNF, IL-1	Local, bone
Haematological malignancies		
Myeloma	Lymphotoxin, TNF-α, IL-1, IL-6	Local, bone
Lymphoma	Lymphotoxin, TNF-α, IL-1	Local, bone
Tumours without bone metastases, humoral effects		
Solid tumours		
Lung, kidney, head and neck	PTHrP	Systemic, bone, kidney
	PG, TGF-α/β, TNF-α, IL-1	Systemic, bone
Haematological malignances		
Hodgkin's lymphoma	1,25(OH)$_2$D	Systemic, gut, bone
T-cell/B-cell lymphoma	1,25(OH)$_2$D	Systemic, gut, bone
	Lymphokines	Bone
	PTHrP	Bone, kidney

1,25(OH)$_2$D, 1,25-dihydroxyvitamin D; IL, interleukin; PG, prostaglandins; PTHrP, parathyroid hormone-related peptide; TGF, transforming growth factor; TNF, tumour necrosis factor.

Probably the most important contribution is made by the renal impairment which is often a feature of myeloma, due to the nephrotoxic effects of immunoglobulin light chains (Bence–Jones protein nephropathy).

The term 'humoral hypercalcaemia of malignancy' (HHM) was suggested first by Martin, to describe the syndrome in which bone metastases were absent or insignificant. The fascinating story, in which the suggestion by Albright in 1941 that hypercalcaemia in some cases of malignancy might be caused by a parathyroid hormone-like factor, finally bore fruit with the characterization of PTHrP in 1987, is beyond the scope of this chapter, but can be read elsewhere [5].

The tumour types associated classically with HHM are squamous cell carcinomas of skin, lung, head and neck. Many breast tumours have also been shown to produce PTHrP, suggesting that osteolytic and humoral mechanisms are not mutually exclusive. Tumour tissue has been used experimentally as the source of mRNAs for PTHrP, enabling cDNAs to be cloned and the protein sequences to be deduced [5].

The amino terminus of PTHrP shows considerable homology with PTH and has eight of the first 13 amino acids in common; the PTH-like actions of PTHrP are associated with the amino terminal region, residues 1–34. PTHrP binds to the same receptors as PTH in classical target organs, stimulating the same adenylate cyclase

response. Animal models of hypercalcaemia have been developed in which the role of PTHrP can be reproduced, and in which antibodies to PTHrP have been effective in correcting the hypercalcaemia [6].

In cell systems *in vitro*, PTHrP appears to be less potent than PTH in renal cells, but equipotent in bone cells. Nevertheless, the renal actions of PTHrP are believed to contribute to the raised plasma calcium in HHM and evidence has been produced for increased renal tubular reabsorption of calcium [7]. Elevated nephrogenous cAMP level is considered by some investigators to be an important factor in the definition of HHM. Enhanced osteoclastic resorption though is usually the major component of the increased plasma calcium and is brought about by PTHrP, probably acting through PTH/PTHrP receptors on osteoblastic cells, which may then produce cytokines that promote osteoclastic activity. In contrast to PTH, PTHrP seems to have no stimulatory effect on osteoblastic activity, and bone histology is quite different in HHM and primary hyperparathyroidism. Other bone resorbing factors besides PTHrP, and which may act in concert with it, have been identified in tumours and tumour cell lines (see Table 78.3); a recent study has shown that IL-6 can enhance the actions of PTHrP on hypercalcaemia and bone resorption [8].

The effects of PTHrP on the renal production of 1,25(OH)$_2$D are controversial. PTHrP might be predicted to stimulate synthesis in the same way as PTH, and there is some support for this in animal experiments and in tissue culture preparations. However, patients with HHM and raised levels of PTHrP tend to have suppressed plasma concentrations of 1,25(OH)$_2$D. Possible explanations for this include the inhibitory effect of raised renal intracellular calcium on the 1α-hydroxylase or the secretion of other tumour factors which may inhibit the enzyme. In some cases, normal or high levels of 1,25(OH)$_2$D have been reported, and it has been suggested that these are determined by PTHrP levels in the absence of demonstrable metastases. This controversy will probably only be resolved when large series of patients with the same type of cancer are studied, rather than the melange of patients reported in most investigations of hypercalcaemia. The roles of PTHrP in the development of hypercalcaemia are illustrated in Fig. 78.3.

It should be noted that although there are similarities between PTHrP and PTH, the syndrome of HHM differs in many ways from that of primary hyperparathyroidism [9]; despite the common receptor pathway, it seems that the response to the two hormones must be modulated in some way by other factors to produce the different outcomes described above. It is possible that other fragments of the PTHrP molecule may have different effects from the PTH-like amino terminal moiety. The more rapid onset of symptoms in HHM may reflect the rapid growth of the tumour or its metastases in contrast to the usually slow-growing parathyroid adenoma. There is no evidence that PTHrP synthesis is controlled by the prevailing calcium level and so the concentration will increase with the number of secreting cells, whereas in primary hyperparathyroidism, the parathyroid gland is still responsive to control by calcium, but is controlled at a higher set-point (the calcium level at which PTH secretion is half-maximal).

An unusual type of HHM is seen in some cases of lymphoma in which the cause is ectopic synthesis of 1,25(OH)$_2$D, either in the lymphoma cells or in associated activated macrophages [3]; the hormone probably raises plasma calcium by effects on both gut and bone. The phenomenon has been demonstrated in both Hodgkin's and non-Hodgkin's lymphoma and, although initially considered to be rare, has been reported to occur in a high proportion of patients in California. The reason for this may be that high levels of sun exposure maintain concentrations of 25-hydroxyvitamin D that can promote extrarenal 1,25(OH)$_2$D synthesis. A recent study supporting this hypothesis indicates that many patients with lymphoma can elevate their serum 1,25(OH)$_2$D level if treated with 25-hydroxyvitamin D, a response not seen in control subjects [3].

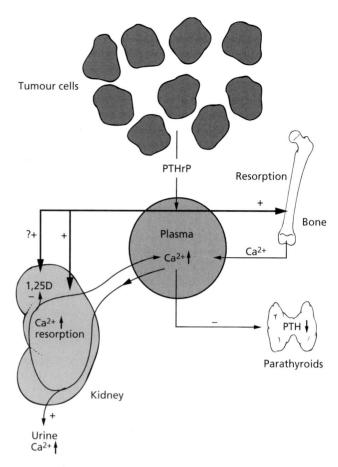

Fig. 78.3 Parathyroid hormone-related protein (PTHrP) secreted by tumour cells stimulates bone resorption and increases the plasma calcium pool. This results in higher urinary excretion of calcium, but the increased filtered load leads to impaired renal function. This together with the stimulatory effect of PTHrP on renal tubular reabsorption of calcium may result in hypercalcaemia. Responses to the increased plasma calcium include suppression of parathyroid hormone (PTH) secretion and impaired synthesis of 1,25-dihydroxyvitamin D (1,25D). The effects of PTHrP on 1,25D synthesis are not clear.

Hypercalcaemia in some lymphomas, especially human T-cell leukaemia virus 1 (HTLV-1), have been associated with the production of PTHrP, while in others, cytokines produced by lymphoma cells may have a direct osteolytic effect in a similar way to that in myeloma.

Current approaches to treatment

The approach to treatment of hypercalcaemia of malignancy will depend upon the severity both of the hypercalcaemia and of the underlying condition. Patients usually become hypercalcaemic at an advanced stage of their disease, often with extensive metastases. Some physicians consider that withholding of treatment may be appropriate in patients who are comatose and for whom no further anticancer therapy is planned.

In theory, if carefully monitored, it should be possible to identify those patients at risk of developing hypercalcaemia; an upward drift of plasma calcium within the normal range, an increase in urinary calcium excretion or a steady rise in plasma PTHrP would all serve as predictors that sooner or later the renal capacity to excrete calcium would be exceeded, with hypercalcaemia as a result. In practice, other investigations are likely to take precedence, and hypercalcaemia usually presents as an emergency.

Severe hypercalcaemia is life-threatening and demands immediate intervention. The main aims are to restore intravascular volume, to promote urinary calcium excretion and to limit the entry of calcium into the extracellular fluid by blocking bone resorption.

Patients are often severely dehydrated because of the inhibitory effects of calcium on the action of ADH in the distal renal tubule, and the nausea and vomiting which restrict oral intake of fluids. The first action is to rehydrate with isotonic saline to the extent of 4–6 l/day. Saline should be used in preference to glucose solutions because calcium reabsorption in the proximal renal tubule is linked to that of sodium, so that saline treatment promotes calcium diuresis and may cause a modest decrease in plasma calcium. Nausea and vomiting should be controlled pharmacologically. Loop diuretics such as frusemide have been used in high doses (80 mg/2 h) in conjunction with saline to promote calcium diuresis, but this approach requires careful monitoring and is not recommended.

When rehydration has been achieved, other agents may be introduced to control the source of increased calcium. These are summarized below and in Table 78.4.

Intravenous phosphate has been used in the past but has now been largely superseded by other treatments. The rationale for phosphate treatment is that a raised concentration of this ion inhibits bone resorption and decreases intestinal absorption of calcium; it probably also reduces $1,25(OH)_2D$ synthesis. The disadvantage is that it causes ectopic precipitation of calcium phosphate. Calcitonin should, theoretically, be useful because of its inhibitory effects on osteoclasts, which possess receptors for the hormone. It is, in practice, less effective than might be predicted because its effects are relatively short term and the calcium-lowering response is not maintained beyond about 48 hours. It may, nevertheless, be useful for short-term therapy, since most patients treated with calcitonin show a response. Mithramycin (plicamycin) is a cytotoxic antibiotic which was found to have calcium-lowering effects by inhibiting osteoclastic activity and

Table 78.4 Treatment of malignancy-related hypercalcaemia

Drug	Dose	Comments
Inorganic phosphorus	1–3 g/day, orally	May cause hyperphosphataemia and ectopic deposition of calcium phosphate, especially in kidney
Calcitonin	4–8 u/kg/day by s.c. or i.m. injection	May cause nausea and vomiting, occasional allergic reaction
Mithramycin	15–25 µg/kg/day for 4–7 days	Nephrotoxic, hepatotoxic, myelotoxic
Glucocorticoids	e.g. Prednisone 40–80 mg/day, orally	Only applicable where tumour is steroid sensitive (myeloma or lymphoma), or producing $1,25(OH)_2D$
Etidronate	7.5 mg/kg per day, slow i.v. infusion, on 3 consecutive days	Maximum effect at 4–6 days, normocalcaemia in up to 40% of patients treated
Pamidronate	30–60 mg, single i.v. infusion, repeated if necessary	Long period of effectiveness, 30 days, normocalcaemia in 80% treated
Clodronate	400–600 mg, single i.v. infusion, oral maintenance of normocalcaemia 400–3200 mg/day	Effective for 10–12 days, normocalcaemia in up to 80% treated

$1,25(OH)_2D$, 1,25-dihydroxyvitamin D.

restricting renal tubular reabsorption of calcium. The extent and duration of the calcium-lowering response are unpredictable and toxicity precludes long-term use. Non-steroidal anti-inflammatory drugs (NSAIDs) have been used to try to control hypercalcaemia on the basis that prostaglandins are implicated in bone resorption, but these have not been found to be effective in practice. Glucocorticosteroids have proved useful in cases where excessive $1,25(OH)_2D$ is the cause of the hypercalcaemia, since they suppress extrarenal synthesis of the hormone.

In the majority of cases where the hypercalcaemia results from excess bone resorption, the most effective agents are the bisphosphonates and this is the treatment of choice. These drugs are analogues of pyrophosphate which differ in the nature of the side-chain substitutions. The mode of action is not fully understood but the overall effect is inhibition of bone resorption. Three bisphosphonates are currently available, etidronate, which is only effective when given by intravenous infusion; pamidronate, a more potent inhibitor of bone resorption, but generally given intravenously, and clodronate which is effective by infusion or by mouth, although oral dosage is more relevant to the maintenance of normocalcaemia once this has been achieved. Clodronate is reported to be more effective in hypercalcaemia resulting from bone metastases rather than the humoral type and may retard progression of bone metastases. Pamidronate appears to be effective for a longer period than either etidronate or clodronate (Table 78.4). A comprehensive review of the use of bisphosphonates in hypercalcaemia of malignancy has been presented by Ralston [10].

Future developments in the treatment of hypercalcaemia will probably include new generations of bisphosphonates with improved potency and more convenient modes of administration. Gallium nitrate has also been shown to be effective in correcting hypercalcaemia in malignant disease, but has to be given as a continuous intravenous infusion; again improvements in administration are being investigated. Most of the therapeutic agents described act at the level of bone resorption; it is to be expected that in the future attempts will be made to control production of PTHrP by tumour cells, so that the adverse effects of this hormone on both bone and kidney can be avoided. A promising finding from this point of view is the report that the somatostatin analogue, octreotide, lowered both PTHrP and calcium in a hypercalcaemic patient with a pancreatic endocrine tumour that was secreting PTHrP. The most effective long-term treatment of malignant hypercalcaemia would, of course, be effective therapy for the underlying cancer.

Conclusion

Hypercalcaemia is an important complication of malignant disease which contributes to the morbidity of seriously ill patients. The causes include metastasis of tumour cells to bone, where they secrete factors which stimulate osteoclastic resorption with the release of calcium into extracellular fluid, or the secretion by tumours of humoral factors which stimulate bone resorption. The most important of these factors is PTHrP, which also promotes renal tubular reabsorption of calcium.

The hypercalcaemia can be severe and life-threatening and requires urgent treatment. After initial rehydration, drugs which inhibit bone resorption should be given to decrease the amount of calcium entering the plasma; of these the most effective are the bisphosphonates. Most treatment for hypercalcaemia of malignancy is palliative, in that patients usually have advanced disease, but where symptoms can be relieved, the patient's remaining quality of life can be improved.

References

1. Mundy GR. Calcium homeostasis — role of the gut, kidney and bone. In Mundy G R. *Calcium Homeostasis: Hypercalcaemia and Hypocal-caemia*. London: Martin Dunitz, 1990:16–27.
2. Mawer EB, Berry JL. The measurement of metabolic bone disease. In Tovey FI, Stamp TCB (eds). *Measurements in Medicine — Metabolic Bone Disease*. London: Parthenon Publishing, 1995:49–76.
3. Davies M, Hayes ME, Yin JAL, Berry JL, Mawer EB. Abnormal synthesis of 1,25-dihydroxyvitamin D in patients with malignant lymphoma. *J. Clin. Endocrinol. Metab.* 1994;78:1202–7.
4. Mundy GR. Hypercalcemia of malignancy revisited. *J. Clin. Invest.* 1988;82:1–6.
5. Martin TJ. Properties of parathyroid hormone related-protein and its role in malignant hypercalcaemia. *Q. J. Med.* 1990;76:771–86.
6. Kukreja SC, Shevrin DH, Wimbuscus SA *et al*. Antibodies to parathyroid hormone-related protein lowers serum calcium in athymic mouse models of malignancy-associated hypercalcemia due to human tumors. *J. Clin. Invest.* 1988;82:1798–802.
7. Bonjour J-P, Guelpa PG, Bisetti A *et al*. Bone and renal components of hypercalcemia of malignancy and response to a single infusion of clodronate. *Bone* 1988;9:123–30.
8. De La Mata J, Uy HL, Guise TA *et al.* Interleukin-6 enhances hypercalcaemia and bone resorption mediated by parathyroid hormone-related protein *in vivo*. *J. Clin. Invest.* 1995;95:2846–52.
9. Stewart AF, Horst RL, Deftos LJ *et al*. Biochemical evaluation of patients with cancer-associated hypercalcemia. *N. Engl. J. Med.* 1980;303:1377–83.
10. Ralston SH. Pathogenesis and management of cancer associated hypercalcaemia. In Hanks GW, Sidebottom E (eds). *Cancer Surveys, Vol. 21: Palliative Medicine: Problem Areas in Pain and Symptom Management*. London: Imperial Cancer Research Fund, 1994:179–96.

Ectopic Adrenocorticotrophic Hormone Secretion

ADRIAN J.L. CLARK AND JOHN NEWELL-PRICE

Definition

Ectopic adrenocorticotrophic hormone (ACTH) secretion is defined as the production and secretion of $ACTH_{1-39}$ and related peptides from extrapituitary tumours. This may lead to overstimulation of the adrenal cortex with production of excess cortisol and the development of Cushing's syndrome.

Prevalence and frequency

Ectopic ACTH syndrome accounts for between 5 and 25% of cases of Cushing's syndrome, depending on the referral centre involved. However unrecognized ectopic ACTH secretion may occur frequently with small-cell lung cancer (SCLC) in which the adverse effects of the tumour obscure a clinical diagnosis of ectopic ACTH syndrome. Clinically apparent ectopic ACTH with Cushing's syndrome may be caused by virtually any type of tumour, although certain histological types, notably carcinoids and SCLC, are more frequent causes (see Table 79.1).

Aetiology

The pro-opiomelanocortin (POMC) gene is primarily expressed in the human anterior pituitary gland, where it is the principal product of the corticotroph cells. However low level expression can also be detected in virtually all other human tissues [1]. The role of this 'peripheral' POMC gene expression is not clear. It is not surprising therefore that low level POMC gene expression can be detected in most tumours, and POMC-derived peptides can be extracted from them. However most tumours do not secrete these peptides, and are not associated with the ectopic ACTH syndrome.

The explanation for this difference between tissues and tumours that express the gene but do not secrete POMC peptides and those that do seems to lie in the nature of the gene transcript. Thus secreting cells express a mRNA of 1150–1250 nucleotides (nt), whereas peripheral cells express an 800 nt mRNA. These mRNAs are the product of different promoters, as indicated in Fig. 79.1. The peptide translation product of the longer mRNA contains the peptide signal sequence which is required for translocation of the peptide across the endoplasmic reticulum membrane. This signal sequence is missing in the product of the shorter mRNA, and we have shown that the short peptide cannot escape from the cell under normal circumstances, and so is probably eventually degraded within the cell [2]. Thus it seems that the factor that determines whether a cell will secrete POMC peptides is the transcription factor or factors that determine which promoter is used.

A further consideration is that it is impossible to know what cell a tumour originates from. It appears that peripheral tissues contain a population of cells that express the short POMC mRNA, and a smaller population of cells that express the full length mRNA. Tumours originating in the latter cell may become typical ectopic ACTH-secreting cells. Alternatively, the tumour may originate in a short POMC mRNA-expressing cell, which then changes its promoter usage, perhaps because of the various neoplastic changes occurring in the cell. These alternatives are represented in Fig. 79.2. The neoplastic events depicted as E1 and E2 may in fact be a series of events, and may differ between tumour types.

The former model might predict that certain tumour types would be associated with ectopic ACTH secretion, whereas the latter might suggest that tumours of any histological origin could secrete POMC peptides; for example, the testis is probably the tissue that expresses the greatest quantities of short POMC mRNA, yet ectopic ACTH-secreting tumours from this tissue are very uncommon. This might suggest that the tumour arises from a cell that already expresses the full-length mRNA.

Table 79.1 The tumours most frequently associated with the ectopic ACTH syndrome in approximate order of frequency

Small-cell carcinoma of the lung
Carcinoid tumours of the bronchus
Carcinoid tumours of the thymus
Carcinoid tumours of the pancreas or gut
Phaeochromocytoma, ganglioma and paraganglioma
Medullary carcinoma of the thyroid

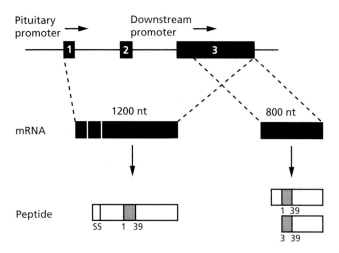

Fig. 79.1 The POMC gene depicted diagrammatically at the top of the figure contains three exons which are transcribed from a promoter upstream of exon 1 in the pituitary and ectopic ACTH-secreting tumours, as shown on the left. The mRNA transcript is 1150–1250 nt long, and encodes a peptide that has a cleavable N-terminal signal sequence (SS). In peripheral tissues the POMC gene is principally transcribed from a 'downstream' promoter located 5' to exon 3, as shown on the right. The mRNA transcript is 800 nt long and encodes a peptide that probably initiates at a position equivalent to methionine 53 or 115 in the pituitary peptide, and which lacks a signal sequence and at least part of the N-POC (N-terminal pro-opiocortin) molecule and possibly the N-terminus of ACTH.

The majority of tumours that secrete ectopic ACTH peptides are of neuroendocrine morphology, that is they have immunohistochemical and cytochemical features revealing a high content of 5-hydroxytryptamine (5-HT), dopamine decarboxylase, neurone-specific enolase (NSE) and tyrosine hydroxylase, and a characteristically high content of secretory vesicles seen on electron microscopy. It seems probable that these early neuroendocrine progenitor cells could also express full-length POMC mRNA, whereas other non-neuroendocrine cell types express the shorter mRNA.

Whichever of these mechanisms operates, a tumour expressing the full-length POMC mRNA clearly arises. Conventional understanding of the regulation of the POMC gene would suggest that this might not be of pathologically great significance, since this gene is normally actively regulated in the pituitary by the negative feedback provided by circulating glucocorticoids. In typical ectopic ACTH-producing tumours, ACTH is secreted despite high cortisol concentrations: the diagnostic basis of the high-dose dexamethasone suppression test. Therefore one would predict that the tumour cell is glucocorticoid resistant either because one or more components of the glucocorticoid signalling pathway are defective, or because the negative action of glucocorticoids is overridden by some other positively acting factor.

Using a number of SCLC cell lines which secrete POMC peptides we have shown that they are indeed markedly glucocorticoid resistant, not just in terms of the POMC gene, but also with respect to other endogenous [3] and introduced glucocorticoid-responsive genes [4], and in contrast to other cell lines such as the mouse corticotroph cell line AtT20. These cells express the glucocorticoid receptor gene, as shown by northern blot analysis, and bind glucocorticoid with normal affinities and in normal numbers per cell. However when these cells are transfected with a glucocorticoid receptor expression vector the glucocorticoid resistance is fully reversed. These findings suggest the existence of either a mutant receptor in these cells, or the presence of some glucocorticoid inhibitor that is overcome in the presence of the high levels of receptor produced following transfection [4].

It remains to be shown that ectopic ACTH-secreting tumours *in vivo* exhibit the same type of global glucocorticoid resistance. If they do, it is interesting to consider why this should be. It seems unlikely that there is a significant advantage to the tumour cell in having the ability to secrete POMC peptides, so it may be that there are other advantages in being glucocorticoid resistant. One possibility is that the tumour cell can avoid an apoptotic death, which may be mediated in part by glucocorticoids. If so, this would provide an interesting example of a situation in which investigation of an endocrine phenomenon provides insights into the mechanisms of oncogenesis in a common and aggressive tumour.

Clinical features

Ectopic ACTH syndrome may present as a typical case of Cushing's syndrome clinically indistinguishable from pituitary-dependent Cushing's disease. The suspicion of an ectopic tumour should be raised in cases with a rapid onset, or associated with marked proximal muscle wasting and weakness, weight loss or skin pigmentation.

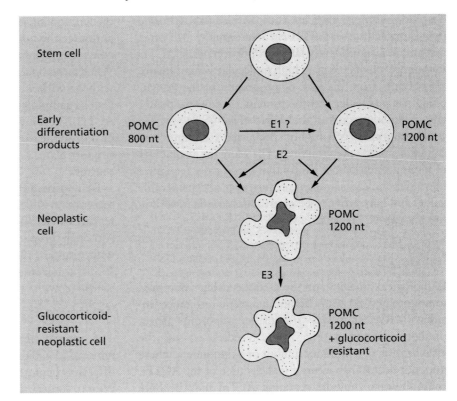

Fig. 79.2 A theoretical model for the genesis of ectopic ACTH-secreting tumours. The principal neoplastic transforming event (E2) may in reality be a series of oncogenic events which transform a cell expressing the pro-opiomelanocortin (POMC) gene into a neoplanocortin cell expressing the full-length mRNA. A previous genetic event (E1) may have converted POMC 800 nt expressing cells into POMC 1200 nt expressing cells. A further event (E3) renders the tumour cell glucocorticoid resistant.

Biochemical features

In the initial biochemical screen the finding of hypokalaemic alkalosis is a valuable and immediate indicator of a greater likelihood of the ectopic ACTH syndrome [5]. This appears to result in part from the excessive mineralocorticoid activity generated by overwhelming the 11β-hydroxysteroid dehydrogenase enzyme by very high levels of cortisol leading to the excessive activity of cortisol on the mineralocorticoid receptor [6].

Endocrine investigations

Formal endocrine testing should reveal the classical features of failure to suppress cortisol during the high-dose dexamethasone suppression test, and an absent response to the corticotrophin-releasing hormone (CRH) test. Neither of these findings are absolute features however, and a frequent problem is the interpretation of borderline or conflicting tests (for review see [7]). Plasma ACTH levels are detectable and may be greatly

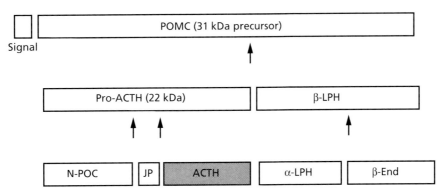

Fig. 79.3 A model for the processing of the pro-opiomelanocortin (POMC) precursor molecule. Successive cleavage of the 31 kDa POMC precursor molecule in anterior pituitary corticotroph cells results in the relatively efficient production of adrenocorticotrophic hormone (ACTH$_{1-39}$) (shaded box). This process is usually very inefficient in ectopic ACTH-producing cells so that the principal products are the 22 and 31 kDa precursor molecules, with little true ACTH$_{1-39}$. JP, joining peptide; LPH, lipotrophin; N-POC, N-terminal pro-opiocortin.

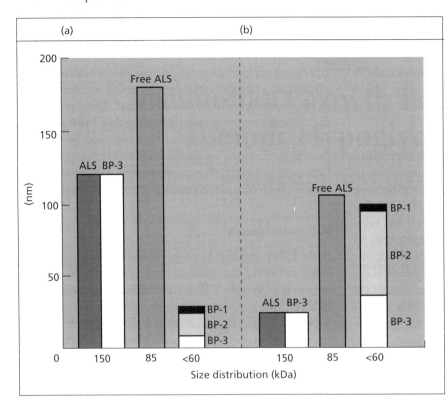

Fig. 80.1 Graphic comparison of the size distribution of insulin-like growth factor binding proteins (IGFBPs) and ALS in (a) normal sera and (b) non-islet cell tumour hypoglycaemia (NICTH) sera based on reported IGFBP-1, -2, -3 and ALS radioimmunoassays in large (150 kDa) and small (< 60 kDa) complexes. In NICTH sera there is a decrease in total IGFBP-3 and ALS and a shift of these components from the large to small complexes. There is also a large increase in IGFBP-2. BP, binding protein.

concentration of free and loosely complexed IGF-2 is increased 4- to 10-fold.

A frequent, if not constant, finding in NICTH is that much of the serum IGF-2 circulates as a partially processed form of proIGF-2 with a 21 amino acid carboxyl extension of the 67 amino acid of the 7.5 kDa IGF-2 [7,8]. Radio-immunoassays directed against this truncated E domain have been developed which have high sensitivity and specificity in the diagnosis of NICTH. In NICTH the big IGF-2 may lack normal O-linked glycosylation required for proper precursor processing. Unlike proinsulin, proIGF-2(E1–21) has equal affinity for the type 1 IGF receptor. It also binds with equal affinity as IGF-2 to serum IGFBPs.

In contrast to the elevated concentrations of IGF-2, the concentrations of IGF-1 in NICTH are reduced frequently to levels found in hypopituitarism. This is attributed to feedback inhibition of GH secretion by tumour IGF-2 (Fig. 80.2).

Other hormonal changes

The concentrations of serum insulin and C peptide are markedly reduced. This would be expected when the patient is hypoglycaemic but even occurs when the blood sugar has been returned to normal. Glucagon fails to rise in the presence of hypoglycaemia. These changes are best explained by direct IGF-2 inhibition of islet hormone secretion (Fig. 80.2). IGF inhibition of islet secretion has been experimentally confirmed when IGF-1 was administered to normal volunteers during a euglycaemic glucose clamp study [9].

GH secretion normally increases in hypoglycaemia but this response is inhibited in NICTH. As mentioned, this is the result of the high levels of free IGF-2 acting on the hypothalamus to increase somatostatin secretion.

The secretions of two other hormonal insulin antagonists are not impaired. In NICTH there are elevations of serum cortisol. If hypoglycaemic attacks are infrequent adrenaline concentrations in the serum rise and adrenergic symptoms are recognized [8]. If hypoglycaemia recurs frequently, the adrenaline response may be lost and neuroglycopenic changes occur without warning adrenergic symptoms. A similar lack of response has been observed also in recurrent insulin hypoglycaemia.

Changes in glucose metabolism

Marked changes in glucose metabolism in NICTH have been described (Fig. 80.3) [3]. In the postabsorptive state normal adults metabolized about 1–2 mg of glucose/kg

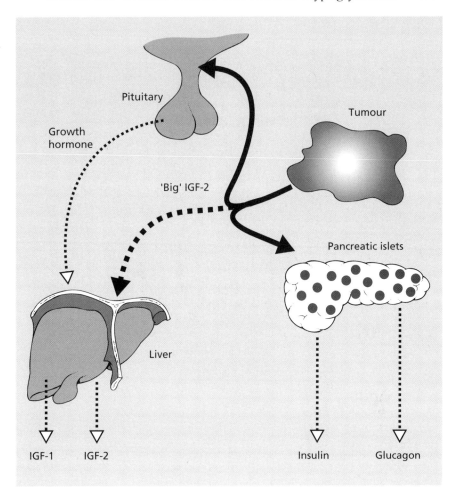

Fig. 80.2 Hormonal changes in NICTH. The increased secretion of insulin-like growth factor-2 (IGF-2) from the tumour suppresses pituitary growth hormone secretion, which, in turn, results in decreased hepatic secretion of IGF-1. Tumour IGF-2 also acts on the pancreatic islets to suppress insulin and glucagon secretion. Hepatic secretion of IGF-2 is also possibly suppressed by tumour IGF-2 as well as by decreased growth hormone.

body weight per minute. This is provided by the liver and maintains blood sugar at normal concentrations. Seventy five percent is provided by gluconeogenesis. Isotopic studies of glucose metabolism in NICTH have shown marked differences from normal. Net splanchnic release of glucose is reduced to about half of normal and peripheral utilization of glucose is increased four to sixfold. Without supplemental glucose hypoglycaemia will result. In some patients 500–1500 g of additional glucose per day is required to maintain tolerable blood glucose concentrations.

A patient with a large extrahepatic recurrence of a hepatoma permitted direct assessment of the glucose utilized by the tumour in comparison to the other sites [3]. Positron emission tomography (PET) scanning was done after administration of labelled glucose. It was calculated that 44% of the glucose was taken up in muscle, 14% by the liver and 15% by the hepatoma. Although the hepatoma utilized significant amounts of

glucose, most of the increased utilization occurred in muscle.

Other changes in fuel metabolism occur. Serum levels of non-esterified fatty acids are lowered with the result that fat oxidation and ketone body formation fall.

The receptors that mediate the IGF-2 metabolic effects changes NICTH are not entirely clear. Muscle is richly endowed with type 1 IGF receptors, which probably accounts for increased glucose utilization. Because human hepatocytes and adipocytes have few type 1 IGF receptors the IGF-2 action on these tissues is possibly mediated by the insulin receptor.

Treatment

Despite the size of some sarcomas associated with NICTH distant metastases may not be present and resection for cure may be possible. If successful, the hypoglycaemia is rapidly corrected and the hormonal abnormalities return

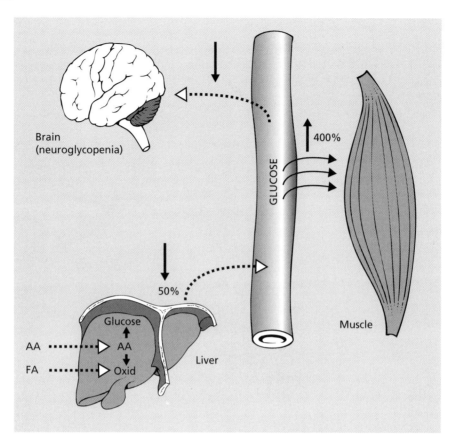

Fig. 80.3 The changes in glucose metabolism in NICTH are shown. Tumour IGF-2 suppresses the rate of glucose release by the liver by inhibiting gluconeogenesis and increases the rate of glucose uptake by muscle even more. Marked hypoglycaemia results and insufficient glucose is available to maintain normal cerebral function (neuroglycopenia). AA, amino acids; FA, fatty acids.

to normal. In other cases of slowly growing tumours with distant metastases, debulking of the primary tumour may result in prolonged remission. In one case this lasted over 6 years before symptoms returned. Few of the tumours associated with NICTH respond well to chemotherapy. One patient with an unresectable hepatoma had a worthwhile remission of hypoglycaemia after injection of Adriamycin into the artery supplying a large hepatoma.

Milder cases of NICTH can be controlled by frequent feedings and carbohydrate-containing liquids. Continuous glucose infusions may be required in the hospital. Some success has been obtained with the administration of high doses of prednisone or GH to antagonize the insulin-like actions of IGFs [6]. In one patient continuous glucagon infusions were beneficial [9]. Octreotide and diazoxide, which are used in the palliation of hyperinsulinism due to malignant insulinomas, are without reported benefit.

References

1. Daughaday WH, Deul TF. Tumor secretion of growth factors. *Endocrinol. Metab. Clin. North Am.* 1991;**20**:539–63.
2. Daughaday WH, Rotwein P. Insulin-like growth factors I and II. Peptide messenger ribonucleic acid and gene structures, serum, and tissue concentrations. *Endocr. Rev.* 1989;**10**:68–91.
3. Phillips LS, Robertson DG. Insulin-like growth factors and non-islet cell tumor hypoglycemia. *Metabolism* 1993;**42**:1093–101.
4. Baxter RC, Daughaday WH. Impaired formation of the ternary insulin-like growth factor binding protein complex in patients with hypoglycemia due to non-islet cell tumors. *J. Clin. Endocrinol. Metab.* 1991;**73**:696–702.
5. Zapf J, Futto E, Peter M, Froesch ER. Can 'big' insulin-like growth factor II in serum of tumor patients account for the development of extrapancreatic tumor hypoglycemia? *J. Clin. Invest.* 1992;**90**:2574–84.
6. Teale JD, Blum WF, Marks V. Alleviation of non-islet cell tumour hypoglycaemia by growth hormone therapy is associated with changes in IGF binding protein-3. *Ann. Clin. Biochem.* 1992;**29**:314–23.
7. Daughaday WH, Trivedi B. Heterogeneity of serum peptides with immunoactivity detected by a RIA for proIGF-II E domain. *J. Clin. Endocrinol. Metab.* 1992;**75**:641–5.

8. Eastman RC, Carson RE, Orloff DG *et al.* Glucose utilization in a patient with hepatoma and hypoglycemia, assessment by a positron emission tomography. *J. Clin. Invest.* 1992;**89**:1958–63.

9. Boulware SD, Tamborlane WV, Rennert NJ, Gesundheit N, Sherwin RS. Comparison of the metabolic effects of recombinant human insulin-like growth factor-I and insulin, dose–response relationships in healthy young and middle aged adults. *J. Clin. Invest.* 1994;**93**:1131–9.

10. Samaan NA, Pham FK, Sellin RV, Fernandez JF, Benjamin RS. Successful treatment of hypoglycaemia using glucagon in a patient with an extrapancreatic tumor. *Ann. Int. Med.* 1990;**113**:404–6.

Cancer Treatment and Hypopituitarism

STEPHEN M. SHALET

Introduction

The evidence that irradiation may damage hypo-thalamic–pituitary function is irrefutable whereas the potential capacity of cytotoxic chemotherapy to induce hypopituitarism is still not established.

Deficiency of one or more anterior pituitary hormones may follow treatment with external radiation when the hypothalamic–pituitary axis falls within the fields of radiation. Hypopituitarism has been described in patients who received radiation therapy for nasopharyngeal carcinoma, tumours of the pituitary gland or nearby structures, and primary brain tumours, as well as in children who underwent prophylactic cranial irradiation for acute lymphoblastic leukaemia or total body irradiation (TBI) for a variety of tumours and other diseases.

The radiobiological impact of an irradiation schedule is dependent on the total dose, number of fractions and duration. The same total dose given in fewer fractions over a shorter time period is likely to cause a greater incidence of pituitary hormone deficiency, than if the schedule were spread over a longer time interval with a greater number of fractions.

The degree of pituitary hormonal deficit is related to the radiation dose received by the hypothalamic–pituitary axis. Thus after lower radiation doses, isolated growth hormone (GH) deficiency ensues, whilst higher doses may produce panhypopituitarism. In the vast majority of children the GH deficiency is isolated; however, in certain centres children with brain tumours or nasopharyngeal carcinoma may receive a higher dose of irradiation to the hypothalamic–pituitary axis leading to other pituitary hormone deficits.

Growth hormone

The greater the radiation dose, the earlier GH deficiency will occur after treatment so that between 2 and 5 years after irradiation, 100% of children receiving ≥ 30 Gy (over 3 weeks) to the hypothalamic–pituitary axis showed subnormal GH responses to an insulin tolerance test (ITT), whilst 35% of those receiving < 30 Gy (over 3 weeks) still show a normal GH response (Fig. 81.1). The prospective studies, however, have concentrated on GH responses to provocative tests: the speed of onset of GH deficiency detected by measurement of spontaneous GH secretion following radiation-induced damage and the natural history of GH deficiency after total body irradiation, however, remain unknown. Furthermore, whilst there is no dispute about the capacity of radiotherapy to render a child GH-deficient, recent prospective studies have suggested that the GH response to an ITT may already be perturbed before radiotherapy, contrary to the findings of earlier studies.

Age and pubertal status

In the human, investigations of GH secretion after cranial irradiation support the experimental animal data, which show the central nervous system (CNS) of young animals to be more radiosensitive than that of older animals. After a mean time of 2.8 years following TBI (10.0–13.2 Gy in 5–6 fractions over 3 days), all 18 adults showed a normal GH response to an ITT, whilst after a mean time of 2.4 years after a similar TBI schedule (11.0–15.2 Gy in 3–8 fractions over 2–5 days) 15 out of 29 children showed subnormal GH responses to an ITT. In three of the 15 children previous cranial irradiation might have explained the GH deficiency, but no irradiation other than TBI had been administered to the remaining 12 children.

Thus the CNS of children appears more radiosensitive than that of adults. Furthermore, there is some evidence in children receiving prophylactic cranial irradiation for acute lymphoblastic leukaemia (ALL) that the younger the child then the greater the susceptibility to radiation-induced GH deficiency.

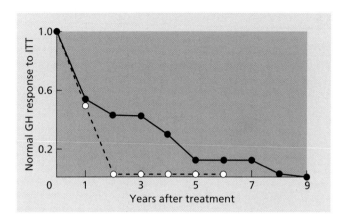

Fig. 81.1 The incidence of growth hormone (GH) deficiency in children receiving 27–32 Gy (●—●) or ≥ 35 Gy (○--○) of cranial irradiation for a brain tumour in relation to time from irradiation.

Growth hormone tests

A further factor influencing the prevalence of radiation-induced GH deficiency will be the type of investigation used to assess GH secretion. Chrousos and colleagues [1] showed in the irradiated primate model that physiological GH secretion could be severely reduced in quantity in an animal which showed a normal GH response to arginine or L-dihydroxyphenylalanine (L-DOPA) stimulation. Similarly normal GH responses to an ITT but subnormal spontaneous GH secretion have been reported in three children who received prophylactic cranial irradiation for ALL. This phenomenon has been described as radiation-induced GH neurosecretory dysfunction. In complete contrast, essentially normal spontaneous GH secretion but blunted GH responses to an ITT have been described in children treated for ALL who had never received any radiotherapy and, in a separate group of children who received cranial irradiation for a variety of malignancies, relatively normal basal insulin-like growth factor binding protein-3 (IGFBP-3, the main intravascular binding protein for IGF) levels in the presence of impaired GH responses to two provocative tests.

It is likely, however, that the higher irradiation doses (≥ 27 Gy) received by the children with brain tumours affect both spontaneous GH secretion and stimulated GH responses fairly equally. Radiation-induced GH neurosecretory dysfunction may only be a real clinical problem in the children treated for ALL who have received a radiation dose in the range of 18–24 Gy. The exact prevalence of this problem is unknown.

Reduced spontaneous GH secretion during 24-hour profiles has been described in both prepubertal and pubertal girls following cranial irradiation for ALL (24 Gy)

with a failure of the expected increase in GH secretion at puberty [2], associated with attenuated pubertal growth. After 1980 the dose of irradiation employed in prophylactic cranial irradiation for ALL was reduced to 18 Gy in an attempt to minimize neuropsychological disturbance and abnormalities of GH secretion.

Results of recently completed studies of GH secretion [3] differ from those earlier studies [2], in that spontaneous GH secretion was normal in the prepubertal children following low-dose cranial irradiation (18 Gy). The pubertal children however, showed abnormalities of spontaneous GH secretion, despite the fact that each underwent puberty spontaneously and showed normal pubertal progression. Apart from a reduction in the total amount of GH secreted there was also a significant disturbance in the periodicity of GH secretion (Fig. 81.2) in the irradiated (18 Gy) pubertal children [3]; a finding which has also been observed in the first year after TBI for childhood leukaemia.

Indications for growth hormone therapy in children treated for brain tumours

To determine whether GH has had a significant impact on growth in children with radiation-induced GH deficiency the growth velocity during the first year of GH therapy has been compared with the pretreatment growth velocity. This will indicate if there has been a significant short-term improvement in growth rate but not if there will be a substantial gain in final height. Thus long-term studies are the most critical and ideally these should include an analysis of the final height and gain or loss in stature (standard deviation score) from initiation of GH therapy until the end of growth in children with radiation-induced GH deficiency, contrasted with the growth pattern in those who did not receive GH therapy.

Our own final height studies indicated that GH therapy was of significant benefit in children with radiation-induced GH deficiency; however, the height gained or rather the 'height loss' that had been prevented, was disappointingly small and much less than that seen in GH-treated children with idiopathic GH deficiency. Similar disappointing results were reported by others.

A number of factors contributed to the suboptimal growth response, including spinal irradiation, precocious or early puberty, the excessively long time interval (mean 5.5–6.7 years) between irradiation and the initiation of GH therapy and the inadequacy of the GH schedule used in the early studies.

Since the first children with radiation-induced GH deficiency treated with GH therapy reached their final height, our clinical criteria for whom to treat and when

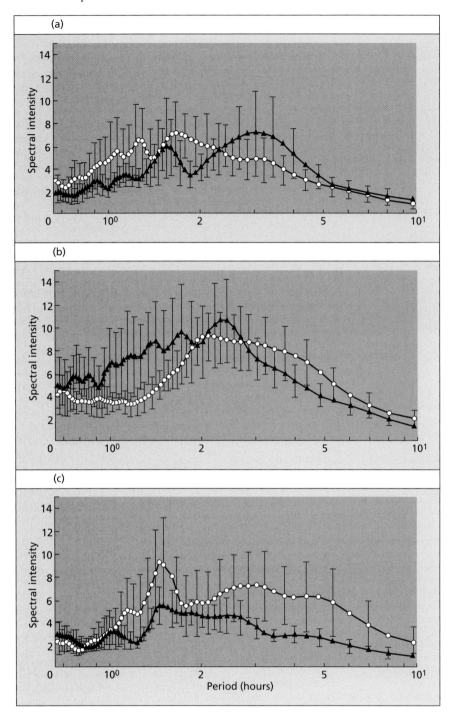

Fig. 81.2 Pooled estimated power spectra for the GH profiles of (a) prepubertal, (b) pubertal and (c) postpubertal groups. Results for both normal children (○) and those treated with low-dose cranial irradiation (18 Gy) (▲) are depicted. Note the spectral flattening for both pubertal and postpubertal irradiated groups. In particular the pubertal irradiated group exhibits increased spectral intensities for all short periods, indicating a randomization of GH pulsing.

to initiate GH therapy have continued to evolve in order to improve the final height prognosis.

The chances of recurrence of a brain tumour are greatest within 2 years of the primary treatment of the tumour. If GH treatment were offered within the first 2 years, it would be associated with a number of tumour recurrences and deaths. Therefore, despite a lack of proof of a causal relationship, many families and doctors would associate GH therapy with tumour recurrence. On the other hand there is no evidence that treatment with GH increased the risk of late recurrence of a brain tumour (≥ 2 years from primary treatment) in children with radiation-induced GH deficiency. A reasonable approach therefore at two years after primary treatment would be to consider for GH therapy all the children with brain tumours treated by standard radiation schedules, including a dose to the hypothalamic–pituitary axis in excess of 30 Gy. By this time they would no longer be receiving cytotoxic chemotherapy, the chance of recurrence of a tumour is low and it is established that most, if not all, will be GH-deficient. In certain centres GH therapy would be offered routinely at 2 years without recourse to GH tests or evidence of impaired growth. Alternatively, others would insist on biochemical evidence of GH deficiency and a subnormal growth rate. In our own centre we establish GH deficiency biochemically but would consider GH therapy independent of the growth rate.

Where the natural history of radiation-induced GH deficiency is less predictable or less well-known, for example, after a radiation dose of 20–30 Gy, standard provocative tests of GH release are performed at 2 years and if the results are abnormal the children receive GH therapy. If GH secretion appears normal and the growth rate is appropriate for pubertal status, then growth is observed and the GH stimulation tests are repeated annually. However, if the growth rate is subnormal in the presence of normal GH responses to pharmacological stimuli, a combination that is very unusual in our centre, then GH neurosecretory dysfunction may be a possible explanation. Alternative approaches would be either an appraisal of physiological GH secretion, such as a 24-hour profile, or an empirical trial of GH therapy. In practice, 24-hour GH profiles are reserved for research studies and not clinical management.

These guidelines assume that in craniospinal-irradiated children, growth is assessed by leg length velocity and that other causes of poor growth such as radiation-induced hypothyroidism, recurrent tumour and malnutrition have been excluded.

In the clinic the timing of the introduction of GH therapy is matched with the special circumstances, age, pubertal status and needs of an individual child. Early treatment is particularly suitable for the craniospinally-treated young child of short parents.

Gonadotrophins

External irradiation of the hypothalamic–pituitary region for treatment of a pituitary adenoma or suprasellar tumour causes gonadotrophin deficiency. Littley and colleagues [4] studied 165 adult patients who underwent external irradiation to the hypothalamic–pituitary region for treatment of a pituitary adenoma (84% of patients) or suprasellar tumour (16% of patients). 140 patients had undergone pituitary surgery before radiotherapy. All patients received external irradiation with a dose of

37.5–42.5 Gy delivered in 15 or 16 fractions over 20–22 days. Before irradiation 79% of patients had gonadotrophin deficiency. Five years after irradiation 91% of the patients had abnormal gonadotrophin secretion; 8 years after irradiation 96% of the patients were gonadotrophin-deficient. This compares with 100% of patients having GH deficiency 5 years after irradiation (82% deficient before irradiation), 84% of patients having adrenocorticotrophic hormone (ACTH) deficiency 8 years after irradiation (41% deficient before irradiation) and 49% of patients having thyroid-stimulating hormone (TSH) deficiency 8 years after irradiation (20% deficient before irradiation).

In the patients who developed multiple pituitary hormone deficiencies following irradiation the most usual order of loss of anterior pituitary hormone function was GH followed by luteinizing hormone (LH)/follicle-stimulating hormone (FSH), ACTH and then TSH (Fig. 81.3). This sequence was seen in 61% of the patients who developed multiple pituitary hormone deficiencies, although 25% of patients with non-functioning pituitary adenomas and 36% of patients with acromegaly who developed multiple deficiencies developed ACTH deficiency before LH/FSH deficiency. Snyder and colleagues [5] demonstrated that gonadotrophin deficiency developed in 50% of patients who had normal gonadotrophin secretion pretreatment, and who had not previously undergone pituitary surgery, 15 years following external

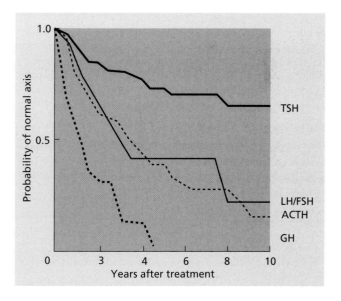

Fig. 81.3 Life-table analysis indicating probabilities of initially normal hypothalamic–pituitary–target gland axes remaining normal after radiotherapy. ACTH, adrenocorticotrophic hormone; FSH, follicle-stimulating hormone; GH, growth hormone; LH, luteinizing hormone; TSH, thyroid-stimulating hormone.

pituitary irradiation at a dose of 44–50 Gy for treatment of a pituitary adenoma.

The development of gonadotrophin deficiency following external pituitary irradiation for treatment of pituitary disease is dose dependent. Littley and colleagues [6], demonstrated that 5 years after irradiation the incidence of LH/FSH deficiency in patients with initially normal gonadotrophin secretion who received 20 Gy delivered in 8 fractions over 11 days was 33%. However, 66% of patients with previously normal gonadotrophin secretion developed LH/FSH deficiency 5 years after receiving 35–40 Gy delivered in 15 fractions over 21 days ($P < 0.05$). Total body irradiation for treatment of a haematological malignancy (10 Gy in 5 fractions, or 12 or 13.2 Gy in 6 fractions, over 3 days) is associated with primary gonadal failure but not with any damage to the hypothalamic–pituitary control of gonadotrophin secretion.

Cranial irradiation for treatment of a cranial tumour, tumours of eye and middle ear, and nasopharyngeal carcinoma [7], can cause gonadotrophin deficiency, if the hypothalamic–pituitary axis lies within the radiation field. Lam and colleagues [7] demonstrated that gonadotrophin deficiency developed in 31% of adult patients 5 years after receiving cranial irradiation at an estimated dose of 39.8 Gy to the hypothalamus and 61.7 Gy to the pituitary for treatment of nasopharyngeal carcinoma. However, 1 year after irradiation men had a significant increase in basal serum FSH, with no change in basal serum LH and testosterone. The integrated serum FSH response to gonadotrophin-releasing hormone (GnRH) was increased, while that of LH was decreased. After 1 year from irradiation there was a progressive decrease in stimulated serum LH, and in both basal and stimulated serum FSH, with increasing time from irradiation. The authors suggest that the fall in serum LH but rise in serum FSH in the first year following irradiation is due to a radiation-induced decrease in the pulse frequency of hypothalamic GnRH secretion. It has previously been proposed that the relative secretion rates of LH and FSH by the pituitary may be regulated by the frequency of pulsatile GnRH secretion from the hypothalamus, and a decreased LH pulse frequency (which suggests a decreased GnRH pulse frequency) has been demonstrated in men with selectively elevated serum FSH levels in the presence of normal serum LH levels. The progressive decrease in secretion of both LH and FSH after the first year following irradiation [7] is in keeping with a progressive reduction in hypothalamic GnRH pulse amplitude.

Precocious or early puberty

Doses of cranial irradiation exceeding 50 Gy to the hypothalamic–pituitary axis may render a child gonadotrophin-deficient. Paradoxically, lesser doses of irradiation may be associated with early puberty. We have recently demonstrated this phenomenon in both sexes in children irradiated with a dose of 25.0–47.5 Gy for a brain tumour [8]. In 46 GH-deficient children previously irradiated for a brain tumour not involving the hypothalamic-pituitary axis there was a significant linear association between age at irradiation and age at onset of puberty. The onset of puberty occurred at an early age in both sexes (mean 8.51 years in girls and 9.21 years in boys plus 0.29 years for every year of age at irradiation); for example, the estimated age at onset of puberty in a boy irradiated at 2 years of age would be 9.79 years and that for a boy irradiated at 9 years of age would be 11.82 years. In the context of GH deficiency, which is usually associated with a delay in the onset of puberty, this is abnormal.

The largest number of children available for the study of pubertal timing after irradiation are those treated for childhood leukaemia (dose of irradiation 18–24 Gy). There is a high incidence of early puberty but predominantly among girls [9,10]. The number of boys entering puberty early is no greater than that anticipated in a normal population. This sexual dichotomy has been attributed to fundamental differences in the interaction between the CNS and hypothalamic function. It has been postulated that the CNS restraint on the onset of puberty is more readily disrupted in girls than in boys by any insult, including irradiation. At the doses of irradiation employed in the treatment of brain tumours (25–47 Gy), however, radiation-induced early puberty is not restricted to girls.

The mechanism for early puberty after irradiation is likely to be related to disinhibition of cortical influences on the hypothalamus. Puberty then proceeds through the increased frequency and amplitude of GnRH pulsatile secretion by the hypothalamus. The impact of early puberty in a child with radiation-induced growth failure is to foreshorten the time available for GH therapy. This has restricted the therapeutic efficacy of GH. Consequently a number of these children are now treated with a combination of a GnRH analogue and GH therapy. It is relatively easy to halt the progression of puberty but it is too early to analyse the impact of this approach on final height.

Adrenocorticotrophic hormone

Adults irradiated for pituitary tumours with a total irradiation dose of between 20 and 45 Gy are at significant risk of developing ACTH deficiency. An impaired cortisol response to an ITT was found in 31% of 25 adults 5 years after low-dose cranial irradiation for pituitary disease (20 Gy in 8 fractions over 11 days). Following an even lower total dose of irradiation, however, there was no evidence of ACTH deficiency in 18 adults who received TBI (10.0–13.2 Gy in 5–6 fractions over 3 days) as part of their treatment for haematological malignancy. In contrast, Sanders and colleagues [11], had reported that 24% of 78 children who had TBI (9.20–15.75 Gy) had subnormal 11-deoxycortisol levels after metyrapone stimulation 1–8 years after transplantation, although further investigations to differentiate between primary and secondary adrenal insufficiency were not performed. Subsequently Ogilvy-Stuart and colleagues [12] demonstrated that, similar to the situation in the adults, very few children showed impairment of pituitary–adrenal responses to an ITT following TBI (11.0–15.2 Gy in 3–8 fractions over 2–5 days).

Definition of a normal pituitary–adrenal axis has relied heavily upon dynamic testing in an attempt to measure the potential response of the axis to a stressful insult such as surgery or an intercurrent illness. It may be, however, that more attention should be directed towards the possibility of subnormal cortisol secretion under basal conditions undetected by dynamic testing. Thus a subtle form of cortisol insufficiency may impair the patient's quality of life under ordinary circumstances with excessive fatigue dominating the clinical picture.

In six adult patients previously treated with external pituitary irradiation for pituitary tumours, symptoms of hypo-adrenalism were reported, which subsequently responded to glucocorticoid replacement. These six patients showed normal cortisol responses to insulin-induced hypoglycaemia, but reduced serum cortisol profiles and 24-hour urinary free cortisol levels. Similar biochemical findings have been described in some patients with isolated ACTH deficiency. These patients showed low 24-hour urinary 17-hydroxycorticosteroids, low or low–normal plasma cortisol levels and a basal plasma ACTH level that was definitely low or, if within the normal range, inappropriately low for the prevailing cortisol concentration. In some patients there was a normal cortisol and ACTH response to an ITT. Similar observations have been reported in a group of 21 patients studied before and 2 years after cranial irradiation for nasopharyngeal carcinoma in whom there was a significant decrease in basal plasma cortisol levels while the integrated cortisol responses to an ITT did not change.

These results indicate that a discordance between physiological ACTH secretion and ACTH responses to pharmacological tests may exist in patients with ACTH deficiency. When associated with radiation damage this discordance may be dose dependent. In childhood, low-dose cranial irradiation (18 Gy in 10 fractions over 14 days) does not appear to affect spontaneous ACTH and cortisol secretion, whilst the six adult patients described earlier received a higher radiation dose of 20–40 Gy in 8–15 fractions over 10–20 days.

Thyroid-stimulating hormone

Our own studies have suggested that of the anterior pituitary hormones TSH is the least vulnerable to radiation damage [4], although others have found a high incidence of TSH deficiency earlier in the evolution of radiation-induced hypopituitarism.

It is possible that irradiation has a more subtle impact upon TSH secretion by modifying the predominant form of TSH secreted, thereby altering the bioactive/immunoreactive TSH ratio. This might explain the high incidence of children with abnormally raised TSH levels and normal thyroxine levels following cranial irradiation alone. With this radiotherapy field effectively no radiation reaches the thyroid gland directly and thus the abnormal thyroid function tests are likely to be a consequence of the radiation to the hypothalamic–pituitary region. There is anecdotal evidence that radiation may modify bioactive TSH adversely in this manner.

Site and nature of radiation damage

Among patients with pituitary adenomas treated by the implantation of yttrium-90 into the pituitary gland with radiation doses of 500–1500 Gy to the pituitary, the combined incidence of TSH and ACTH deficiency was 39% at 14 years [13], as compared with an incidence of over 90% at 10 years among patients who underwent external irradiation at doses ranging from 37.5 to 42.5 Gy [4]. The most likely explanation for the difference in the incidence of hypopituitarism after the two types of irradiation is that the fields for external irradiation included the hypothalamus, which was relatively unaffected by yttrium-90 treatment.

Further evidence that the hypothalamus is the site of radiation-induced damage comes from studies in patients who received cranial radiation. These demonstrated: delayed anterior pituitary hormone responses to releasing hormones in those with deficiencies of gonadotrophin and TSH; increased basal serum prolactin concentrations; normal serum GH responses to single bolus doses of GHRH in those with subnormal serum GH responses to the administration of arginine or insulin-induced hypoglycaemia; and reduced spontaneous secretion of GH despite normal serum GH responses to pharmacological

Cancer Therapy and Gonadal Dysfunction

STEPHEN M. SHALET

Introduction

It is important to remember that in the same cancer patient, for example a child with a brain tumour, the reproductive axis may be damaged at several different sites by the primary therapies, external irradiation and cytotoxic drugs administered for the malignancy. Cranial irradiation may damage the central nervous system (CNS) including the hypothalamic–pituitary axis leading to hyperprolactinaemia and/or gonadotrophin deficiency. In children cranial irradiation may cause early or precocious puberty. Irradiation to the gonads included in abdominal, pelvic and spinal fields or direct testicular irradiation schedules or cytotoxic chemotherapy may induce gonadal dysfunction manifested by infertility and impaired sex steroid production. In this chapter the consequences of direct gonadal damage are reviewed as radiation-induced disorders of the hypothalamic–pituitary axis are covered elsewhere.

Radiation and the testis

The testis is one of the most radiosensitive tissues with a direct radiation dose of as low as 0.15 Gy causing a significant depression in the sperm count and temporary azoospermia occurring after doses of 0.3 Gy [1]. The germinal epithelium is far more radiosensitive than the Leydig cells. Differentiating spermatogonia are very radiosensitive and after doses as low as 1 Gy both their numbers and that of their daughter cells, the preleptotene spermatocytes are severely reduced. The doses of irradiation required to kill spermatocytes are higher than for spermatogonia (2–3 Gy results in an inability to complete maturation division, with a resultant decrease in spermatid numbers). Spermatids show no overt damage but after 4–6 Gy the resultant spermatozoa are significantly decreased in number, signifying covert spermatid damage. Thus during the first 50–60 days after low-dose irradiation (1.5–2.0 Gy), sperm production remains above 50% of control values and then drops dramatically with temporary oligo- or azoospermia. Higher radiation doses cause a more rapid onset of oligo- and azoospermia by a direct effect on the later stages as well as earlier stages of sperm production.

Recovery takes place from the surviving stem cells and proliferation of stem cells results in regeneration of stem cell numbers [1]. With single-dose exposures, complete recovery takes place within 9–18 months after less than 1 Gy, 30 months for 2–3 Gy and 5 or more years after 4–6 Gy.

Irradiation of the testis during radiotherapy usually involves fractionated exposures. Under certain conditions fractionation causes more stem cell killing than do single treatments, although this has not been proven in humans. Serial semen examinations were carried out in 11 cancer patients who had received large pelvic field irradiation or interstitial ^{125}I seeds implanted in the prostate with a total calculated dose to the testes of 1.18–2.28 Gy delivered in 24–35 fractions. All patients suffered temporary azoospermia beginning at about 3 months postirradiation. Recovery of spermatogenesis was first noted between 10 and 18 months after irradiation in five patients. In a follow-up study, a cohort of patients was studied in whom a total fractionated radiation dose of 0.09–1.78 Gy was received by the remaining testis following unilateral orchidectomy for seminoma [2]. Azoospermia occurred in ten out of 14 patients who received more than 0.65 Gy to the testis. Sperm reappeared in the semen within 30–80 weeks after the start of treatment. Similar findings have been described in males receiving abdominal irradiation (inverted Y abdominal, pelvic and inguinal fields) for Hodgkin's disease and in whom the testes received a scatter dose of irradiation.

Following fractionated courses of irradiation, azoospermia has been induced by a testicular dose as low as 0.35 Gy. After a radiation dose of between 2 and 3 Gy, the primary impact of the damage is on the germinal epithelium with recovery of spermatogenesis sometimes delayed for 10 years or more. Leydig cell function is intact as judged by a normal serum testosterone concentration, although in some patients this may be maintained only by a rise in the circulating luteinizing hormone (LH) level [3]. As the testicular irradiation dose is increased tenfold, to 30 Gy, the serum testosterone often becomes frankly subnormal and androgen replacement therapy is required.

Radiation and the ovary

When girls and adult women are irradiated the response of the ovary involves a fixed population of cells which, once destroyed, cannot be replaced. Effects on fertility are most readily explained on the basis of a reduction in the fixed pool of oocytes. While a permanent menopause can be caused by a total radiation exposure of about 6 Gy in women aged 40 years or more [4], radiotherapists' estimates of the 50% probability level for permanent sterility is approximately 20 Gy over a 6-week period in young women. If the radiation dose is delivered over a greater number of fractionated doses, the damage to the ovary and consequent chance of infertility is likely to be less.

The treatment of patients with Hodgkin's disease is influenced by the extent of the disease. Certain patients receive irradiation to the lymph nodes along the iliac vessels. Since the ovaries lie in this area, they receive a dose of about 35 Gy, which inevitably causes ovarian failure.

Transposition of the ovaries (oophoropexy) before irradiation, with a consequent reduction in the dose delivered to the shielded ovaries to a maximum of 6 Gy over 12–45 days decreased the incidence of amenorrhoea by over 50%. Nonetheless, the exact benefit to be derived from oophoropexy is controversial. The extent of the disease needs to be carefully staged before considering oophoropexy and then the procedure needs to be performed with great accuracy and care.

Studies of ovarian function following abdominal irradiation in childhood remain few. After 20–30 Gy over 25–44 days to both ovaries, ovarian failure is almost universal [5]. Morphological studies have revealed marked inhibition of follicular growth and severe reduction in the number of oocytes. Recent studies have indicated that the spinal component of craniospinal irradiation for the treatment of brain tumours and total body irradiation (TBI) for bone marrow transplantation may cause ovarian dysfunction due to radiation-induced ovarian damage. The patients present with either failure to undergo or to complete pubertal development, or later in adult life with

a premature menopause. On occasions the ovarian failure may prove reversible. The LD_{50} for the human oocyte has been estimated not to exceed 4 Gy and in conjunction with information about the position of the ovaries in relation to the radiation field, the predicted age at ovarian failure can be calculated approximately [6].

Radiation and the uterus

In those women irradiated during childhood in whom ovarian function is preserved but in whom the uterus has been included in the radiation field, there is evidence that radiation changes to the uterus result in failure to carry a pregnancy. The risk of miscarriage or low birthweight infants is greatly increased.

Following an irradiation dose in childhood of 20–30 Gy to the whole abdomen, these women have a significant reduction in uterine length and an endometrium which is unresponsive to physiological serum levels of oestradiol and progesterone attained by exogenous administration [7]. Doppler signals from the uterine arteries are absent in most cases. It is not yet clear whether this is a consequence of primary damage to the microvasculature of the uterus and associated blood supply. As appropriate vascularization and subsequent growth of the endometrium are essential, however, for implantation and successful continuation of pregnancy, it is unlikely that women who have received a significant dose of abdominal irradiation in childhood will be able to sustain a pregnancy to term. This has implications for *in vitro* fertilization with donor oocytes in irradiated women with concomitant ovarian failure.

Chemotherapy and gonadal damage

In humans, gonadal damage has most frequently been described following the use of alkylating drugs such as mustine, cyclophosphamide and chlorambucil; however, nitrosoureas, procarbazine, vinblastine, cytosine arabinoside and cisplatinum have all been incriminated.

Testis

The extent of the damage and the potential for recovery are dependent on the nature of the drugs received and the dosage. Recovery of spermatogenesis has been described in many but not all males previously treated with single cytotoxic drugs. Following certain combinations of cytotoxic drugs, however, azoospermia is usually permanent, although the possibility of recovery is still dose-dependent. After six or more courses of MVPP (mustine, vinblastine, procarbazine and prednisolone) for Hodgkin's disease, less than 5% of males will have a normal sperm count 5 years later and virtually all will have been rendered azoospermic after the first course of chemotherapy [8,9].

The prognosis for recovery of spermatogenesis is better after other schedules of combination chemotherapy such as cisplatinum, vinblastine and bleomycin for metastatic testicular cancer. Azoospermia is very common after completion of chemotherapy but within 3 years the sperm count is normal in 50% of patients.

There is no doubt that the cytotoxic drugs which damage the testis predominantly affect the germinal epithelium. More detailed studies in men treated with MVPP for Hodgkin's disease, however, have suggested a subtle impairment of Leydig cell function. The circulating testosterone concentration and the steroidogenic response to an acute bolus injection of human chorionic gonadotrophin (hCG) are normal. The basal LH concentration is frequently raised and the LH response to a gonadotrophin-releasing hormone (GnRH) test is exaggerated. The bioactive to immunoreactive LH ratio is normal and there is no disturbance of LH pulse frequency; however, the amplitude of the LH pulses is significantly elevated. Due to this compensatory process, androgen replacement therapy is rarely indicated following chemotherapy-induced testicular damage.

Gynaecomastia has been reported following the use of busulphan, vincristine, nitrosoureas and various combinations of cytotoxic drugs. It appears to be a clinical manifestation of Leydig cell dysfunction associated biochemically with a subtle alteration in the circulating oestrogen : androgen ratio. It may be transient and is more likely to occur in those prone to developing gynaecomastia, such as the elderly.

Ovary

In the female most information is available on the effect of cyclophosphamide on reproductive function. Typically the ovarian damage results in amenorrhoea with all the usual clinical features associated with oestrogen deficiency and characterized biochemically by an undetectable oestradiol level and grossly elevated gonadotrophin levels. In a minority of patients the ovarian damage is less severe, evidenced by less elevated gonadotrophin levels, a mid-follicular phase oestradiol level and, other than amenorrhoea, a lack of symptoms.

The amenorrhoea may or may not be permanent. Furthermore the total dose of the drug received will determine how soon after initiation of treatment the amenorrhoea will develop and whether the amenorrhoea is reversible.

The susceptibility of women to develop cytotoxic-induced ovarian failure is age dependent. In studies of women with breast carcinoma, who had been treated with different cytotoxic drugs including cyclophosphamide, the average dose of cyclophosphamide given before the onset of amenorrhoea in patients in their forties, thirties and twenties was 5.2, 9.3 and 20.4 g, respectively [10]. It might be predicted that cytotoxic-induced ovarian failure would rarely occur in the prepubertal and pubertal female. Clinical and morphological studies, however, indicate that the young girl is not totally resistant to such damage.

Following the marked reduction in the mortality rate from gestational trophoblastic tumours and Hodgkin's disease, there has been increasing interest in the impact of chemotherapy on reproductive function. Out of 314 women successfully treated for gestational trophoblastic tumours between 1962 and 1977, 159 subsequently achieved a pregnancy despite previous treatment with methotrexate, 6-mercaptopurine, actinomycin D and 6-azauridine [11]. The incidence of amenorrhoea following MVPP or MOPP (mustine, vincristine, procarbazine and prednisolone) therapy for Hodgkin's disease is reported to range from 15 to 62%. The progression from regular menses to amenorrhoea is variable; in some it is abrupt, while in others there is a slow transition phase of oligomenorrhoea followed by a premature menopause. The amenorrhoea may prove to be reversible but there is no established diagnostic test that will allow selection of those women with a better reproductive prognosis from those without hope.

With occasional exceptions women with chemotherapy-induced ovarian failure under the age of 50 years should receive sex steroid replacement therapy with a preparation containing oestrogen and progestogen in order to prevent osteoporosis, reduce the mortality from ischaemic heart disease and to alleviate symptoms in the symptomatic.

Strategies to preserve fertility

As a consequence of the high incidence of azoospermia following MVPP/MOPP therapy for Hodgkin's disease and cisplatinum, vinblastine and bleomycin for testicular teratoma, sperm storage facilities have been offered to some male patients before they start chemotherapy. Sperm storage is likely to be useful only if the sperm concentration, morphology and motility are not severely affected by the disease process itself. Unfortunately a significant proportion of patients with Hodgkin's disease or those who have had a hemicastration for testicular tumour are oligospermic before chemotherapy. Thus sperm banking will offer little hope for future reproduction in such patients.

Alternative modalities of therapy are being sought to provide similar 'cure' rates to established regimens associated with a reduced incidence of gonadal toxicity. It has been suggested that ABVD (Adriamycin, bleomycin, vinblastine and decarbazine) chemotherapy fulfils this aim when compared with MOPP for the management of Hodgkin's disease in adults [12].

More recently there have been attempts to suppress hormonally the pituitary–gonadal axis to prevent chemotherapy-induced gonadal damage in humans. The attempts to achieve gonadotrophin suppression have been via GnRH agonist analogues in both sexes or oestrogen therapy in the female. In neither sex has there been any convincing evidence of protection utilizing this approach. In the rat model, however, there is evidence that GnRH agonist and antagonist analogues or testosterone may protect, at least partially, the spermatogenic epithelium from procarbazine damage [13].

References

1. Rowley MJ, Leach DR, Warner GA, Heller CG. Effect of graded doses of ionising irradiation on the human testis. *Radiat. Res.* 1974;59:665–78.
2. Hahn EW, Feingold SM, Simpson L, Batala M. Recovery from aspermia induced by low dose radiation in seminoma patients. *Cancer* 1982;50:337–40.
3. Tsatsoulis A, Shalet SM, Morris ID, de Kretser DM. Immunoactive inhibin as a marker of Sertoli cell function following cytotoxic damage to the human testis. *Hormone Res.* 1990;34:254–9.
4. Doll R, Smith PG. The longterm effects of x-irradiation in patients treated for metropathia haemorrhagica. *Br. J. Radiol.* 1968;41:362–8.
5. Wallace WHB, Shalet SM, Crowne EC, Morris Jones PH, Gattamaneni HR. Ovarian failure following abdominal irradiation in childhood: natural history and prognosis. *Clin. Oncol.* 1989;1:75–9.
6. Wallace WHB, Shalet SM, Hendry JH, Morris Jones PH, Gattamaneni HR. Ovarian failure following abdominal irradiation in childhood: the radiosensitivity of the human oocyte. *Br. J. Radiol.* 1989;62:995–8.
7. Critchley HOD, Wallace WHB, Mamtora H et al. Abdominal irradiation in childhood: the potential for pregnancy. *Br. J. Obstet. Gynaecol.* 1992;99:392–4.
8. Chapman RM, Sutcliffe SB, Rees LH, Edwards CRW, Malpas JC. Cyclical combination chemotherapy and gonadal function. *Lancet* 1979;1:285–9.
9. Whitehead E, Shalet SM, Blackledge G et al. The effects of Hodgkin's disease and combination chemotherapy on gonadal function in the adult male. *Cancer* 1982;49:418–22.
10. Koyama H, Wada T, Nishizaw Y et al. Cyclophosphamide-induced ovarian failure and its therapeutic significance in patients with breast cancer. *Cancer* 1977;39:1403–9.
11. Walden PAM, Bagshawe KD. Pregnancies after chemotherapy for gestational trophoblastic tumours. *Lancet* 1979;2:1241.
12. Viviani S, Santoro A, Ragni G et al. Gonadal toxicity after combination chemotherapy for Hodgkin's disease. Comparative results of MOPP versus ABVD. *Eur. J. Cancer Clin. Oncol.* 1985;21:601–5.
13. Morris ID, Shalet SM. Protection of gonadal function from cytotoxic chemotherapy and irradiation. *Clin. Endocrinol. Metab.* 1990;4:97–118.

83

Radiation-induced Thyroid Tumours

ARTHUR B. SCHNEIDER

Introduction

Radiation-related thyroid cancer was first described in 1950 by Duffy and Fitzgerald. Subsequent work confirmed the relationship between thyroid cancer and radiation and showed that the thyroid gland was among the most sensitive organs with respect to radiation's neoplastic effects.

While many studies have focused on thyroid cancer following radiation exposure, most of these have involved patients who received relatively small doses to treat benign head and neck conditions. Much less is known about the effects of the larger doses administered to treat malignancies in the head and neck area. Knowledge is limited for the following reasons:
1 the difficulty of studying a large enough sample of patients over a sufficiently long time;
2 the relatively high frequency of thyroid neoplasms and thyroid cancer, especially at older ages, in the general population;
3 the variable ascertainment caused by the fact that most thyroid neoplasms are asymptomatic and discovered by careful medical evaluation.

There are several very carefully documented case reports of thyroid cancer following radiation treatment of cancer, but these cannot be taken as proof of a relationship. However, they do indicate that a variety of thyroid cancers may occur. Well-differentiated thyroid cancers have been described most often, but reports of anaplastic cancers and a thyroid lymphoma have appeared.

The most convincing data comes from the Late Effects Study Group [1]. They followed 9170 patients who had survived 2 or more years after the diagnosis of a childhood cancer. With a mean follow-up of 5.5 years (range 2–48 years) they observed 23 cases of thyroid cancer. Compared to the general population, this was a 53-fold increased risk (34–80, 95% confidence interval). By selecting controls without thyroid cancer from among the study population, they confirmed a dose-response relationship. This relationship is very convincing evidence of a radiation effect. In a study designed to assure uniformity of clinical follow-up, Kaplan and colleagues [2] examined 95 patients who received radiotherapy to the neck region for childhood cancer 5 to 34 years earlier. Palpable thyroid nodules were present in 26 of these patients and three papillary carcinomas were found in the ten patients who had surgery. However, no relationship to the estimated thyroid dose was found.

Radiation treatments for malignancies in other parts of the body also result in thyroid exposure [3]. In an international cooperative study of cancer of the cervix, a twofold increased risk of thyroid cancer was observed with average thyroid dose of 0.11 Gy (although this was not significant).

Dose–response relationships

For many years it was felt that the dose–response relationship for thyroid cancer decreased significantly at higher doses. This was deduced, in part, from the well-documented observation that thyroid cancer does not occur as a result of radioactive iodine treatment for Graves' disease. This generated the hypothesis that at higher doses radiation leads to cell killing rather than to damage and subsequent neoplasia. However, it is now well accepted, even if it remains enigmatic, that the effects of external and internal radiation exposure are very different.

The shape of the dose–response curve for external radiation to the thyroid has been considered in previous reviews [4,5]. Uncertainty exists at the low end where it is not clear whether there is a threshold and which model fits the relationship best. At the high end of the dose–response curve it now appears, in part from the data cited above [1], that a risk remains, but whether the trend continues to increase, flattens out, or declines remains

514

to be determined. By pooling the data from several large studies, it now seems most likely that the relationship levels off (E. Ron, personal communication).

Modifying risk factors

Latency

The time between radiation and the occurrence of thyroid cancer (latency) has been studied most carefully after childhood exposure. Five years is generally considered the shortest interval between radiation and detectable thyroid cancer. However, with newer methods, particularly thyroid ultrasound, this time may be reduced.

The latency in adults is less well known. At the time of radiation exposure many adult patients already have subclinical thyroid neoplasms. Surveys of thyroid glands in adults, using sensitive ultrasound imaging, indicate that this may apply to approximately one-third of the population. In theory a shortened latency could be observed if radiation transforms a benign neoplasm into a malignant one or a slow-growing malignant one into an aggressive one.

Age at exposure

One of the most consistent findings in studies of radiation and thyroid cancer is that age of exposure is a significant modifying factor. Most of the data come from studies of childhood exposure and show that younger age at exposure is associated with a higher risk of developing thyroid cancer [6]. This trend also appears to apply to high-dose radiation exposure. Radiation treatment of Hodgkin's disease in adults was followed by fewer thyroid cancers than compared with children with Hodgkin's disease [1].

Dose fractionation

The effects of external and internal (iodine-131) radiation of the thyroid, even at comparable doses, are very different. One potential explanation is that the two modes have different rates at which the dose to the thyroid is delivered. This raises the question as to whether dose fractionation may alter the risk of developing thyroid cancer. Fractionated doses, allowing for DNA repair in the intervals between the treatments, would be associated with a lower risk of thyroid cancer. Unfortunately, there are no data at any level of thyroid exposure, which verify or refute this possibility.

Thyroid function

A clear relationship exists between the use of radiation to treat head and neck malignancies and the subsequent development of hypothyroidism: a relationship that is much clearer than the one for thyroid cancer [7,8]. The ability to detect impaired thyroid function is greatly facilitated by the measurement of thyroid-stimulating hormone (TSH). Clinical hypothyroidism is easily recognized by a markedly elevated TSH, decreased thyroid hormone levels, and characteristic clinical findings. However, this constellation is not frequent after radiation, except when treatment also requires partial thyroidectomy.

A damaged thyroid gland may continue to produce sufficient thyroid hormone, but only after receiving additional stimulation from an elevated TSH. This is the most common finding following head and neck cancer radiation, that is, normal thyroid hormone levels, an elevated TSH, and the absence of clinical findings [8].

The modifying effect on the risk for hypothyroidism of age at radiation is not clear. In one study, from Stanford University, the risk increased with increasing age up to 16 years and decreased thereafter [7]. However, multivariate analysis, including the effect of dose, eliminated the effect of age at treatment over the age of 16 years. Subtle changes in the thyroid function may be even more prevalent than revealed by the TSH measurements [9]. The intrathyroidal content of iodine was measured in 54 patients 1 to 17 years after external radiation to the neck for Hodgkin's disease. The prevalence of 44% for elevated TSH levels was exceeded by the prevalence of reduced intrathyroidal iodine content. Even in the patients with normal TSH, the intrathyroidal iodine content was reduced by approximately 50%. Also, 53% of the patients had elevated serum thyroglobulin levels. These could be an indication of early functional or neoplastic changes in the thyroid.

The data supporting the relationship between radiation and hypothyroidism are convincing for two reasons:
1 the proportion of individuals developing hypothyroidism is strikingly high;
2 the results of various studies have been uniform.
In an illustrative study, 81 patients who had received mantle field radiation for Hodgkin's disease were examined 10–18 years later. Elevated levels of TSH were found in 47 (58%) of these patients. The time course for developing hypothyroidism, defined as an elevated TSH, was reported in the Stanford study. Of 1730 patients with Hodgkin's disease whose treatment included radiation therapy, hypothyroidism was found in 513 patients. It occurred most frequently during the first 3 years, but continued to occur until 20 years after exposure. In this study the

frequency of hypothyroidism was related to the dose of radiation. In the examination study cited above [2], the TSH levels measured at follow-up were positively correlated to the dose of thyroid radiation. In the Stanford study, 32 patients developed Graves' disease. This finding has not been widely recognized and remains to be confirmed.

Diagnosis and treatment

From the information presented above it is clear that patients exposed to therapeutic radiation in the neck area should have periodic examinations of their thyroid glands. This should occur approximately every year and should include careful palpation of the gland. Whether imaging of the thyroid gland is necessary is difficult to decide. In favour of imaging is the observation, in other settings, that thyroid scanning and thyroid ultrasound are both more sensitive than thyroid palpation. The concern, particularly with thyroid ultrasound, is that many abnormalities are detected, even in individuals with no radiation exposure. Therefore, if these methods are used, the response to a positive finding must be carefully considered to prevent overtreatment and its attendant morbidities.

Fine needle aspiration cytology (FNAC) of thyroid nodules has taken the central role in management. However, two studies in the literature demonstrate that additional caution must be used in interpreting the FNAC results from nodules in patients after radiation treatment for head and neck cancer [10,11]. These aspirates are marked by cellular and nuclear atypia, which make the interpretation more difficult than usual. Another problem, seen at all levels of radiation exposure, is the increased frequency of multiple lesions within the thyroid, including mixtures of benign and malignant nodules.

The treatment of thyroid cancer is discussed in Chapters 16–18. In a previous review of thyroid cancer following radiation treatment of Hodgkin's disease, it was observed that many of the cases in the medical literature are associated with a poor prognosis [12]. This would suggest a more aggressive approach to treatment than might apply to comparable thyroid cancers not associated with radiation. However, it is likely that selection bias is entered into the initial reports in the literature, and more observations are necessary. For thyroid cancers following lower levels of radiation exposure, no differences in the behaviour of these cancers compared with the cancers in non-irradiated patients were found [13].

In addition to thyroid cancer, other radiogenic neoplasms should be considered in the following patients. For radiation in the head and neck area, these should include

Table 83.1 Evaluation and management of patients after radiation treatment of head and neck cancers

Thyroid palpation
1 Annually
2 For uncertain or abnormal findings:
  (a) Ultrasound (± scan) to delineate anatomy and function
  (b) Fine needle aspiration; atypia very common

Thyroid function
1 Every 6–12 months, more frequently at first
2 Treat elevated thyroid-stimulating hormone level with levothyroxine

Routine imaging
1 Every 3–5 years with normal palpation (controversial)
2 Interpret with caution

Observe for other radiation-related neoplasms
1 Salivary gland: palpate
2 Hyperparathyroidism: serum calcium
3 Schwannomas and acoustic neuromas: history and physical examination
4 Meningioma: history and physical examination

Treat thyroid cancer as in non-irradiated patients. Evidence for increased aggressiveness needs to be confirmed

hyperparathyroidism (parathyroid adenomas), benign and malignant salivary gland tumours, Schwannomas including acoustic neuromas, and possibly meningiomas.

It has been suggested that prior to administering radiation to treat head and neck cancers, thyroid hormone prophylaxis should be started [14]. While there would be little risk in this approach, provided that the dosage was carefully monitored, there are no data supporting this suggestion. However, in animal studies it is clear that radiation and TSH stimulation act synergistically. Therefore, it is prudent to start thyroid hormone replacement in any patient who develops an elevated TSH level. A summary of these clinical recommendations is given in Table 83.1.

Acknowledgements

This work was supported, in part, by grant CA21518 from the National Cancer Institute, NIH. I thank Phyllis Gallegos for help with the preparation of the manuscript.

References

1. Tucker MA, Jones PHM, Boice JD Jr *et al.* Therapeutic radiation at a young age is linked to second thyroid cancer. *Cancer Res.* 1991;51:2885–8.
2. Kaplan MM, Garnick MB, Gelber R *et al.* Risk factors for thyroid abnormalities after neck irradiation for childhood cancer. *Am. J. Med.* 1983;74:272–80.

3. Boice JD Jr, Engholm G, Kleinerman RA *et al*. Radiation dose and second cancer risk in patients treated for cancer of the cervix. *Radiat. Res.* 1988;**116**:3–55.
4. Maxon HR, Thomas SR, Saenger EL, Buncher CR, Kereiakes JG. Ionizing irradiation and the induction of clinically significant disease in the human thyroid gland. *Am. J. Med.* 1977;**63**:967–78.
5. Shore RE. Issues and epidemiological evidence regarding radiation-induced thyroid cancer. *Radiat. Res.* 1992;**131**:98–111.
6. Schneider AB, Ron E, Lubin J, Stovall M, Gierlowski TC. Dose–response relationships for radiation-induced thyroid cancer and thyroid nodules: evidence for the prolonged effects of radiation on the thyroid. *J. Clin. Endocrinol. Metab.* 1993;**77**:362–9.
7. Hancock SL, Cox RS, McDougall IR. Thyroid disease after treatment of Hodgkin's disease. *N. Engl. J. Med.* 1991;**325**:599–605.
8. Peerboom PF, Hassink EAM, Melkert R *et al*. Thyroid function 10–18 years after mantle field irradiation for Hodgkin's disease. *Eur. J. Cancer* 1992;**28A**:1716–18.
9. Schlumberger M, Sebagh M, De Vathaire F *et al*. Thyroid iodine content and serum thyroglobulin level following external irradiation to the neck for Hodgkin's disease. *J. Endocrinol. Invest.* 1990;**13**:197–203.
10. Pretorius HT, Katikineni M, Kinsell TJ *et al*. Thyroid nodules after high-dose external radiotherapy. *JAMA* 1982;**23**:3217–20.
11. Carr RF, LiVolsi VA. Morphologic changes in the thyroid after irradiation for Hodgkin's and non-Hodgkin's lymphoma. *Cancer* 1989;**64**:825–9.
12. Robinson E, Neugut AI. The clinical behavior of radiation-induced thyroid cancer in patients with prior Hodgkin's disease. *Radiother. Oncol.* 1990;**17**:109–13.
13. Schneider AB, Recant W, Pinsky SM *et al*. Radiation-induced thyroid cancer: Clinical course and results of therapy in 296 patients. *Ann. Intern. Med.* 1986;**105**:405–12.
14. McHenry C, Jarosz H, Calandra D *et al*. Thyroid neoplasia following radiation therapy for Hodgkin's lymphoma. *Arch. Surg.* 1987;**122**:684–6.

84

Neuroimmunoendocrinology

PAUL J. JENKINS AND ASHLEY GROSSMAN

Introduction

The constancy of homeostasis requires precise integration of the different interdependent systems of an organism. Over the last two decades it has become increasingly apparent that this includes the immune and endocrine systems which communicate with each other using common chemical messengers, resulting in a bidirectional flow of information [1]. The principal endocrine system involved is the hypothalamic–pituitary–adrenal (HPA) axis, and it is now clear that the immune system affects this at all levels, while conversely adrenocorticotrophic hormone (ACTH) and glucocorticoids have wide ranging effects on the immune system. What is less certain, and subject to a great deal of controversy, is the putative existence of ultrashort feedback loops in which cells of the immune system synthesize and secrete ACTH and the ACTH precursor pro-opiomelanocortin (POMC) to act in a paracrine or autocrine fashion. The significance and purpose of this bidirectional communication is also under debate. In general, it may be that activation of the immune system, in addition to producing a co-ordinated local inflammatory reaction, also activates the endocrine system such that immunological function is modified to prevent an overexuberant immune response. An alternative hypothesis is that the two systems act together to *localize* inflammatory reactions; it is only when the immune system becomes overwhelmed and there is generalized production of cytokines that the HPA axis is activated in order to maintain vascular integrity [2].

This immunoendocrine interaction is known to be important in many human disease states. Much work has focused on the autoimmune diseases such as rheumatoid arthritis, juvenile diabetes mellitus and Hashimoto's thyroiditis, which result from tissue destruction by cells of the body's own immune systems [3]. Since the treatment of such disorders often involves immune suppression by the administration of glucocorticoids,

there is the suggestion that the HPA axis might also play a role in their pathogenesis. A model that has been used when studying this question is that provided by the Lewis rat, which is particularly susceptible to the development of a form of chronic arthritis. It has been shown that these rats lack corticotrophin-releasing hormone (CRH) responsiveness, and thus are able to mount only a poor cortisol response to various stressors. Injection of streptococcal cell wall polysaccharide into these rats results in the development of a form of arthritis, resembling human rheumatoid arthritis, which can be prevented by the prior administration of glucocorticoids. Furthermore, normal rats which have an intact HPA axis do not develop arthritis following similar injections but do so after bilateral adrenalectomy or the administration of the glucocorticoid antagonist RU-486. Circumstantial evidence for a pathogenetic role of the HPA axis in rheumatoid arthritis is also provided by human studies, as patients with this condition have both a less pronounced diurnal rhythm in cortisol production compared to those with osteoarthritis and less pronounced pituitary and adrenal responses to surgery.

Further information on the functional significance of immunoendocrinology comes from work on the obese strain (OS) chickens which have been used as a model for Hashimoto's thyroiditis. Such chickens have massive infiltration of the thyroid gland by T-cells and this is associated with glandular dysfunction. Marked elevations in circulating glucocorticoid-binding globulin are also observed, which decrease the amount of free corticosterone, and there are also deficiencies in the HPA axis such that a suboptimal cortisol response to stressors is given. The development of this autoimmune thyroid disease can be prevented by the administration of hydrocortisone to neonatal OS chickens.

In human oncology, the role of interactions between the immune and endocrine systems remains controversial. We have recently shown that patients with lymphoma and other malignancies have significant bilateral adrenal hyperplasia that is unrelated to their overall health or the stage of their disease. Functional studies on these patients have shown that many fail to suppress their cortisol after a low-dose dexamethasone suppression test (0.5 mg, 6-hourly for 48 hours) but have undetectable or very low circulating levels of plasma ACTH. This suggests that these patients have biochemical Cushing's syndrome due to an as yet unidentified adrenal stimulating substance, possibly a cytokine. The functional significance of these observations remains to be determined, although it is interesting to speculate about their potential oncological significance. The development of a cancer and the associated antigenic changes may result in activation of the immune system with subsequent cytokine stimulation; in addition to their potential cytotoxic effects on the cancer, these cytokines may also stimulate the HPA axis (see below). One hypothesis is that this activation in some way represents an attempt by the body to potentiate its defence mechanisms, an idea that is supported by our observation of adrenal hyperplasia and increased cortisol levels, as high-dose steroids are an effective treatment for lymphoma. Alternatively, the adrenal activation may suppress all but the most intense inflammatory reactions thereby possibly aiding tumour growth by inhibiting immune surveillance mechanisms. That there is a critical balance between the two is suggested by the fact that the prognosis of patients with ectopic ACTH resulting from oat cell carcinomas is worse than that of non-ACTH secretors: furthermore, ACTH secretors show increased susceptibility towards overwhelming infections [4,5]. Further circumstantial evidence in support of an interaction is provided by several studies which suggest that behavioural and psychological factors may exert a profound adverse effect on the progress of malignancy, and patients undergoing marked life-event changes show a more rapid progression of tumour growth.

Activation of the HPA axis by the immune system

One of the most controversial aspects of the interaction between the immune and endocrine systems is whether cells of the immune system are capable of synthesizing and secreting POMC and its derivatives, especially ACTH. Support for this idea has mainly come from studies by Blalock and associates, who suggested that human peripheral blood mononuclear cells (PBMCs) were able to secrete ACTH and endorphin-like peptides when stimulated *in vitro* with α-interferon-induced Newcastle disease virus lipopolysaccharide (LPS) endotoxin and CRH. However, their methods for detecting these sub-

stances in the medium utilized antiserum affinity columns, which are unreliable and much of their work has not been corroborated by other centres. Nevertheless, ACTH-like immunoreactivity has been demonstrated *within* cells of the immune system using specific antiserum to ACTH (1–24) and (1–39), although in order to demonstrate the *functional* significance of such immunoreactivity it is necessary to demonstrate that the expression of POMC mRNA varies according to functional state. Careful work by van Woudernberg and colleagues [6] has shown that in PBMC full-length POMC mRNA (1200 nt) is undetectable, and there is no increase after stimulation by LPS, concanavalin-A (Con-A) or CRH. However, a short transcript of 800–900 nucleotides was detected in cultured PBMCs which was increased after Con-A stimulation. Such a short transcript represents transcription from exon 3 only and although it can also be detected in virtually all tissues, it is unlikely to be of physiological importance. While monocyte secretion of ACTH and related peptides remains unproven [7], there is considerable evidence that such cells may synthesize and secrete other neuroendocrine peptides such as prolactin and growth hormone.

Immunological modulation of the HPA axis

The idea that the immune system could activate the HPA axis was first suggested by work in the 1950s which showed that injection of bacterial endotoxin or pyrogen increased plasma concentrations of adrenal corticosteroids, both in humans and rats. It was subsequently shown that such effects did not occur in the absence of an intact hypothalamopituitary unit. However, it was not until work by Besedowsky and colleagues in the mid1970s that the mechanisms for this effect began to be elucidated. It was demonstrated that the infusion of medium from Con-A stimulated leucocytes resulted in the prompt elevation of plasma corticosteroid levels. The active factor present in the medium was subsequently shown to be interleukin-1 (IL-1). It is now clear that IL-1 is one of the major mediators of HPA axis stimulation in response to inflammatory and immunological challenges (Fig. 84.1). Although IL-1 has some direct actions on the adrenal gland and at the pituitary level, the majority of work suggests that its major site of action is via the hypothalamus, certainly in terms of acute stimulation [8]. *In vivo* injection of IL-1 results in depletion of hypothalamic CRH as well as an increase in its mRNA expression, while *in vitro* IL-1 has been shown to cause direct release of CRH from the rat hypothalamus. It should be noted that IL-1 exists in two isoforms, IL-1α and IL-1β, with IL-1β as the principal secreted product.

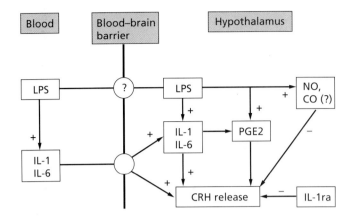

Fig. 84.1 The effects of lipopolysaccharide (LPS) in stimulating corticotrophin-releasing hormone (CRH) release may be mediated via the peripheral induction of interleukin-1 and -6 (IL-1 and IL-6) which then cross the blood–brain barrier (BBB). Alternatively, LPS may directly cross the BBB to act centrally via the induction of hypothalamic IL-1 and IL-6. Prostaglandins (PGE$_2$) are involved in this central pathway, either under the direct influence of LPS or secondary to IL stimulation. An inhibitory role has been postulated for the labile gases nitric oxide (NO) and carbon monoxide (CO), and possibly IL-1ra.

Although they are only around 30% structurally homologous, it is probable that the majority of their activity is exerted at a common receptor.

IL-1 is produced by a number of immune cells in response to antigenic stimulation, and in particular LPS (endotoxin). The stimulatory effects of IL-1 on CRH release are now thought not to be direct but to be mediated via the prostaglandins, in particular prostaglandin E$_2$ (PGE$_2$) (Fig. 84.1). Microinjection of PGE$_2$ into the pre-optic area of the hypothalamus produces a marked increase in plasma ACTH, an effect that can be counteracted by the administration of indomethacin (an inhibitor of the cyclo-oxygenase pathway) or the injection of a PGE$_2$ receptor antagonist into the anterior hypothalamus. Pretreatment with CRH antiserum can also counteract the increase in plasma ACTH observed after intrahypothalamic injection of PGE$_2$, while pretreatment with indomethacin significantly antagonizes the rise in plasma ACTH produced by intravenous injection of IL-1. Taken together, these *in vivo* experiments appear to show that PGE$_2$ mediates the effects of IL-1 on the HPA, a conclusion that has generally been supported by *in vitro* experiments. On the basis of a number of further studies, a picture is generally being drawn that PGE$_2$ might mediate this interaction at two separate sites: these would include the organ vasculosum lamina terminalus (OVLT), a vascular structure devoid of the blood–brain barrier situated within the anterior wall of the third ventricle and the anterior hypothalamus,

and second, directly on CRH neurones in the paraventricular nucleus (PVN; or possibly the median eminence), where cytokines interact with their specific receptors to produce the acute release of CRH [9]. It has been shown that intravenous injection of IL-1 results in a marked increase in PGE$_2$ levels within the OVLT, although the exact mechanism by which this increased PGE$_2$ mediates CRH release within the PVN remains unknown.

In addition to IL-1, IL-6 is also now known to be involved in the interaction between the immune and HPA axes. Within the central nervous system, IL-6 is produced mainly by astrocytes in response to tumour necrosis factor (TNF) and LPS but is probably also present within scattered, neurones. IL-6 is also produced in the pituitary by folliculo-stellate cells, suggesting a possible paracrine role for its modulation of anterior pituitary hormone secretion, and has been shown to stimulate directly the HPA by activating both CRH and vasopressin release. IL-6 has wide-ranging neuroprotective and neurone growth-stimulating actions, and it can be envisaged that in response to noxious stimuli, such as LPS, both IL-1 secretion, with consequent immunosuppressive activation of the HPA axis, and IL-6 secretion, with consequent neuroprotective and neurotrophic effects, is stimulated [9].

As mentioned above, LPS is a major inducer of the actions of IL-1 on the HPA. In rats, LPS produces significant increases in both plasma ACTH and corticosterone as little as 30 minutes after injection, a similar time course to that following the intravenous injection of cytokine itself. This identical time course for both LPS and cytokine-induced HPA stimulation suggests that LPS might also have a direct action on the hypothalamus. Some evidence in support of this is that selective depletion of macrophages (the major source of IL-1) does not completely prevent the HPA activation by LPS, although high doses are required for this macrophage-independent effect, which itself is thought to involve local hypothalamic IL-1 and PGE$_2$ synthesis.

There is evidence that IL-6 is also involved in HPA stimulation via LPS, having an additive effect to that of IL-1. Other cytokines that are induced by LPS include TNF and the interferons, in addition to central catecholamines and serotonin. Noradrenaline in particular has been shown to be involved in the subacute stimulation of CRH by LPS, as increased levels of this catecholamine have been found in the rat hypothalamus as early as 90 minutes after intraperitoneal injection of LPS.

In spite of its stimulatory effect on CRH *in vivo*, LPS shows an inhibitory effect on CRH release *in vitro*. It is now increasingly probable that the gaseous neurotransmitters nitric oxide (NO) and carbon monoxide (CO) play such an inhibitory role. LPS has been shown to up-regulate the expression of inducible NO synthase (NOS) leading to increases in systemic NO synthesis. This effect has also been demonstrated in astrocytes and NOS activity has been detected within the hypothalamus. *In vitro* experiments have shown that increased NO and CO both inhibit depolarization and IL-1β-induced CRH and vasopressin release from hypothalamic explants; furthermore, inhibition of NOS by α-arginine methylester has been found to potentiate the rise in plasma ACTH levels induced by IL-1β. Thus, these evanescent gases may act as counter-regulatory inhibitors to the HPA in response to inflammatory stimuli, the net output reflecting the coordinated balance of stimulators and inhibitors [10].

Conclusion

In conclusion, therefore, there is a complex interaction between the immune system and HPA axis. Inflammatory and immunological challenges result in stimulation of CRH and vasopressin release via IL-1 and IL-6 with consequential activation of ACTH and glucocorticoids, hence producing partial immunosuppression. Local inhibitors of CRH release by LPS allow for fine tuning. Thus, homeostasis is maintained, although the pathophysiological significance of these interactions remains to be fully determined, particularly with regard to chronic inflammatory and oncological stimuli. Modulation of these processes may allow for therapeutic deceleration in the progression of tumour growth.

References

1. Reichlin SR. Neuroendocrine–immune interactions. *N. Engl. J. Med.* 1993;**329**:1246–53.
2. Grossman A. The regulation of human pituitary responses to stress: a description and a suggested model. In Brown MR, Rivier C, Koob G (eds). *Neurobiology and Neuroendocrinology of Stress.* New York: Marcel Dekker, 1991.
3. Derijk R, Berkenbosch F. The immune–hypothalamo–pituitary–adrenal axis and autoimmunity. *Int. J. Neurosci.* 1991;**59**:91–100.
4. Dimopoulos MA, Fernandez JF, Samaan NA, Holoye PY, Vassilopoulou-Sellin R. Paraneoplastic Cushing's syndrome as an adverse prognostic factor in patients who die early with small cell cancer. *Cancer* 1992;**69**:66–71.
5. Shepherd FA, Laskey J, Evans WK *et al.* Cushing's syndrome associated with ectopic corticotropin production and small-cell lung cancer. *J. Clin. Oncol.* 1992;**10**:21–7.
6. Van Woudenberg AD, Metzelaar MJ, Van der Kleij AAM *et al.* Analysis of proopiomelanocortin (POMC) messenger ribonucleic acid and POMC-derived peptides in human peripheral blood mononuclear cells: no evidence for a lymphocyte-derived POMC system. *Endocrinology* 1993;**133**:1922–33.
7. Sharp B, Linner K. What do we know about the expression of proopiomelanocortin transcripts and related peptides in lymphoid tissue. *Endocrinology* 1993;**133**:1921A–1921B.
8. Busbridge NJ, Grossman AB. Stress and the single cytokine: interleukin modulation of the pituitary–adrenal axis. *Molec. Cell. Endocrinol.* 1991;**82**:209–14.
9. Navarra P. Schettini G, Grossman AB. Neuroendocrine responses to immunological challenge: the role of cytokines, autacoids and astrocytes. In Buckingham JC, Gillies G, Cowell A (eds.) *Stress, Stress Hormones and the Immune System.* Chichester: John Wiley, 1995.
10. Navarra P. The effects of endotoxin on the neuroendocrine axis. *Curr. Opin. Endocrinol. Diabetes* 1995;**2**:127–33.

Cytokine-responsive Tumours

JAMES S. MALPAS

Introduction

The clinical effects of cytokines on human tumours have been studied for just over a decade. Their use in clinical practice has been made possible by recombinant DNA technology, allowing the production of adequate pure material. Interferon (IFN), the most frequently-used cytokine, has proved highly beneficial in hairy cell leukaemia and chronic myeloid leukaemia, but less so in solid tumours. Interleukin-2 (IL-2) has occasionally produced major responses in solid tumours, but has also been noted for its toxicity. New cytokines are being developed and alternative strategies devised for established agents [1].

Cytokines

Cytokines are proteins produced by cells in response to a variety of stimuli. They are secreted by a wide range of cells present in various tissues, and affect the behaviour of target cells by binding to specific receptors on their surface. Signal transduction across the cell surface membrane then gives rise to a variety of biological effects, usually due to a change in gene expression in the nucleus.

Three types of cytokine–cell interaction have been described and these are autocrine, paracrine and endocrine (Fig. 85.1).

Cytokines are low molecular weight proteins of some 15–30 kDa. The structures and molecular weights of cytokines with antitumour properties are given in Table 85.1.

Properties of major cytokines involved in tumour growth or suppression

Before considering the clinical applications of cytokines, a brief review of the major properties of cytokines of proven clinical use, or those that could possibly be used as targets for manipulation in various cancers, is given.

Interleukin-2

IL-2 was known as T-cell growth factor because its principal source is T lymphocytes. It is unusual in being controlled by one gene in humans, located on chromosome 4q26-28, producing a 15–16 kDa glycoprotein. It is mainly produced by T-helper cells after the T-cell receptor has engaged a major histocompatibility complex on the antigen-presenting cell. There now appear to be three receptors: IL-2Rα, β and γ. The α receptor binds with high affinity, whilst the β and γ receptors associate to form an intermediate affinity receptor. IL-2's regulating activities are listed in Table 85.2.

The generation of lymphokine-activated killer (LAK) cells has been thought to be an important component of the anti-tumour activity of IL-2. This has been demonstrated in animal studies, but results in human cancers have been equivocal. Major toxicities have been seen in patients treated with IL-2, the most dangerous being those associated with vascular permeability leading to pulmonary oedema, and a decrease in systemic vascular resistance causing hypotension. The major toxicities are listed in Table 85.3.

These toxicities are all readily reversible on cessation of IL-2 infusion, but they may necessitate a patient's transfer to an intensive care unit. IL-2 is rapidly cleared from the blood, with a half-life of 7 minutes, and is almost completely cleared by 30 minutes. Its clinical activity has been explored mainly in renal cell carcinoma and melanoma, and details of these studies and results are given below.

Interleukin-6

IL-6 was previously known as interferon β2, β-cell differentiating factor, or BSF2. The gene controlling its production is on human chromosome 7 p21–22. IL-6 has a molecular weight of 21–28 kDa. The IL-6 gene is

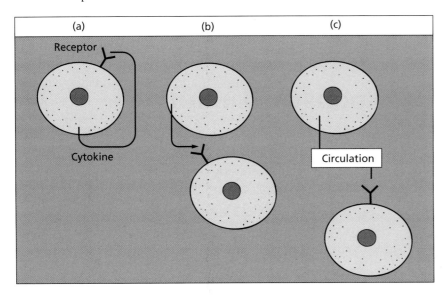

Fig. 85.1 Cytokine–cell interactions: (a) autocrine, (b) paracrine, (c) endocrine.

Table 85.1 Structure and properties of cytokines affecting tumours

Type of cytokine	Number of amino acids	Molecular weight	Principal sources	Activity
Interleukins				
IL-2	133	15 400	T lymphocytes	Increases antigen-specific T-cell and NK/AK cell cytotoxic effect on function
IL-6	184	*c.* 21 000–28 000	T lymphocytes, monocytes, fibroblasts	Promoter of malignant cell growth, e.g. in myeloma by paracrine activity
IL-12	–	–	–	Enhances activity of NK cells inhibiting cell-mediated immunity
Interferons				
IFN-αs	166–172	16 000–27 000	T lymphocytes, B lymphocytes	Inhibitors of malignant cell proliferation; down-regulate oncogene activity
IFN-β	166	*c.* 20 000	Fibroblasts	Enhance or induce host immune response to tumour
IFN-γ	143	*c.* 50 000 (dimer)	T lymphocytes	Produce other anti-tumour cytokines

AK, activated killer; NK, natural killer.

Table 85.2 Main cell-regulating activities of IL-2

Stimulation of activated T-cell growth and differentiation
Generation of lymphokine-activated killer activity
Stimulation of proliferation and immunoglobulin production in B cells
Stimulation of macrophage cytotoxic activity

Table 85.3 Major toxicities associated with IL-2

Hypotension
Hypervolaemia and pulmonary oedema
Renal failure
Myelosuppression
Pyrexia
Neuropsychiatric complications

expressed by a variety of lymphoid cells, and also by fibroblasts and monocytes. It can be induced by IL-1 and IFN-β. Its cell regulatory activities are given in Table 85.4.

One of the most interesting features of IL-6 is that it acts as an autocrine growth factor for plasmacytoma and myeloma cells. Evidence for autocrine and paracrine

Table 85.4 Cell regulating activities of IL-6

Stimulates immunoglobulin production by B cells
Stimulates liver cells to produce acute phase protein
   C-reactive protein
Stimulates IL-2 production by some T cells
Autocrine growth factor for plasmacytoma and myeloma

stimulation from local bone marrow fibroblasts is accumulating. Its promoting activity can be countered by anti-IL-6 antibody, both in tissue culture and in human tumours [2]. The possibility of blocking or down-regulating IL-6 receptors as a means of inhibiting growth of these tumours is now being explored. These programmes are now at the stage of initial clinical pilot trials [3].

Interferon

IFN was first identified by Isaacs and Lindemann [4] as a protein produced in response to viral infection. In addition to antiviral properties, interferons were found to be important in the immune response, and to be involved in the control of cell growth and differentiation. Recombinant DNA technology allowed large quantities of the pure substance to be produced, and IFN-α, -β and -γ are now available for clinical use. Their structure and origins are given in Table 85.1. IFN-α and -β genes are clustered on human chromosome 9 pter-q12. There is a single gene for IFN-β, and IFN-γ is also regulated by one gene. Leucocytes are the main source of IFN-α, and fibroblasts that of IFN-β, contrasting with IFN-γ which can be produced by all subsets of T cells. There are tumour receptors for IFN type 1, which binds IFN-α and -β, and for type 2, which specifically binds IFN-γ.

When IFN became available, it was tested unsuccessfully as a therapy for acute myeloid leukaemia. Subsequent studies showed a high response rate for the rare hairy cell leukaemia, and the more commonly occurring chronic myeloid leukaemia (when it is at an early stage). In hairy cell leukaemia, cessation of therapy was accompanied by relapse, and it was found that in patients in the later stages of chronic myeloid leukaemia there was generally a poor response.

Results in solid tumours have been less satisfactory, with the exception of carcinoid tumour, where objective responses have been seen in as many as 50% of patients treated, and where in the case of midgut carcinoid tumours the 5-year survival has approached 70% (the best results seen so far).

Toxicity of interferon

Although IFN was heralded as being a non-toxic treatment for cancer, this proved to be untrue. Toxicity was dose-dependent, and side-effects tended to diminish after the first few weeks of treatment. Many of these side-effects could be abolished by the use of paracetamol.

The most common side-effect is a flu-like syndrome which is transient. Varying degrees of fatigue have been reported. More serious events such as bone marrow suppression, hypotension and neuropsychiatric symptoms have been described. The toxicities are listed in Table 85.5.

IFN has been extensively investigated in all its forms, using several routes, in conditions where conventional chemotherapy has been unsatisfactory [5]. Treatment with α-IFN has resulted in objective responses in 22% of 350 patients with renal cell carcinoma, with a response range of 7–56% (Table 85.6). Although modest, these are better than the results of chemotherapy or hormonal therapy. Patients with prior nephrectomy, prolonged survival between nephrectomy and recurrence of disease, and those with a low tumour burden of lung metastases were most likely to have a good response.

Another malignancy which shows resistance to primary chemotherapy is malignant melanoma. In 11 studies (Table 85.6) 286 patients showed an average objective response rate of 13%, with a range of 3–23%, similar to most chemotherapeutic trials. However, some patients had complete remission which lasted several years. There were no particular features in the responding patients.

Table 85.5 Major toxicities of interferon

Fever
Headache
Muscle pain
Fatigue
Bone marrow suppression
Depression

Table 85.6 Response rates in solid tumours when interferon is given by intramuscular, intravenous or subcutaneous administration in low or high dose (after [5])

Tumour	Number of studies	Total no. of points	Objective response (%)	Range
Melanoma	11	286	13	3–23
Renal cell carcinoma	16	350	22	7–56
Kaposi sarcoma	7	192	27	3–67

Response occurred in both previously treated and untreated patients, and the site of primary disease did not affect response [5].

With the increasing incidence of Kaposi sarcoma as a complication of the autoimmune deficiency syndrome (AIDS), much attention has been given to new methods of treating this condition. The further immune suppression caused by many chemotherapeutic agents has led to the exploration of the use of cytokines, and encouraging results have been seen in some series treated with IFN.

IFN-α has been used in ovarian cancer. Studies have been performed in heavily pretreated patients, and either i.v. or i.m. routes have resulted in disappointing response rates. In contrast, IFN-α given intraperitoneally produced complete or good partial remissions in 5/11 (45%) of surgically re-staged patients. These good responses were seen in those women who had tumour nodules < 5 mm in size. IFN-β is less active, and IFN-γ is inactive [6].

Local high-dose therapy has also been shown to be effective for the treatment of *in situ* bladder cancer, although the response rate has been lower than that achieved by bacille Calmette–Guérin (BCG). However, IFN therapy was not associated with the serious side-effects seen with BCG.

Combination therapy

The use of IFN-α and IL-2 is now being explored in chemoresistant tumours such as renal cell cancer and colon cancer. Reports have shown variable efficiency. Ilson and colleagues [7], using IL-2 and IFN-α, found minimal activity in renal cell cancer. Bergmann and colleagues [8], using alternate administration of high-dose IFN-α and IL-2, achieved a 25% complete response rate in renal cell cancer. Atzpodien and colleagues [9] added 5-fluorouracil (5-FU) to IL-2 and IFN-α, and obtained an overall response rate of 48% in this condition, which must be amongst the highest response rates recorded. Similar studies in colon cancer and malignant melanoma would suggest that the use of cytokines and chemotherapy may be synergistic. A summary of response rates in colon cancer is given in Table 85.7.

Cytokines have recently been combined with retinoids. These latter possess similar antiproliferative, differentiative and immunomodulatory activities, and are relatively non-toxic. IFN-α and 13-cis retinoic acid (13cRA) have been shown to be synergistic in tissue culture systems. When used together to treat squamous cell carcinoma of the skin, an overall response rate of 68% has been seen. Similar response rates have been found in cervical cancer, and the potential for this combination has been reviewed

Table 85.7 Phase II clinical trials of 5-fluorouracil (5-FU) and interferon (IFN) in colon cancer (after [5])

Institution	Number of patients	Response (%)
Albert Einstein	32	63
M.D. Anderson	52	35
ECOG	38	42
N.E. Deaconess	8	38
Memorial	34	26

ECOG, Eastern Co-operative Oncology Group; N.E., New England. More recently, large randomized controlled trials have failed to confirm any survival benefit when IFN is added to 5-FU in colon cancer. In fact the quality of life was poorer for the IFN-treated group [10].

by Bollag and Holdener [11] and Lippman and colleagues [12].

It is only just becoming apparent why some of these unlikely combinations may be successful. In the combination of IFN and 5-FU, IFN inhibits the uptake and phosphorylation of thymidine to give thymidilate. 5-FU is converted to 5-fluorodeoxyuridilate in the cells, which inhibits the enzyme thymidilate synthetase. Hence, both agents are acting synergistically in inhibiting thymidilate production. If thymidilate is reduced, then DNA production (and therefore cell division) is inhibited [13].

The reason for the apparent synergy between retinoic acid and IFN is currently under investigation. It is probable that retinoic acid increases the expression of receptors for IFN.

Summary of results in solid tumours

Enough experience has now accumulated to state that there is a definite, although modest, effect of cytokines on a number of solid tumours, including renal cell carcinoma, melanoma, Kaposi sarcoma, and carcinoid tumours. When used in combination with chemotherapy there seems to be synergy, and an improved response rate, but little effect on survival (for example, in colon cancer). Local therapy in particular circumstances has been demonstrated to be as effective in ovarian cancer and bladder cancer (for example). The roles of combinations of cytokines, cytokines and chemotherapy, and cytokines and retinoids remain to be elucidated, and their place in current management defined.

Future prospects

In addition to the use of combinations of cytokines and other agents, the use of cytokines in the future will depend on the discovery of more effective members of this family.

An example of this is the recent identification of IL-12 also known as natural killer cell-stimulating factor (NKSF), originally purified and cloned from a line of B-lymphoblastoid cells. It is a very potent growth factor for T and NK cells, and is therefore a critical component in the development of cell-mediated immunity [14]. Initial studies of NKSF in renal cell cancer, melanoma and colon cancer in mouse models have shown marked tumour regression [15], but whether this will be translated into effective treatments in humans will be shown by the phase I and II trials now beginning.

Another approach would be to inhibit promoters of cancer cell proliferation. This has already been done in patients with plasmacytomas, who have been treated with IL-6 [2]. Ten patients were treated with murine monoclonal antibodies directed at IL-6. Complete inhibition of plasmablastic proliferation was seen in 6/10 patients, and there were no major side-effects apart from thrombocytopenia. These interesting preliminary results were obtained in heavily pretreated and refractory patients, and although clinical response was short-lived, this imaginative new approach may lead to the identification and inhibition of other growth-promoting cytokines.

The potential for manipulating the complex cytokine network to suppress and destroy tumour cells is in its infancy, but the prospects are encouraging.

References

1. Balkwill FR. *Cytokines in Cancer Therapy*. Oxford: Oxford University Press, 1989.
2. Klein B, Bataille R. Cytokine therapy in myeloma. In Malpas JS, Bergsagel D, Kyle RA (eds). *Myeloma*. Oxford: Oxford University Press, 1995:307–13.
3. Bauer J, Herrmann F. Interleukin-6 in clinical medicine. *Ann. Haematol.* 1991;**62**:203–10.
4. Isaacs A, Lindenmann J. Virus interference. I. The interferon. *Proc. R. Soc. Lond. [Biol]* 1957;**147**:259–67.
5. Wadler S. The role of interferons in the treatment of solid tumours. *Cancer* 1992;**70**:949–58.
6. Bookman MA, Berek JS. Biologic and immunologic therapy of ovarian cancer. *Hematol. /Oncol. Clin. North Am.* 1992;**6**:941–65.
7. Ilson DH, Motzer RJ, Kradin RL *et al*. A phase II trial of interleukin-2 and interferon alfa-2a in patients with advanced renal cell carcinoma. *J. Clin. Oncol.* 1992;**10**:1124–30.
8. Bergmann L, Fenchel K, Weidmann E *et al*. Daily alternating administration of high-dose alpha 2b interferon and interleukin-2 bolus in metastatic renal cancer. *Cancer* 1993;**72**:1733–42.
9. Atzopodien J, Kirchner H, Hanninen EL *et al*. Interleukin-2 in combination with interferon-α and 5-fluorouracil for metastatic renal cell cancer. *Eur. J. Cancer* 1993;**29A**(Suppl. 5):S6–S8.
10. Hill M, Norman A, Cunningham D *et al*. Royal Marsden phase III trial of fluorouracil with or without interferon alfa-2b in advanced colorectal cancer. *J. Clin. Oncol.* 1995;**13**:1297–302.
11. Bollag W, Holdener EE. Retinoids in cancer prevention and therapy. *Ann. Onocol.* 1992;**3**:513–26.
12. Lippman SM, Glisson BS, Kavanagh JJ *et al*. Retinoic acid and interferon combination studies in human cancer. *Eur. J. Cancer*, 1993;**29A**(Suppl. 5):S9–S13.
13. Clemens MJ. *Cytokines*. Oxford: BIOS Scientific Publishers, 1991.
14. Scott P. IL-12 — initiation cytokine for cell mediated immunity. *Science* 1993;**260**:496–7.
15. Brunda MJ, Luistro L, Warrier RR *et al*. Antitumour and antimetastatic activity of interleukin-12 against murine tumours. *J. Exp. Med.* 1993;**178**:1223–30.

86

Endocrine-responsive Tumours

JONATHAN WAXMAN

Introduction

Endocrine-responsive tumours constitute approximately one-fifth of all cancers occurring in the West and are uncommon in the developing world. The most important numerically of these tumours are breast and prostate cancer. Both tumours have increased in incidence over recent years and at present in the USA, breast cancer is the most common tumour of women, and prostate cancer the most prevalent malignancy of men and the second commonest cause of male cancer deaths. It is probable that there are many reasons for this increase but the most clearly important is diet. These tumours are uncommon in the Far East where diets are low in animal proteins. The migration of populations to the West, with subsequent changes in dietary patterns, has been associated with a concomitant increase in incidence of breast and prostate cancer. The incidence of cancer of the breast and prostate in vegetarians is half that of meat eaters. It may be that one potentially successful way of dealing with the pandemic of breast and prostate cancer would be to concentrate on public health measures.

The management of breast and prostate cancer has radically changed over the last decade and these clinical advances have led to significant improvements in patients' life quality and expectancy. This chapter will review clinical developments in prostate and breast cancer.

Prostate cancer

Prostate cancer is androgen dependent. Anti-androgen treatment leads to a subjective response in 80% of patients and an objective response in 50% of patients and this response has a median duration of approximately 1 year. The median duration of survival of patients with metastatic prostate cancer is between 2.5 and 3 years. Prior to the 1980s the standard treatments offered to patients with prostate cancer were castration or oestrogen therapy.

Castration is a psychologically unacceptable procedure and oestrogen therapy is associated with an increased risk of cardiovascular death as well as a number of other side-effects.

Gonadotrophin-releasing hormone agonists and the concept of complete androgen blockade

In the 1980s gonadotrophin-releasing hormone (GnRH) agonists were introduced into the treatment of prostate cancer, providing a safe medical alternative to orchidectomy which was without significant side-effects. Depot preparations were developed which allowed the patients to be minimally inconvenienced by treatment. In the early 1980s the concept of so-called 'complete androgen blockade' was introduced into oncological practice. It was argued that in a disease that is androgen sensitive, it is important to remove all sources of androgen. In the medically castrated male, approximately 45% of all tissue androgen is derived from the adrenal gland and to limit the peripheral availability of androgenic metabolites, anti-androgens such as flutamide were used in combination with GnRH agonists.

Currently there are only two published randomized studies that provide details of response and survival, the first study out of as many as 26 studies that are in progress was carried out by the National Cancer Institute (NCI) in Maryland, and involved just over 600 patients with metastatic prostate cancer who were treated with leuprorelin (a long-acting luteinizing hormone-releasing hormone (LHRH) agonist) with or without flutamide. The progression-free survival of patients treated with combination endocrine therapy was 16.5, versus 13.9 months for those patients treated with monotherapy. The median survival of the combination treatment group was 35.6 months as compared with 28.3 months for the monotherapy group. Both variations were significantly different [1].

The second study to be completed was published on behalf of the European Organization for the Research and Treatment of Cancer (EORTC). Three hundred and twenty seven patients with metastatic prostate cancer were randomized to treatment with goserelin acetate (another long-acting LHRH agonist) and flutamide or orchiectomy. The median progression time for patients treated by orchiectomy was 46 weeks and for patients treated with combination endocrine therapy 71 weeks. The median duration of survival was 27 months for patients treated by orchiectomy and 34.4 months for patients treated by combination therapy and both these differences were statistically significant [2].

Both these studies provoke an unequivocal conclusion that combination endocrine therapy offers a significant advantage over single-agent therapy. There are a number of complicating issues; for example, in breast cancer there have been many studies comparing combination endocrine therapy with sequential endocrine therapy. In these investigations there is an advantage in terms of initial response rates to patients treated with combination therapy. However, the overall survival is identical, so it may be that if patients with prostate cancer were treated with an LHRH agonist until they relapsed and were then prescribed an anti-androgen, the survival of these patients might be similar to those given initial combination therapy. The second complicating issue comes from recent observations of the effects of flutamide withdrawal in relapse prostate cancer. Responses are seen in approximately 30% of patients for a median of 5 months [3].

Both the NCI and EORTC trials were carried out on patients with metastatic prostate cancer. Approximately 40% of patients with prostate cancer have locally advanced disease without evidence of metastases on presentation. The median survival of this group of patients is 4.5 years and it is not known currently whether combination endocrine therapy offers an advantage over monotherapy in this patient group. All these issues need to be considered and confound and confuse the relatively simple concept of the advantage of combination endocrine therapy in the treatment of metastatic prostate cancer.

New anti-androgen treatments

Although combination endocrine therapy has led to an improvement in the median survival for patients with prostate cancer, the basic problem remains and this is that all patients inevitably relapse and die of their disease. This provides a powerful impetus for the development of new treatments for this condition. Casodex is a non-steroidal anti-androgen which is structurally similar to flutamide. Preclinical testing has shown that it is a more potent anti-androgen than flutamide. Early clinical trials established dosage regimens for treatment [4]. No phase III studies have yet been published; however, initial information from phase II studies suggests a similar response rate to conventional therapies.

Testosterone is converted in tissue to its active metabolite dihydrotestosterone. Dihydrotestosterone has 100 times more androgenic activity than testosterone and so peripheral conversion is extraordinarily important in the control of prostate cancer.

In this context, the pharmaceutical industry has enthusiastically proceeded with the development of inhibitors of the enzyme responsible for the peripheral conversion of testosterone. This enzyme, 5-α-reductase, is inhibited by a variety of pharmacological agents. The first drug to be clinically developed has been finasteride. This agent, marketed for the treatment of benign prostatic hypertrophy, has been used to treat patients with prostate cancer. As yet there are no reports of clinical efficacy. However prostate-specific antigen (PSA) levels have been reduced by approximately 20% over a 6-week period of observation [5]. Although it is possible that this agent may have activity in prostate cancer, this possibility is regarded with some scepticism. The reason for this is that due to a lack of feedback inhibition, tissue testosterone levels increase. Since testosterone is an active androgen, the presence of increasing tissue levels of testosterone cannot be good in a disease that is androgen-sensitive. It may be that other 5-α-reductase inhibitors do not have this problem associated with their use, but no trials have yet been published.

Breast cancer

There have been spectacular advances in the treatment of breast cancer over the last decade. These advances have not come as a result of remarkable curative developments but rather from a re-evaluation of the effects of existing treatments and a greater understanding of the biochemistry of action of these agents. The latter has led to the introduction of non-toxic treatments.

Tamoxifen

The effects of adjuvant treatment with tamoxifen was analysed by the Early Breast Cancer Trialists Collaborative Group. This Oxford-based study was a meta-analysis of 133 randomized trials involving 75 000 women. The trialists showed that adjuvant treatment with tamoxifen led to a significant reduction in the risk of local recurrence and death. This benefit occurred in all women, regardless of menopausal status. The trialists estimated that if all of the women with breast cancer in the world were treated with adjuvant therapy with tamoxifen then 100 000 women's lives would be saved worldwide over the next 10 years. No advantage was found to dosages of tamoxifen over 20 mg a day, nor for treatment that extended beyond 2 years [6]. In previous individual reports a trend to an advantage of higher dosage adjuvant therapy, for longer periods has been reported. As a result of their careful study the Oxford Trialists have modified clinical practice.

Tamoxifen has disadvantages associated with its use. The most important of these is endometrial carcinoma, probably stemming from the oestrogenic agonist effects of this compound. Reports of the relative risk vary greatly but in a recent analysis by the National Surgical Adjuvant Breast Cancer Group this risk was rated at approximately two cases per 10 000 women years of use of tamoxifen.

The development of analogues of tamoxifen with less oestrogenic activity has been encouraged by this observation. Toremifene was one of the first agents to be investigated but unfortunately endometrial carcinoma has also been reported with this agent. The use of less oestrogenic compounds is further complicated by the fact that oestrogenic activity is of value. For example, in postmenopausal women, tamoxifen has been found to increase the bone protein content, decreasing the risk of subsequent osteoporotic fracture.

Aromatase inhibitors

Aminoglutethimide is considered to be conventional second-line therapy for breast cancer. It was introduced into clinical practice for the treatment of epilepsy some 30 years ago. It was subsequently withdrawn from use because of the development of hypo-adrenalism in some patients. This side-effect was used to the advantage of women with breast cancer as a medical alternative to adrenalectomy.

Unfortunately, aminoglutethimide is toxic and between 40 and 60% of patients develop significant side-effects from treatment. An analysis of the endocrinological effects of aminoglutethimide has shown that its effects upon the adrenal gland are transient. The most important activity of aminoglutethimide is its effect upon the peripheral aromatase system of enzymes. This enzyme system converts the main adrenal androgen, androstenedione, to oestrone by hydroxylation. The second step is the conversion of oestrone into oestradiol and oestrone sulphate, which is undertaken by the sulphatase system of enzymes.

A series of competitive inhibitors of the aromatase system were developed by Brodie in the late 1970s and early 1980s [7]. These were found to effectively reduce blood levels of oestrogenic steroids in animals and humans and to inhibit the growth of breast cancer in animal models. The first clinical studies were published in 1984 but the introduction into clinical practice of formestane, the first aromatase inhibitor, took another 8 years. This delay was the result of problems in manufacture.

Formestane is currently given as a 2-weekly injection. Response rates are equivalent to aminoglutethimide but treatment is without the considerable toxicity of this agent [7]. No phase III clinical studies have been performed, so the comparative activity of this agent is not known. Recently, orally active aromatase inhibitors which include vorazole and arimidex have entered clinical trial. Phase III trials are currently underway and hopefully these orally active aromatase inhibitors will be as successful a treatment of breast cancer as formestane [8].

We await with interest the development of sulphatase inhibitors which may offer further advances over the aromatase inhibitors as treatments for breast cancer. These are at a very early stage of investigation and are currently in preclinical testing.

It is not yet known how it is that a tumour can respond to so many different hormonal therapies. The same patient may respond to anti-oestrogens, oestrogens, androgens, anti-androgens and progestogens, and in this context, the biology of the hormonal response elements of the steroid receptors is a mystery.

In the search for new treatments for breast cancer a new group of agents have recently been introduced into clinical trials. Antiprogestogens such as RU38486 or mifeprastone have recently been evaluated in phase I/II trials. In one series, one of 11 postmenopausal women was seen to respond to this agent [9].

Conclusion

The treatment of hormone responsive tumours is unendingly fascinating but complex. Over the last decade, significant new treatments for these malignancies have been developed and piece by piece the role of the various therapies has been established. It is to be hoped that an understanding of the molecular basis for response and relapse will lead to cure rather than palliation of these endocrine-responsive malignancies.

References

1. Crawford ED, Eisenberger MA, McLeod DG *et al.* A controlled trial of leuprolide with and without flutamide in prostatic carcinoma. *N. Engl. J. Med.* 1989;**321**:419–24.

2. Denis LJ, Whelan P, Carneiro de Moura JL *et al.* Goserelin acetate and flutamide versus bilateral orchidectomy: a phase III EORTC trial (30853). *Urology* 1993;**42**:119–30.

3. Scher HI, Kelly WK. Flutamide withdrawal syndrome: its impact on clinical trials in hormone-refractory prostate cancer. *J. Clin. Oncol.* 1993;**11**:1566–72.

4. Lunglmayr G. Casodex (ICI 176 334), a new, non-steroidal anti-androgen. Early clinical results. *Horm. Res.* 1989;**32**:77–81.

5. Presti JC Jr, Fair WR, Andriole G *et al.* Multicenter randomized, double blind, placebo controlled study to investigate the effect of finasteride (MK-906) on stage D prostate cancer. *J. Urol.* 1992;**148**:1201–4.

6. Early Breast Cancer Trialists' Collaborative Group. Systemic treatment of early breast cancer by hormonal, cytotoxic, or immune therapy. *Lancet* 1992;**339**:1–15.

7. Coombes RC. 4-Hydroxyandrostenedione treatment for post-menopausal patients with breast cancer. *J. Steroid Biochem. Molec. Biol.* 1992;**43**:145–8.

8. Raats JI, Falkson G, Falkson HC. A study of fadrozole, a new aromatase inhibitor, in postmenopausal women with advanced metastatic breast cancer. *J. Clin. Oncol.* 1992;**10**:111–16.

9. Klijn JGM, de Jong FH, Bakker GH *et al.* Antiprogestins, a new form of endocrine therapy for human breast cancer. *Cancer Res.* 1989;**49**:2851–6.

Oestrogen Therapy: Benefits and Risks

MARTIN P. VESSEY AND EDEL DALY

Introduction

This chapter provides a brief overview of the effects of combined oral contraceptives (including biphasic and triphasic preparations) and hormone replacement therapy (HRT). Attention is confined to major morbidity and mortality as revealed by epidemiological studies with special reference to the balance of benefits and risks.

Combined oral contraceptives

Combined oral contraceptives (COCs) contain both an oestrogen and a progestogen. They have been available since 1960 and have been taken by millions of women. Only two oestrogens, ethinyl-oestradiol and mestranol, have been used in the UK but seven progestogens are currently available (norethisterone, norethisterone acetate, ethynodiol diacetate, levonorgestrel, desogestrel, gestodene, norgestimate), while others have been used in the past. Early COCs contained high doses of oestrogen and pro-gestogen. These have been gradually reduced over the years to the present low levels.

Most of the research on the benefits and risks of COCs (which is very extensive) has been conducted in Western countries, particularly the UK and the USA. Unfortunately, a large-scale randomized controlled trial of the effects of Enovid (an early COC) in comparison with the effects of a vaginal contraceptive, which was commenced in Puerto Rico in 1961, was a failure. Consequently, information has been derived from observational studies, with all their shortcomings. The case-control approach has been very widely used, but since the mid-1970s, four large-scale cohort studies (the Royal College of General Practitioners' study, the Oxford Family Planning Association study, the Nurses Health study and the Walnut Creek study) have also made major contributions. It should be stressed that these cohort studies have largely been concerned with the early COCs containing 50 μg or more of oestrogen.

Information about the benefits and risks of COCs in developing countries is very sparse. The reader is cautioned not to extrapolate the findings discussed in this chapter to parts of the world to which they may not apply.

Established benefits

The most important benefit of COCs concerns their high level of effectiveness and acceptability. Used conscientiously, the failure rate is well below one per 100 women per year. If pills are accidentally missed, which is not uncommon, the failure rate may be appreciably higher than this.

From the earliest days of COC use, it has been known that the preparations protect against menstrual bleeding problems, including menorrhagia. As a consequence, they also reduce the risk of iron-deficiency anaemia which may be of considerable importance in developing countries.

Many studies have shown that COCs reduce the risk of biopsy for a benign breast lump. There is uncertainty about what this implies in terms of underlying breast pathology. The effect is largely confined to current users, increases with duration of use and is probably attributable to the progestogen component of the pill. Few data are available about modern low-dose COCs but there is some evidence that they may be less beneficial in this respect than earlier preparations.

COCs reduce the risk of pelvic inflammatory disease, an important benefit in the young. This effect may not extend to disease caused by chlamydial infection.

Corpus luteum cysts and follicular cysts of the ovary may cause symptoms and signs which lead to surgical intervention. As a consequence of suppression of ovulation, such cysts occur infrequently in users of COCs.

The protective effects of COCs against epithelial cancer of the ovary and cancer of the endometrium are of major importance, not only in the context of this chapter, but also in terms of public health [1]. The results of epidemiological studies (both of case-control and cohort design) have been remarkably uniform, while vital statistical trends are also consistent with the postulated benefits. Overall, COC users have about half as great a risk of developing either cancer as non-users, but the protective effect increases with duration of COC use (especially with respect to ovarian cancer) and persists for at least 15 years after stopping.

Possible benefits

COCs may offer some protection against rheumatoid arthritis, uterine fibromyomas and endometriosis. There is currently considerable interest in the possibility that COC users may establish a greater peak bone mass than non-users but the existing cross-sectional studies have not yielded clear-cut results.

Established risks

Many early studies demonstrated that high-dose COCs can cause venous thromboembolism, acute myocardial infarction, thrombotic stroke and (possibly) haemorrhagic stroke [2]. Relative risks for some of these conditions were high, around six for venous thromboembolism, for example. In recent years, however, modern low-dose pills have been generally adopted, while doctors are more selective about the prescription of COCs and keep users under closer surveillance than in the past. Perhaps not surprisingly, a recent study of all deaths from cardiovascular disease during the years 1986–88 in England and Wales, found much lower relative risks (around or below two for each condition) than those previously accepted. This study, however, included very few women using COCs containing the 'third generation' progestogens, gestodene, desogestrel and norgestimate. In late 1995, results were published from an international collaborative study organized by the World Health Organization (WHO) which suggested that COCs containing gestodene and desogestrel were about twice as likely to cause venous thromboembolism as COCs containing 'second generation' progestogens (such as levonorgestrel) [3]. The findings in the WHO study have been confirmed by other investigations conducted in the UK and elsewhere in Europe. It should be noted that in most studies, increased cardiovascular risks have been confined to current COC users and unrelated to duration of use.

The mechanisms underlying adverse cardiovascular reactions to COCs are uncertain. However, COCs have effects on coagulation and fibrinolysis, on serum lipids, on carbohydrate metabolism and on blood pressure; any or all of these factors may be relevant.

There is clear evidence that long-term use of the older, higher-dose COCs increases the risk of hepatocellular adenoma. Case-control studies of women in Western countries strongly suggest that the same is true for hepatocellular carcinoma, but a WHO study concerned with developing countries found no effect. It must be stressed that both types of liver tumour are very rare in countries such as the UK.

Temporary impairment of fertility may follow COC use, especially in those over the age of 30 trying to have a first baby.

Possible risks

The epidemiological literature on COCs and breast cancer is extensive and confusing. Fortunately, an important overview has been published recently which takes into account the findings in almost all the epidemiological studies of oral contraceptives and breast cancer in the world literature [4]. The main conclusion is that there is about a 25% increase in breast cancer risk in current oral contraceptive users which tails off after discontinuation of use and is back to baseline about 10 years after cessation.

With regard to cancer of the cervix uteri, the majority of investigations have suggested that there is a positive association with long-term COC use. Even though most studies have adjusted for the influence of age at first sexual intercourse and number of sexual partners, residual confounding by sexual factors (such as human papilloma virus (HPV) infection) may well be responsible for the observed effect.

Recent findings suggest that chronic inflammatory bowel disease occurs with increased frequency in COC users. Various other adverse effects, such as an increased risk of malignant melanoma, chromophobe adenoma of the pituitary, depression, urinary tract infection and fetal malformation if taken inadvertently during pregnancy, have been suggested, but the findings are, in general, unconvincing.

Balance of benefits and risks

Various authors have used a variety of methods to investigate the balance of benefits and risks of COCs. We refer here to three approaches. It is important to note that all the material in this section antedates the

Table 87.1 Morbidity (in terms of hospital admissions) experienced by women aged 25–39 years using either combined oral contraceptives (COCs) or the condom to try to prevent pregnancy for 1 year. The data relate to preparations containing 50 µg oestrogen and are derived from the Oxford Family Planning Association contraceptive study supplemented by other epidemiological data

	Number of hospital admissions*	
Reason for hospital admission	COCs	Condom
Beneficial effects of COCs		
Menstrual problems	375	500
Anaemia	22	30
Benign breast disease	115	230
Pelvic inflammatory disease†	60	60
Functional ovarian cysts	15	60
Ovarian cancer	5	10
Endometrial cancer	2	4
Harmful effects of COCs		
Acute myocardial infarction	10	5
Thrombotic stroke	50	10
Haemorrhagic stroke	7	5
Venous thromboembolism	100	20
Hepatocellular adenoma	2	0
Hepatocellular carcinoma	0	0
Accidental pregnancy‡		
Term birth	300	3040
Spontaneous abortion	63	640
Extrauterine pregnancy	3	20
Induced abortion	134	1300

* Number of hospital admissions in 1 year among 100 000 women relying on either COCs or condoms.
† These rates are equal because both COCs and condoms offer protection against pelvic inflammatory disease.
‡ The failure rate for COCs has been taken to be 5/1000 per year and for the condom to be 50/1000 per year.

Table 87.2 Assumptions made about relative risks associated with combined oral contraceptive (COC) use in mortality analysis. For sources of relative risks see Vessey [5]

Condition	Assumptions
Ovarian cancer	Protection increases with duration of use and persists in ex-users. Duration of use ≤ 2 years, 0.7; 3–4 years, 0.6; 5–9 years, 0.4; ≥ 10 years, 0.2
Endometrial cancer	Protection increases with duration of use and persists in ex-users. Duration of use < 1 year, 1.0; 2 years, 0.7; ≥ 3 years, 0.4
Hepatic cancer	Risk increases with duration of use and persists in ex-users. Duration of use ≤ 7 years, 1.0; ≥ 8 years, 4.5
Breast cancer	Risk increased up to age 35, no increased risk thereafter. Duration of use ≤ 4 years, 1.0; 5–8 years, 1.4; ≥ 9 years, 1.75
Cervical cancer	Risk increases with duration of use and persists in ex-users. Duration of use ≤ 2 years, 1.0; 3–5 years, 1.25; ≥ 6 years, 1.5
Cardiovascular disease	Risk increased in current users only. Acute myocardial infarction, 1.5; subarachnoid haemorrhage, 1.5; thrombotic stroke, 2.0; venous thromboembolism, 2.0
Unplanned pregnancy	Failure rate for COCs 5/1000/year, for the condom 50/1000/year. Pregnancy associated mortality per million maternities age < 20, 82.3; 20–24, 57.6; 25–29, 85.7; 30–34, 107.1

publication of WHO study on venous thromboembolism and the collaborative group study on breast cancer [3,4]. Nonetheless, the data still provide a reasonable overview of the issues that have to be considered when balancing benefits and risks.

First, hospital in-patient morbidity data from the Oxford Family Planning Association contraceptive study, supplemented where necessary by other epidemiological data, have been used to make a comparison over a 1-year period between women using either COCs or the condom for contraception. The findings are summarized in Table 87.1. It should be noted that the data presented relate to the older 50 µg pills; this explains the substantial relative risks for cardiovascular disorders. The analysis throws into relief the serious morbidity associated with unplanned pregnancies. When this is taken into account, the results are quite favourable with respect to COCs.

To examine the possible effects of COCs on mortality,

we used a rather more ambitious model [5]. It was assumed that a cohort of one million women started to use COCs at age 16 and that a similar cohort decided to rely on the condom. These two cohorts then continued with their chosen method of birth control to age 35 when they were sterilized. Follow-up in the analysis continued, however, to the age of 50. We examined the mortality experience of these two cohorts with regard to cancers of the ovary, endometrium and liver; with regard to cardiovascular disease; and with regard to unplanned pregnancies. In a second analysis, we added in cancers of the breast and cervix as well to see what effect they might have if, in fact, they were associated with COC use. The assumptions made about relative risks are shown in Table 87.2 and the results of the analyses in Table 87.3. If there are no adverse effects of COCs on breast or cervical cancer, the COC cohort clearly fares best. If there is an effect on breast cancer up to age 35 and an effect on

Table 87.3 Difference in mortality (number of deaths) by cause between combined oral contraceptive cohort and condom cohort, from age 16 to 50 years

Cause of death	Number of deaths
Ovarian cancer	−1400
Endometrial cancer	−97
Hepatocellular cancer	202
Acute myocardial infarction	33
Subarachnoid haemorrhage	96
Thrombotic stroke	20
Venous thromboembolism	37
Unplanned pregnancy	−131
Total	−1240
Breast cancer	311
Cervical cancer	764
Total	−165
Breast cancer, persistent risk	4157
Total	3992

cervical cancer, there is little to choose between the cohorts. A persistent effect on breast cancer beyond age 35 (for which there is little or no evidence) would, however, alter the picture markedly.

Finally, mortality data have been published from all four major cohort studies. The largest number of deaths (2879) has been reported from the Nurses Health study [6]. In this study, the overall relative risk of death in women who had ever used oral contraceptives in comparison with those who had never done so was 0.93 (95% CI, 0.85–1.01). It should be noted, however, that very little of the observation period in this study concerned current users of COCs and that there was little information about oral contraceptive use at an early age.

In conclusion, on the basis of the available evidence, the continued use of COCs seems entirely justified. Continued monitoring of modern, low-dose COCs, however, is still required.

Hormone replacement therapy

There are two main kinds of HRT: oestrogen alone (ORT), which is generally given to women who have had a hysterectomy, and progestogen–oestrogen (PORT), which is generally given to women in whom the uterus is intact. Although HRT has been available for several decades, there has been a rapid increase in levels of use in the UK during the last few years and some studies suggest that up to 25% of women aged 45–64 years may now be taking it. Administration of HRT is generally by

mouth or transdermally, although other routes are sometimes used. In the UK oestradiol, conjugated oestrogens, mestranol, oestriol and oestrone are used as the oestrogen component of HRT, while norethisterone, norgestrel and levonorgestrel are used as the progestogen component.

Most of the research on HRT comes from the USA, where conjugated oestrogens administered alone as ORT have dominated the market. Information on PORT, consisting of conjugated oestrogens with medroxyprogesterone acetate, is beginning to emerge from that country, while data on other preparations are becoming available from European countries and Scandinavia.

Although many randomized controlled trials concerned with the influence of HRT on menopausal symptoms and on bone density have been published, no large-scale trial capable of providing reliable information about long-term effects has yet been reported. A number of such trials are being planned; they will be difficult to conduct because compliance with HRT is poor, while an unknown proportion of the women in the control group would be expected to request HRT at some time after randomization. In the meantime, as with oral contraceptives, we have to rely on the findings in numerous observational studies both of case-control and cohort design. Of the cohort studies, the Nurses Health study and a community-based investigation carried out in Uppsala in Sweden have been of particular value. A valuable overview of all disease endpoints has been provided by Grady and colleagues [7].

Epidemiological information about HRT from developing countries is essentially non-existent. Accordingly, as was the case with oral contraceptives, the reader is cautioned against inappropriate extrapolation of the findings summarized here.

Benefits

Both ORT and PORT are highly effective in relieving the menopausal syndrome, especially the vasomotor symptoms and the symptoms associated with genital atrophy. Generally, however, this may require only short-term therapy, lasting, say, from 6 months to 3 years. Accordingly, when HRT is administered for this purpose alone, the question of long-term effects does not arise.

Long-term HRT is usually given to prevent postmenopausal osteoporosis with a view to reducing the risk of osteoporotic fractures, especially of the femoral neck, the vertebral column and the wrist. Numerous studies, including randomized controlled trials, have shown that available preparations, both ORT and PORT, are effective in preventing osteoporosis for as long as they are continued. Bone loss starts once again, however, once the preparations have been stopped. Studies of the risk of fracture in relation to HRT are fewer than those concerned with osteoporosis and are of the observational type. They uniformly show a protective effect while HRT is in current use, but they tend to suggest that the protective effect may wear off completely some time after discontinuation. This point, which urgently requires further research, is of crucial importance, because HRT tends to be taken by women in their 50s, while femoral neck fractures tend to occur among women in their 70s and 80s.

Apart from the effect of HRT on osteoporosis, long-term treatment is increasingly being considered for the prevention of ischaemic heart disease. A large number of epidemiological studies of both case-control and cohort design have suggested that conjugated oestrogens may reduce the risk of myocardial infarction by up to 50% [8]. This reduction in risk may be mediated partly through beneficial changes in serum lipids, and partly through favourable effects on arterial wall tone. The same effect might be expected to apply to other forms of ORT, but it has been suggested that the progestogenic component of PORT, particularly if it is androgenic, might tend to reduce or even eliminate the benefit attributable to oestrogens. This suggestion has been hotly disputed and it may be noted that the limited empirical data available at present suggest that PORT, as well as ORT, is cardio-protective [9].

Unfortunately, existing epidemiological studies have largely been concerned with the comparison between women ever using HRT and those never doing so. There is little information about the effect of current use versus past use, of duration of use, or of dose. Furthermore, many of the studies have been criticized as being subject to selection bias. Thus, for example, HRT has tended to be used by healthy women from the higher social classes, that is by women with a low intrinsic risk of ischaemic heart disease. Although a number of studies have included detailed information about risk factors for ischaemic heart disease and about social class, and have still shown a beneficial effect after allowing for these factors, the results of one or more large-scale randomized controlled trials would clearly be of great value.

Finally, there is some evidence that HRT may reduce the risk of stroke as well as that of ischaemic heart disease. The available data do not, however, enable a firm conclusion to be drawn.

Risks

It has been known for 20 years that conjugated oestrogens administered to women with intact uteri are a cause of endometrial cancer. The risk, which is substantial, is closely related to dose and to duration of use and almost certainly applies to all forms of ORT. The addition of an adequate dose of a progestogen for 10–12 days during each cycle of ORT protects against the excess risk of endometrial cancer; this, of course, is why PORT is given to women requiring HRT who have intact uteri.

An enormous amount of careful epidemiological research has examined the possible relationship between HRT and breast cancer. For the most part the data relate to conjugated oestrogens but there is limited information about other forms of ORT and about PORT as well. It seems clear that conjugated oestrogens have, at most, a modest adverse effect on breast cancer risk; although the findings in some studies have been positive, the results of others are negative and the data generally are heterogeneous. Nonetheless, some meta-analyses have come to the conclusion that there is a small rise in the incidence of breast cancer with prolonged therapy with conjugated oestrogens, such that the relative risk for 15 years use or more is around 1.5. In addition, the Nurses Health study, which has provided by far the largest amount of information on a prospective basis, has suggested that the increased risk is confined to current users [10]. Epidemiological studies carried out in Europe have tended to show higher breast cancer risks after shorter periods of HRT use than studies carried out in the USA. Whereas users in the latter are mainly concerned with the use of unopposed conjugated oestrogens, subjects in the European studies were more likely to be users of other oestrogens and of PORT. Further information about these newer forms of HRT is urgently required.

Balance of benefits and risks

We have conducted a detailed analysis of the balance of the benefits and risks associated with HRT using a model with some similarities to that described earlier for oral contraceptives [11]. In the HRT model it was assumed that there were two treatment cohorts, one consisting of hysterectomized women entering the menopause at age 50 and treated with ORT for 10 years, and the other consisting of women with intact uteri entering the menopause at age 50 and treated with PORT for 10 years. Compliance of 100% was assumed for both groups. Morbidity and mortality in these hypothetical cohorts were then compared with the patterns observed in the general population.

Table 87.4 shows the standard assumptions about disease risk changes. It should be noted that in addition to the effects already discussed, it is assumed that bleeding

Table 87.4 Standard assumptions about disease risk changes following 10 years' use of hormone replacement therapy (HRT) starting at age 50

Risk of	Therapy	Comments
Fractures	ORT/PORT	20% reduction in risk during first 5 years of use, 60% reduction in risk following 5 years' use
Ischaemic heart disease	ORT	25% reduction in risk after 5 years' use, 50% reduction in risk after 10 years' use
	PORT	Protection assumed to be halved
Stroke	ORT	12.5% reduction in risk after 5 years' use, 25% reduction in risk after 10 years' use
	PORT	Protection assumed to be halved
Breast cancer	ORT/PORT	30% increase in risk following 10 years' use
Hysterectomy/D and C	PORT	Risk of intervention increased by 25% during treatment period only
Endometrial cancer		No increase in risk in PORT users

Unless otherwise stated, relative risk returns to baseline 10 years after treatment is stopped.
ORT, oestrogen HRT; PORT, progestogen–oestrogen HRT.

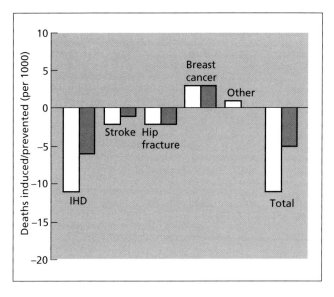

Fig. 87.1 Deaths induced or prevented by cause in patients aged up to 69 years, following 10 years' hormone replacement treatment with oestrogen alone (□) or oestrogen–progestogen (■). IHD, ischaemic heart disease.

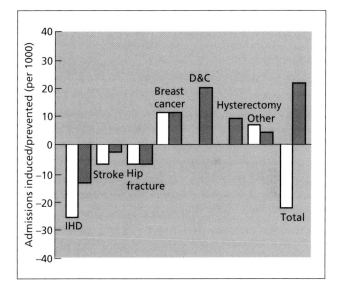

Fig. 87.2 Hospital admissions induced or prevented by cause in patients aged up to 69 years, following 10 years' hormone replacement treatment with oestrogen alone (□) or oestrogen–progestogen (■). D & C, dilatation and curettage; IHD, ischaemic heart disease.

disturbances associated with PORT lead to a 25% increase in the risk of dilatation and curettage and of hysterectomy.

Figure 87.1 shows the deaths induced or prevented by cause to age 69 in the two treatment cohorts. There is a reduction in mortality in both cohorts but this is much more substantial in the ORT cohort than in the PORT cohort. Figure 87.2 provides the corresponding data for hospital admissions. Here there is a net advantage for users of ORT but a net disadvantage for users of PORT. A substantial part of the latter is attributable to admissions for dilatation and curettage and for hysterectomy.

Calculations were also undertaken to estimate the average life years gained per woman when the members of the two cohorts were followed through to death. Values of 0.2 and 0.1 years, respectively, were obtained for ORT users and PORT users. Extension of the treatment period from 10 to 20 years increased these two figures to 1.1

and 0.5 years, respectively. Additional sensitivity analyses were conducted in which individual components of the model were varied while the remaining components were held constant. It was concluded that benefits in relation to ischaemic heart disease overshadowed adverse effects; for example, with 10 years' treatment, a permanent 50%

reduction in the risk of ischaemic heart disease would increase average life-expectancy by 1.2 years.

All the above calculations were conducted on the basis of treating asymptomatic women. Clearly, a woman suffering from menopausal symptoms would gain additional benefit, in quality of life terms, from having her symptoms relieved. Additional analyses, which involved the computation of quality adjusted life years, were undertaken but the findings are too complex to summarize here.

In conclusion, on the basis of existing knowledge, the use of HRT seems justified, both to treat menopausal symptoms and, perhaps, to prevent chronic disease, especially in hysterectomized women. However, the available epidemiological information is incomplete; results from large-scale, long-term, randomized, controlled trials would, of course, be invaluable, but for reasons stated earlier, there has to be serious doubt about their feasibility.

References

1. Vessey MP. Oral contraception and cancer. In Filshie M, Guillebaud J (eds). *Contraception: Science and Practice*. London: Butterworths, 1989:52–68.
2. Thorogood M. Oral contraceptives and cardiovascular disease: an epidemiologic overview. *Pharmacoepidemiol. Drug Safety* 1993;2:3–16.
3. World Health Organization Collaborative Study of Cardiovascular Disease and Steroid Hormone Contraceptive. Effect of different progestagens in low oestrogen oral contraceptives on venous thromboembolic disease. *Lancet* 1995;346:1582–8.
4. Collaborative Group on Hormonal Factors in Breast Cancer. Breast cancer and hormonal contraceptives. *Lancet* 1996;347:1713–27.
5. Vessey MP. The Jephcott Lecture, 1989: an overview of the benefits and risks of combined oral contraceptives. In Mann RD (ed). *Oral Contraceptives and Breast Cancer*. Carnforth: Parthenon Publishing, 1990:121–32.
6. Colditz GA. Oral contraceptive use and mortality during 12 years of follow-up: the Nurses' Health Study. *Ann. Intern. Med.* 1994;120:821–6.
7. Grady D, Rubin SM, Petitti DB *et al*. Hormone therapy to prevent disease and prolong life in postmenopausal women. *Ann. Intern. Med.* 1992;117:1016–37.
8. Stampfer MJ, Colditz GA, Willett WC *et al*. Postmenopausal estrogen therapy and cardiovascular disease: ten-year follow-up from the Nurses' Health Study. *N. Engl. J. Med.* 1991;325:756–62.
9. Falkeborn M, Persson I, Adami H-O *et al*. The risk of acute myocardial infarction after oestrogen and oestrogen-progestogen replacement. *Br. J. Obstet. Gynaecol.* 1992;99:812–18.
10. Colditz GA, Egan KM, Stampfer MJ. Hormone replacement therapy and risk of breast cancer: results from epidemiologic studies. *Am. J. Obstet. Gynecol.* 1993;168:1473–8.
11. Daly E, Roche M, Barlow D, Gray A, McPherson K, Vessey M. Hormone replacement therapy: an analysis of benefits, risks and costs. *Br. Med. Bull.* 1992;48:368–400.

Index